AF731670

Bhave's Textbook of Adolescent Medicine

Second Edition

Editor-in-Chief

Swati Y Bhave (Lele)

Academic Editors

PSN Menon
A Parthasarathy

Guest Editor

Donald E Greydanus

Foreword by

MKC Nair
Bruce Dick

Appreciation by

Padmabhushan Awardee Dr RD Lele

PEEPEE

PUBLISHERS AND DISTRIBUTORS (P) LTD.

Bhave's Textbook of Adolescent Medicine

Published by
Pawaninder P. Vij and Anupam Vij

Peepee Publishers and Distributors (P) Ltd.
Head Office: 160, Shakti Vihar, Pitam Pura
Delhi-110 034 (India)

Correspondence Address:

7/31, First Floor, Ansari Road, Daryaganj
New Delhi-110002 (India)

Ph: 65195868, 23246245, 9811156083

e-mail: peepee160@yahoo.co.in

e-mail: peepee160@gmail.com

www.peepeepub.com

Second Edition: **2016**

ISBN: 978-81-8445-194-8

This book is dedicated to

My Husband, Yashwant,

who has supported me all these years

to devote to the cause of adolescent health

Dr Swati Y Bhave
Editor-in-Chief

EDITOR-IN-CHIEF

Dr Swati Y Bhave (Lele)

MD, DCH, FCPS, FIAP, FAAP (HON)

Executive Director: AACCI (Association of Adolescent and Child Care in India) (2007 to date)
Head and In-charge: Adolescent Wellness Clinic, Jehangir Hospital, Pune (2014 to date)
Visiting Consultant: Indraprastha Apollo Hospital, New Delhi (2003-2014)
Senior full time Consultant and PG teacher: Bombay Hospital Institute of Medical Sciences, Mumbai (1991-2001)
Professor of Pediatrics: B.J. Medical College and Sasson Hospital (1989-91)
President IAP: Indian Academy of Pediatrics (2000)
Regional Vice President IAAH: International Association of Adolescent Health (2009-13 and 2013-17)
Technical Advisor: Adolescent Health–International Association of Pediatrics (IPA) (2008-2013)
Member: WHO TSC Committee of Child and Adolescent Health (2009-10) and HPV Vaccine (2010)
Regional Advisor: (APPSSEAR) Asia Pacific Pediatric Association (APPA) (2000-03)
Member: Governing Council NCD Child (2014 to date)

ACADEMIC EDITORS

Dr PSN Menon

MD, MNAMS, FIAP, FIMSA
Consultant and Head, Department of Pediatrics, Jaber Al-Ahmed Armed Forces Hospital, Kuwait
Former Sub-Dean and Professor of Pediatrics, All India Institute of Medical Sciences, New Delhi
Consultant Incharge of the Pediatric Endocrinology and Officer-in-charge WHO SEARO Regional Research and Training Centre in Genetics, AIIMS, New Delhi
President of the Indian Society for Pediatric and Adolescent Endocrinology (ISPAE) (2010-2011)
Member of the Executive Council of the Asia Pacific Pediatric Endocrine Society (APPES) (2009-2011)
Editorial board member–prestigious journals in the field of pediatrics, diabetes and endocrinology
Over 150 original research publications in reputed and indexed journals
Edited IAP and other textbooks in the field of pediatrics and pediatric endocrinology including 'IAP Textbook of Pediatrics', 'PG Textbook of Pediatrics' and 'Pediatric Endocrine Disorders'

Dr A Parthasarathy

MBBS, DCH, MD (Ped), DSc (Honoris Causa), FIAP
Retd Senior Clinical Professor of Pediatrics, Madras Medical College and Deputy Superintendent, Institute of Child Health and Hospital for Children, Chennai
Ex-Distinguished Professor of Pediatrics–TN Dr MGR Medical University
National President of Indian Academy of Pediatrics (IAP) 1997
Regional Adviser APPSSEAR (APPA) 1997-99
Founded the Indian Journal of Practical Pediatrics and IAP Infectious Diseases Chapter in 1997
Founding Editor-in-Chief of >5 IAP and >10 Partha's series of books for last 18 years
International Associate Editor for AAP publication 2009
IAP Infectious Diseases chapter has instituted Annual National Oration titled A. PARTHASARATHY ORATION in the Annual 'National Conferences of Pediatric Infectious Diseases'(NCPIDs) since 2007

GUEST EDITOR

Dr Donald E Greydanus

MD, Dr HC (ATHENS), FAAP, FSAM (Emeritus), FIAP (HON)
Professor and Founding Chair and Program Director, Department of Pediatrics
Western Michigan University School of Medicine (Kalamazoo, Michigan, USA)
Published extensively in the field of adolescent medicine
Received numerous honors and awards from various organizations
Doctor Honoris Causa–University of Athens (Greece) as a "distinguished scientist who through outstanding work has bestowed praise and credit on the field of Adolescent Medicine (Ephebiatrics)"
Outstanding Achievement in Adolescent Medicine Award from SAM Society for Adolescent Medicine "as a leading force in the field of adolescent medicine and health" 2010

Foreword for the Second Edition

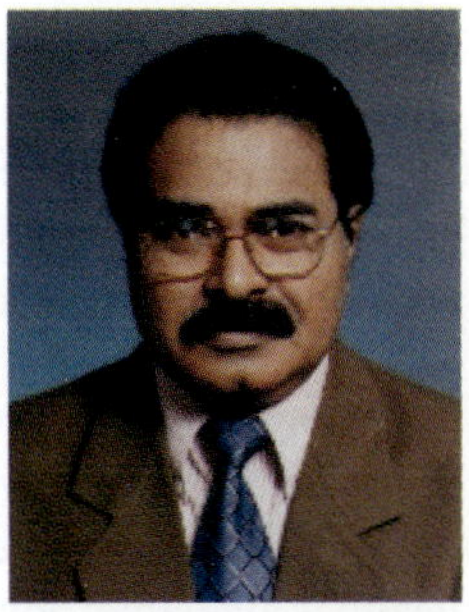

It is a great privilege and honor to write the foreword for the 2nd edition of **Bhave's Textbook of Adolescent Medicine,** published by Peepee Publishers and Distributors (P) Ltd., New Delhi. My association with Dr Swati Bhave in the Indian Academy of Pediatrics for the last 30 years has helped us to develop a personal bond beyond academics. Together we were able to develop adolescent pediatrics as a distinct sub-specialty of pediatrics in India.

A person with a poetic disposition would describe adolescence, as the most fascinating period of life, full of fun and frolic. But parents, who have an 'adolescent child', would probably define it, as the most stressful period of parenting lifecycle, wherein; at one moment you feel that children have grown up and at the next, you realize that they are worse than small kids. This is also the period when they start experimenting with their first smoke, and skips meals as they are extremely figure conscious but at the same time have the bad habit of eating out often. Lots of infatuations and broken hearts are not rare as they also show emotional lability, finding it difficult to handle the rapid physiological and associated physical and mental changes.

We pediatricians are privileged to be able to care for the adolescents between 10 and 19 years, yet, only few of us are formally trained and confident to manage adolescent issues. Fortunately, the large majority of adolescents do not have serious medical problems, having passed the stage of childhood illnesses and not yet reached the stage of adult lifestyle diseases. But, they do have issues related to their growth and development, nutrition, emerging sexuality, physical reproductive and mental health, special senses, sports and recreational activities and risk taking behavior.

I am happy to note that the second edition has fewer pages, to serve as a desktop reference for physicians of all specialties, who are seeing adolescent patients. The eminent authors and editors have tried to put matter which is very adolescent specific and not reproduce what is already available in pediatric and adult textbooks.

My best wishes.

MKC Nair
Hon'ble Vice Chancellor
Kerala University of Health Sciences
Thrissur, Kerala

Foreword for the Second Edition

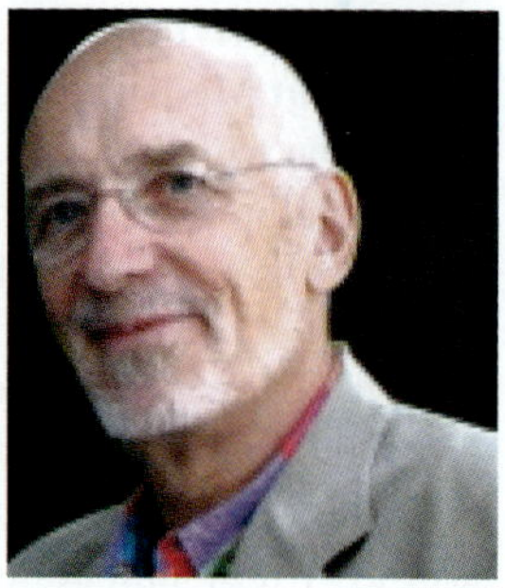

There is growing appreciation from all regions of the world that the health and development of adolescents is a central building block for health across the life-course, for this generation and the next. Furthermore, we know that it is not only important for public health, but also for adolescents' ability to learn, and for them to make successful transitions to adulthood, with all the implications that this has for wider social and economic development.

Many things need to be done to improve the health of adolescents, and a range of different sectors and partners will need to be involved. Naturally, the heath sector has a central role to play, ensuring that the strategic information needed for planning and monitoring adolescents' health is available; advocating for the development and implementation of a range of protective and enabling policies; mobilising and supporting the essential contributions of other sectors; and, of course, providing health services.

Ensuring that health systems are responsive to the needs of adolescents and being clear about how to apply the principles and practices of universal health coverage to this phase of the life-course will be crucial for improving the health of adolescents, and to improving public health more generally. At the core of such developments is the need to have health workers who understand, and are able to respond to the prevention, screening, treatment and care of the health problems that arise during the adolescent years–to be clear about the ways in which adolescents differ from small children and adults, and to be able to use this understanding to respond effectively to their health needs.

The second edition of **Bhave's Textbook of Adolescent Medicine** will make an important contribution to ensuring that when adolescents do reach health services, the clinicians that they encounter are competent and credible, and the services that they provide are of high quality. There is growing attention being paid to the importance of achieving core competencies for adolescent health through pre-service training and continuous professional training programmes. The new edition of this textbook will be a useful addition to achieving these ends, primarily for health workers who have a specific focus on adolescents, but also for clinicians in other fields of medicine who encounter adolescents in their clinical settings: the health of adolescents is everybody's business.

The previous edition of this book, published in 2006, was the first textbook on adolescent medicine published in India, with contributions from a range of experts working in the field of adolescent health, most of them practicing in India. It focused primarily on clinical medicine but also included some key aspects of public health. This second edition is a significantly condensed version, intended more as a desktop reference for practicing physicians. It benefits from Dr Swati Bhave's many years of clinical and public health experience, during which time I have had the pleasure to be associated with her work as a respected colleague, both in India and also internationally.

Bruce Dick
Independent Consultant (Adolescent Health)
Senior Associate, Johns Hopkins Bloomberg School of Public Health
President, International Association for Adolescent Health

Foreword for the First Edition

भारत सरकार
स्वास्थ्य एवं परिवार कल्याण मंत्रालय
निर्माण भवन, नई दिल्ली - 110011
Government of India
Ministry of Health & Family Welfare
Nirman Bhavan, New Delhi - 110011

Prasanna Hota
Health & FW Secretary
Tel.: 23061863 Fax : 23061252
e-mail :secyfw@nb.nic.in

Today's generation of young people is the largest in known history. Half of the world's population (almost 3 billion) is under the age of 25. By the 2015 deadline, today's 10-year-old will be 20 and ready to fully take on the role as agents of development. For the next 10 years, today's adolescents will be active participants in helping us to achieve the Millennium Development Goals. Policy decisions regarding the education, health, employment and human rights of today's young people will also affect the next wave of 1.2 billion children who will be adolescents in 2015. Decisions taken or opportunities missed today will reverberate for generations to come.

The youth of a country are crucial to its development, and their impressionable minds can be molded very easily. It is specially important for our country where there are 225 million adolescents that include 12% in the 10-14 years and 10% in the 15-19 age group (according to the census 2001). The Ministry of Health recognizes the public health impact of the growing number of teenage pregnancy contributing to high MMR, IMR and LBW babies. There is also concern about the high incidence of HIV and STDs and nutritional deficiencies: specially anemia in adolescents (70% girls). Hence, delivery of services related to Adolescent Reproductive and Sexual Health (ARSH) is a priority and has been included in the RCH II program.

In the Western medical world adolescent medicine is a well established specialty. In India adolescence is not a special subject in the undergraduate medical curriculum and currently no postgraduate degree exists which is recognized by Medical Council of India. Professional organizations need to promote this subject and come out with training programs and appropriate literature. I have learnt that there is no dedicated textbook of adolescent medicine in our country today. To respond to this need, a group of senior and experienced professionals from the fields of Pediatrics, Gynecology and Obstetrics, Mental Health, Public Health and some super-specialties have come together to publish this textbook. Some well-known international experts have also contributed a number of chapters. This book has been written to provide professional support to the doctors, mental health professionals, paramedical, social and community workers dealing with adolescents. It will also be very useful to postgraduate medical students in various specialties focusing on adolescent areas.

I am happy to know that this book covers every aspect of adolescent health including growth and development, common diseases, immunization, mental health issues including anxiety, depression and suicide, adolescent reproductive and sexual health with special focus on teenage pregnancy and HIV-AIDS; impact of the internet and media, benefits of yoga and meditation. Some chapters are unique for this type of book such as positive health which includes parenting, positive discipline, stress management and anger control.

I am pleased to see that this book goes beyond hospitals, into the community, to discuss adolescent-friendly health services, Government and NGO programs for adolescents; importance of school mental health programs, issues of street children and child labor and juvenile crime.This makes it immensely useful to large strata of people.

I congratulate Dr Swati Y Bhave and her dedicated team for working hard to bring out this excellent book and wish them all success in this commendable endeavor.

Prasanna Hota
Secretary to the Government of India

From the Desk of the Guest Editor

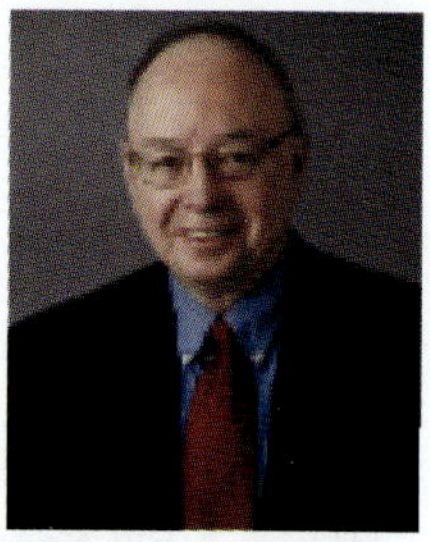

The time of adolescence has typically been turbulent since recorded history. Adults of all ages seemed to be perturbed by their youth and find ways to stop them from disobeying adult rules that included not disobeying parents and not being sexually active. In the ancient Western world the original legal rule book, the Code of Hammurabi (1796 BC to 1750 BC) had one stern warning and rule for youth: "*Cut off the hand of a son if he slaps his father*." The ancient Hebrews were also concerned with behaviors of their adolescents and the writer of the Old Testament Pentateuch book, Leviticus (1450 BC) warned its youth: "*If anyone curses his father or mother, he must be put to death* (Leviticus 20:9)." In the Western world, the ancient Greeks were also worried about their adolescents as noted by the words of the famous Greek poet, Hesiod (700 BC): "*I see no hope for the future of our people if we are dependent on the frivolous youth of today....for certainly all youth are reckless beyond words*." This was a major statement since the ancient Greeks were rarely at a loss for words and seemed to have a word for everything.

This consternation about frivolous, reckless youth in Western civilization has continued until the present 21st century. One of the West's most famous writers, William Shakespeare (1564-1631 AD) wrote in his "A Winter's Tale" (1623 AD): "*I would that there were no age between ten and three and twenty or that youth would simply sleep out the rest; for there is nothing in-between but getting wenches with child, wronging the ancestry, stealing, and fighting.*"

After millennia of worry and anger at youth, Western science and medicine began to study this age group in the 20th century led by many pioneers, such as G. Stanley Hall (1844-1924), J.R. Gallagher MD, Adele D. Hofmann MD (1926 to 2001) and others. I was an adolescent medicine fellow of Professor Adele D. Hofmann at New York University School of Medicine (New York, USA) and was honored to write with her about adolescent medicine seeking to influence others around the world in this important field.

In this regard it was my high honor and pleasure to meet Dr Swati Bhave in 2001 when she came to my institution in the United States for postgraduate training in adolescent medicine. I lead an international group that came to India in 2002 for a PG certificate course in adolescent medicine conducted by the IAP adolescent chapter in collaboration with my Institute and Michigan State University which was a week-long course and attended by nearly 200 pediatricians. In this course, I had the honor of working with Dr Bhave and also meeting many wonderful pediatricians in India with an interest in adolescent medicine that was ignited by the Professor S Bhave's passion for adolescent health care. I was also deeply privileged to be a Guest Editor for the 2006 **Bhave's Textbook of Adolescent Medicine** with Swati Y Bhave as Editor-in-Chief and also the Academic Editors—MKC Nair, A Parthasarathy and PSN Menon.

Since then I have seen Dr Bhave at various international meetings where her passion for adolescent medicine and her genius for organization was on display. I told people that I was the one to ignite this passion but, in reality, it was there all along! I was happy that she again came for a refresher course at my institution in 2008. Her passion for learning and updating herself does not stop. After a long and challenging journey, here is the Second Edition of this book to teach additional pediatricians the importance and the technical aspects of adolescent health care for the teenagers of India and beyond! I am again deeply grateful to be a Guest Editor for this Second Edition.

Donald E Greydanus
MD, Dr HC (ATHENS), FAAP, FIAP (HON)
Professor and Founding Chair
Department of Pediatric and Adolescent Medicine, Western Michigan University
Homer Stryker MD School of Medicine
1000 Oakland Drive, Kalamazoo, MI 49008-1284
E-mail: donald.greydanus@med.wmich.edu

Experts Speak.....

International Experts in Adolescent Health

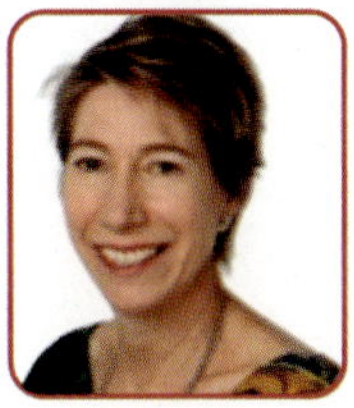

Across the world, it is being realized that health services are not meeting the needs of adolescents, and health professionals need specific competencies to practice more effectively with the young. Nowhere is this more apparent than in India, given its huge population of adolescents whose health and wellbeing will be powerfully influenced by the social determinants created within their communities, shaped by their experiences of health services. The expert editors and authors of this 2nd edition of **Bhave's Textbook of Adolescent Medicine** are warmly congratulated for their efforts in helping make visible the health needs of Indian adolescents, and the ways in which health professionals can respond. Bravo!

Professor Susan Sawyer MBBS, MD, FRACP

Prof Sawyer co-led the 1st (2007) and 2nd (2012) series on Adolescent Health for The Lancet, and is a commissioner for the 2016 Lancet Commission on Adolescent Health and Wellbeing. For the past 4 years, she has chaired the Technical Steering Committee for the World Health Organization's Department of Maternal, Newborn, Child and Adolescent Health.

She is the Geoff and Helen Handbury Chair of Adolescent Health, Department Pediatrics, University of Melbourne, and Director, Centre for Adolescent Health, Royal Children's Hospital Melbourne, Australia

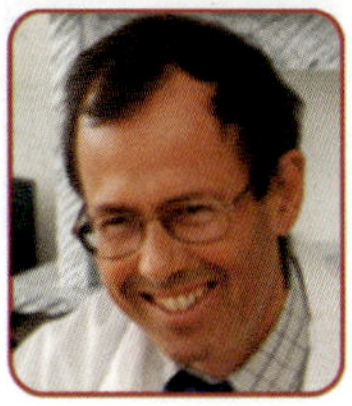

Bhave's Textbook of Adolescent Medicine is a timely comprehensive tool which will assist health care professionals in addressing most of adolescents' health problems and diseases. Not only does it provide sound knowledge on frequent and concerning situations which practitioners have to deal with, but it also focuses on the ingredients of adequate health care to young people, including communication skills and adequate care setting (e.g. adolescent friendly health services). The release of this volume attests of the importance of the health of young people in India as well as the vitality of the field of adolescent medicine and health in this country and part of the world.

Professor Emeritus Pierre-André Michaud MD
Coordinator, Program EuTEACH/European Training in Effective Adolescent Care and Health
Independent Consultant in School and
Adolescent Health and in Medical Education
Former Head, Multidisciplinary Unit for Adolescent Medicine
Division of Pediatrics, University Hospital of Lausanne
Former Vice Dean for Medical Education
Faculty of Biology and Medicine, Lausanne, Switzerland

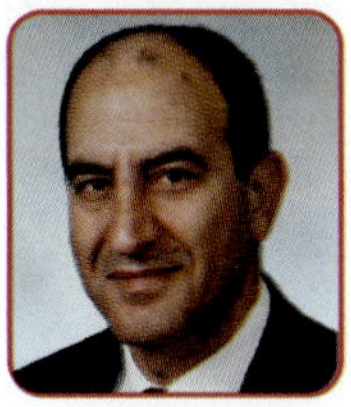

Mortality and morbidity in adolescents is mostly the result of preventable causes. Understanding teen development and the psychosocial issues contributing to the problems adolescents face is crucial in improving health outcomes of teens and societal health as a whole. The second edition of **Bhave's Textbook of Adolescent Medicine** will provide health care practitioners and public health leaders with an invaluable resource toward accomplishing these goals. It addresses every topic related to adolescent health in a comprehensive, easy to use and up-to-date way that will make it a great resource for anyone dealing with young people. I am confident it will be a great success.

Professor Hatim Omar, MD
Professor, Pediatrics & Obstetrics/Gynecology
Division of Adolescent Medicine Chief | Children's Miracle Network Chair
UK Healthcare | Department of Pediatrics
Division of Adolescent Medicine and Young Parents Program
KY Clinic, Lexington, KY UNITED KINGDOM

Public Health Specialists

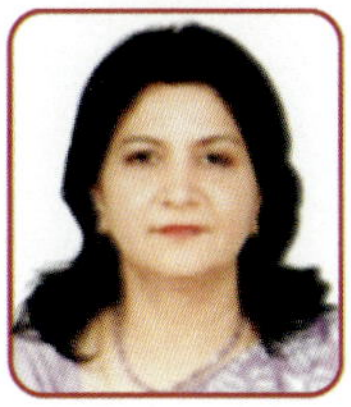

The 2nd edition of **Bhave's Textbook of Adolescent Medicine** includes important reference materials for physicians of all specialties who deal with adolescent patients. Issues of public health importance like preconception care, non-communicable diseases and mental health are included. The inclusion of flowcharts and tables format makes it user friendly and will serve its purpose of being a desktop reference. Having trained Dr Swati Bhave in adolescent health to become a master trainer in WHO adolescent health programs, it is heartening to note her contributions and commitment towards building capacities of physicians. I wish this book all success!

Neena Raina
Regional Advisor
Child and Adolescent Health
World Health Organization
Regional Office of South-East Asia, New Delhi

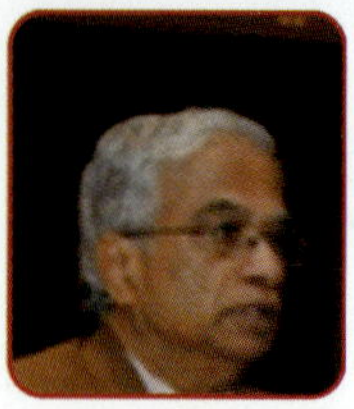

My association with Dr Swati Bhave, began since 2000 as President of IAP, and in the last 15 years it has developed into a personal bond beyond academics. I was faculty in the first training program of IAP Adolescent chapter. International Training Program–ITPAH-2002. There is need to have health workers who understand the special needs of adolescents and the ways in which they differ from small children and adults. This 2nd edition of **Bhave's Textbook of Adolescent Medicine** will be most useful for primary and secondary health care workforce and clinicians in other fields of medicine dealing with adolescents to make them competent to ensure that the services that they provide are of high quality. Dr Bhave is fortunate to get the unstinted support of her husband Yashwant Bhave throughout her professional journey.

K Suresh
MD, DIH, DF, FIAP, FIPHA, FISCD
Public (Child) Health Consultant
Retired Senior Program Officer-Health
UNICEF India Country Office, New Delhi

Presidents of Indian Academy of Pediatrics

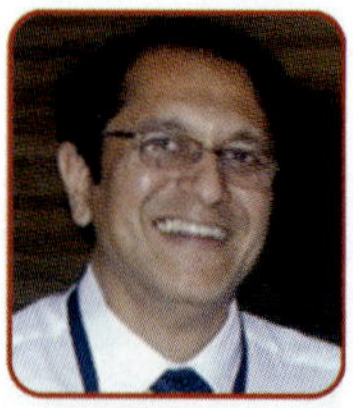

Adolescence is one of the most beautiful and poignant phase of one's life, yet it is also one of the most difficult and turbulent phases. We, the pediatricians, as gatekeepers, have the pleasant responsibility of making this journey better and easier for both the teens and their parents and teachers by empowering them. We can be that someone whom they can trust and confide in, someone who can guide and is non-judgmental. **Bhave's Textbook of Adolescent Medicine** will accomplish this task. It will serve as a desktop reference and equip all pediatricians and also clinicians of all specialties to deal with adolescents.

Professor Pramod Jog
MD, MNAMS, FIAP
President IAP, 2016
Professor of Pediatrics, DY Patil Medical College
Consultant Pediatrician Pune, Maharashtra

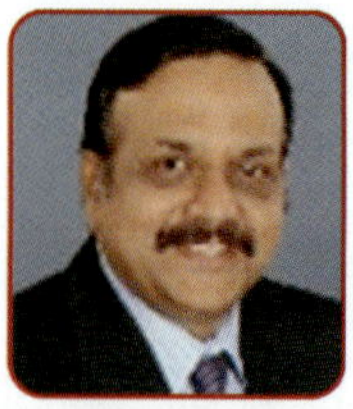

IAP was a pioneer in adolescent health training and had declared the year 2000 as the "IAP Year of Adolescent Health". The IAP adolescent health leaders, Dr Swati Bhave (President IAP, 2000), Dr MKC Nair (President IAP, 2004) with Dr Parthasarathy (President IAP, 1997) and Dr PSN Menon brought out the first **Textbook of Adolescent Medicine in India in 2006**–endorsed by the IAP Adolescent Chapter. This second edition is a desktop reference for practicing clinicians of all specialties who are catering to adolescent clients. Such a concise book covering all possible clinical aspects was the need of the hour and I congratulate the editors for their painstaking effort of choosing useful contents and wish the book all success.

Dr S Sachidananda Kamath
MD, FIAP
President IAP, 2015
Medical Director, Welcare Hospital, Kochi, Kerala

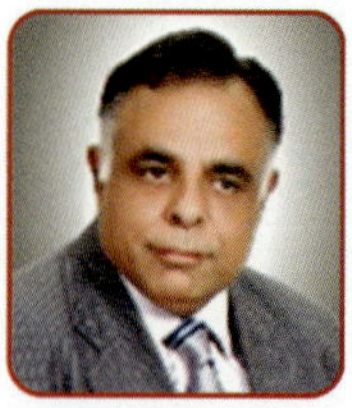

Adolescent medicine in India still is not a recognized degree by any University or by the Medical Council of India. The problems of adolescents are interdisciplinary; thus there is a dire need for training in adolescent medicine. This book which caters to the unique aspects of adolescent patients will indeed fill the gap that exists. Since it is brought out by an editorial team who were pioneers in bringing out the first **Textbook of Adolescent Medicine in India in 2006**, the credibility is well established. Having been an integral part of the first edition, I wish this book all success.

Anupam Sachdeva
MBBS, DCH, MD
President Elect IAP, 2017
Chairman, Department of Pediatrics and Academics
Director, Pediatric Hematology Oncology
and Bone Marrow Transplantation
Sir Ganga Ram Hospital, New Delhi

IAP Presidents

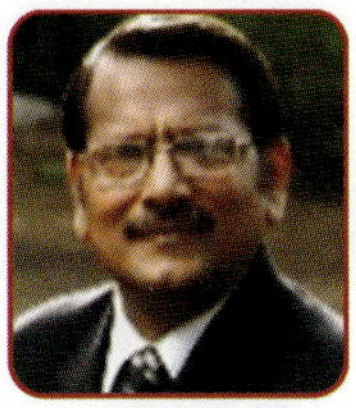

I am very happy to know that the 2nd edition of **Bhave's Textbook of Adolescent Medicine** is being released. I was an integral part of the holistic first edition published in 2006. It is very heartening to note that this version is catering to the practicing clinicians of not only adolescent pediatrics but for clinicians of all specialties. The contents show the efforts made by the editorial team to cover all aspects of clinical practice. I find that this book will be indeed very useful in practice and wish them all success.

CP Bansal
MD, FIAP, PGDAP, FICMCH
President IAP, 2013
President, South Asia Pediatrics Association (SAPA)
Former Chairperson, Adolescent Health Academy India, Gwalior
Consultant Pediatrician, Gwalior
Madhya Pradesh

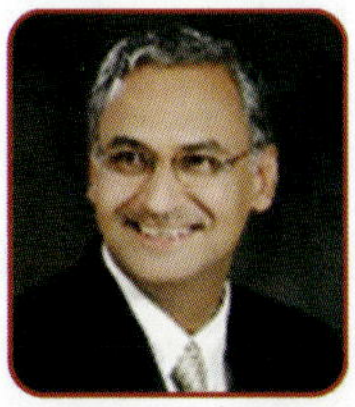

The second edition of **Bhave's Textbook of Adolescent Medicine** is a perfect book for all the pediatricians. The book has knowledge embedded by its expert and experienced authors and it will be helpful for the readers. I congratulate all the contributors and editors who have worked immensely for preparing this textbook which will be a guide for pediatricians.

Naveen Thacker
MD, FIAP
President IAP, 2007
President–Asia Pacific Pediatric Association (APPA), 2016-2018
Coordinator of Development, International Pediatric Association (IPA)
CSO representative–GAVI Alliance Board
Director, Deep Children Hospital and Research Centre
Kutch–Gujarat

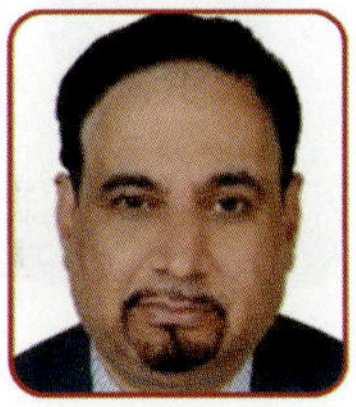

The second edition of **Bhave's Textbook of Adolescent Medicine** is intended as a desktop reference for practicing physicians of all specialties, who are consulted for adolescent problems in daily practice. The eminent authors and editors have tried to put matter which is very adolescent specific and user friendly. It benefits from Dr Swati Bhave's many years of clinical and public health experience, during which time I have had the pleasure to be associated with her work as a respected colleague, both in IAP and in academic field. I congratulate Dr Swati Bhave and the dedicated team for working hard to bring out this excellent book and wish them all success in this commendable endeavor.

Uday Bodhankar
MD, DCH, FIAP
President IAP, 1994
International President, Commonwealth Association for Health and Disability (COMHAD), UK
International Council Member–Asian Society Pediatric Research (ASPR), Japan
Consultant Pediatrician, Nagpur, Maharashtra, India

Adolescent Pediatrician

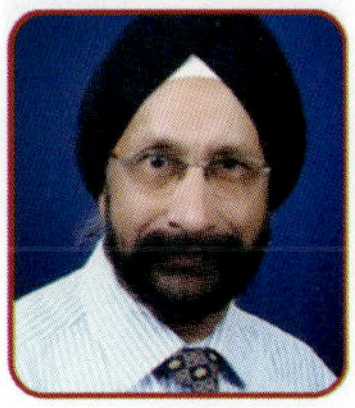

This book was a critical requirement given the growing number of adolescent issues in our country. It would definitely be useful for the practicing adolescent physicians as well. A lot of useful articles have been included in the 2nd edition of this book.

JS Tuteja
MD, DCH, PGDAP, FIAP
Chairperson, Adolescent Health Academy–IAP 2012-15
Mission Kishore Uday 2013 President Action Plan-2012
National Convener–IAP Difficult Adolescent
Consultant Pediatrician, Indore
Madhya Pradesh

Consultant Pediatric Gastro-Enterologist And Hepatologist

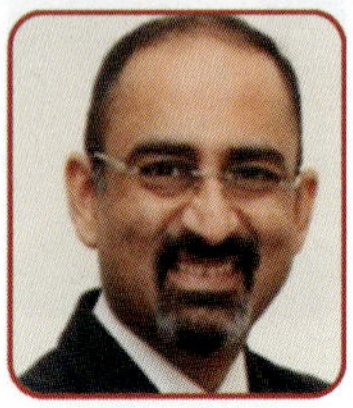

The Textbook of Adolescent Medicine focuses on a clinical approach to adolescent development and the conditions commonly seen during adolescence. A very well written book by Dr Swati Y Bhave and the editorial team, Dr Parthasarathy and Dr PSN Menon. This book is a must read for everyone linked to adolescent health.

Professor Anupam Sibal
MD, FIMSA, FIAP, FRCP (Glasg), FRCP (Lon), FRCPCH, FAAP
Group Medical Director, Apollo Hospitals Group
Senior Consultant Pediatric Gastroenterologist and Hepatologist, Indraprastha Apollo Hospital, New Delhi
Clinical Professor, Faculty of Medicine and Health Sciences Macquarie University, Sydney, Australia

Community Medicine Physician

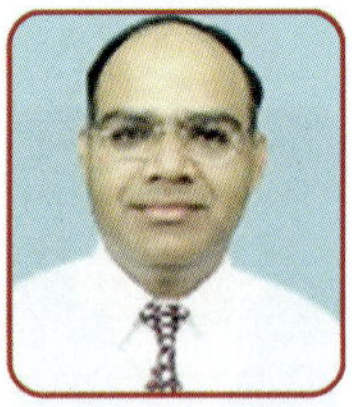

Adolescent Medicine is urgently required to harness the maximum benefit of young population in India. The 2nd edition of **Bhave's Textbook of Adolescent Medicine** deserves appreciation for its scientific contents, variety of topics and authorship and also approach to the problem. It is commendable work of editors. Topics for example, on Non-communicable Diseases, Nutrition, Karyakram (RKSK) are satisfying the academic need of the not only students of pediatrics, obstetrics and gynecology, social welfare but also public health. My best wishes for its success. STD, teen pregnancy, contraception, environmental issues, WHO pre-conception care and Rashtriya Kishor Swasthya Karyakram.

Jugal Kishore
MBBS, PGCHFWM, PDGEE, MSc, MD, PhD, FNAMS, FIMSA, FIPHA, FIAPSM, FIMAAMS
Secretary General of Indian Association for Adolescent Health (IAAH), Head of Community Medicine
Vardhman Mahavir Medical College and Safdarjung Hospital, New Delhi

Endocrinologist

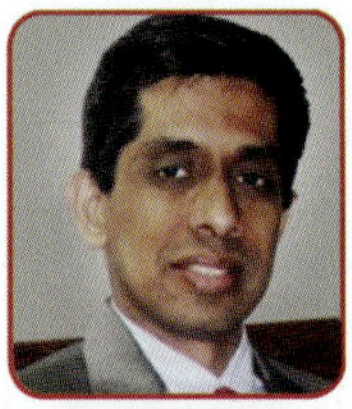

The release of the second edition of **Textbook of Adolescent Medicine** itself speaks volume about the quality of the book content. The experts have left no topic uncovered that will help the practicing physicians. One of the topics which demand current attention is nutrition, because of the changing times. With the advent of technology, mental health is a key area of interest associated with the well-being of the adolescent. I think this book on health of the adolescent can contribute majorly in the growing economy of India. My heartiest congratulations for this step and best wishes for success.

Shashank R Joshi
MD, DM, FICP, FACP (USA), FACE (USA), FRCP (Glsg & Edin)
Padma Shri Awardee 2014
President, Endocrine Society of India and Indian Academy of Diabetes
Endocrinologist, Joshi Clinic, Lilavati and Bhatia Hospital Mumbai, Maharashtra, India

Internal Medicine Physician

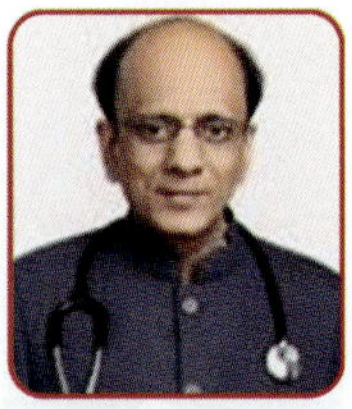

Adolescent Medicine is the need of the day. The 2nd edition of **Bhave's Textbook of Adolescent Medicine** is full of scientific evidence-based contents. It covers all topics like non-communicable diseases, nutrition, STD, teen pregnancy, contraception, environmental issues, WHO pre-conception care and Rashtriya Kishor Swasthya Karyakram. This edition will be like a textbook for the practicing doctors and has inputs of Dr Bhave's years of experience in public health. I congratulate Dr Swati Y Bhave and her dedicated team for this academic feat.

KK Aggarwal
Honorary Secretary General, Indian Medical Association (IMA)
Editor-in-Chief, IJCP Group of Publications and eMedinewS
Sr Consultant Medicine and Cardiology, Dean Board of Medical Education
Moolchand Hospital, New Delhi

Obstetrician and Gynecologist

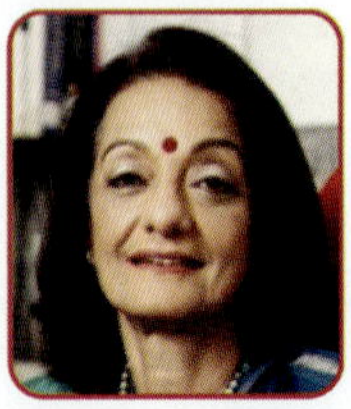

Dr Swati Bhave has once again created a masterpiece–a book focusing on adolescent health, an area which is neglected, by physicians for both adults and children. This very much needed book will assist physicians in offering better health care to our youth as it covers every aspect of adolescent health in a very practical manner for clinicians to follow. I wish Swati Bhave all the best for this venture.

Duru Shah
MD, FRCOG, FCPS, FOCS, FICOG, FICMCH, DGO, DFP
President, The PCOS Society (India), 2015
President, Federation of Obstetric and Gynecological, Societies of India (FOGSI) 2006
Chair of the Indian College of Obstetrics and Gynecology (ICOG) (2009-2011)
Consultant Gynecologist–Breach Candy Hospital, Jaslok Hospital Gynaecworld, Mumbai

Preface to the Second Edition

We were fortunate to be the pioneers in bringing out the first textbook of adolescent medicine in India in 2006 and now again working together for this second edition.

We are honored to have a two forewords for this book from very illustrious personalities: from one of our own team of editors from the first edition, Dr MKC Nair who is one of the pioneers of adolescent health in the country and is now the Vice Chancellor of the Kerala University of Health Sciences and Dr Bruce Dick who is the President of the IAAH–International Association of Adolescent Health and is an internationally acclaimed adolescent health expert who had worked in WHO, Geneva in the child and adolescent section for many years. We are privileged to have an appreciation from Padmabhushan Awardee Dr RD Lele known as the "Father of Nuclear Medicine in India", and author of many outstanding books in medicine and non-medical subjects. He is now 87 years old and had also given us an appreciation for the 1st edition.

We are fortunate to again have as our Guest Editor, Dr Donald E Greydanus, who is an internationally renowned, American Adolescent specialist, who has authored innumerable books on various aspects of adolescence.

The last edition was a voluminous book with more than 1200 pages. It was the need of the hour as adolescent medicine was in its infancy in our country and we wanted to cover as many topics as possible which would be of value to all stakeholders in adolescent health. So many topics were included in addition to clinical medicine relevant to adolescent health — school mental health, life-skill training, parenting, positive discipline, stress and anger management, gender issues, dating violence, risk-taking behaviors, sports medicine, disaster management, public health issues, field experience of NGOs and many more.

This edition is now focusing only on clinical adolescent medicine and the aim is to cater to physicians of all specialties who see adolescents in their clinical practice. We have tried to make it a desktop reference which highlights adolescence-specific issues in clinical medicine which may not be available in other pediatric or adult medicine textbooks. Our aim is not to provide detailed disease descriptions; but highlight those diseases and health issues that present in adolescent age group for the first time or get aggravated in adolescent age group. We have also spent a lot of pages on chapters which are very important to practicing clinicians—setting up an ideal adolescent-friendly health clinic, understanding neurodevelopment to learn how to deal with the adolescent age group, specialized history taking, approach to adolescent patients and handling parents. Some important new topics like WHO preconception care, screening and prevention of non-communicable diseases and palliative care are added.

Some annexures for practical use have IAP growth charts which are useful standards for height, weight and BMI; drug dosages, and various questionnaires and proformas which should be of help for practicing adolescent specialists. We also have added information on the prestigious RKSK program of Government of India and a resource list of important documents of WHO on adolescent health.

The format used is more of tables and figures and less of text matter.

We hope the readers like this format and this book is even a bigger success than the first edition.

Swati Y Bhave
PSN Menon
A Parthasarathy

Preface to the First Edition

We are fortunate to be the pioneers in bringing out a Textbook of Adolescent Medicine which was a much felt need in India today.

We are honored to have the foreword from none other than Mr PK Hota, The Secretary of Health, Government of India, a man who has done so much for the adolescent health in India and is actively involved in the implementation of adolescent friendly health services and adolescent reproductive and sexual health programs in RCH II, which is a prime need today.

We are privileged to have a message from Padmabhushan Awardee Dr RD Lele known as the "Father of Nuclear Medicine in India" and author of many outstanding books in medicine and non-medical subjects.

We are fortunate to have as our Guest Editor, Dr Donald E Greydanus, who is an internationally renowned, American adolescence specialist, who has authored innumerable books on various aspects of adolescence. Our Editorial Advisory Board consists of Dr Dilip R Patel, a sports medicine and adolescence specialist and Dr Helen D Pratt, a clinical adolescent psychologist from USA. Both have co-authored books and various PCNA issues along with Dr Greydanus. The other eminent members include a popular psychiatrist Dr Jitendra Nagpal, Clinical psychologist, Dr Anuradha Sovani and the President of FOGSI, Dr Duru Shah, all from India.

Adolescent care requires team work and specialists from all fields. Our senior editors and editorial board members are reputed in their field and their contributions have made this book the state-of-the art. We have some young contributors, bringing contemporary ideas into the book.

We wanted this book to be of use to all persons dealing with adolescent health and so in addition to the growth, development, puberty and medical issues we have also covered a large number of social and community issues. We have gone beyond the walls of the hospitals to cover street children, child labor, violence and juvenile crime.

A large number of problems adolescents face are due to their risk taking behaviors which can easily be prevented by appropriate information education, preventive counseling and anticipatory guidance. We have covered a large number of issues like school mental health, life skill training, parenting, positive discipline, stress and anger management, impact of internet and media. We have an excellent section on Psychiatric and Behavioral Disorders and Substance Abuse.

Reproductive and sexual health of adolescents is vital issue and we have reviewed HIV/AIDS, STIs, contraception, teenage pregnancy, nutrition, anemia, gender issues, dating violence, rape, sexual abuse, etc. with a focus on adolescence.

Participation in sports competitions is on the rise and we have a whole section devoted to this. We also have covered the impact of disasters and effects of environmental hazards in this vulnerable age.

Some annexures for practical use have common laboratory values, drug dosages, various questionnaires and proformas which should be of help for practicing adolescent specialists.

Just as a rose bud needs adequate watering to slowly bloom into a beautiful rose, an adolescent child requires adequate physical, mental and emotional nourishment to develop into a healthy, strong and beautiful young adult. Most of us became pediatricians because we love children. This textbook is for those who love adolescents and want to be part of making their transition into adulthood rich and rewarding.

This being the first edition and being brought out in a record time of six months, may have some lacunae and may not be a perfect copy. But the felt need was great and time was of essence. We request you to read and point out the lacunae so that we make the future editions even better and we do hope that this Textbook of Adolescent Medicine would meet the expectations of one and all.

Swati Y Bhave
MKC Nair
A Parthasarathy
PSN Menon

From the Desk of the Chief Editor
Second Edition

Dear Readers,

It was 10 years ago that we published the first textbook of adolescent medicine in the country. The first edition was very holistic and covered every aspect of adolescent health from clinical medicine, public health perspective, school mental health, psychological and behavioral medicine etc as it was aimed at creating a universal awareness of this speciality of adolescent medicine which was in its nidus in 2006 in our country.

In the last 10 years there have been tremendous advances in the field of adolescent medicine. Newer imaging techniques like functional MRI (fMRI) and PET scan have given a tremendous insight on the neurodevelopment of the adolescent brain. In the past it was thought that at 18 years a human being is a mature adult and hence most countries at this age, one is given the right to vote, right to drive, legal permission to consume alcohol and tobacco products etc. It is now realised the adolescent brain is still under development and is only completely mature between 25–30 years! Hence we have added a new chapter of neurodevelopment in this edition. It is now known that the adolescent is functioning at the limbic level of the brain as the prefrontal cortex is the last to mature. Thus unlike an adult who has top down regulation from the prefrontal cortex the adolescent brain has a bottom up approach of regulation by the hypothalamus and responds with hot cognition i.e. emotions. This has given us insight into the adolescent behavior that is reward seeking and experimentation and results in high risk behavior. It has also shown that adolescent brain is very vulnerable to substance abuse and exposure to tobacco and alcohol in adolescent age not only has adverse effect on the developing brain but has very high chance of long time addiction lasting into adult life.

Non-communicable diseases (NCD) i.e. lifestyle diseases are now the main global burden in both developed and developed countries. It has also been realised that behaviors that begin in adolescence like sedentary lifestyle and reduction in physical activity, addiction to high sugar, high salt, processed food with high levels of transfat and exposure to tobacco and alcohol are the nidus of lifestyle diseases in adults and hence prevention and screening has to begin in adolescence. We have added a new chapter on NCD in this edition.

A group of like-minded doctors and other adolescent stakeholders have come together in 2008 to form an Association of Adolescent and Child Care in India–AACCI (www.aacci.in). We have been working to promote healthy lifestyle for prevention of lifestyle diseases using the approach of life skill education devised by WHO. We conduct workshops for students of all ages, teachers and parents on various adolescence related issues and also conduct multicentric behavioral research.

One of the definition of adolescence was a period which began with puberty and ended with either financial independence and/or parenthood. With higher education and advanced age of marriage and delaying the first offspring, the *"period of adolescence"* has now extended far beyond the WHO definition of 10–19 years, to now also include young people, youth or young adults which can be upto 25–30 years. This is called *"extended adolescence"*. This has important implications for health care workers and policy makers. The global community is now increasingly aware of the opportunities of investing in adolescence and hence a new Global Strategy for Women's, Children's and Adolescents' Health has recently been launched.

Hence, it is very important for those clinicians working for adolescents to keep updating themselves with new knowledge of adolescent health to keep abreast of the advances in this fascinating field of adolescent medicine. I have had the opportunity to get a refresher course in adolescent medicine in 2008 under our Guest Editor Dr Greydanus at Kalamazoo Center of Learning, Michigan State University in USA. I have done a certificate course on Adolescent Health and Counseling from Indira Gandhi National Open University in 2013-14. In September-November 2015, I also did an 8-week online course on Adolescent Global Health designed by stalwarts in this field Dr George Patton and Dr Susan Sawyer from Australia.

In the last 10 years I have also expanded my horizon in adolescent health. I was fortunate to work and as a member of WHO, Geneva TSC–Technical Steering Committee on Child and Adolescent Health in 2009-10. WHO HPV Vaccine Advisory Committee in 2010. I am the regional vice president for IAAH–International Association for Adolescent Health for South East Asia from 2009 to 2017. I have worked as Technical Advisor in Adolescent Health in International Pediatric Association (IPA) from 2008 to 2013. I have worked in various capacities in IPA from 2001 to 2013 and I was IPA representative to work with WHO, Geneva on adolescent health for many years. This gave me multiple opportunities to attend many WHO meetings and make presentations on various aspects of adolescent health in many international conferences where I could interact and share experiences with world class international experts on adolescent health which has really enriched my outlook on adolescent health.

Having been extremely busy professionally I could not spend time to come out with a second edition of this book though it was always at the back of my mind and many people kept asking me about it. I have edited three handbooks on topics related to adolescent health during 2006 to 2010 on Adolescent Gynecology and Adolescent Reproductive and Sexual Health (ARSH), Sports Medicine and Immunization. I have been fortunate to be one of the advisory consultants in the final phase of development of WHO "Adolescent Job Aids" in 2009, for teaching clinical approach for adolescents and also helped in the field of testing in India. I have also worked as one of the resource persons for developing training manuals for various prestigious national programs over last decade–WHO manual for psychosocial support for children and adolescents in disaster situations, AEP–Adolescent Education Program, RKSK–Rashtriya Kishor Swasthya Karyakram.

In last 10 years adolescent medicine has got due recognition as a specialty in India and Dr MKC Nair has started a PG diploma course at Kerala University and many pediatricians have been trained in adolescent medicine and doing clinical practice. DY Patil Medical College, Pune is also planning to start a certificate course in adolescent pediatrics.

Many physicians of all specialties now understand the concept of well adolescent monitoring and not just looking at the medical illnesses of adolescents. A lot of my clinician friends working for adolescent health have expressed the need to have some clinical book in adolescent health and I have been thinking about coming out with a book that specifically highlights what is different in an adolescent patient compared to a pediatrics or adult patient. I wanted this to be a smaller book with totally a clinical approach which practicing clinicians could use as a desktop reference when dealing with an adolescent patient. We have highlighted the aims and objectives of this 2nd edition in the preface of this book.

I am extremely fortunate that even though it has been 10 years I could gather together the same team that worked for the 1st edition. Dr Greydanus an internationally renowned adolescent physician from USA, who was the Guest Editor in the first edition, again agreed to come on board and it has been a privilege to once again have his guidance. Dr A Parthasarathy, who is doyen in pediatric book publishing in India and whom I consider one of my gurus in IAP agreed to come as the Academic Editor. He is a constant guiding force and his expertise in publishing books has been invaluable. Dr PSN Menon a great academician and a valuable friend also agreed to be in the team and has worked meticulously as an Academic Editor for this edition also. His perfectionism has raised the standard of our chapters. The fourth editor of the previous team, Dr MKC Nair has now become Vice Chancellor of the Kerala University of Health Sciences, Thrissur and we are honored that he has written a foreword for this book. We are also fortunate that we have got a foreword from Dr Bruce Dick, President of IAAH–International Association of Adolescent Health.

We had a huge editorial team for the last edition as it was a book over 1200 pages but we have just kept the core editorial team for this smaller version. The last team had honored me by deciding to call it as **"Bhave's Textbook of Adolescent Medicine"** and we have continued the same title. I am also fortunate that most of the senior authors of the last edition have again rewritten their chapter for this edition. We have some new senior authors and to infuse new ideas we have also taken some young authors.

Last edition had an appreciation page by Dr R.D. Lele, my father and also my role model in the field of medicine. I am fortunate he is still active even at the age of 87 years with all his faculties intact. He was able to write an appreciation for this 2nd edition and has also contributed to the chapter on nuclear medicine in this book along with my brother Dr Vikram Lele who had contributed to the first edition.

Last edition was dedicated to the loving memory of my dear mother, who passed away in 2003. She was of immense support to me all through her life and had always motivated me in my academic pursuits, especially in writing. She would have indeed been very proud to see the 2nd edition. This book is dedicated to my husband, Yashwant, who sacrificed many hours of our family life by allowing me to work hours together on my passion of adolescent medicine and editing this book in the last six months. But for his support, this book would not have seen the light of the day.

I hope this book proves to be of value to all those working with adolescents. Needless to add, all the credit goes to the editorial team and contributors while I remain responsible for the shortcomings!

Swati Y Bhave
Adolescent Pediatrician and Head of Adolescent Wellness Clinic
Jehangir Hospital, Pune, Maharashtra (2014 to date)
Executive Director, AACCI (2007 to date)
Association of Adolescent and Child Care in India, Mumbai, Maharashtra
Regional Vice President SE Asia
International Association of Adolescent Health (IAAH) (2009-13 and 2013-17)
Member Governing Council NCD Child (2014 to date)

From the Desk of the Chief Editor First Edition

Dear readers,

It has given me a great sense of fulfillment and joy to have finally realized my dream of writing a comprehensive textbook of adolescent medicine for our country.

In 1999, as President Elect IAP, I began planning my IAP presidential program with Dr MKC Nair. The year 2000 was declared as "IAP Year of Adolescent Health" and an IAP national task force was formed under my chairpersonship to focus on Adolescent Health for next five years. The IAP adolescent chapter was formed in the year 2000. I worked as its chairperson from 2002-05. It has over 1000 members today and has been in the IAP best award chapter category in three consecutive years 2003, 2004 and 2005.

I met Dr Greydanus, the guest editor of this book, at a conference of the American Academy of Pediatrics in 1999. He is considered as the doyen of adolescent medicine, having written innumerable books on adolescent health. We discussed the development of Adolescent Pediatrics as a specialty in India. He was gracious to promise all help including spending quality time by coming to India and conduct training programs with his team. I did a short postgraduate training in adolescent medicine under him at the Kalamazoo Center, Michigan State University, USA in 2001. I consider him my mentor for my work on adolescent health.

In December 2002, the IAP adolescent chapter held a certificate course training program in collaboration with his university which was attended by nearly 200 pediatricians from all over the country. This week-long course was paid by the participants themselves without any sponsorship. We brought out two large volumes for this course: Part I on US scenario and Part II on the Indian scenario. These are popular even today and are being used as course material for the IAP adolescent chapter training programs. From the feedback by the participants, it is gratifying to note that a majority of them have involved themselves in adolescent health care delivery either by starting adolescent clinic or by allocating separate slots exclusively for adolescents in their pediatrics clinics.

This experience made us feel the need of a good textbook for adolescent medicine in India. I deeply appreciate the help given by Dr Parthasarathy in his persistent motivation to me and approaching Jaypee to start the administrative process in 2003. But all good things take time and it was only in June 2004 that I started working on this book. We have brought it out in a record time of six months. I am conscious of the slips that may have cropped in, for which I request the indulgence of the readers. Critical appraisal from the readers will go a long way in shaping the future editions in a better format.

I am overwhelmed by the love and affection of the editorial team by deciding to call it **"Bhave's Textbook of Adolescent Medicine".** I thank Dr TS Jain and Dr CP Bansal, the Chairperson and Secretary for the IAP adolescent chapter and its executive board members for giving this book an endorsement of the chapter. I thank all the members of the editorial team and the contributors and specially the Delhi Group of Adolescent Pediatricians, Rajesh Mehta, Harish K Pemde, Sangita Yadav for their continuous help and motivation.

I am honored that Mr Prasanna Hota, The Secretary to Government of India, Ministry of Health and Family Welfare graciously consented to write the Foreword. I am fortunate to have the appreciation of Dr RD Lele who is my father and also my role model in the field of Medicine. I dedicate this book to the loving memory of my dear mother, who passed away two years ago. She was an immense support to me all through her life and has always motivated me in my academic pursuits, especially in writing. She would have indeed been very proud to see this book. My husband Yashwant sacrificed many hours of our family life by allowing me to work hours together, editing this book in the last six months. But for his support this book would not have seen the light of the day.

My two sons Ajinkya and Aditya made my experience of parenting of adolescents a period of joy, to cherish and remember and inspired me to branch out of pediatrics into the field of adolescent medicine. Most of us became pediatricians because we love children. This textbook is for those who love adolescents and want to be part of making their transition into adulthood rich and rewarding.

I hope this book proves to be of value to all those working with adolescents. Needless to add, all the credit goes to the contributors while I remain responsible for the shortcomings!

Swati Y Bhave
Convener, International Pediatric Association (IPA) Interest Group on Adolescent Health
Member, WHO Regional Technical Committee on Adolescent Health
Chairperson, Indian Academy of Pediatrics (IAP) Task Force on Adolescent Health 2000-04
Chairperson, IAP Adolescent Chapter 2002-05 and
IAP Adolescent Chapter Research and Training Wing 2006-08
Member: Governing Council NCD Child (2014 to date)

Appreciation

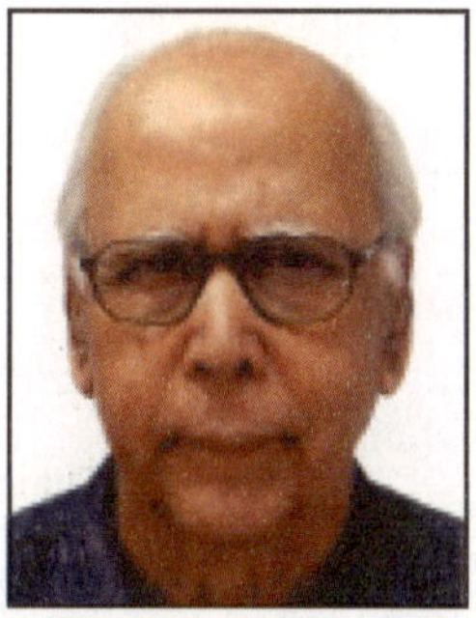

I am very happy to be able to write the appreciation for the 2nd edition of **Bhave's Textbook of Adolescent Medicine**. I had written the appreciation for the 1st edition published 10 years ago in 2006, which was the first textbook of adolescent medicine in the country and has been widely appreciated. In the last 10 years adolescent medicine has progressed a lot with many clinicians wanting to work exclusively for this specialty. The Government of India also has given adolescent health due recognition by launching the RKSK–Rashtriya Kishor Swasthya Karyakram Program.

Care of adolescent girls in the last many years has helped in reducing the widely prevalent gender discrimination against females, and has put major emphasis on the care of the mother and the female child and adolescent girl, e.g. nutrition, menstrual hygiene, provision of sanitary napkins, prevention of iron deficiency, sex education and prevention of STD/HIV, emergency contraception, women's reproductive health and promotion of breastfeeding. According to a report by AC Nielsen 2011, "88% of Indian women use unhygienic methods for menstrual discharge as a result of which 70% women have infection of the genital tract". Arunachalam Muruganantham from Coimbatore–Tamil Nadu, a school drop-out resolved to produce low cost affordable sanitary napkins, using cellulose from pinewood bark in place of cotton. He invented a machine costing Rs. 75000 which can be used by village women to produce 200-250 sanitary pads per day and provide work for ten women. His aim is to increase the usage of sanitary pads in villages to 100%. The 2014 Time magazine included Muruganantham's name among the "Most Influential People". Anil Virmani made a documentary on the "Menstrual Man" which got an award in 2013.

India still has a large number of adolescent pregnancies which adds to the high maternal and infant mortality in the country. Care of the pregnant adolescent has to be ensured to see that no baby is born with a birth weight of less than 2.5 kg. But much more still needs to be done on this front to reduce the stagnant IMR in our country. Hopefully the NKSK–Navjath Shishu Swasthya Karyakram would change the scenario.

Adolescent health has been given due recognition in India since ancient times. It is interesting to note that *Kaumarabrhrutya* (pediatrics) was one of the eight components of Ayurveda and the word "*Kumar*" includes adolescents, not just children. Ayurveda divides the early human life-span into (1) *Balya* upto 10 years, (2) *Kaumarya* upto 16 years, (3) *Vivardhamana* (growth 16-20 years), and (4) *Youvana* youth (20-30 years).

By this concept–it is logical to include the *Kaumarya* extending upto 16 years and *Vivardhamana* 16-20 age group into the adolescent group–adulthood beginning with the 21st birthday!

India has a long tradition of comprehensive health care, extending over more than 2500 years. *Ayurveda* (literally meaning 'Science of Life') emphasizes that "health is not a commodity that can be purchased–it is an asset which has to be assiduously maintained with care by following rules of conduct regarding diet, exercise and behavior". Diseases occur in those who do not observe the rules of healthy living; viz. "*Swastha Vrutta* for the body and *Sad Vrutta* (ethical conduct) for the mind". Ayurveda clearly states that, the aim of medicine is three-fold: (1) Promotion of positive health, (2) Prevention of disease, and (3) Treatment of disease when it arises. These three aims remain as important today as in the past. One new component that has been added as part of treatment is rehabilitation. Non-communicable diseases (NCDs) in adults are known to have their nidus in not following healthy lifestyle from the adolescent age group. In this respect adolescent screening and prevention of these lifestyle disorders is of vital importance. These behavioral factors are sedentary lifestyle and lack of exercise, consumption of 'High salt, high fat' and 'High fat processed food' that contribute to obesity and high risk of NCDs and tobacco and alcohol consumption. Preventive counseling and anticipatory guidance to reduce high risk behavior and related issues from the pediatric and adolescent age group is the need of the hour if we want to reduce the adult burden of these diseases.

Parents willingly pay doctors' fees for various childhood illnesses and also pay for visits to "well baby clinics". In adolescent age group the physical illness is much less and parents in India have yet to understand the concept "well adolescent monitoring" and hence do not avail of whatever "adolescent services" that are available. Parents are reluctant to pay for these services and adolescents do not have a paying capacity. Physicians and stakeholders of adolescent health have a great role to play to ensure that adolescents get the comprehensive health care–promotive, preventive and curative– so well emphasized in this book.

This book has a focus of serving as a desktop reference for physicians from all specialties who are dealing with adolescent patients. The topics covered are very comprehensive and the table format is very user friendly and I am sure it will serve a great purpose in clinical adolescent medicine.

Padmabhushan Awardee RD Lele
MBBS (Osm) DTM&H (Eng), MRCP (Edin), FRCP (Lon), FNAMS, Hon DSc, Hon D Litt
Hon Chief Physician and Director of Nuclear Medicine and
Ex-Medical Director, Jaslok Hospital and Research Centre, Mumbai
Hon Director of Nuclear Medicine, Lilavati Hospital and Research Centre, Mumbai
Emeritus Professor of Medicine (for life) and Ex-Dean JJ Hospital and Grant Medical College, Mumbai
Emeritus Professor of the National Academy of Medical Sciences, India
Chairman Scientific Advisory Committee, Haffkine Institute of Research, Training and Testing, Mumbai

Acknowledgements

- To our Guest Editor, Dr Donald E Greydanus for his guidance, Dr MKC Nair and Bruce Dick for the forewords and Padmabhushan Awardee Dr RD Lele for his appreciation.

  To all the eminent experts who spared valuable time to give an opinion on this book.

- To all the learned contributors for sparing time to write on the various topics in the short period given.
- Shri Pawaninder P Vij, Chairperson and Managing Director and Mr Anupam Vij, Peepee Publishers and Distributors (P) Ltd. for their cooperation.
- We are grateful to Mr SK Sharma and Mr Pawan Sharma, staff of Peepee Publishers and Distributors (P) Ltd., for their hard work in production of this book.
- Our families for accepting the deprivations of their family time and allowing us to work on this book for last six months.
- God Almighty for giving all our team motivation when at times we thought the task was impossible.

Swati Y Bhave
PSN Menon
A Parthasarathy

Acknowledgements for front and back cover:

We thank the following young people (in alphabetical order) and their parents who kindly provided us their photographs and gave permission for publication.

Front Cover Collage:

Aditya Y Bhave, Akshaya Sagane, Dhanashree Nagare, Gopika Gopidas, Jyothilakshmi, Kavya Balaji, Mahiya Balaji, Muthu Manikandan Ramalingam, Sabarinathan Chelian, Sanjana Chelian, Shilpa Sachdeva, Supriya Sachdeva and Urvashi Lele.

Back Cover Photo Strip:

Aditya Y Bhave, Ajinkya Y Bhave, Isha Dixit, Preshit Sonavane, Sharvari Sagane, Shruthi Pavana, Swathi Pavana and Urvashi Lele.

The collage was designed by Dr Swati Y Bhave.

Contributors

Ambrish Dharmadhikari DPM
Senior Resident
Department of Psychiatry
HBT Medical College and
Dr RN Cooper Municipal General Hospital, Mumbai
ambrish30@gmail.com

Ankur Kumar MD
Senior Resident (DM 1st Year)
Pediatric Clinical Immunology and Rheumatology
Allergy Immunology Unit, Advanced Pediatrics Centre
Post Graduate Institute of Medical Education and Research
Chandigarh
ankurjindal11@gmail.com

Anuradha Sovani M Phil, PhD
Professor and Head
Department of Psychology
SNDT Women's University, Mumbai
anuradhasovani@gmail.com

A Parthasarathy MD (Ped), DCH, DSc (Hons), FIAP
Ex-Distinguished Professor of Pediatrics
The Tamil Nadu Dr MGR Medical University
Retd Senior Clinical Professor of Pediatrics
Madras Medical College and Deputy Superintendent
Institute of Child Health and Hospital for Children, Chennai
apartha2030@gmail.com

Arun Kumar Gupta MD, FAMS
Professor and Head
Department of Radiodiagnosis
All India Institute of Medical Sciences, New Delhi
arunk676@gmail.com

Ashish Kakar BDS, MSc (London), FICOI
DICOI, FICD (USA)
Senior Consultant
Indraprastha Apollo Hospitals, New Delhi
kakar.ashish@gmail.com

Ashwini Bhalerao Gandhi MD, DGO, DFP
FCPS, DNB, FICOG
Consultant Gynecologist
PD Hinduja Hospital and Hinduja Healthcare Surgical, Mumbai
ashwinibgandhi@rediffmail.com

Bharat R Agarwal MD, DCH, DNB, MNAMS
Head, Department of Pediatric Hematology and Oncology
BJ Wadia Hospital for Children
Institute of Child Health and Research Centre
Parel, Mumbai
parulbrat@gmail.com

Bindusha S MD, DNB
Associate Professor, Department of Pediatrics
SAT Hospital and Government Medical College
Thiruvananthapuram
drbindusha@gmail.com

Deepak K Jumani MBBS, ACS (USA), FIAMS, PhD, FACS
Diplomate American Board of Clinical Sexology
AASECT Certified Sex Therapist, Consultant
Sexual Health Physician, Counsellor and Ex-Clinical Associate
Department of Sexual Health Medicine
KEM Hospital, Mumbai
deepak.jumani@gmail.com

Dimple Shastri MBBS, DPM
Consultant Psychiatrist
Dr Shastri's Clinic, Andheri West, Mumbai
Honorary Psychiatrist, Child Development Centre
Haji Ali, Mumbai
dimplej5@hotmail.com

Devendra K Gupta MS, MCh, FAMS,
FRCS (Glas and Edin), DSc (HC)
Professor and Head, Department of Pediatric Surgery
All India Institute of Medical Sciences, Ansari Nagar, New Delhi
profdkgupta@gmail.com

Devika Malhotra MD
Department of Pediatric and Adolescent Medicine
Western Michigan University
Homer Stryker MD School of Medicine
Kalamazoo, Michigan, USA
devika.malhotra@med.wmich.edu

Dilip R Patel MD, MBA, FACSM
Professor, Department of Pediatric and Adolescent Medicine
Western Michigan University
Homer Stryker MD School of Medicine
Kalamazoo, Michigan, USA
dilip.patel@med.wmich.edu

Divya Prabhat MS, DORL, DNB, FICS
Head, Department of ENT
Wadia Children's Hospital, Mumbai
divyaprabhat@gmail.com

Donald E Greydanus MD, Dr HC (ATHENS), FAAP, FIAP (HON)
Professor and Founding Chair
Western Michigan University
Homer Stryker MD School of Medicine
Kalamazoo, Michigam, USA
donald.greydanus@med.wmich.edu

Elizabeth KE MD, PhD
Professor and Head, Department of Pediatrics
SAT Hospital and Government Medical College
Thiruvananthapuram
drelizake@gmail.com

Elyska De Sa MBBS, DCH
Fellow in Developmental and Behavioral Pediatrics
New Horizons Research Foundation, Mumbai
desaelyska@gmail.com

Gitanjali Pillai MA
Clinical Psychologist and Clinical Coordinator
New Horizons Child Development Centre, Mumbai
gitanjalipillai@enablemychild.org

Harish K Pemde MD, FIAP
In-charge, Centre for Adolesent Health and
Professor of Pediatrics, Lady Hardinge Medical College and
Kalawati Saran Children's Hospital, New Delhi
harishpemde@gmail.com

Himabindu Singh MD, FIAP, PGDAP
Professor of Pediatrics
Institute of Child Health
Niloufer Hospital for Women and Children
Osmania Medical College, Hyderabad
dr.himabindusingh@gmail.com

Jay P Shastri MBBS, DPM
Consultant Psychiatrist
Shrimati Motibai Thakersey Institute for Research in
Field of Mental Retardation, Mumbai
jai31@hotmail.com

Jayakar Thomas MD, DD, MNAMS, PhD, FAAD
FIAD, FIAP, FRCP (Edin), FRCP (Glasgow), FRCP (London)
FRCP (Ireland), FRCPCH (London)
Professor and Head, Department of Skin and STD
Sree Balaji Medical College, Chennai
jayakarthomas@gmail.com

Jeeson C Unni MD Pediatrics
Consulting Pediatrician
Dr Kunhalu's Nursing Home, Kochi
jeeson@asianetindia.com

Kamlesh Harish MD
Head, Department of Pediatrics
ESI Hospital, Rohini, Delhi
kamleshharish1@gmail.com

Kaviya Lakshmipathy MBBS
Resident, Department of Pediatrics
Maulana Azad Medical College and Lok Nayak Hospital
New Delhi
drkaviya89@gmail.com

Kevin W Cates MPH
Medical Student
Homer Stryker MD School of Medicine
Kalamazoo, Michigan, USA
kevin.cates@med.wmich.edu

Kumar Abhishek MBBS, MPH, CCPPM
Palliative Care Physician–CanKids-KidsCan
Advocacy Officer–Pallium, Thiruvananthapuram
kumarabhishek2003@rediffmail.com

Mahesh Baldwa MBBS, MD, DCH, FIAP, MBA, LLB
LLM, PhD (Law)
Senior Pediatrician and Medico-Legal Advisor
Former Assistant Professor of Pediatrics
TN Medical College and Nair Hospital, Mumbai
drbaldwa@gmail.com

Malathi Sathiyasekaran MD, DCH, MNAMS, DM
Consultant Pediatric Gastroenterologist
Kanchi Kamakoti CHILDS Trust Hospital and
Sundaram Medical Foundation Hospital, Chennai
mal.bwcs@gmail.com

Manisha Jana MD, DNB, FRCR, MNAMS
Assistant Professor, Department of Radiodiagnosis
All India Institute of Medical Sciences
New Delhi
manishajana@gmail.com

Mathew Varghese MBBS, DNB
Senior Resident
Pushpagiri Institute of Medical Sciences
Thiruvalla, Kerala
revin_6@hotmail.com

Mona P Gajre MD
Professor of Pediatrics
Lokmanya Tilak Municipal Medical College
Sion, Mumbai
monapote@yahoo.co.in

M Vijayakumar MD, DCH, DNB, FIMSA
Additional Professor, Department of Pediatrics
Institute of Maternal and Child Health
Government Medical College
Kozhikode, Kerala
drmvijaycalicut@gmail.com

Neelkamal S Soares MD
Developmental-Behavioral Pediatrician
Geisinger Health System
Lewisburg, PA, USA
nssoares@geisinger.edu

Nehal Kothari BASLP, MA (USA), CCC-SLP (USA)
Speech Language Therapist and Audiologist
Let's Talk Speech Therapy Rehabilitation Centre
Mumbai
nehalslp@gmail.com

Newton Luiz MD (Ped), DCH, DNB
Consultant Pediatrician
Dhanya Mission Hospital
Potto PO, Thrissur District, Kerala
newtonluiz@gmail.com

Parimalam Kumar MD, DD, Dip NB, FRCP (Glasgow)
FIAD
Professor and Head, Department of Dermatology
Villupuram Medical College
Tamilnadu
drparimalam@gmail.com

Pramod Jog MD, DNB, FIAP
Professor of Pediatrics
DY Patil Medical College, Pune
dr_ pramodjog@yahoo.co.in

Prashant P Patil MD
Fellow in Pediatric Endocrinology (PDCC)
Bharati Vidyapeeth Medical College, Pune
dr_prash4u@yahoo.com

Preeti M Galagali MD, PGDAP
Director and Consultant, Adolescent Health Specialist
Bangalore Adolescent Care and Counseling Centre, Bangalore
drpgalagali@gmail.com

Preeti Singh
Assistant Professor Department of Pediatrics
Lady Hardinge Medical College and Kalawati Saran Children's Hospital, New Delhi
drpreetisingh3@gmail.com

PSN Menon MD, MNAMS, FIAP, FIMSA
Consultant and Head, Department of Pediatrics
Jaber Al-Ahmed Armed Forces Hospital, Kuwait
Former Professor of Pediatrics
All India Instute of Medical Sciences, New Delhi
psnmenon@hotmail.com

Quresh B Maskati MS, FCPS, DOMS, FICS
Consultant Eye Surgeon
Maskati Eye Clinic, Mumbai
qureshmaskati@gmail.com

Rajani Vaidya MS
Clinical Assistant
PD Hinduja National Hospital, Mumbai
dr.rajanivaidya@gmail.com

Rajeev Seth MD, FIAP, FAAP (USA)
Senior Consultant, Developmental Pediatrician and
Head, Department of Pediatrics, Rockland Hospital, New Delhi
sethrajeev@gmail.com

Rajesh Mehta MD
Medical Officer, Child and Adolescent Health
WHO-SEARO, New Delhi
Former Consultant in Pediatrics, Safdarjang Hospital, New Delhi
drrajeshmehta@gmail.com

RD Lele MBBS (Osm), DTM&H (Eng)
MRCP (Edin), FRCP (London)
Head Nuclear Medicine Department
Lilavati Hospital and Research Center, Mumbai
Former Dean of Grant Medical College and JJ Hospital, Mumbai
nuclearmedicinedept@gmail.com

RN Srivastava FRCPE (Ed), FIAP, FAMS
Consultant, Pediatric Nephrologist
Indraprastha Apollo Hospital, New Delhi
Former Professor of Pediatrics AIIMS, New Delhi
drrnsri@gmail.com

Ruth Etzel MD, PhD, FAAP
Professor, Joseph J Zilber School of Public Health
University of Wisconsin, Milwaukee, USA
retzel@earthlink.net

Samir H Dalwai MD, DCH, FCPS, DNB, LLB
Director and Developmental Pediatrician
New Horizons Child Development Centre
Honorary Consultant, Neurodevelopmental Clinic
Lokmanya Tilak Municipal General (Sion) Hospital and Medical College, Mumbai
samyrdalwai@enablemychild.org

Sandra G Hassink MD, MS, FAAP
Medical Director
AAP Institute for Healthy Childhood Weight
Elk Gove Village, Illinois, USA
shassink@aap.net

Sangeeta Yadav MD
Director Professor and Head
Department of Pediatrics
Incharge Pediatric and Adolescent Endocrinology
Maulana Azad Medical College and Lok Nayak Hospital
New Delhi
sangeetayadava@gmail.com

Satinder Aneja
Director Professor, Department of Pediatrics
Lady Hardinge Medical College and Kalawati Saran Children's Hospital, New Delhi
drsaneja@gmail.com

Sharad Agarkhedkar
Professor and Head
Department of Pediatrics
Dr DY Patil Medical College, Hospital and Research Centre
Pimpri, Pune
agarkhedkar@gmail.com

Shilpa Sharma MS, MCh, DNB, PhD
Assistant Professor, Department of Pediatric Surgery
All India Institute of Medical Sciences, New Delhi
drshilpas@gmail.com

Smriti Rana MSc
Holistic Psychological Counselling
Programme Director, Children's Palliative Care Project (CPCP)
Consulting Psychologist, Pallium, India, Thiruvananthapuram
smiriti@palliumindia.org

Sonia Joychan MD
Instructor, Department of Pediatric and Adolescent Medicine
Western Michigan University
Homer Stryker MD School of Medicine
Kalamazoo, Michigan, USA
sonia.joychan@med.wmich.edu

Subik Nagi BDS, MDS
Consultant in Pediatric Dentistry
E 79 Kalkaji, New Delhi
subiknagi@gmail.com

Sujata Kanhere MBBS, DCH, DNB, MNAMS, RCPCH
Fellowship in Pediatric Neurology (UK)
Professor and Head of Unit
Incharge Pediatric Neurology
KJ Somaiya Medical College and Hospital, Mumbai
drsujatakanhere@yahoo.co.in

Sumathi Bavanandam MD, DCH, DM
Senior Assistant Professor of Pediatric Gastroenterology
Institute of Child Health and
Hospital for Children, Chennai
drbsumathi@rediffmail.com

Supriya Phanse Gupte MD, FICMCH
Fellowship (Ped Endocrinology), ESPE Fellowship, UK
Consultant Pediatric Endocrinologist, Columbia Asia Hospital
and Panel Consultant, Deenanath Mangeshkar Hospital, Pune
supriya.r.phanse@gmail.com

Surjit Singh MD, DCH (London), FRCP (London)
FRCPCH (London), FAMS
Professor of Pediatrics and Incharge Allergy Immunology Unit
Advanced Pediatrics Centre
Post Graduate Institute of Medical Education and Research
Chandigarh
surjitsinghpgi@rediffmail.com

Suyog V Jaiswal MD
Assistant Professor
Department of Psychiatry
HBT Medical College and
Dr RN Cooper Municipal General Hospital, Mumbai
suyogjaiswal@gmail.com

Swati Y Bhave MD, DCH, FCPS, FIAP, FAAP (HON)
Senior Consultant in Adolescent Pediatrics and
Head and Incharge of Adolescent Wellness Clinic
Jehangir Hospital, Pune
Former Professor of Pediatrics
BJ Medical College and Sasson Hospital, Pune
sybhave@gmail.com

TU Sukumaran MD, DCH; MNAMS, M Phil, FIAP
Professor of Pediatrics
Pushpagiri Institute of Medical Science, Thiruvalla, Kerala
tusukumaran@gmail.com

Vaman Khadilkar MD, DNB, MRCP (UK), DCH (London)
Pediatric and Adolescent Endocrinologist
Jehangir Hospital, Pune and Bombay Hospital, Mumbai
Head, Division of Pediatric Endocrinology
Bharati Vidyapeeth Medical College, Pune
vamankhadilkar@gmail.com

Vasudha A Mashankar MD, MRCPCH
Consultant Pediatrician
Mumbai
vasudha_17@yahoo.com

Vikas Kohli MD, FAAP, FACC
American Board Certified, Pediatric Cardiology
Director, Pediatric Cardiology
Delhi Child Heart Center, New Delhi
vkohli_md@yahoo.com

Vikram R Lele MD, DNB, DRM
Director, Department of Nuclear Medicine and PET-CT
Jaslok Hospital and Research Center, Mumbai
vikram.lele@gmail.com

Vinod Gunasekaran MD
Senior Fellow, Institute for Child Health
Sir Ganga Ram Hospital, New Delhi
anupamace@yahoo.co.in

Contents

Section 4—SEXUALITY

Section 5—SYSTEMIC ILLNESSES IN ADOLESCENCE

Section 6—OTHER MEDICAL ISSUES

Section 7—SPECIAL ISSUES IN ADOLESCENCE

Section 8—MENTAL HEALTH IN ADOLESCENTS

Section 9—IMAGING

Section 10—ADOLESCENT PHARMACOLOGY

Section 11—ANNEXURES

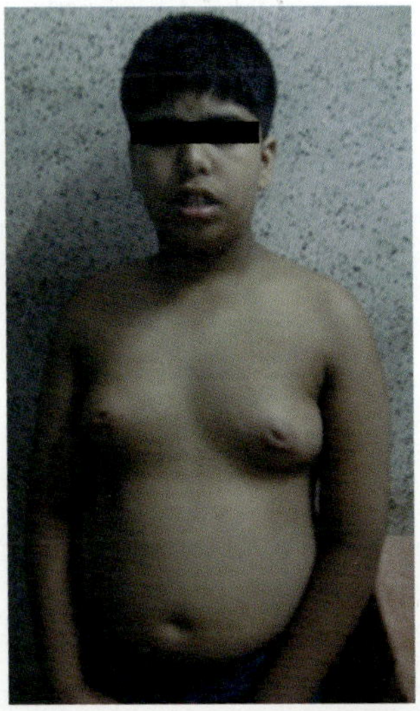

Figure 2.2.2.1: A 4-year-old boy with delayed puberty and gynecomastia. The karyotype was suggestive of Klinefelter syndrome (47,XXY) (Page 76)

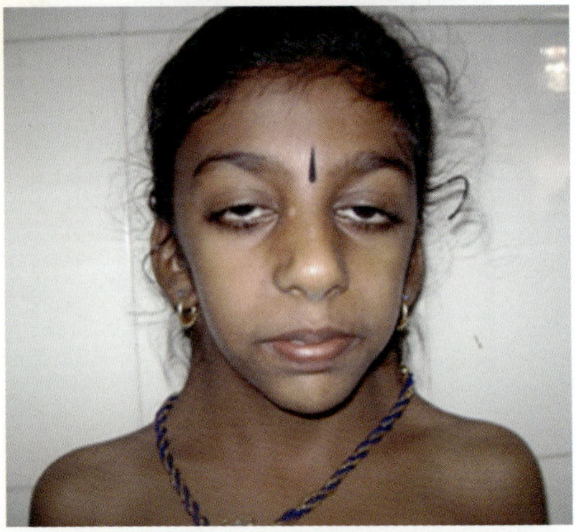

Figure 2.2.2.2: An adolescent girl with primary amenorrhea with hypergonadotropic hypogonadism. Note the features of Turner syndrome including webbing of neck, bilateral partial ptosis and low-set and abnormal ears (Page 76)

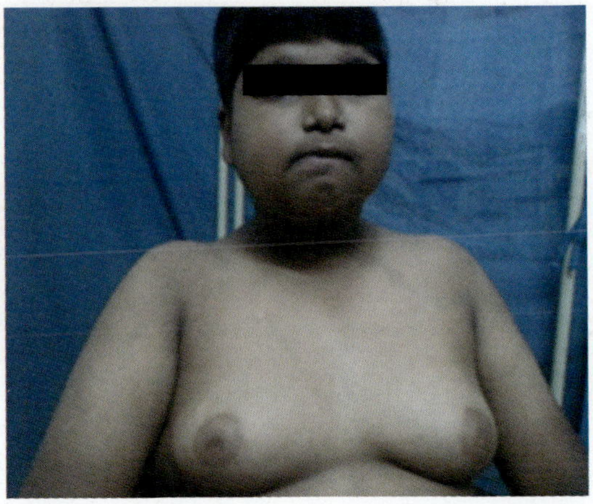

Figure 2.2.2.3: Adolescent idiopathic gynecomastia (Page 79)

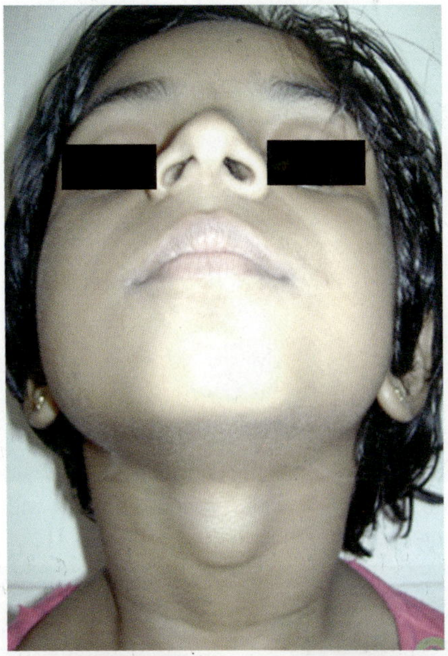

Figure 5.6.1.1: Adolescent girl with enlarged ectopic thyroid (Page 193)

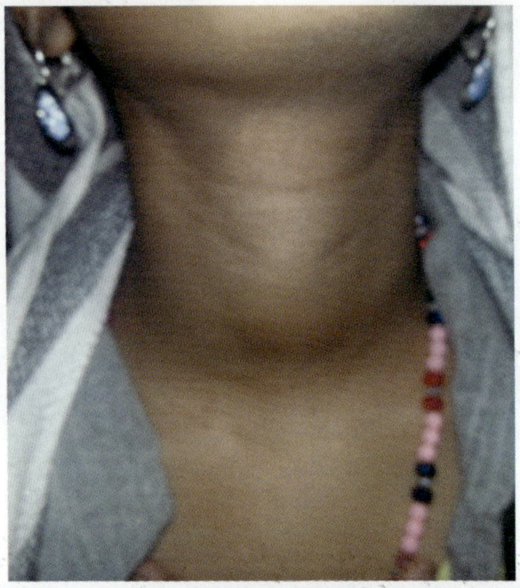

Figure 5.6.1.2: Adolescent girl with autoimmune thyroiditis (Page 193)

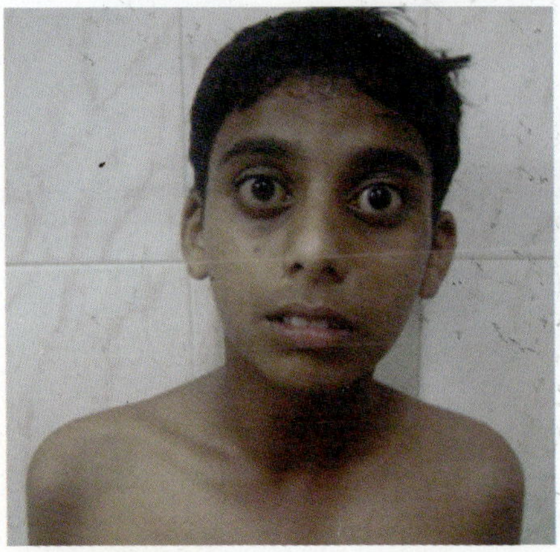

Figure 5.6.1.3: Graves disease in an adolescent boy with ophthalmoplegia (Page 195)

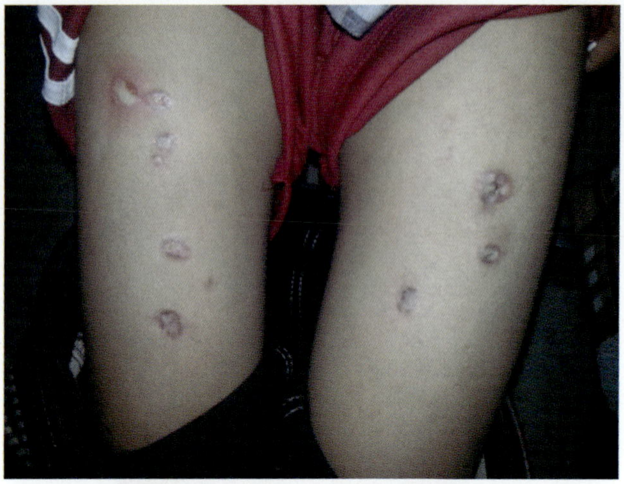

Figure 5.6.2.1: A boy with Type 1 diabetes with scars of infected injection sites (Page 202)

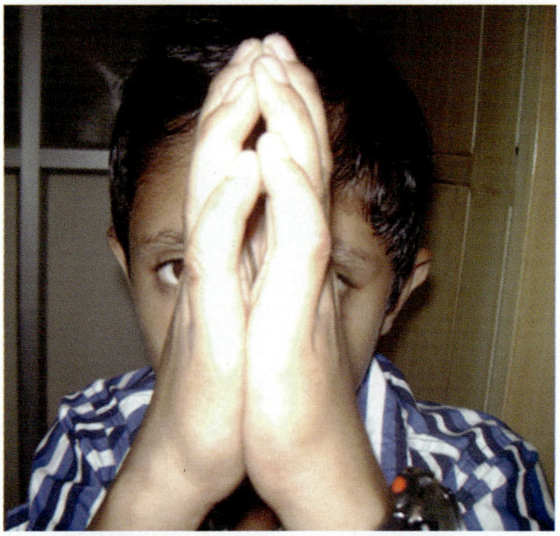

Figure 5.6.2.2: "Prayer sign", bilateral painless contracture of finger joints, a complication of type 1 diabetes due to limited joint mobility (Page 204)

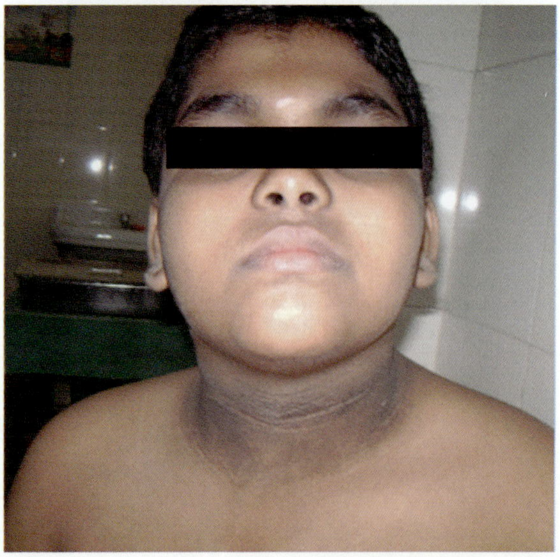

Figure 5.6.2.3: An adolescent with type 2 diabetes. His father is a known diabetic. Note acanthosis nigricans around neck (Page 205)

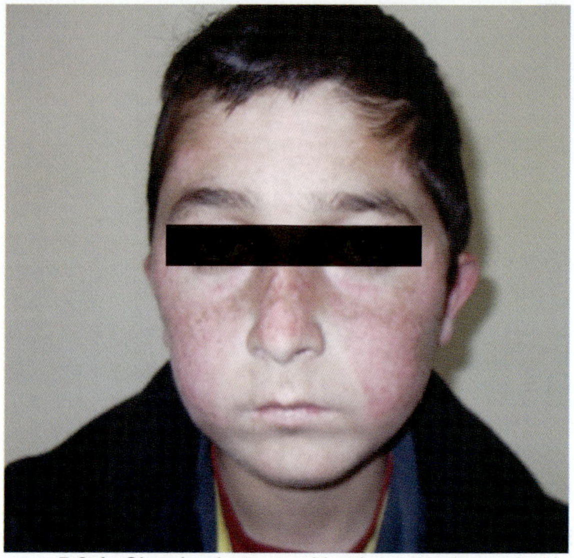

Figure 5.8.1: Classic photosensitive lupus malar rash. Note the distinct sparing of nasolabial folds (Page 217)

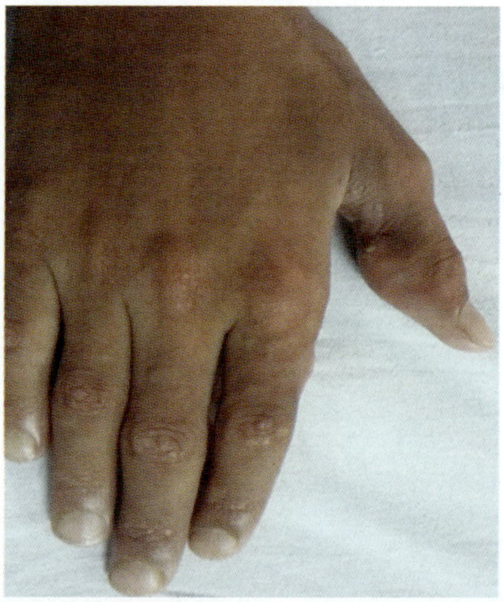

Figure 5.8.2: Gottron papules over proximal and distal interphalangeal joints in an 11-year-old with juvenile dermatomyositis. Also visible over the thumb is calcinosis with extrusion of calcium crystals (Page 217)

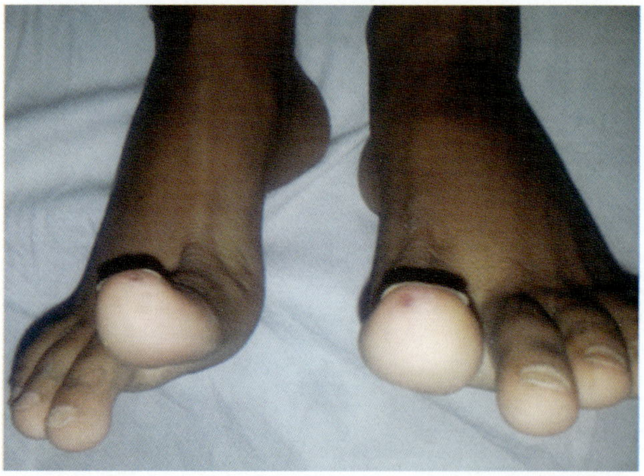

Figure 5.8.3: Vasculitic ulcers at tip of digits of lower limb (Page 217)

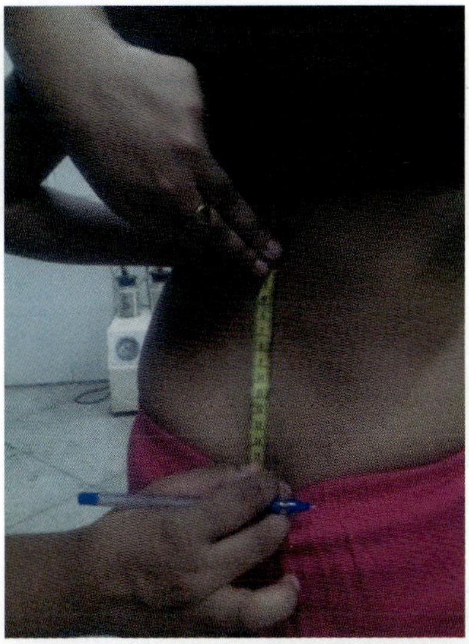

Figure 5.8.4: Demonstration of Modified Schober test in a 12-year-old with suspected enthesitis related arthritis (Marks are first put 10 cm above and 5 cm below lumbosacral junction and the child is then asked to bend forward) (Page 218)

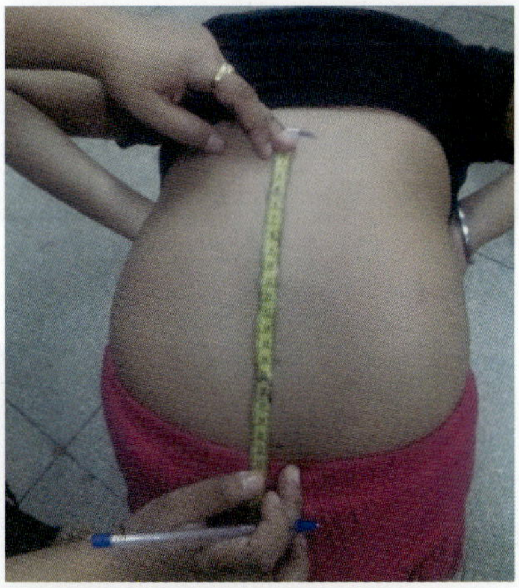

Figure 5.8.5: Demonstration of Modified Schober test. An increase of 6 cms. or more is considered normal (Page 218)

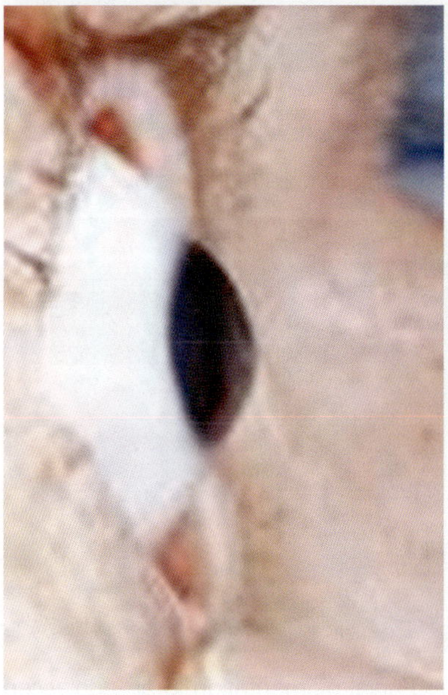

Figure 6.1.1: Keratoconus (Page 226)

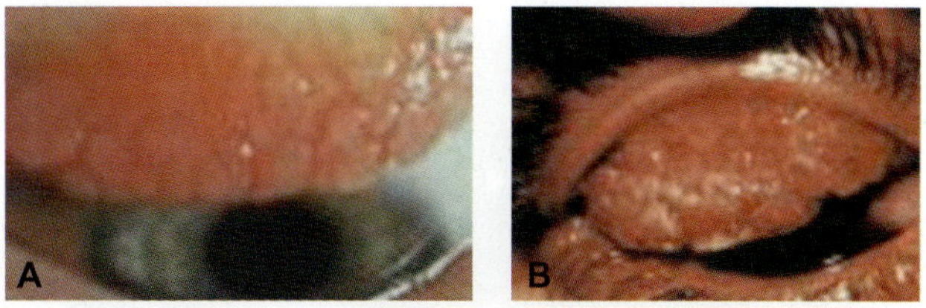

Figure 6.1.2A and B: Giant or cobblestone papillae on tarsal conjunctiva–Palpebral allergic conjunctivitis (Page 228)

A

B

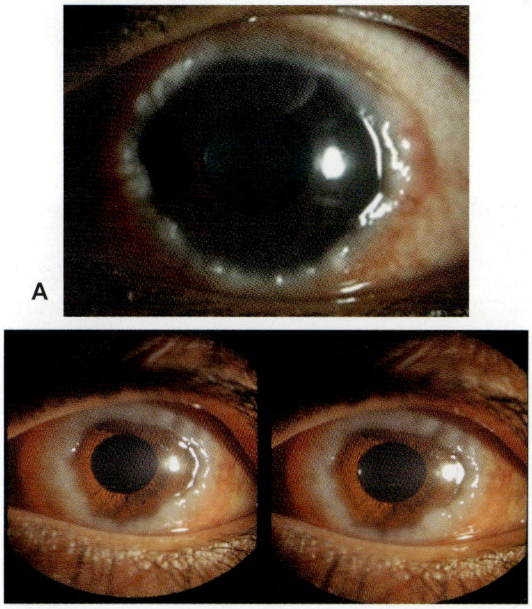

Figure 6.1.3A and B: Confluent papillae at limbus–Bulbar allergic conjunctivitis (Page 228)

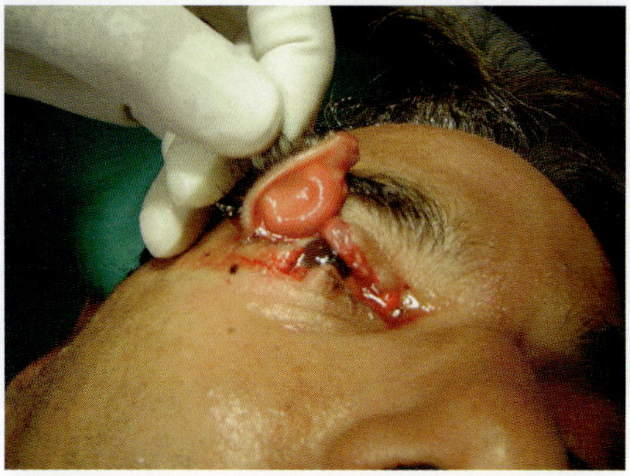

Figure 6.1.4: Upper eyelid avulsion due to road accident (Page 229)

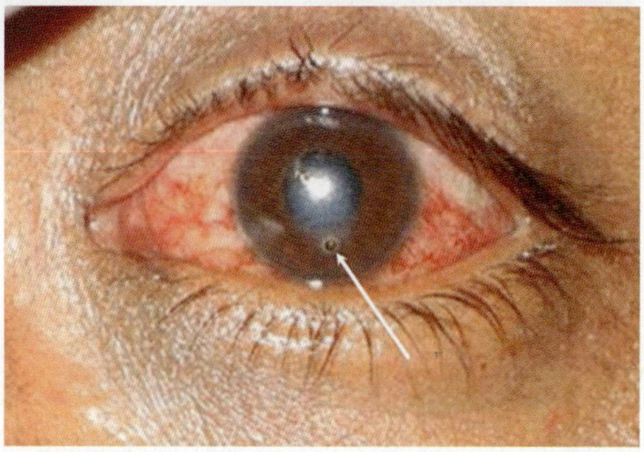

Figure 6.1.5: Corneal foreign body (white arrow) (Page 229)

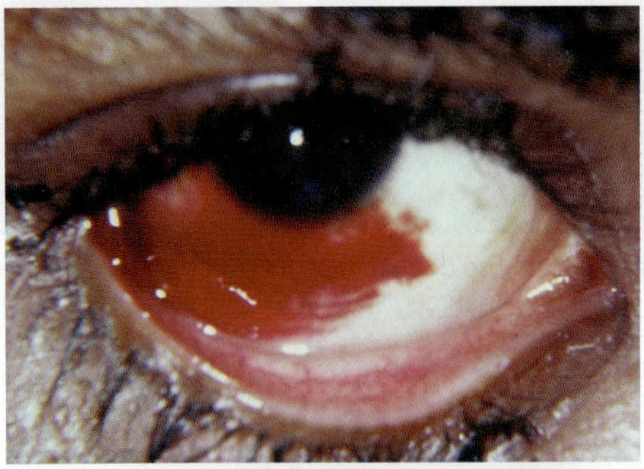

Figure 6.1.6: Sub-conjunctival hemorrhage due to injury (Page 229)

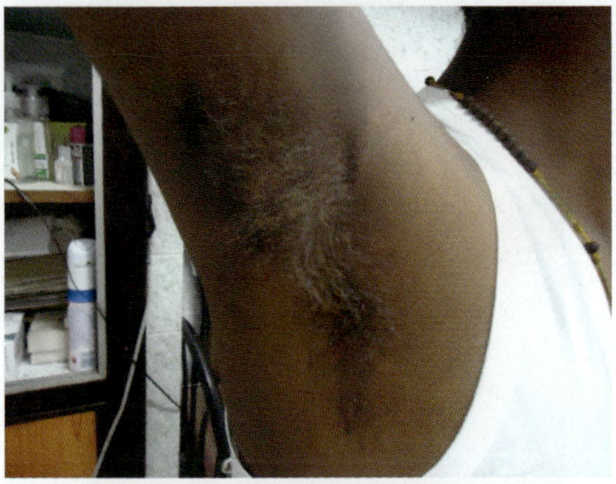

Figure 6.4.4: Trichomycosis axillaris caused by *Corynebacterium tenuis* (Page 241)

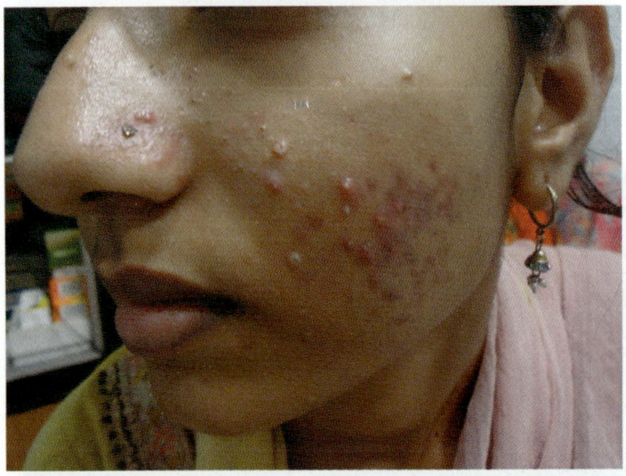

Figure 6.4.1: Grade I acne vulgaris (Page 241)

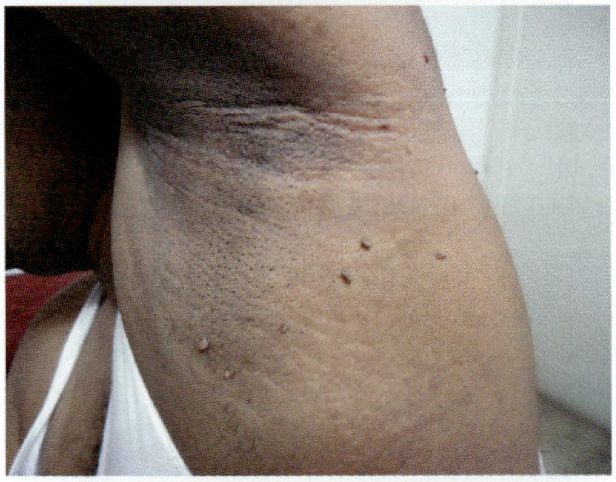

Figure 6.4.5: Acanthosis nigricans with velvety appearance over axilla (Page 242)

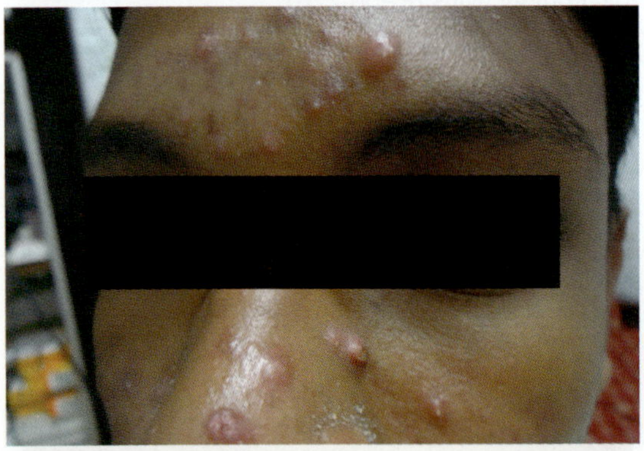

Figure 6.4.2: Grade IV nodulocystic acne (Page 241)

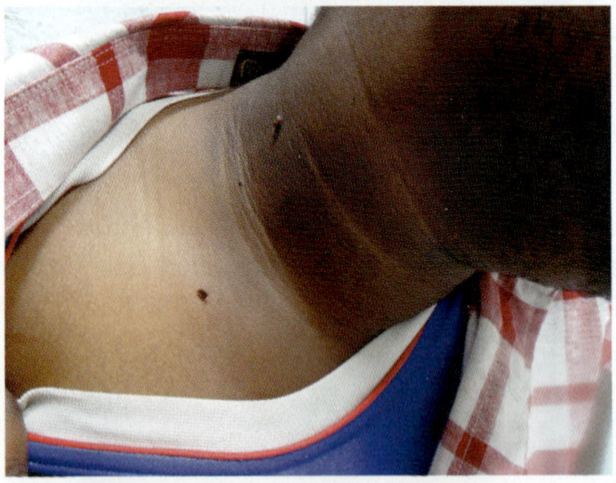

Figure 6.4.6: Acanthosis nigricans over neck (Page 242)

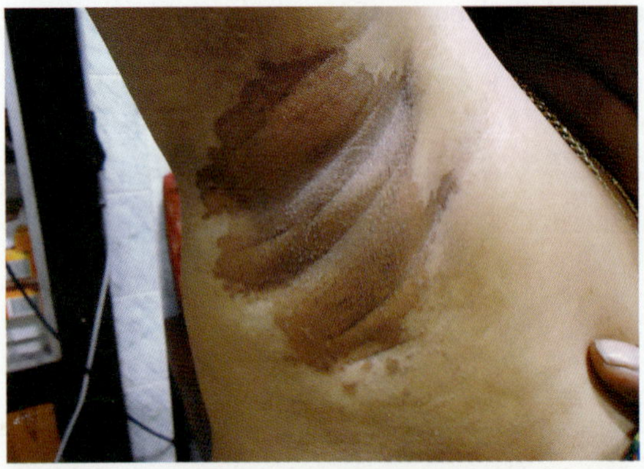

Figure 6.4.3: Erythrasma caused by *Corynebacterium minutissimum* (Page 241)

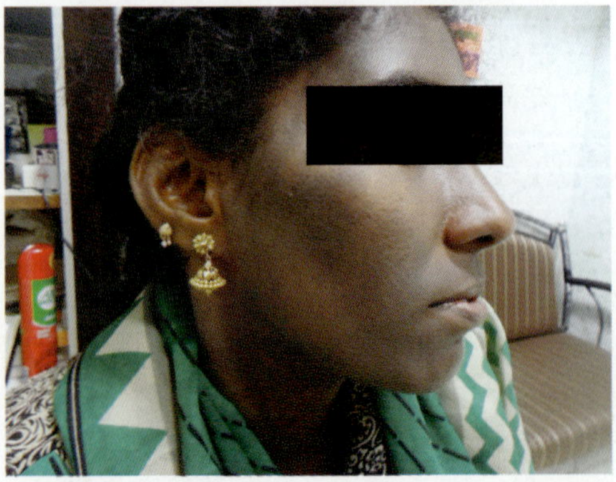

Figure 6.4.7: Facial pigmentation in an adolescent girl due to overexposure to sunlight (Page 242)

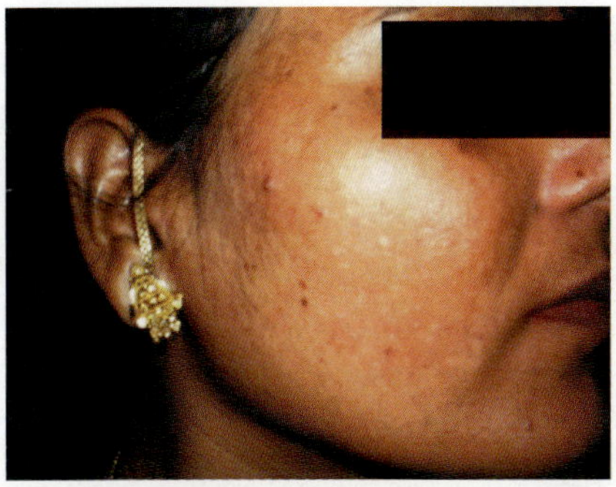

Figure 6.4.8: Melasma in an adolescent girl (Page 242)

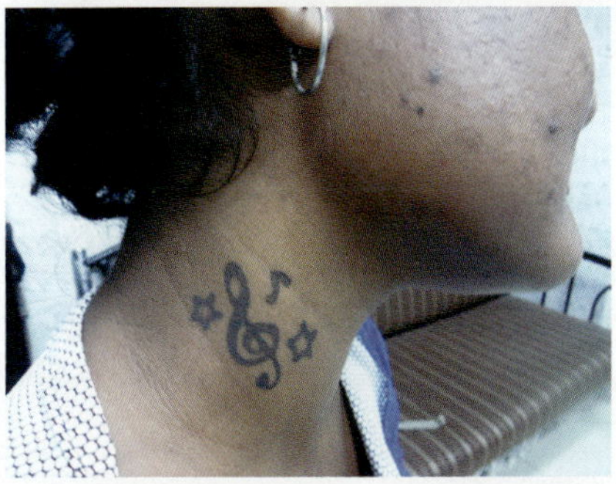

Figure 6.4.9: Depiction of tattoo in an adolescent female (Page 243)

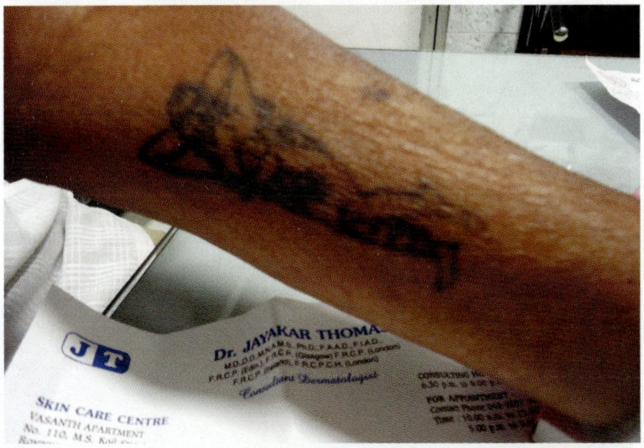

Figure 6.4.10: Depiction of tattoo in an adolescent male (Page 243)

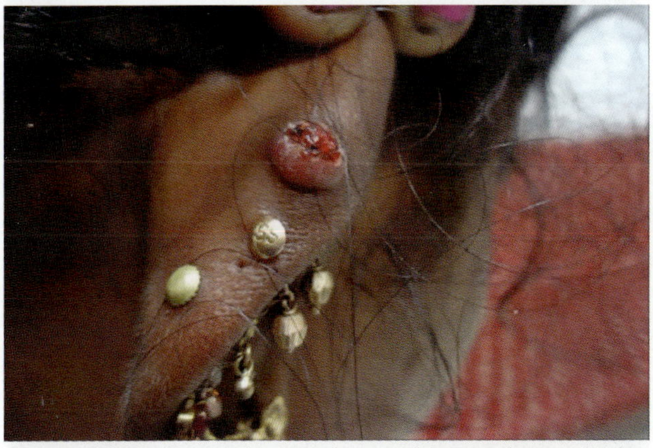

Figure 6.4.11: Pyogenic granuloma arising at the ear-boring site (Page 244)

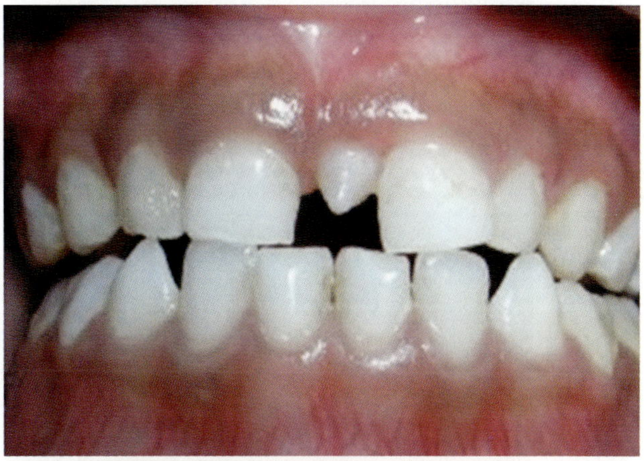

Figure 6.5.1: Mesiodens (Page 247)

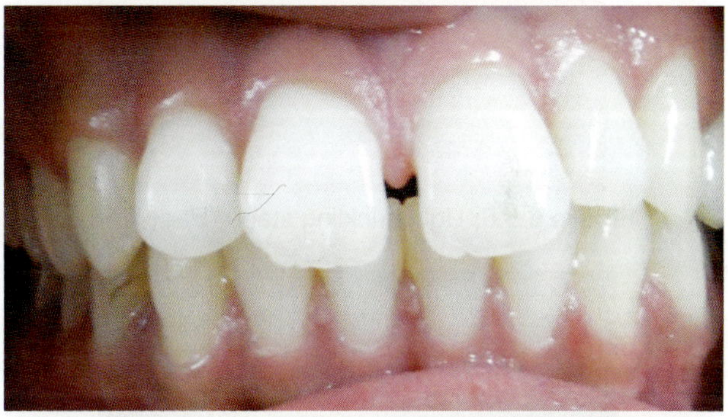

Figure 6.5.2: Midline diastema (Page 247)

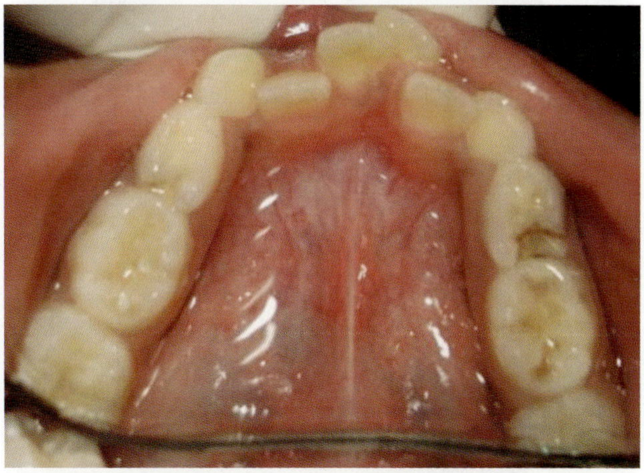

Figure 6.5.3: Crowding (Page 248)

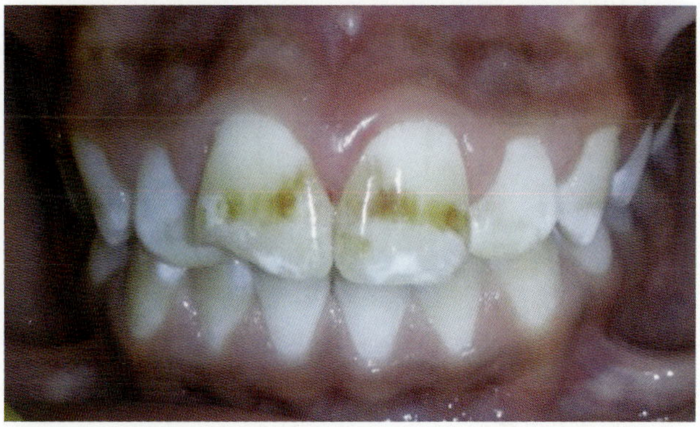

Figure 6.5.4: Dental fluorosis (Page 248)

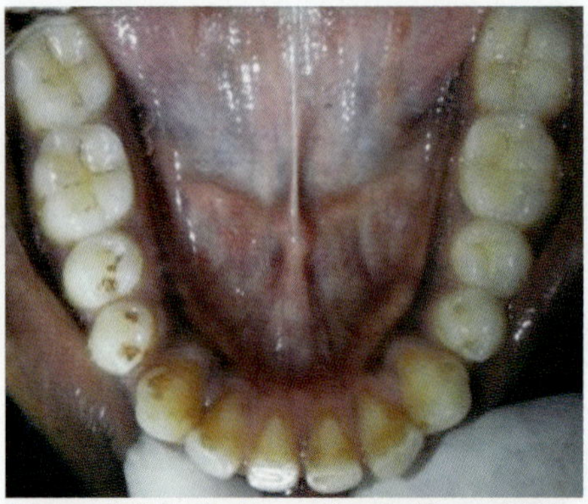

Figure 6.5.5: Stains on teeth (Page 248)

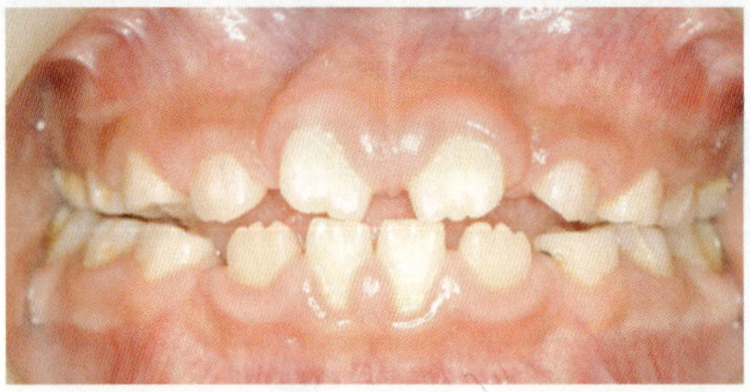

Figure 6.5.6: Ugly duckling stage (Page 248)

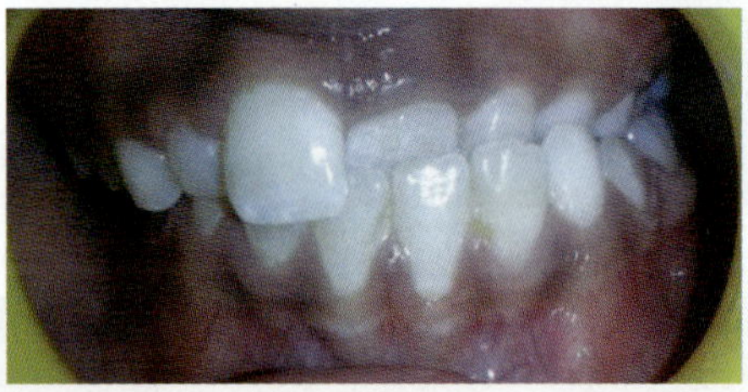

Figure 6.5.7: Cross bite (Page 248)

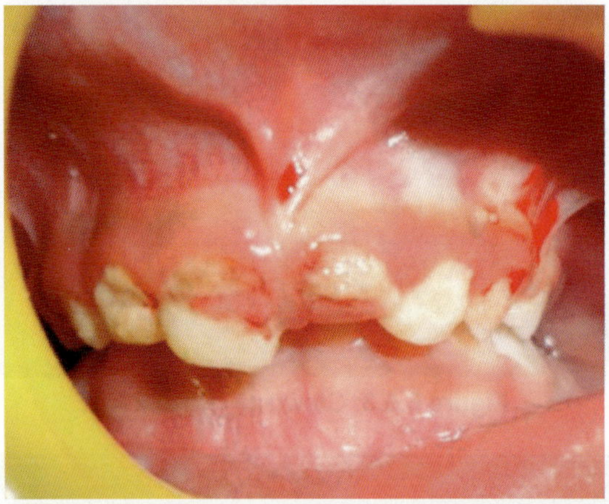

Figure 6.5.8A

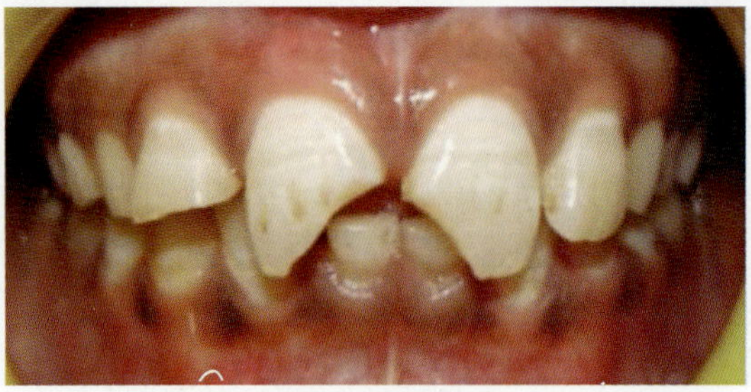

Figure 6.5.8B
Trauma leading to tooth fracture (Page 248)

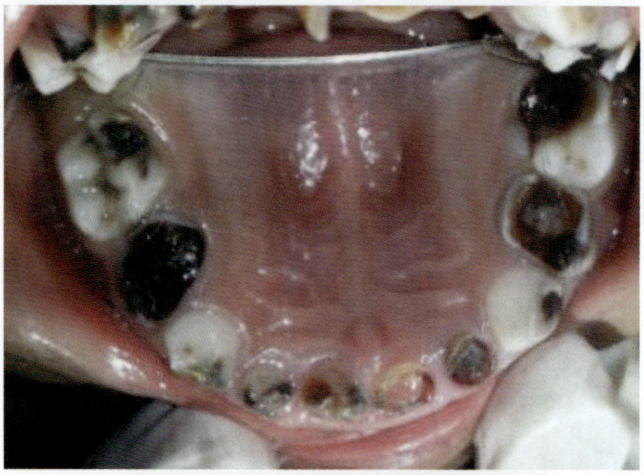

Figure 6.5.9: Rampant caries (Page 248)

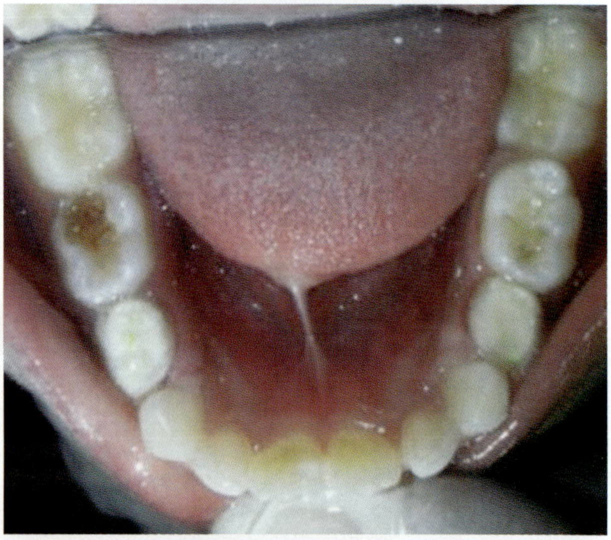

Figure 6.5.10: Tongue tie and high frenum (Page 249)

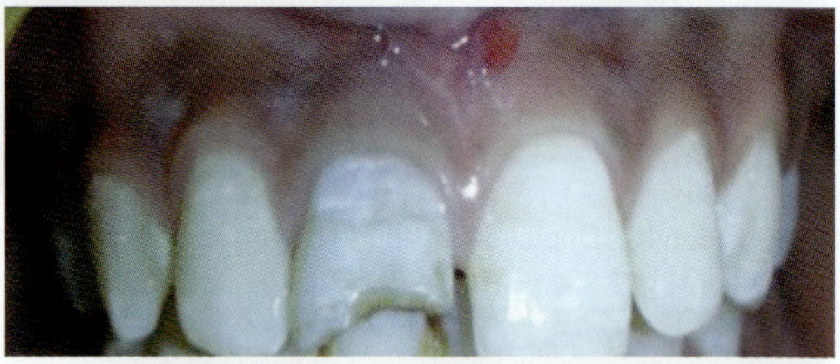

Figure 6.5.11: Sinus tract (Page 249)

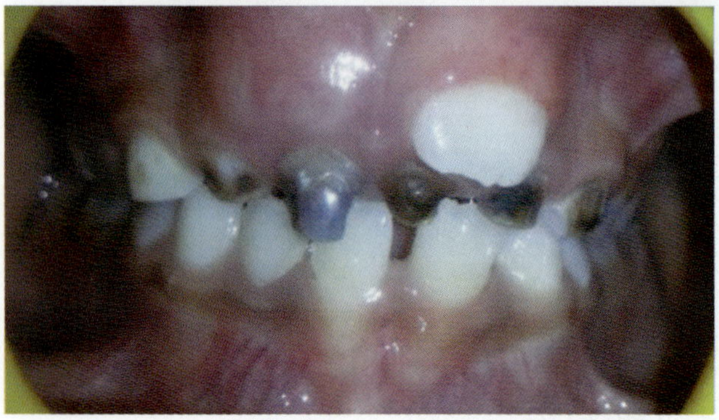

Figure 6.5.12: Black necrosed tooth (Page 249)

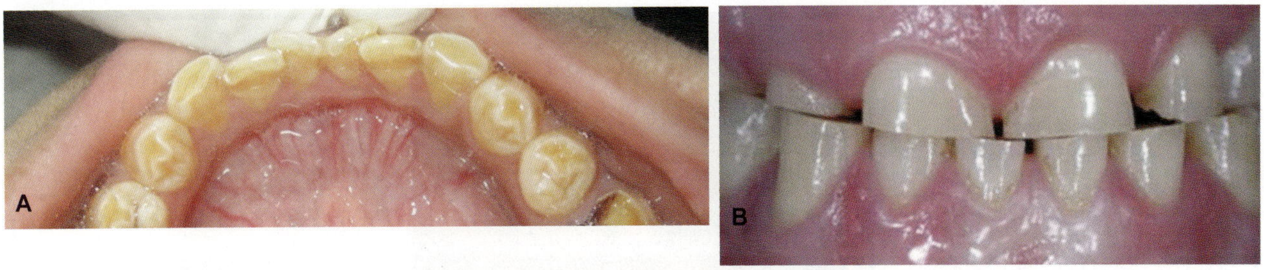

Figures 6.5.13A and B: Attrition/Erosion (Page 249)

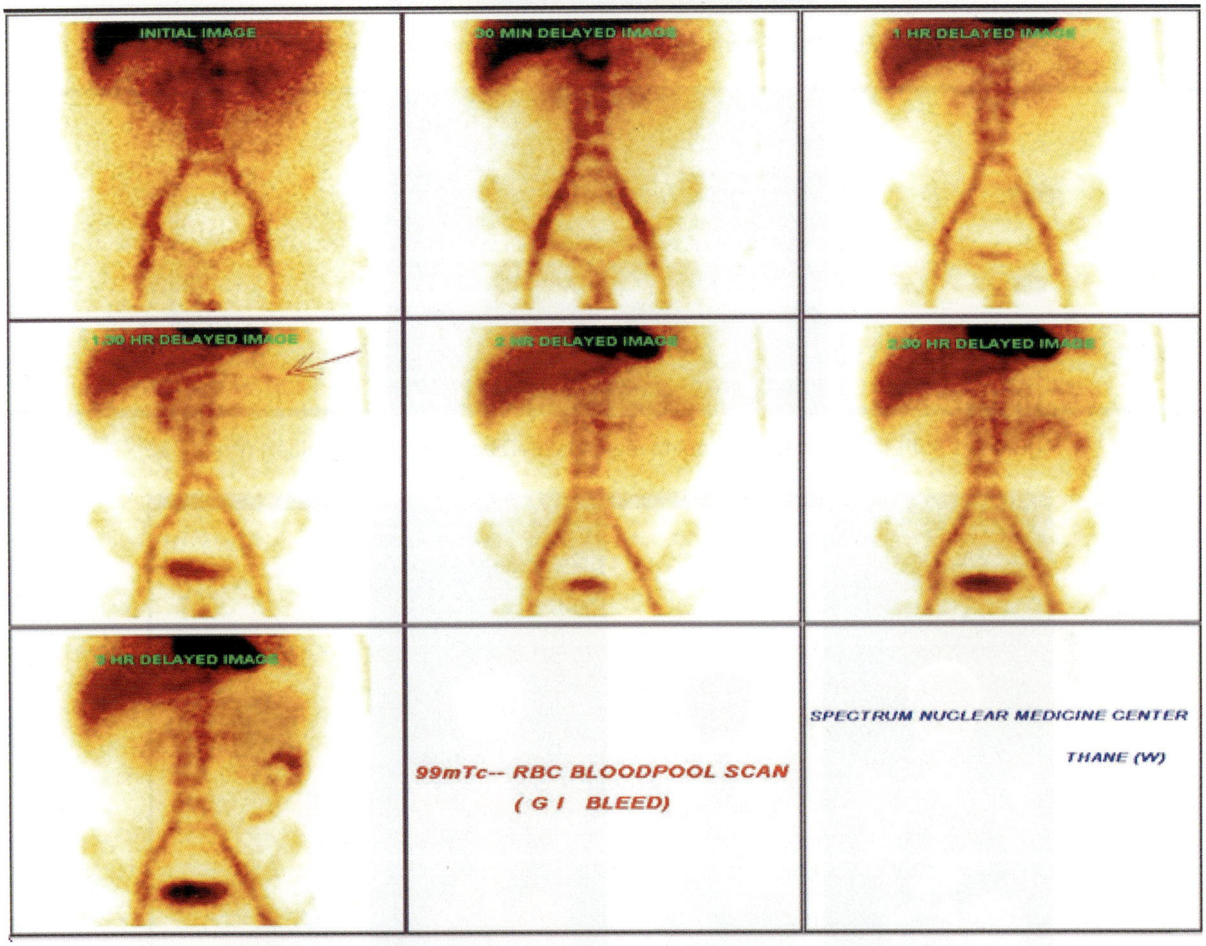

Figure 9.1.2: Labelled red blood cell scan showing normal hepatic and large vessel blood pool. A site of small bowel bleeding is seen in left hypogastric region (arrow) increasing over time (Page 330)

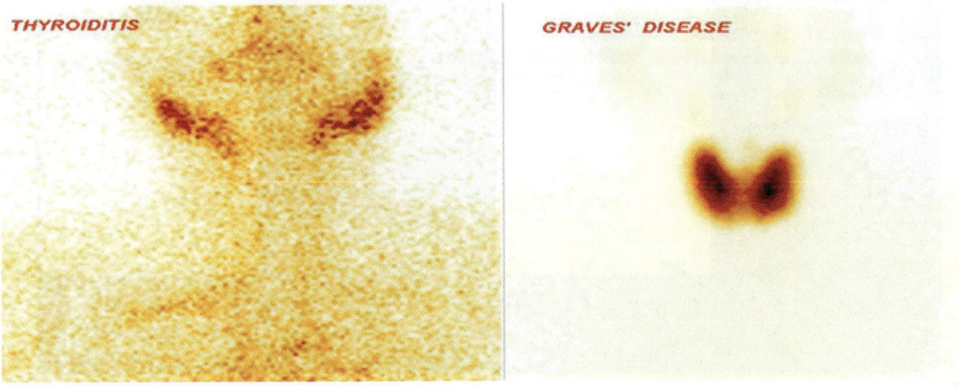

Figure 9.1.3: 99mTc-pertechnetate scans showing absence of uptake in the thyroid gland in thyroiditis (left) and intense uptake in the thyroid in Graves' disease (right) with similar clinical presentation (Page 330)

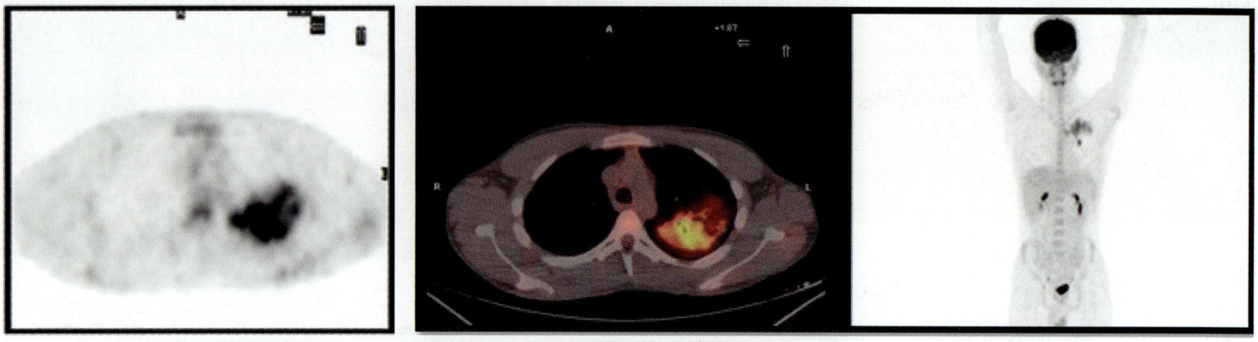

Figure 9.1.4: FDG PET CT images–Showing uptake in the lung lesion (Page 332)

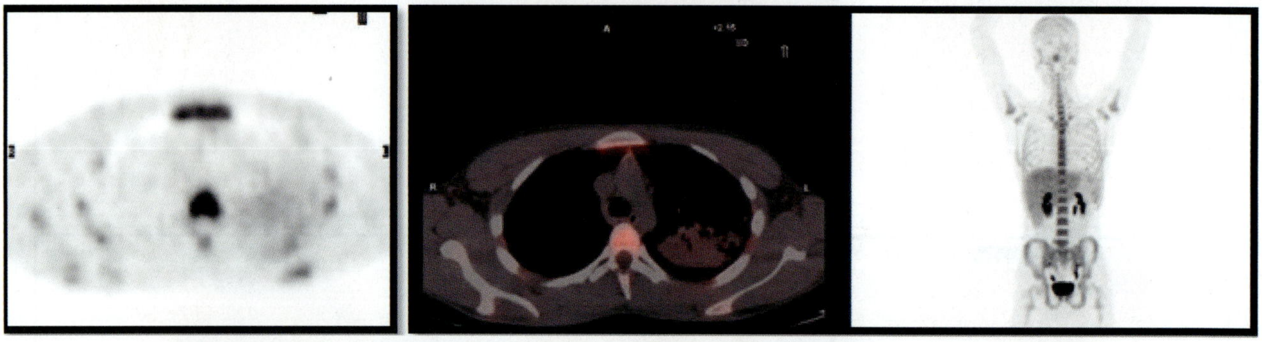

Figure 9.1.5: FLT PET images do not reveal uptake–Diagnosis of tuberculosis (Page 332)

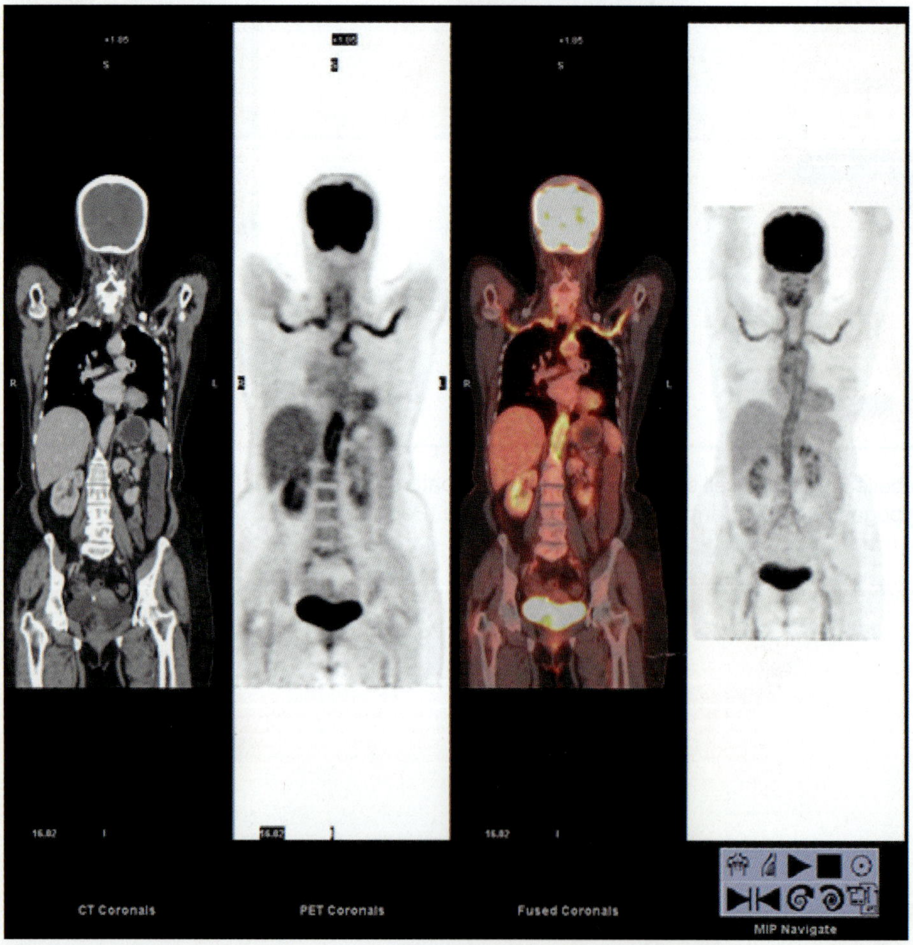

Figure 9.1.6: PET-CT scan with 18F-FDG showing uptake in large arteries (carotids, subclavian, abdominal aorta) in a case of large vessel vasculitis (Page 333)

Why Adolescent Medicine?

1.1

Donald E Greydanus

INTRODUCTION

Adolescence is the life-changing stage of human life that starts in childhood and ends with the onset of adulthood. Events of childhood and adolescence set the stage for a successful or dysfunctional adulthood and thus, attention by clinicians in practice can play a major part in helping youth become healthy adults contributing positively to their families and society.

Those of us in clinical practice are privileged to help these ambassadors of the future who will be around long after we have made our own journey from this existence. It is a challenging yet vital role that adolescent pediatricians in practice can accomplish.

The sheer numbers of youth in the world is enough to make us realize how important it is to help these persons who will shape the future of the world as this 21st century continues. There are over 1.2 billion adolescents (10-19 years of age) in the world and half of the world's population is now under age 25 years.

All of these teenagers need health care and adolescent pediatricians and clinicians of all other specialties in practice can screen for factors that induce considerable morbidity and mortality in this population. Many health problems can be treated in the office setting much to the gratitude of this patient and the family. Youth can receive mixed and error-filled views on health from peers, the internet, and other societal elements.

The clinicians can provide reassurance to a worried teenager (and family), identify health issues before they become damaging problems, give health education that can be utilized for decades to come, and refer this young patient to the proper consultants in health (mental or medical). Patterns of health maintenance are established in adolescence that last the lifetime of this person and clinicians can help make this a positive development. This is an awesome yet gratifying responsibility shared by millions of clinicians around the world.

ADOLESCENT STAGES

- It is important for the clinician to understand about stages of development in adolescence so that one can understand what is normal versus abnormal development. The view that teens will simply mature out of their problems without help is not substantiated by research.
- Narcissism is normal in the young adolescent (10-13 years of age) as is homosexual experimentation.
- The young person whose body is changing rapidly needs reassurance that these changes are normal or what to do if abnormalities are present. Puberty can be a difficult process for many teens, and the caring clinician can be there with them from beginning to end serving as a trusted guide and teacher.
- Social skills are important for all youth but certainly for the young teen that is transitioning from a family milieu to an environment where close friends become important. Advice on social skills training can be lifesaving for this young patient.
- The caring clinician will understand that sexual behavior is normal for adolescents and is typically initiated in the middle adolescent (14-16 years of age) when heterosexual experiences are common.
- Thus, education regarding responsible sexual behavior should be conducted by the caring clinician then if not sooner to prevent unwanted pregnancy and sexually transmitted infections. Mental health issues can occur at any time but prevalence of many disorders (i.e., depression, anxiety, others) approximates that of adults. For more details see section 8.

- Though the older (late) adolescent (17-21 years of age) becomes more adult-like, as noted below, clinicians must understand that the adult brain (i.e., maturation of the prefrontal cortex) does not occur until the mid-twenties in many persons. Thus, youth can make many mistakes based on immaturity and constant education by the clinician regarding health issues remains a paramount part of adolescent health care that is so vital to the present and future of this patient.

CNS MATURATION

Maturation of the central nervous system involves complex changes in the child and adolescent brain in the journey to adulthood. Just as the child cannot talk until sufficient maturation occurs in the Broca's area for speech, the youth cannot understand many principles of adult living until the child brain matures into the adolescent brain and the adolescent brain matures into the adult brain.

A final step in this process is maturation of the prefrontal cortex which is the brain structure key to understanding normal adult reasoning and functioning—*the executive function.* Such function allows the adult to differentiate between thoughts that are conflicting, understand what is "good" and "bad", how to work toward a defined goal, and suppression of desires for what the adult world consider socially unacceptable results. This usually does not occur until the twenties—often in the mid-twenties and often earlier in females than males. It is important for caring clinicians to understand such principles of maturation to provide effective guidance to their vulnerable adolescent patients. More on brain development is discussed in Chapter 1.2.

GUIDANCE IN SEXUALITY

Sexuality is a complex phenomenon that has been developed over millions of years of life for, among other purposes, the survival of the human species. Sexual urges begin early in adolescence and millions of youth are sexually active—indeed, the onset of coital behavior (i.e., sexarche) is in adolescence in all populations around the world. Caring clinicians must recognize this normal aspect of adolescent development and it is vitally important for practitioners to provide advice regarding abstinence, contraception, condoms, and sexually transmitted infection screening as well as management. More details in section 4.

It is unfair to our youth for pediatricians to ignore such advice at a time when these vulnerable patients do not understand the consequences of their CNS-driven drive for sexual behavior. Adolescents can make tragic mistakes with negative lifelong consequences. Though most youth are involved in heterosexual activity, a minority of youth become homosexual and they need advice regarding safe sex as well as screening for societal negativity toward homosexuality that includes bullying leading to depression, anxiety and suicide. Caring for the gay, lesbian, and bisexual youth is part of the professional obligation of practicing clinicians and such care is vital to the health of these persons.

CHRONIC ILLNESS

The importance of adolescent medicine for clinicians also becomes evident when considering that one-third of youth have chronic illness or disability in which 21% of this group have two conditions, and 9% have three or more. The impact is not only medical but also behavioral. Millions of youth in India are affected by chronic illnesses that includes asthma, epilepsy, diabetes mellitus, obesity, impaired vision as well as hearing, cardiac disease, renal disease, and many others.

Illness not identified in adolescence will worsen in the adult years resulting in considerable preventable complications as well as unnecessary premature mortality in this adult. The examples are many and include hypertension, hyperlipidemia, obesity, diabetes mellitus and more. More on screening and prevention of NCD in adolescents is discussed in Chapter 1.8.

Over 90% of children with chronic illness reach age 20 in many countries if clinicians carefully care for these children and it is a moral imperative from any national or religious perspective to take care of these precious individuals to maximize their potential as children, adolescents and adults.

Screening and management are vital functions of adolescent pediatricians, other clinicians and all are important including careful evaluation of vital signs, thorough physical examination, astute differential diagnosis, and up-to-date management of illness.

Sensitive management of issues the clinician might not consider serious (i.e., mild acne vulgaris) can be major problems for the sensitive teen patient. Sound advice on diet and physical activity can extend the life of obese youth as well as improve their quality of life. More details in section 3.

Mental Illness

A unique type of chronic illness is mental illness which involves 20% or more of adolescents and, though the individual can be physiologically healthy, their quality of life can be devastated by depression, anxiety, psychosis, and other problems with psychiatric disorders. Millions of our youth have additional complications from the violence milieu of the world including wars and homicide.

The presence of depression complicated by the pressures of life can lead to many youth contemplating, attempting, and completing suicide—most of which are preventable deaths if proper screening and management principles are implemented by caring clinicians. Mental illness has much co-morbidity including other mental illnesses and substance abuse disorder. Clinicians can seek to identify and manage substance use issues early and seek to prevent worsening drug problems that can result in a lifetime of devastating drug abuse in adulthood. Mental illnesses are discussed in detail in section 8.

Encouraging family therapy is an important part of the clinician's message to help behavioral dysfunctions in youth. Such work is why practicing pediatricians must care about the adolescent patient and why application of adolescent medicine principles is so vital to implement in practice. Lives are saved and quality of life can be expended for decades—well into this century and perhaps beyond!

YOUTH VIOLENCE

The practice of adolescent medicine is vital to help blunt the impact of a violent world that produces untold youth violence with resultant tragic consequences of physical and psychosocial morbidity and mortality in the youth of the world. Globally there are millions of incidents of physical attacks, sexual assaults (including dating violence) and homicides. The medical cost as well as the psychological cost from such violence is staggering around the world and it is vital that clinicians respond by caring for these youth in their offices as well as getting governments to unite in methods to curb such violence. The youth of the world are exposed to constant violence in many ways and developing youth are vulnerable to such environmental toxicities. Thus, it is critical and even mandatory for clinicians to care for these youth in their offices and seek to blunt the impact of violence for the sake of these youth and society in general—now and into the future.

MORTALITY

The cost in morbidity is staggering but perhaps more sobering is the realization that violence results in three-quarters of deaths in youth 15 to 24 years of age. In many countries the leading cause of death is the motor vehicle accidents which in the United States causes 30% of deaths versus unintentional injuries at 16%, homicide at 16%, and suicide at 12%. Morbidity and mortality that finds its conclusion in our youth can also be from abuse at the hands of family and society. These factors can also lead to millions of youth in the world who are runaways and homeless as well as being incarcerated subject to ever greater violence and maltreatment. Clinicians can understand the risk factors that lead to these deaths and provide screening as well as management options for their patients. It is part of the message regarding why caring for youth is so vital to these youth and to their world that they will inherit if they remain alive.

PREVENTION

Clinicians who care for children and adolescents are in an excellent position to provide principles of prevention to their patients who come to their offices and clinics for a variety of reasons. A classic way to provide this is with the annual well child (teen) visit but any visit can serve as a way for caring clinicians to help youth in their area. A classic manner for prevention is the judicious and widespread use of principles of immunization. Care for this age group can focus on dealing with the majority of factors leading to adolescent morbidity and mortality: drug use (alcohol, tobacco, cannabis, others), sexual activity, psychosocial issues (leading to suicide, motor vehicle accidents and homicides), limited physical activity and poor diets.

In addition to screening and treating medical conditions as well as providing anticipatory guidance, the caring clinician can serve as a trusted advisor to the youth at a time when this patient may not wish to share confidential data with parents but needs a qualified adult for confidential advice and guidance. This is a major reason for the importance of adolescent medicine in clinical practice. Counseling can involve a limited number of sessions and be goal-directed to get a youth to stop using drugs, to stay in school, to increase communication with parents, and many others. Issues of confidentiality are discussed elsewhere in this publication. Interaction with youth should be in a manner that is friendly, respectful, confidential and safe. More details in Chapters 1.3 and 1.4.

It is important for clinicians to receive training in the tenets of caring for adolescents with the understanding that adolescent medicine is important for the well-being of these ambassadors to the future. Such care cannot take place in a hospital setting but in the outpatient or clinic milieu. It is a duty for clinicians charged with the privilege of responsibility of caring for youth and we can serve as conveyors of medical care, advisors of prevention, and committed counselors to take these precious humans and help this precious cargo become successful adults in the potentially perilous and turbulent times that await them as this 21st century hurls into the future.

"To keep a lamp burning, we have to keep putting oil in it."—***Mother Teresa***

SUGGESTED READING

1. Britto MT, Tivorsak TL, Slap GB. Adolescents' needs for health care privacy. Pediatrics 2010;126(6):e1469-76.
2. Ford C, English A, Sigman G. Confidential health care for adolescents: Position paper for the Society for Adolescent Medicine. J Adolesc Health 2004;35:160-67.
3. Greydanus DE, Hutchins TA. Adolescent Health. In: Wallace HM, G Green G, Jaros KJ, eds. Health and Welfare for Families in the 21st Century, 3rd edition. London; Jones and Bartlett, London; 2014.
4. Greydanus DE, Patel DR, Reddy VN, Feinberg AN, Omar HA: Handbook of Clinical Pediatrics: An Update for the Ambulatory Pediatrician. Singapore: World Scientific Publishing and Imperial College Press, 758 pages, 2010.
5. Greydanus DE, Patel DR, Omar HA, Feucht C, Merrick J. Adolescent Medicine: Pharmacotherapeutics in General, Mental and Sexual Health. Berlin: De Gruyter, 417 pages, 2012.
6. McPherson A. Adolescents in primary care. BMJ 2005; 330(7489):465-67.
7. Newacheck PW, Rising JP, Kim SE: Children at risk for special health care needs. Pediatrics 2006;118:334-42.

Neurodevelopment

1.2

Swati Y Bhave, Preeti M Galagali

INTRODUCTION

In the past it was thought that the human brain matures by the age of 18 years and hence most countries have made this the legal age for permission of voting, driving, drinking and consent. It was also assumed that high-risk taking behavior and experimentation would be over by this age and then the individuals could be considered as responsible adults. Continuation of such behavior by youth beyond the age of 18 years was assumed to be wayward behavior. Since 2000 with various imaging techniques like functional MRI, PET scans and diffuse tensor imaging MRI as well as mammalian experiments and postmortem studies, the adolescent brain has been studied in detail. It is now evident the human brain is not fully mature till the age of 25 years. Due to limited sample sizes and laboratory constraints, as of now, causal relationships are difficult to establish and confirm.

Adolescent brain development is the result of a very fascinating interplay of genes, hormones and environment. This involves complex neuronal growth, reorganization and myelination in limbic system, amygdala, corpus callosum, cerebellum, pineal gland and finally in frontal lobes (Table 1.2.1).

The plasticity of the brain helps the adolescent to adapt, change and survive the challenges of the current era. To a large extent, preliminary results have offered neurobiological basis of adolescent behavior. Puberty triggers hormone dependent changes in reward circuitry of brain, increased sex drive and aggression. Risk taking behavior prepares the adolescent to face difficulties and crisis in life; sex is important for reproduction and aggression for protection of species. Hence changes in adolescent brain have an evolutionary basis and are essential for adapting to the existing living environment. Testosterone stimulates aggressive behavior while estrogen favors a nurturing response.

The various factors that affect the adolescent neurodevelopment are heredity, pre- and post-natal insults, sex, nutrition, sleep, exercise, media exposure, stress and drugs. Adolescent brain is very vulnerable to substance abuse and other addictive behaviors (Box 1.2.1). For more details please see Chapters 7.4 and 8.2.

Clinical Implications

Due to extensive neurodevelopmental changes in adolescence, it is often termed as a period of both opportunity and vulnerability. Adolescent neurodevelopment has wide ranging implications on the following clinical issues:

1. Approach to an adolescent
2. History taking
3. Physical examination
4. Investigations
5. Management
6. Counselling: Preventive and therapeutic

Most of these are covered in detail in other chapters (1.3, 1.6 and 2.3) and only the neurodevelopmental aspects will be discussed here.

HISTORY TAKING

History should be taken from the parents and from adolescents in private. For more details see Chapter 1.3. The neurodevelopment aspects relevant to history taking are given below.

Birth and Development Record

Taking a detailed birth history and developmental history should not be missed in every adolescent whatever problem they come with. One should ask for the antenatal history and antenatal card for maternal factors and the neonatal card for birth history and the well baby card to see the development and other illnesses.

Table 1.2.1: Adolescent neurodevelopment: Key issues

Areas	*Development*	*Results*
Synaptic pruning	Major "rewiring" The principle–"Use it or lose it" Grey matter decreases–inverted U shaped curve Peak at 11 years in girls and 13 years in boys	The synaptic connections that are used the most get 'hardwired' and persist into adulthood while the others are lost Brain efficiency improves Opportunity to influence adolescents for adopting healthy lifestyles for a lifetime
Myelination	Integration of neural circuitry	Increased cognitive ability and information processing Gradual shift from concrete operational thinking to formal logical operation
Frontalization	Myelination of the brain begins from posterior to anterior Prefrontal lobes are the last to mature The 'top down' control system is relatively weak Complete maturity of the frontal lobe is achieved by 21-24 years	Weak executive functions: organization, time management, controlling emotional urges, judgment, decision making and problem solving
Highly developed limbic system	Highly responsive 'bottom up' system Complex emotional situations result in increased activity in amygdala and less in prefrontal cortex Increased activation of amygdala Amygdala less sensitive to aversive stimuli and slow reaction time Adult decision making possible by 15 years of age, but in stressful and emotional periods this ability is compromised due to a highly reactive amygdala	"Hot cognition"–High emotive response to stressful situation e.g. peer pressure and emotionally arousing situations The propensity to impulsive behavior Cold cognition–Calm response during non-intimidating situations Experience adverse effects of excessive alcohol intake like 'black outs' much later than adults Poor response to harsh discipline techniques
Reward circuitry: Dopaminergic neurotransmitter system and its projections into ventral striatum	Greater activation in ventral striatum compared to children and adults while receiving rewards Weak top down control also results in intense reward seeking behavior	This results in increased tendency towards novelty and sensation seeking behavior
Hypothalamic-pituitary-adrenal axis	Immaturity results in large surges of cortisol under stress	High prolonged levels of cortisol are neuro-toxic and can also compromise cardio-vascular and immune systems Adolescents should learn stress management techniques
Corpus callosum	Myelination	Improves creativity, vocabulary, visuo-spatial skills and psychomotor functions
Cerebellum	Maturation	Enhances coordination and motor skills
Pineal gland	Later onset of melatonin secretion	Results in resetting of the circadian rhythm and delayed sleep onset

Prenatal insult in the form of severe maternal stress can alter the fetal neuroendocrine stress response and results in changes in amygdala and orbitofrontal tracts in utero. These individuals are prone to cardiovascular diseases and anxiety disorders in adolescence and adulthood. Postnatal insult in the form of hypoxia can alter neurodevelopment.

Going through childhood records also helps to understand if the onset of the problem is of recent origin or present since childhood. Attention deficit hyperactivity disorder (ADHD) is known to have weak orbitofrontal neural circuitry. In these cases the 'adolescence phase' is particularly prolonged and the individual tends to be more impulsive and reward seeking until late thirties due to impaired 'top down' control.

Box 1.2.1: Adolescent brain is very vulnerable to substance abuse and other addictive behaviors

- Poorly developed control of prefrontal cortex with a highly responsive amygdala in this age makes the adolescent to 'give in' easily to negative peer pressure and thereby into substance use and addiction.
- An adolescent who does not have a high self-esteem and does not get rewards or appreciation from trustworthy elders and friends or from involvement in academic and extra-academic activities may resort to drugs to seek a dopamine high.
- Drug use in adolescence can 'hijack' the reward circuitry of the brain resulting in lifelong addiction.
- The drugs bind on dopamine receptors, inhibit reuptake of dopamine and flood the synaptic junctions resulting in a 'high'– a feeling of thrill and pleasure.
- These adolescents cease to get enjoyment from their involvement in academics, extracurricular activities and sports and get a 'high' only with drugs.
- The adolescent brain is less sensitive to aversive effects of drugs paving the way to excessive substance use.
- Neurotoxins like drugs can damage the immature adolescent brain permanently leading to defective cognition, poor learning due to a smaller hippocampus and increased impulsivity due to impaired development of frontal lobe.
- Gambling, internet and compulsive consumption of high calorie food also stimulate the reward circuitry of brain and are known addictive disorders.

Family History

Genetics affects neurodevelopment. Many mental disorders e.g., depression, bipolar disorder, substance abuse and schizophrenia have a genetic propensity.

Past History and History of Chronic Disorders

- It is important to take a history of acute illnesses like traumatic brain injury or meningitis and chronic disorders e.g., diabetes mellitus, asthma, epilepsy and juvenile idiopathic arthritis that may have implications on neurodevelopment.
- The clinician should reassess the current degree of control of chronic diseases such as epilepsy and diabetes mellitus. Control is dependent on adolescent adherence to therapy.
- Due to conflicts with authority figures and anxiety about its effect on peer affiliation, adolescents may detest taking regular medication. Hence they need one on one counselling for ensuring therapeutic compliance. Poor control of chronic disorders has a deleterious effect on brain development.

Psychosocial History Taking

Excessive stress results in increased levels of cortisol which can hamper the neuronal growth especially in the hippocampus which is the main seat of learning and memory. Hence eliciting stressors in various domains of an adolescent's life are essential, especially if there is a recent history of problem behavior.

It is important to assess positive personality traits of the adolescent for strength based counselling. The acronym, HEEADSSS is used for taking psychosocial history regarding home, education, eating, depression, substance use, sexuality and safety respectively. Details of HEEADSSS are given in Chapter 1.3.

In this chapter we will discuss only the neurodevelopment aspects.

Home: Abusive upbringing and poor attachment with caregivers have adverse effects on brain neurodevelopment. Authoritative parenting style keeps brain development on track.

Education: Bullying and teasing from peers may impair neurodevelopment.

Eating: A very detailed history of diet needs to be taken as junk food is addictive and leads to obesity and metabolic syndrome (Chapters 3.3 and 3.4).

Diets rich in omega 3 fatty acids promote myelination. Its deficiency has been implicated in development of ADHD and schizophrenia. This is of special significance to adolescence when important areas of brain like the prefrontal cortex are in the process of maturation and myelination.

Deficiency of iron impairs neural and cognitive development.

As adolescents are emotionally labile, a negative body image may result in onset of eating disorders.

Activities: Details of exercise, sleep, media usage and hobbies should be taken as these greatly affect the developing brain. *It is important to promote a healthy lifestyle.*

Sleep: It is important to take a sleep history to explain to the adolescents the importance of sleep and sleep debt. Adolescents need at least 8 hours of sleep. Most of them sleep very late due to excessive usage of electronic gadgets and prolonged study hours. Sleep deprived adolescents have a hyper-responsive amygdala and so do the ones who watch excessive violent media. This heralds the onset of impulsive behavior and also sleep deprivation syndrome.

Physical activity: A very detailed history should be taken about the physical activity and sedentary habits to explain to them the high risk of non-communicable diseases (NCD) (for more details see Chapter 1.8). Exercise improves blood flow to parietal and temporal lobes of the brain. It also stimulates release of brain-derived neurotrophic factor (BDNF) that stimulates neuronal growth and myelination.

Extracurricular activities: Participation in extra academic activities like dance, music, social service and sports stimulates the reward center of the brain that is a neurodevelopmental 'need' in adolescence which keeps 'risky rewarding behavior' like drugs, violence and gambling at bay. Both adolescents and their parents should be encouraged to participate in healthy activities.

Details of peers and related activities should be noted as peer influence in adolescence as peers are known to influence adolescent behavior to a great extent. They have an intense impulsive response to emotional cues due to a highly reactive amygdala. Positive peer pressure is encouraged and negative discouraged.

Substance Use: History should be taken of experimentation with gateway drugs like tobacco and alcohol. Substance abuse adversely affects neuro-development and can result in long term brain damage and high chance of lifelong addiction (Box 1.2.1). For more details, please see Chapter 8.2.

Safety Issues: Impulsive and reward seeking behavior may result in speed driving especially under the influence of alcohol and in violent behavior. Due to relative immaturity of the cerebellum, the chances of road traffic accidents are high in adolescence. It is important to take a history regarding these safety issues.

CLINICAL EXAMINATION

Neurodevelopmental aspects during clinical examination are covered here (for other details see Chapter 1.3).

- Due to emerging autonomy in adolescence, privacy is essential during clinical examination.
- Due to enhanced cognition, a prior explanation about the details of the procedure of examination would improve cooperation from the adolescents.
- While examining, an ongoing conversation regarding 'normative' physical changes and 'sensitive observations' regarding abnormal ones will put the adolescent at ease.

INVESTIGATIONS

Adolescent brain development has the following implications on investigations:

- Consent should be taken from the adolescent and procedural details should be explained before performing any investigative procedure. Adolescents can be very reactive to pain, hate being pricked and hence the reasons for blood testing and vaccinations have to be explained in detail for getting their cooperation. For more details see Chapters 1.2 and 1.5.
- Depression and anxiety are common mental health issues in adolescents which also can be due to organic causes and hence tests for anemia, thyroid screening and investigations for chronic diseases like diabetes, arthritis etc. should be done.
- History and clinical suspicion of high risk behavior should prompt the clinician to perform specific investigations like blood and urine levels for drug screening and pregnancy testing and screening for sexually transmitted diseases.
- Due to their emotional reactivity, adolescents have poor compliance to medical treatment. Hence while treating chronic diseases, investigations need to be done to monitor compliance e.g. lung function tests for asthma, serum levels of antiepileptic drugs for seizure disorders, blood glucose monitoring for juvenile diabetes.

MANAGEMENT

A major role clinicians dealing with adolescents have to play is in imparting is anticipatory guidance and preventive counseling. More details are given in Chapter 1.3.

Explaining to teens about neural plasticity and the principle of 'use it or lose it' of pruning and 'hardwiring' will help them to understand the importance of inculcating good habits and skills at this age. A good rapport with the adolescent will ensure a lifestyle change for a lifetime.

Parental Guidance Based on Neurodevelopment

- Emotional reactivity, poor executive functions and predilection for high risk behavior of the adolescent can be explained on the basis of a 'reactive' mature limbic system and an immature of 'control' of frontal lobe.

- This scientific explanation would help 'distraught' parents to empathize with the adolescent and handle them with increased sensitivity.
- If neuronal connections for 'good' judgement are used often in adolescence, they would persist in adulthood. Encourage parents to expose their teens to life skill education.
- A 'nurturing environment' is very important for healthy neurodevelopment.
- Due to their propensity towards high risk behavior, adolescents need careful monitoring of their activities and peer group.

More on handling parents is given in Chapter 1.6.

LEARNING POINTS

- In the last decade there has been increased understanding of the neurodevelopment of adolescents that gives a better understanding of their emotions and behavior.
- Educating all adolescent stake holders will improve their understanding of "normal adolescent behavior" and prevent labeling of many normal adolescents as "abnormal or difficult adolescents".
- Health professionals can understand the importance of dealing with adolescents in a different manner as compared to child or adult patients.
- Policy makers will learn to make more adolescent appropriate policies.
- It will also help parents and teachers to understand the importance of having caring, trustworthy, non-judgemental adults to help nurture the developing brain of adolescents and keeping the brain development trajectory on tract by promoting self-esteem and guiding and counselling in an age appropriate manner.

SUGGESTED READING

1. Arian M, Haque M, Johal L, *et al.* Maturation of the adolescent brain. Neuropsychiatric Disease and Treatment 2013;9:449-61.
2. Briones DF, Wilcox JA, Mateus B, Boudeinah D. Risk factors and prevention in adolescent substance abuse: A biopsychosocial approach. Adolesc Med 2006;17(2)335-52.
3. Geidd J. Structural magnetic resonance imaging of adolescent brain. Ann NY Acad Sci 2004;1021:77-85.
4. Geidd JN. The digital revolution and adolescent brain evolution. J Adolesc Health 2012;51:101-05.
5. Nelson EE, Leibenluft EE, McClure E B and Pine DS. The social re-orientation of adolescence: A neuroscience perspective on the process and its relation to psychopathology. Psychol Med 2005;35(2):163-74.
6. Sowell ER, Siegel AW, Siegel DJ. Adolescent brain and cognitive changes. In: Fisher MM, Ed. Textbook of adolescent health care. American Academy of Pediatrics 2011;32-38.
7. Spear LP. Adolescent Neurodevelopment. J Adolesc Health 2013;52(S): S7-13.
8. Steinberg L. Cognitive Transitions. In: Steinberg L. Ed. Adolescence, 9th edition. New York; McGraw Hill. 2011; 57-86.
9. Tarokh L, Raffray T, vanReen E, Carskadon MA. Physiology of normal sleep in adolescents. Adolesc Med2010; 21(3):401-17,vii.
10. White AM. Understanding adolescent brain development. Adolesc Med 2009;20:73-90.

History Taking and Approach to An Adolescent Client 1.3

Swati Y Bhave, Rajesh Mehta

INTRODUCTION

Clinicians who are not trained in understanding psycho-social development of adolescents find it rather difficult to establish a rapport and elicit history from adolescents. Clinicians need to understand that because of inadequate concrete thinking ability at this age, young adolescents have poor ability to understand and have a modest perspective of future happenings. They also lack in self-confidence and can be very shy and self-conscious. Interviewing adolescents is a complex skill that requires in-depth knowledge about developmental stages of this age group, good interpersonal communication skills and a very flexible attitude. Adolescents are very sensitive to body language and hence the physician must develop both verbal and non-verbal communication skills as well as the ability to recognize emotions by understanding non-verbal expressions of the adolescent clients. In addition, parental involvement in the interview is a judgment that needs to be individualized in each case.

It is important to assess the young person's developmental level. The physical appearance and chronological age may be misleading as measures of cognitive development. An adolescent with early puberty may look very mature in physical stature but may not be emotionally mature; conversely an adolescent with late puberty (though within the normal range) may be very mature with good cognitive development but look childish due to less physical maturity. Clinician must study well the normal psychosocial development during the phases of early, middle and late adolescence (Chapter 2.3). This will enable the physician to evaluate the mental capacity of the adolescent clients and deal with them differently across these age groups. In addition, it is important to appreciate that the needs of young adolescents are different from older adolescents, e.g. you need to discuss and inform a 10-13-year-old about growth and development, menarche, nutrition and hygiene etc., whereas with a 16-19-year-old you would like to discuss about sexual behavior, contraception, pregnancy, safe sex etc. to enable them to make informed choices and protect themselves.

In addition to competence of the physician, the adolescent clinic should fulfil the criteria of being adolescent friendly which includes adolescent friendly ambiance which will put the adolescent at ease so that the clinical interaction is effective and result-oriented (Chapter 1.4).

Approach to Adolescent Who are Specially Challenged/with Special Needs/with Chronic Diseases

Clinicians dealing with adolescents will also have to train themselves for dealing with adolescents who have chronic problems and special needs, which are very challenging during this phase of life (Table 1.3.1). Such adolescents bear a double burden as they have to deal with the problems of their chronic diseases and also with the challenges that they have to face due to the transition. The chronic diseases have an adverse effect on self-esteem and identity formation and makes them especially liable for high risk health behavior which can worsen or complicate disease. As children the onus of managing

Table 1.3.1: Chronic diseases in adolescents

Childhood disabilities	Cerebral palsy
Congenital malformations	Congenital heart diseases
Neurological conditions	Spina bifida
Childhood onset diseases continuing into adolescence	Bronchial asthma Juvenile diabetes Chronic arthritis
Childhood diseases with better survival–into adolescence	Thalassemia Cystic fibrosis Childhood cancers HIV/AIDS Renal diseases
Diseases manifesting in adolescence and likely to become chronic	Asthma Type 2 diabetes Arthritis Bronchial asthma Musculoskeletal disorders

the medications and modification of lifestyle for chronic diseases is on the parent, while during adolescence there is a shift on making the adolescents responsible for their own monitoring. This is difficult due to the immaturity of their developing brain and the high emotional drive. Many adolescents become non-compliant with medications and the restrictions in lifestyle and thus land in poor disease control and worsening of their symptoms, e.g., bronchial asthma and juvenile diabetes.

Dealing with specially challenged adolescents is not easy for parents, nor for adolescents themselves. Clinicians have to spend more time in assessing such adolescents, as they need to go beyond the medical condition and also address the functional impairment, effect on cognitive development and associated psychosocial issues which can have an impact on the normal development of the adolescent and his/her mental status. The management is not complete unless all these issues are examined and assessed and appropriate interventions put in place. Specially challenged adolescents will have lot of difficulties in the transition through puberty and this can result in mental health comorbidities like anxiety, depression, suicidal feelings, and substance abuse. Often the sexuality aspects of these young people are forgotten as everyone is focusing on their physical status. One has to remember that these adolescents will have all the normal sexual desires and not being able to express them can lead to lot of frustration.

HISTORY TAKING

A rigid structured approach to history taking as taught in medical schools may not work in an adolescent interview. Establishing a working therapeutic relationship is most important in the initial interview. This can help in diagnosing of many hidden or underlying health concerns and problems. Hence, a functional approach to interview, which is more *patient-centered* than *physician-centered* and allows flexibility, is important to establish the patient's trust and compliance.

These are basic and essential elements of a successful interview with the adolescent clients (Box 1.3.1).

Box 1.3.1: Guidelines for communication in an adolescent interview
1. Establish rapport
2. Create an appropriate atmosphere
3. Maintain confidentiality
4. Obtain complete information
5. Recognize and adjust to barriers in doctor-patient communication
6. Summarize the interview session

Establishing Rapport

Many adolescents may not have come willingly to the clinic, but brought against their wishes by the parents or referred by school. Hence, it is important to establish a rapport with the adolescent in the very first visit (Box 1.3.2). The physician must convey the message that s/he considers the adolescent, and not the parent, his/her primary client. To deal with the accompanying parents, the physician can follow either of the two techniques:

(i) First receive both the parent/s and adolescent together. Explain that the adolescent will be considered as the primary client and interactions with him/her will not be revealed to the parents. Then, spend most of the initial interview with the adolescent after gently informing the parents to wait outside till they are called in after finishing with the adolescent.

(ii) See the parents first and the adolescent next, when the adolescent must be asked his/her opinion on what his/her parents may have told the doctor.

It is also important to remember two points:

(a) First, it is important to continue keeping the parents as allies in the management of their adolescent. Alienated parent may sabotage the physician-adolescent relationship and also stop allowing or bringing the adolescent for follow-up visits.

(b) Second, the adolescent must have the opportunity to decide the course of action and must feel that he or she is being treated as an individual and not an extension of their parents.

While establishing rapport, the physician must not over-identify with the patient. Trying to act like a teenager by wearing similar dress or using similar language is not necessary. Such a behavior is quickly perceived and repulsed by most adolescents. Adolescents have come to seek expert advice to a technically resourceful person; hence, the physician must act and behave like an expert.

The physician also, must not act like the adolescent's parent. He/she must stay objective and must not project aspiration and hopes for their own children on to their patients. It is important for the physician to remember that s/he should avoid being judgemental and *should not impose his/her own value system* upon the patient as a parent or give advice based on his/her own adolescent experiences. S/he must remain detached while expressing empathy with the client.

Creating an Appropriate Atmosphere

Privacy and minimal interruptions are very important elements that contribute to an adolescent friendly atmosphere. Make sure that you provide for auditory and visual privacy and do not allow others to walk into the room when a session is on. If brought by parents or accompanied by a friend allow time and space to speak privately with the adolescent client.

One can begin the interview by chatting informally about friends, hobbies or school etc. and letting the adolescent talk freely for a while. This will decrease the tension and enable the clinician to gain insights into the adolescent's personality and thought content. One must use good skills of communications, both verbal and non-verbal, like eye contact, friendly demeanor, active listening, clear and appropriate language, asking open-ended questions etc. Adolescents are more responsive to a physician, who is warm, understanding and attentive (Box 1.3.2).

A physician also should have the insight about the underlying cause of the reactions of the adolescent patient. A frightened adolescent usually responds with hostility and physician should understand this defence mechanism and handle him or her gently. Similarly a silent, non-communicative adolescent is often hiding worry, fear or anger and can best be reached by a warm, caring attitude.

Maintaining Confidentiality

The following points are important regarding confidentiality at your clinic:

- Familiarize yourself with the law regarding confidentiality in your city, state and country.
- Establish that your clinic follows the policy of confidentiality.
- Make sure that adequate procedures and checks are in place for confidentiality. For example, how is the diagnosis recorded, when linked with name, and who all have access to the register, files or records?
- Make sure all staff understand adolescents' legal rights (age of consent, policies on confidentiality).

Explaining about confidentiality to the adolescent and the parents:

- It may be good policy to speak with parents and adolescents together for some time and explain to them the clinic policy of maintaining confidentiality.
- Decide with the adolescent which issues should be discussed in the presence of parents or accompanying friends.
- Adolescents must be told early in the relationship that anything that they share with you will remain with you.
- But one must also explain to the adolescents, that it is in the interest of his or her welfare, that certain situations will require the involvement of parents or elders like in a case of abuse, rape, unwanted pregnancy, suicidal ideation, homicidal feelings, conflict with law etc. Confidentiality cannot be guaranteed in these situations.
- When the physician feels it is necessary to involve parents for support or if parents insist on knowing the content of the patient-doctor conversation, the adolescent must be informed in advance.

For ethical and legal aspects see Chapter 1.5.

Obtaining Complete Information

With some adolescent clients, it is a challenge to obtain complete information. Many adolescents report to the clinic for somatic complaints while the actual concern or health problem remains camouflaged or hidden. He/she may present with abdominal pain while they have underlying concerns related to small breasts (girls), poor facial hair (boys), masturbation, sexual abuse or unplanned sexual encounter, or use of tobacco and alcohol. It is important to uncover the actual or real problem being experienced by the adolescents.

During the interview medical history and psychosocial history, which evaluate the youngster's coping abilities in three spheres, i.e., school, family and peer-group should be elicited. Many structured interview tools or questionnaires/checklists have been in use to obtain complete information on the individual context of the adolescent client and about the common health-risk behaviors/activities that are known to bother adolescents or occur among them. Examples of such questionnaires/checklists include the screening tools developed by the American Medical Association (Guidelines for Adolescent Preventive Services, or GAPS) and the American Academy of Pediatrics. A popular tool used is the HEEADSSS approach. "Adolescent Job Aid", a WHO publication includes the HEEADSSS approach (see Table 1.3.2) that captures the most important domains for adolescent health. The most recent version of the HEEADSSS 3.0 can be obtained from contemporary pediatrics.com/HEEADSSS resource center.

While using such screening tools the art is to use open-ended questions as far as possible so that the adolescent can express himself/herself freely. It is recommended to use third person approach rather than the direct first person approach to ask specific behaviors. For example:

(a) Rather than straight away asking if s/he smokes or drinks, you may initially ask if any of his/her friends or parents use tobacco or alcohol. If the answer is yes, you should follow-up to ask if s/he ever joined them in this and how frequently.

Box 1.3.2: Communication skills for interaction with adolescent client
In general, adolescents do not always admit to health problems On initial questioning, adolescents, particularly young and unmarried adolescents, may not admit to having had sex, the possibility of having HIV or being pregnancy, or provide information on important signs and symptoms of these.
Be open and approachable • Use a gentle, reassuring tone of voice. • Be positive, respectful, calm and reassuring. • Explain what to expect during the visit.
Convey respect • Listen, be empathetic and non-judgmental (even if you disagree with the lifestyle or values of the adolescent). • Treat adolescents as individuals who are entitled to have an opinion like adults and have human rights. • Be on time for appointment or inform the adolescent clients if you are getting late.
Special communication skills for history taking may be necessary • Offer privacy for interaction. • Assess developmental attributes and level of the adolescent client. • Be aware that you communicate verbally and non-verbally. • Use simple questions in plain language. • Repeat questions, rephrase or come back to it later. • Probe sensitively. • Offer options even when s/he has denied the problem. • Reassure about confidentiality.
Avoid moralizing and judging • Be understanding of the adolescent's situation. • Overcome your discomfort (if any) with adolescent's value system. • Learn to discuss puberty and sexuality comfortably and effectively.
Be patient • Be aware that adolescents may have limited experience in talking to adults and using health services. • Adolescents may need time to tell you their problem or make a decision. • You may have to repeat the question to clearly understand and keep asking open-ended questions and listen carefully, as there may be more than what meets the eye. • It may be difficult to uncover the actual problem of the adolescent in a single session; several sessions may be necessary. • Adolescents tend to focus on the present. They often do not think about making long-term future plans. Therefore, concentrate on the immediate future (next 1-2 weeks).
Adolescent may appear difficult and non-communicative This can be due to a variety of reasons. It might be because of embarrassment or fear of parental discovery of sexual activity, adult or peer disapproval of her/his behavior or relationships, social stigma related to her/his health concern etc. *Some ways to handle this are:* • Explain why you are asking certain specific questions, e.g., on sex or substance abuse. • Tell the adolescent that s/he may not answer a specific question if s/he does not want to. • Convey that no question or answer is wrong and encourage the adolescent to ask questions or express fears or concerns even if it is uncomfortable or embarrassing. • Give simple, direct answers in clear language. Explore the option of having a trusted friend or family member present with them during the visit.
For adolescents with disabilities (mental or physical): • Remember that it is often difficult for them to access services. • Take extra care and patience in attending to them. • Be careful not to regard them with pity. • An adolescent with a disability is first and foremost an adolescent and wants what adolescents generally want in life such as happiness, fulfilling relationships, independence, meaningful occupation, being trusted in and being accepted by others. • Do not excessively focus on the disability unless it is part of the presenting complaint. • Bear in mind that disabled adolescents have the same rights as their able-bodied peers. Never violate their rights.

Table 1.3.2: Information that can be obtained from a HEEADSSS assessment	
Home	Where they live With whom they live Whether there have been recent changes in their home situation How they perceive their home situation
Education/Employment	Whether they study/work How they perceive how they are doing How they perceive their relation with their teachers and fellow students/employers and colleagues Whether there have been any recent changes in their situation What they do during their breaks
Eating	How many meals they have on a normal day What they eat at each meal What they think and feel about their bodies
Activity	What activities they are involved in outside study/work What they do in their free time–during week days and on holidays Whether they spend some time with family members and friends
Drugs	Whether they use tobacco, alcohol, or other substances Whether they inject any substances If they use any substances, how much do they use; when, where and with whom do they use them
Sexuality	Their knowledge about sexual and reproductive health Their knowledge about their menstrual periods Any questions and concerns that they have about their menstrual periods Their thoughts and feelings about sexuality Whether they are sexually active; if so, the nature and context of their sexual activity Whether they are taking steps to avoid sexual and reproductive health problems Whether they have in fact encountered such problems (unwanted pregnancy, infection, sexual coercion) If so, whether they have received any treatment for this Their sexual orientation
Safety	Whether they feel safe at home, in the community, in their place of study or work; on the road (as drivers and as pedestrians) etc. If they feel unsafe, what makes them feel so
Suicide/Depression	Whether their sleep is adequate Whether they feel unduly tired Whether they eat well How they feel emotionally Whether they have had any mental health problems (especially depression) If so, whether they have received any treatment for this Whether they have had suicidal thoughts Whether they have attempted suicide

(Reproduced with Permission from WHO Adolescent Job Aid)

(b) Instead of asking directly if he/she has had sexual experience you could say that you receive some clients of his/her age who have had sexual experience and if s/he has any such concerns. This way you help normalize the issue and decrease the stigma associated with such issues. It is important to periodically check that the client has understood correctly by asking them to rephrase their understanding of the question or the issue. Even if you use a standard screening tool in your clinic there should be some flexibility in the sequencing of the questions according to the need of the situation.

HEEADSSS screening starts with least sensitive, day-to-day issues before proceeding to more personal and threatening issues like drugs, sexuality and suicide etc. Sexuality issues may be difficult for both the adolescent and the doctor to discuss. The physician may herself/himself feel the discomfort and the patient timidity or inhibition. However, it is physician's responsibility to explore the client's sexual behavior and plans knowing fully well that some of them would already be sexually active during late adolescence.

At times patients are non-communicative and at other times patients may use a constant flow of words to avoid discussing the actual problem. In such situations, the interview needs structure and the physician should gently remind the patient of the purpose of the meeting. Some experienced physicians are able to use the HEEADSSS screening to concurrently provide anticipatory or preventive guidance while they are eliciting information in each domain. With experience one can evolve this higher level of use of the health screening opportunity to promote health behaviors and prevent risky behaviors among the adolescents.

Recognize and Adjust to Barriers in Doctor-Patient Communication

While talking to an adolescent client, the physician must pay attention to non-verbal communication of the client, e.g., facial expressions, fidgeting etc. and look for underlying feelings of depression in patients with repeatedly vague somatic complaints, in order to bring out the actual (but hidden) concerns of the adolescent to the surface. Sometimes the non-verbal cues are more informative than verbal expressions.

At the same time one should be able to recognize barriers in communication and make adjustment to obtain the required information. Recognizing the barrier is the single most important step towards overcoming it (Box 1.3.3).

Box 1.3.3: Barriers in communication with adolescent patients
Verbal-non-verbal mismatch: An adolescent, who on being asked about family problems, may say everything is fine, while looking sad.
Cognitive dissonance: This is illustrated by a patient who does not feel well yet denies any stress, even when there has been a recent death in the family.
Unexpected resistance: A patient, on show of sympathy by the doctor, may respond angrily.
Non-compliance to management: Sometimes the only clue to a barrier may be that the treatment is not working. Non-compliance to the agreed upon management plan may be due to unresolved conflicts or barriers between physician and patient.
A physician, may also have unexpected feelings that act as a communication barrier, e.g., strong negative feelings towards a patient with alcoholism, because of his/her feelings towards his/her own alcoholic mother, or may have homophobia etc.

Summarizing the Interview Session

Once the interview is over the physician must gather his/her inputs and summarize them. S/he should end on a positive note with emphasis on the adolescent's strengths and should also explain his/her assessment and outline the treatment plan, first to the adolescent and then to the parent (while assuring confidentiality of the client), and agree to the plan of action.

Time Requirement for the Interview

Usually 30 minutes is sufficient for the initial visit. The first 5 minutes can be spent with the adolescent and the parent, then 10 minutes for an interview with the adolescent, 10 minutes for physical examination and 5 minutes for discussion of findings and treatment with the adolescent. In follow-up visits, 15 minutes are sufficient.

For complex bio-psychosocial problems, two or three sessions of 30 minutes each, one week apart are more productive, rather than one long session in the beginning. This way, both the physician and the adolescent can look back and think about their assessment and responses given in the previous session.

History Taking in Adolescent Who are Specially Challenged/with Special Needs/with Chronic Diseases

In such group of adolescents it is first important to access the effect the disease or condition has had on the adolescents by taking a detailed history with the parents before asking questions to the adolescents themselves. The following points are important:

- How long has the disease/condition been present?
- Is it well controlled or are there any issues?
- Was it well controlled before and now problems have occurred after child has entered adolescence?
- What is the attitude of the adolescent towards his/her disease?
- Is s/he in a state of denial, anger, depression, or acceptance? Any other?
- Or his/her mental status fluctuates? Which mood is more dominant?
- What is the relationship with peers?

- Has s/he been a victim of bullying or ragging related to his/her condition?
- Is the disease affecting his/her cognitive ability?
- Is s/he having any difficulty in vision, hearing, speech impairment that is affecting his/her cognition or day-to-day activities?
- Is s/he having any difficulty in locomotion or movements that prevent him/her from normal daily activities without assistance, e.g., physical support wheel chair etc?
- Is there any contraindication for him/her taking part in sports, or outdoor activities like trekking etc?
- Has s/he developed any behavioral problems due to the chronic health issue?
- Has s/he developed mental health problems like aggression, violence, depression, substance abuse or any addiction due to inability to cope up with the disease?
- What are their own feelings towards the adolescent and his/her condition?
- Have they got a good network and support system to share their feelings or are they feeling isolated?
- How is their relationship with the adolescent?
- What is the relationship of the adolescent with the siblings and other family members?

PHYSICAL EXAMINATION

One has to be very careful legally and be sensitive to the feelings of adolescents when subjecting him/her to a physical examination.

- Discuss with the adolescent if he/she wants the accompanying person to be present during the physical examination.
- Explain to the adolescent what you are planning to do during the examination and its purpose. Adolescents especially in the early- and mid-adolescence are undergoing various body changes due to puberty. They are extremely self-conscious about being physically examined by a stranger. The physician should first explain what is going to take place during the examination in a relaxed manner utilizing simple, non-technical words and take permission for touching and examining the adolescents.
- Ideally the same sex doctor should conduct the physical examination; if not one must have a chaperone available during the examination. It is best to have a nurse or another staff member from the clinic that is the same gender as the adolescent.
- One should always guard against the claim of inappropriate touching during a physical examination. Presence of a third person decreases the intimacy in the room. Also, the patient may relate to the non-threatening chaperone more easily.
- This is very important when you are examining for secondary sexual character development for Tanners staging.
- This also protects the physician from a youngster's fantasies of sexual invasion and minimizes flirtation, which can occasionally happen.
- It is very important to do the physician examination only when the physician has developed a rapport. If you are faced with a very shy adolescent it is better to postpone the physical examination in a well adolescent to a second visit if possible, unless the physical examination is urgent for the medical problem.
- The examination should be done in a separate room reserved specifically for this purpose and the adolescent should be appropriately draped. Breasts and genitalia should be exposed only during actual inspection, palpation or auscultation. Frequent comments about normal findings are also most appreciated.

It is good idea to keep talking during the physical examination to put the adolescent at ease. This also helps to elicit whatever issues have remained in the history taking.

Physical Examination in Adolescents Who are Specially Challenged/with Special Needs/with Chronic Diseases

In addition to the routine general and systemic examination, based on detailed history taking an assessment needs to be done for the following:

1. If the chronic disease is well controlled or inadequately controlled.
2. Does the adolescent have any functional impairment related to the disease or condition?
3. Does the adolescent have any psychosocial problems that are related to his/her chronic diseases? Use screening questionnaires, e.g., to personality screening, anxiety and depression (Chapter 8.7).

INVESTIGATIONS

Whatever investigations you order are going to be done and paid for by the parents but have to also be accepted by the adolescents themselves. It is important that you explain to both the adolescent and the parent why you are asking for the tests and how the results will help in management. Adolescents may hate being tested specially pricked for blood collection.

Investigations in Adolescents Who are Specially Challenged/with Special Needs/ with Chronic Diseases

If the chronic disease is inadequately controlled then appropriate investigations should be done for assessment.

TREATMENT

- Make special efforts to educate about the illness and prepare the adolescent for self-management as appropriate. It is especially important for them to feel competent and in control.
- Unlike the pediatric age group when all instructions were given to the parent, in case of adolescents both have to be involved–the adolescents themselves to learn self-monitoring and the parents to supervise and ensure compliance.
- Adolescents are often less tolerant of medication and their side effects and are at risk of stopping these before completion of treatment. Therefore, they need to be well informed of the possibilities of side effects.
- Explain about the treatment, adherence and completion of the regimen. Discuss fixing a specific time during the day for the adolescent to take medicine to help compliance.
- Be aware of her/his weight and dosage. You may have to use a smaller dose of medication, especially with very young adolescents or those very small in stature.
- Discuss storage of drugs because of concerns of privacy and safety.
- Extra effort is required to achieve adherence to treatment of chronic illness:
  - Denial of the disease and denial/lack of recognition of symptoms of complication are common among adolescents.
  - Concerns about peer pressure and being different may impair use of medication and other forms of treatment such as the inhaler for an asthmatic adolescent or insulin injections for diabetes.
  - Make sure to plan for ways to permit sports, exercise and other activities as appropriate.

Clinicians dealing with adolescents need to be well aware of various phases of adolescence (Chapter 2.3) as the approach to an adolescent patient, the health messages to be delivered, as well as management of various adolescent issues have to be customized as per the stage of development, to be really effective.

Management in Adolescents Who are Specially Challenged/with Special Needs/ with Chronic Diseases

1. If the disease is inadequately controlled then one has to focus on the specific issues of the disease or condition which is discussed in the various chapters in sections 5 and 8.
2. If the adolescent has any psychosocial problems that are related to his/her chronic diseases it is very important to address and adequate referrals to mental health professionals should be done for appropriate counseling, psychotherapy and/or medications as the need be.
3. The adolescent should also be encouraged for self-management wherever feasible in chronic diseases to improve self-confidence and self-image and feel more in control of their lives.

ANTICIPATORY GUIDANCE AND PREVENTIVE COUNSELING

Adolescents often lack knowledge about pubertal changes, nutrition and physical activities, sexual maturation, contraception, physiology of conception and signs of pregnancy, dangers of unprotected sex and the risk of pregnancy, human immunodeficiency virus (HIV) infection and sexually transmitted infections (STIs) and dangers of use of tobacco and alcohol. Hence age-appropriate guidance and preventive counseling must be provided to adolescent clients during all contacts, if possible. In addition, the adolescent health physician should be able to provide generic and specific guidance to accompanying parents on how they support their adolescents during health and sickness (Box 1.3.4).

For best results knowing the cognitive stage of development of the adolescent is important as one has to give customized age appropriate messages for it to be effective (Table 1.3.3).

LEARNING POINTS

- History taking of an adolescent or *interview* as it is called is a skill that needs to be acquired with good training and practice. A respectful, non-judgmental and a conversational style of communication rather than an interrogative style is recommended.
- A physician's success in adolescent care depends on positive attitude towards adolescents and not only on the specialized training. The physician must possess knowledge of developmental attributes of adolescents,

Box 1.3.4: Anticipatory guidance and preventive counseling

Provide age appropriate information on:

- Normal development and anatomy
- Puberty
- Menstruation
- Sexual and reproductive function
- Dangers of sexual predators and abuse
- Convey the message of delaying sexual debut. If adolescent chooses to be sexually active, reinforce the message of reduced number of sexual partners and protection against pregnancy, STI, HIV and unwanted sex
- Contraception: Use of condom and other contraceptive methods including emergency contraception
- Pregnancy: Physiology of conception and unsafe sex
- HIV/STIs, prevention, signs and symptoms
- Cigarettes, drugs, or other substance use/abuse

From the history taking and interview access and provide information and guidance about specific concerns

- Does s/he have concerns about puberty, social acceptance, peer pressure, forming relationships, possibility of stigma and violence?
- Explain options to resolving problems at hand
- Educate on the advantages of saying 'No' to sex like preventing unwanted pregnancy, STI, HIV
- Demonstrate condom use. Reinforce these skills if taught in school
- If you cannot do this, refer the adolescent to organizations that teach life skills

Table 1.3.3: Cognitive development and health implications

Stages	*Cognitive ability*	*Results*	*Implications*
Early (10-13 years)	Concrete thinking immediate and short term consequences Cognitive abilities are also dominated by egocentrism and impulsive behavior	Poor abstract reasoning limits their capacity to comprehend complex health messages like healthy nutrition and lifestyle at this age and long term positive impact on health or adverse long term impact of tobacco To manipulate their ideas and concepts, we need to use concrete representation	Lack the skills and ability to appreciate why behavior change is important for future health status and hence can't make changes Can be improved by WHO life skill education (LSE)
Middle (14-16 years)	Abstract reasoning skills begin to emerge Can start understanding that there can be multiple outcomes of their action In calm state of mind will understand and accept adult advice Under stress and if emotionally disturbed the thinking becomes concrete and they can make wrong decisions	Conflicts over personal choices, like food, etc. become increasingly common Lifestyle choices are more influenced by what the peers are doing rather than what the family is doing or advising Hence very often they experiment with and indulge activities which are high risk for health Likes use of mnemonics to remember	Consider themselves invincible Often indulge in risky impulsive behaviors This is the right time to give messages that their health behavior at present can affect their health status in future But this knowledge alone does not help them to make the right choices Negative peer pressure may prevent them from putting this knowledge into practice Can be improved by WHO life skill education (LSE)
Late (17-19 years)	Maturation of frontal lobes facilitates regulatory competence The expansion of formal operational abstract reasoning skills continues May still go back to concrete thinking under stress and pressure	Strong personal identity. Less body image problems Less affected by peer pressure and conflict over personal issues, such as food choices, also decreases Able to suppress impulsive behavior Able to manage increasingly sophisticated social situations They are less dependent on family for emotional and financial support	They can now understand that their lifestyle choice just now will result in good health in adult life also This helps adolescent girls to understand about risky sexual behavior They can now develop the skills for solving problems and be able to make change in behavior These can be enhanced by LSE

and have sincere fondness for youth, willingness to listen, the self-security and maturity to be non-judgmental and empathetic.

- Time required for an adolescent client is more than what you need with a child, so enough time should be provided to adolescent client to complete the interaction. Rapport building is crucial in the initial stage as most adolescents will not be forthcoming with crucial aspects in the history unless they feel comfortable with the physician and are assured privacy and confidentiality.
- It is better to use standardized screening tools like HEEADSS which help explore the psychosocial domains, identify any risk situations or behaviors and help uncover the actual and underlying concern/ issue.
- Appropriate care should be taken during physical examination and treatment planning.
- It is prudent to appropriately involve the parents in patient care and support without compromizing confidentiality of the adolescent who is your primary client. This is especially important in case of young adolescents below 18 years.
- Specially challenged adolescents and those with chronic diseases need a sensitive approach and holistic management that takes into account all aspects of their disease in addition to challenges of normal adolescence.

SUGGESTED READING

1. Adolescent Job Aid: A handy desk reference tool for primary level health workers. World Health Organization, Geneva, 2010.
2. Coupey SM. Interviewing Adolescents: Pediatr Clin North Am 1997;14(6):1349-62.
3. Goldenring JM, Rosen DS. Getting into adolescent heads: An essential update. Contemp Pediatr 2004;21(1):64-90.
4. Hagan JF, Shaw JS, Duncan PM, eds. Bright Futures: Guidelines for Health Supervision of Infants, Children and Adolescents, Third Edition. Elk Grove Village, IL: American Academy of Pediatrics.
5. Kaplan DW, Mammal KA. In: Merenstein GB, Kaplan DW, Rosenberg AA, Eds. Handbook of Pediatrics. Prentice Hall International Inc 1997; 217.
6. Levenberg PB, Elster AB. Clinical Evaluation and Management Handbook. Guidelines for Adolescent Preventive Services (GAPS). Chicago; American Medical Association, 1995.
7. Ministry of Health and Family Welfare; Government of India. Facilitator Guide for Rashtriya Kishore Swasthya Karyakram, 2014.
8. Patton GC, Viner R. Pubertal transitions in health. Lancet 2007;369(9567):1130-39.
9. Sawyer SM, Drew S, Yeo MS, Britto MT. Adolescents with a chronic condition: Challenges living, challenges treating. Lancet 2007;369(9571):1481-89.
10. SkillscascadeCom. Communicating with children, adolescents and more than one patient at a time. Available at http://www.skillscascade.com/special.htm accessed on 16 Aug 2015.
11. The Royal Children's Hospital, Melbourne. Engaging with and assessing the adolescent patient. Available at http://www.rch.org.au/clinicalguide/guideline_index/accessed on 16 Aug 2015.

Setting up Adolescent Health Clinics in Private Health Sector

1.4

Swati Y Bhave, Preeti M Galagali

INTRODUCTION

The need of the hour is to set up adolescent friendly clinics to deliver holistic health care. Adolescent friendly clinic is a set-up where the adolescents and their parents feel comfortable to discuss their problems and have confidence and trust in the professional skills of the health care provider to fulfil their needs. Since adolescent medicine is not a well-established specialty in India, delivery of comprehensive adolescent health services in a private set-up exists in very few centres. Unlike the widely acceptable concept of well baby clinic, the community and many health professionals have not yet recognized the need of routine well adolescent monitoring.

Adolescent health has now received due recognition in India. In 2014, Government of India (GOI), Ministry of Health and Family Welfare launched the National Adolescent Health Strategy named RKSK–Rashtriya Kishore Swasthya Yojana under which adolescent specific health clinics would be established in many districts of India. WHO has also published standard guidelines for setting up adolescent friendly health services.

Most of the contemporary health problems amongst the adolescents are related to personal behavior and are potentially preventable. It has been observed that consistent health promotional messages from parents, teachers and doctors can significantly decrease mortality and morbidity among the youth. Adolescent clinics are apt for conveying such messages. The other aims of setting an adolescent clinic are enumerated in Box 1.4.1.

Box 1.4.1: Aims of setting an adolescent clinic

1. To reinforce and encourage health-promoting lifestyles
2. To detect physical, emotional and behavioral problems and to intervene early
3. To give age appropriate preventive counseling for common issues
4. To provide anticipatory guidance against risk taking behavior
5. To immunize
6. To provide parental guidance

Setting up of an adolescent center is not difficult, however it is a major challenge to get sustained clientele to access available services as it is not a felt need. Common barriers to delivering and accessing comprehensive health services to adolescents include lack of confidentiality, need of consent from parents or guardians, unfriendly atmosphere and social stigma. Health professionals can easily overcome these are barriers by stringently following the WHO criteria of Adolescent Friendly Health Services (AFHS) elucidated in Box 1.4.2. Global research has identified two key common characteristics of 'friendly' health services as perceived by adolescents. These are protection of confidentiality and to be treated with respect by the health care provider.

Box 1.4.2: AFHS–Adolescent friendly health services (WHO Guidelines adapted by GOI)

- Adolescent friendly facility and ambience
- Adolescent friendly staff
- Adequate space
- Convenient timings
- Lucid privacy and confidentiality rules
- Health education material (e.g. charts and pamphlets) on adolescent health issues and concerns
- Counseling services
- Outreach programs to generate need and awareness amongst adolescents and community

CRITERIA OF ADOLESCENT FRIENDLY HEALTH SERVICES

The physician in charge of the adolescent clinic should be familiar with the basic principles of establishing adolescent friendly health services that are enumerated in Box 1.4.3.

Box 1.4.3: Hoffman's basic principles of adolescent services

- Availability
- Accessibility
- Approachability
- Acceptability
- Appropriateness
- Affordability

Availability

The first principle of establishing adolescent services is that these should be easily available to the teenage population otherwise their desire to utilize these services would be minimal. In private setup these can be set-up in individual clinics or polyclinics or can be hospital based. The best setting to establish such services is either in a corporate hospital or a polyclinic where all the required services and specialties are easily available under one roof. This is because looking after adolescents entails team work, between the adolescent physician, mental health professional, gynecologist, ophthalmologist, dentist, orthopedic surgeon, and dermatologist and so on. If adolescents have to be sent elsewhere for a referral, there is a possibility that they may not go or they may be lost for future follow-up. Establishing an adolescent clinic in a small private setup is possible but involves a lot of hard work to establish a local network of adolescent friendly consultants from other specialties for efficient referral services.

Community-based adolescent services work very well as the adolescent does not feel conscious or stigmatized while accessing such a health service. The best example of this is in Thailand. Adolescent centers there have been established in shopping malls. These centers have help lines, individualized counseling services and classes for training in dancing and public speaking.

Accessibility

For adequate utilization of services, it is essential to ensure that the clinic timings are suitable for the adolescents. Hence holding clinics on weekdays during school or college hours is definitely not going to make for good attendance at the clinic.

Various favorable time schedules can be:

1. Evening hours from 6 to 8 PM. Apart from being after-school hours, this timing has the advantage that it is after office hours and is suitable for parents if they need to accompany the adolescent.
2. Saturday afternoons is also a good time since many schools are closed or have half-day timings.
3. Sunday mornings are suitable for both adolescents and parents but have the disadvantage of everyone missing out on the weekly cherished holiday and may prove to be counter-productive.

Location

The clinic should be at a location that is easily accessible by public transport, which is primarily used by unaccompanied adolescents.

Approachability

Adolescents are very sensitive to the atmosphere in a clinic and will not return if it makes them uncomfortable. A lot of planning should be done to decide what would be a welcoming and comfortable ambience related to the culture and the class of adolescent clientele. A very posh atmosphere would make middle or lower social class diffident and a shabby atmosphere would drive all adolescents away.

Create an Adolescent Friendly Atmosphere

A pediatrician starting an adolescent clinic should remember that adolescents have graduated from the 'baby doctor' and want to be treated as an adult. They will therefore not be comfortable with an atmosphere of baby toys and pictures; neither would they like to stand in front of height charts that are not suitable for their stature. It is important to make an extra effort to change the clinic ambience from that of a 'baby clinic' to 'to an adolescent friendly atmosphere' with suitable posters and magazines.

Adolescents are usually not sure on what topics or to what extent questions can be asked in this clinic. A good way to get this message across is to keep pamphlets on various subjects in the waiting room e.g. obesity, diet, exercise, stress management, sexually transmitted disorders, use of condom, menstrual hygiene, masturbation, etc. This serves a dual purpose—it educates them in a non-threatening manner and it also gives a signal to them that it is okay or 'done' to ask questions on these issues. Magazines or other reading material on these aspects also should be kept in the waiting room.

Acceptability

The teen should be accepted as an adult and not as a child brought to the clinic by parents. Hence they should be addressed and questioned directly. They will come to the clinic only if a good rapport is established with them. The staff should not be judgmental or moralistic. They should remember that they are in the clinic to help and to guide the adolescent through their problems, which could include delicate issues like sexuality and substance abuse.

Scheduling of Appointments

- The appointment should not be forced upon them but it should be set up with their consent and preferences so that it does not overlap with their important academic assignments and other activities such as hobbies, and sports.

- Waiting time should be kept to a minimal.
- The length of the visit may vary from 30 to 45 minutes.
- As adolescents prefer to be with others of the same age, it is advisable not to see younger patients at the same time.
- Individual files of the patient's medical records should be maintained but this should not be accessible to everyone in the clinic to maintain confidentiality.

Appropriateness

For Physician

- Adolescent clinics should not be established for generating 'extra income', in order to get more patients or because it is the 'latest fad'.
- Teenagers are not the easiest to handle unless the service provider has the skills for it. Hence it not just enough to undergo training in adolescent care before venturing into starting a clinic but it is equally important that the service provider must genuinely like teenagers. After all most pediatricians chose pediatrics because they like kids.
- The health personnel should treat the adolescent with respect, display warmth, unconditional positive regard and offer counseling without criticizing or being judgmental.
- When advice is given for sensitive issues like sexuality, it is important to keep in mind the teen's upbringing, sociocultural aspects, mental and emotional capacity. For example, ideas about dating and pocket money in higher socioeconomic groups could be quite different from those of a conservative middle class ideology that emphasizes moral values. The advice has to be based on individuals and generalized advice on these issues may not yield the desired results.

Affordability

As in other areas of pediatric or medicine practice, the service provider needs to keep the fees flexible. Efforts should be made not to deprive needy teenagers just because they cannot afford the clinic fees. In case the adolescents cannot afford the clinic fees, they should be referred to centers which have free services, especially in cases of prolonged treatment. In a Western setup where teenagers start earning at an early age, they pay for their consultations.

WHO in its recently published guidelines has based its definition of adolescent friendly health services on the Hoffman's principles. WHO considers health services to be adolescent friendly if they are accessible, acceptable, equitable, appropriate and effective.

ESTABLISHING ADOLESCENT FRIENDLY HEALTH SERVICES

First, Be Safe

The Ministry of Health has still not accepted the Indian Academy of Pediatrics (IAP) proposal that recommends that pediatricians look after children till 18 years of age. If a pediatrician has received training in adolescent issues and if the hospital authorities give permission, to see children between 12 to 18 years, it is possible to set up adolescent clinics in private institutions. Private clinics or nursing homes will have to bear in mind the problems involved in starting on their own. It is best to start with an outdoor practice of well adolescents. Indoor practice can have medico-legal implications. In the Government setups, pediatricians trained in adolescent care through various governmental training programs on adolescent health are delivering services in the adolescent clinics in medical colleges and district hospitals.

Keeping in view the aims, anticipated barriers and basic principles of organizing adolescent clinics, the suggested steps for establishing adolescent clinics are tabulated in Box 1.4.4. The services that should be delivered are in Box 1.4.5.

Box 1.4.4: Steps in organizing adolescent health services

1. Survey the available adolescent services in the neighborhood.
2. Determine the needs of the adolescents by conducting a survey in the existing pediatric clinic.
3. The physician in-charge of the adolescent clinic to undergo training in adolescent medicine.
4. Train ancillary staff in handling delicate sensitive adolescent issues.
5. Identify school and community referral networks to increase the scope and reach of the services.
6. Set up a multispecialty adolescent friendly referral network specialties for comprehensive management of adolescent problems.
7. Establish an adolescent clinic, based on the surveys and inputs received.

THE LAYOUT OF THE CLINIC

If a new adolescent clinic is being constructed, it is very important to plan it properly. If the clinic is being laid out in an already established setup, care should be taken to reorganize it in such a way that will make the adolescents

Box 1.4.5: Suggested services at adolescent clinic

- Annual health check-ups and issuing an adolescent health card
- Monitoring normal growth and development
- Immunization
- Anticipatory guidance
- Family life education
- Life skill education
- Promoting positive mental health
- Personality development
- Nutritional assessment and counseling
- Risk behavior screening
- Screening and counseling for psychosocial problems
- Assessment and counseling for scholastic issues
- Sports pre-participation evaluation
- Sexual and reproductive health education and counseling
- Pre-marital counseling
- Transition to adult health care
- Referral services

feel comfortable and they will feel like utilizing its services in times of need. The layout of the adolescent clinic is described in detail below.

RECEPTIONIST AND WAITING AREA

Both the receptionist and waiting area should be adolescent friendly. The receptionist and other staff should be sensitive towards adolescent issues. Rude or judgmental receptionists will put-off the adolescent patient who may not return for a follow-up. As discussed earlier, if the adolescent clinic is in a pediatric clinic, baby posters and toys should be removed from the waiting area. Health education material, pamphlets and magazines should be kept in the waiting area. The recommended services to be provided by the clinic are listed in Box 1.4.5. The available services could be prominently displayed on the notice-board in the clinic.

Consultation Room and Examination Room

If space permits, the consultation and examination rooms should preferably be separate to allow for privacy.

Laboratory Facilities

The laboratory facilities should be easily accessible to perform screening tests as needed. Hemoglobin estimation and a urine microscopy should be done at least once in adolescence. Lipid profile and blood sugar measurements could be done for all obese adolescents and those with a positive family history of premature coronary artery disease, diabetes mellitus and hypercholesterolemia. Screening for pregnancy, acquired immunodeficiency syndrome and sexually transmitted diseases should be done in high risk cases.

Seminar Room

It is important to do group counseling for conveying preventive health messages. If possible one should have access to a seminar room with audio-visual facilities. It could be used to conduct health awareness programs and group discussions with the adolescents.

Medical Personnel

Apart from an adolescent pediatrician, other personnel ideally required are a clinical psychologist, and counsellor. If they cannot be present in the clinic, they should be available for ready referral. A referral network should be set up with other specialists such as an adult physician, a gynecologist, an otolaryngologist, an ophthalmologist, an orthopedic surgeon, a dentist, a dermatologist, a physiotherapist, etc. The adolescent physician should refer to only 'adolescent friendly' specialists to ensure compliance with referrals.

Equipment

While setting up an adolescent clinic it is very important to make a list of equipment that includes the following:

- Appropriate weighing machines and height measurement charts are required. A stadiometer and a standardized electronic weighing machine would give accurate height and weight measurements respectively. Teenagers do not like the awkwardness of a pediatric setup being used on them.
- Appropriate sizes of blood pressure cuffs and peak flowmeters are a must.
- Blood pressure and peak expiratory flow rate percentile charts should be readily available.
- An adult size stethoscope is essential.
- Snellen chart for testing acuity, a tuning fork and an otoscope for doing an ear examination are also essential.
- For assessing growth quickly and accurately, height, weight and body mass index (BMI) charts should be available. It is important to track BMI.
- A chart for Tanner staging to assess puberty should be placed in each file along with the growth and height charts for future follow-up of the individual teen.
- Standardized questionnaires for adolescents and

parents may be used for screening and assessment of various problems like Beck's Depression Inventory for depression and SCARED (Screening for childhood anxiety and related emotional disorders) tool for anxiety and the newly released DSM-5 questionnaires that can be freely downloaded from www.dsm5.org

- Region specific waist circumference charts are useful in defining metabolic syndrome.
- Orchidometer is essential to assess pubertal staging in boys.
- The table size should be a minimum of six and a half feet to accommodate the teenager. They are typically not happy lying on baby tables with their legs sticking out.
- Privacy during examination is essential. If a separate room is not available, the examination table should be cordoned off with a screen or a curtain.

WELL ADOLESCENT MONITORING

Adolescents need to be monitored for their growth, development and preventive counseling on the lines of a 'well baby clinic'.

Monitoring of Growth

Height, weight and BMI measurements should be taken at appropriate intervals with at least one routine visit to the adolescent clinic in a year.

The examination should be done for an adolescent boy in the presence of a male attendant and for a girl in the presence of a female attendant if the treating clinician is of the opposite sex. While eliciting a history and performing a physical examination, the opportunity to provide anticipatory guidance should not be missed. The details of the physical examination are covered in the Chapter 1.3.

With media publicity on sports and beauty pageants, teenagers and parents are enamored by a tall thin body stature and a zero figure. In fact, one of the reasons for coming to an adolescent clinic is for advice on increasing the height. An approach to this problem is discussed in detail in the chapter problems of growth and development (Chapter 2.1). This is the right opportunity to emphasize the importance of proper diet, healthy media usage and exercise. Depending on the weight, appropriate advice needs to be given for obesity, eating disorders and malnutrition. These are detailed in Chapters 3.2, 3.3 and 8.4.

Due to a sedentary lifestyle and unhealthy dietary habits, obesity in teenagers is on the increase in many cities of our country. Due to various body image concerns amongst teenagers, we have an increase in incidence of eating disorders and abuse of anabolic steroids. Monitoring of weight provides a good opportunity to deal with these issues.

Monitoring of Puberty

Parents and teenagers are often anxious about early or late puberty. A proper Tanner staging and reassurance (if within normal limits) and appropriate investigations and management when necessary are important services to be provided at an adolescent clinic.

Immunization

Booster doses, catch-up immunization and vaccines for special circumstances should be given. These are detailed in Chapter 7.1 on immunization. The important vaccines to be given according to the IAP schedule in adolescence are Tdap and HPV. Varicella, MMR, typhoid, hepatitis B, meningococcal and hepatitis A vaccines could also be given in select cases.

Anticipatory Guidance

- While eliciting a history and doing an examination, anticipatory guidance should be given for high risk behavior, school performance, eating disorders, nutritional status, physical activity, media usage, sleep, emotional well being, relationships with peers, family and teachers, high blood pressure and visual defects.
- Adolescents also need to be educated about their normal physical, emotional and social development in various phases of adolescence.
- Safety practice knowledge is also imparted like wearing seat belts and helmets while traveling by motorized vehicles and not to drive under the influence of alcohol and below the legal age of driving.
- Anticipatory guidance should also be given to all parents at least once in early, middle and late adolescence for healthy parenting skills.

Preventive Counseling

Adolescent clinics are good avenues to provide preventive counseling in groups on lifestyle modification, stress management, prevention of reproductive tract infections, teenage pregnancy, etc. These are discussed in detail in sections 2, 3 and 4.

Community Programs of Adolescent Clinics

To reach out to the community and thereby improve clientele attendance in the clinic, it is a good idea to design and conduct programs that have been outlined in Box 1.4.6.

Box 1.4.6: Outreach programs of adolescent clinic

- Regular programs for teenagers, teachers and parents through schools and colleges
- Providing information and education to community by linking up with clubs like Rotary, women's group and youth groups like Nehru Yuvak Kendra Sangathan (NYKS) and National Service Scheme (NSS)

LEARNING POINTS

- Aims and basic principles of setting up an adolescent friendly clinic in a private setting
- AFHS as per WHO guidelines adapted by Ministry of Health and Family Welfare, Government of India
- Steps to be taken in the planning process, details about the equipment needed, staffing as well as referral issues
- List of services to be provided by the adolescent clinics to ensure delivery of holistic health care to the youth of our country
- Monitoring and preventive counseling in practice
- Parental guidance and community outreach programs

SUGGESTED READING

1. Adolescent friendly health services: An agenda for change. World Health Organization 2003 http://apps.who.int/iris/bitstream/10665/67923/1/WHO_FCH_CAH_02.14.pdf Accessed on 1 September 2015.
2. Bhave SY, Galagali PM. Setting up Adolescent Health Clinics in Private and Public environment. In:Bhave SY. Chief Editor. Bhave's Textbook of Adolescent Medicine; 2006. New Delhi: Jaypee Brothers Medical Publishers Pvt Ltd 2006; 9-16.
3. Bhave SY. Setting up Adolescent Services in Private Setting. In: Bhave SY. Chief Editor.CourseManual for Adolescent Health. Part 2 2002; IAP-ITPAH; 32-35.
4. Elster AB, Kuzkents NJ. AMA Guidelines for Adolescent Preventive Services. Williams and Wilkins, USA, 1994.
5. Elster AB, Levenburg P. Integrating Comprehensive Adolescent Preventive Services into routine Medical Care. Pediatr Clin North Am 1997;4:1365-77.
6. Kaul P, Kaplan DW. Caring for Adolescents in Office. In: Greydanus D, Pratt H, Patel DR, Eds. Essential Adolescent Medicine, New York; McGraw Hill 2006;17-27.
7. Making health services adolescent friendly: Developing national quality standards for adolescent health services. World Health Organization; 2012 http://www.who.int/maternal_child_adolescent/documents/adolescent_friendly_services/en/ Accessed on 1 September 2015.
8. Marks A. The adolescent friendly practice. In: Fisher MM. Chief Editor. Textbook of Adolescent Health Care. American Academy of Pediatrics 2011;210-15.
9. Quality assessment guidebook: A guide to assessing health services for adolescents clients. World Health Organization;2009 http://www.who.int/maternal_child_adolescent/documents/fch_cah_9789241598859/en/ Accessed on 1 September 2015.
10. Strategy Handbook. Rashtriya Kishor Swasthya Karyakram. Adolescent Health Division, Ministry of Health and Family Welfare, Government of India; 2014 http://www.nhp.gov.in/health-programmes/national-health-programmes/rashtriya-kishor-swasthya-karyakram-rksk Accessed on 1 September 2015.

Ethical and Legal Issues 1.5

Donald E Greydanus, Mahesh Baldwa

INTRODUCTION

Adolescent pediatricians have the important role of helping young patients for a safe and effective transition from childhood to adulthood. This chapter reflects on some of the ethical dilemmas clinicians may encounter while caring for adolescents and youth that can be complicated by legal standards, which vary from country to country. This chapter also reflects on the western and Indian perspectives with regard to issues such as confidentiality, emancipated vs mature minor, health record privacy (applicable to health records as well as unrecorded oral communications), and some specific circumstances (i.e. sexuality-related issues, substance abuse, mental health, emergency treatment, and end-of-life decisions). Finally comments regarding conducting research on youth are also discussed.

ISSUES INVOLVED IN DOCTOR-PATIENT CARE

Medical care has evolved as a contract between a health care provider (HCP) and the patient. If patients do not agree with treatment recommendations, they may sabotage treatment efforts in many ways.

A medical contract involves a clinician seeking consent of a patient for health care and also providing a consent that is informed—i.e. what are the risks and benefits of the proposed treatment for the patient? Even if a patient is not able to provide consent (e.g. being a minor), it is important for the patient to provide assent to the treatment. The patient should be willing to agree to the management and also asked about his/her preferences in this regard.

The scenario of doctor-patient relationship is quite different in India as compared to the western world and are reviewed briefly in Box 1.5.1.

Box 1.5.1: Societal perceptions about the role of a doctor in India

- India is a traditional caste and class based society where there is greater acceptance of social distance between medical professionals and patients in general. The doctor is identified as a person belonging to a superior class.
- Patients usually assume submissive position vesting authority to take decisions in physician; thus even affluent and educated patients often want the doctor to make decisions for them.
- Most patients are unaware of their rights or are culturally conditioned not to exercise their own choices.
- The social structure is such that the adolescent patients welcome participation of family members in decision making in contrast to the western society where they put high emphasis on individual autonomy.
- The authority of the parents is near absolute. The adolescent is not given chance to exercise any consent/opinion in normal course.
- Thus, adolescents often, find it hard to give their opinion and look up to the parents for their decision.
- Urban adolescents are a new emerging group of patients with wide awareness about consent and confidentiality forcing doctors to change, whereas rural adolescents still believe in traditional approach.

LAW AND MEDICAL ETHICS

Law as applicable to medical profession: Application and action under law may be operative from the moment allegations of improper, unskilled, or negligent treatment are hurled by the patient against physician/HCP as explained in detail below.

Medical ethics: This is an ideology of just criteria that implements values and perceptions to medical practice. Tenets of medical ethics are based on four principles:

1. Autonomy (i.e. rights of patients to choose or refuse treatments)
2. Beneficence (i.e. clinicians must act in the best patient interest)
3. Non-maleficence (i.e. *primum, non nocere*—first of all, do not harm the patient)
4. Justice (i.e. all patients receive equal treatment—fairness and equality in treatment of patients)

Consent and confidentiality are all about personal autonomy of choosing what is good for an individual especially in matters of privacy related to health as disclosed to a medical professional (see Box 1.5.2).

Box 1.5.2: Ethics and law
Ethics and law have considerable overlap. But both share the common goal of creating and maintaining social good. • **Ethics** is more about expected conduct: *What ought to be?* It is the identification of values, which should be prevailing in society. • **Law** says: *What has to be?* Law has the following important functions: • It lays down the established rule for conduct, the violation of which creates criminal or civil liability. • It forces citizens to adhere to a minimum standard expected by society. • It gives expression to such values to remedy the wrong behavior of citizens, so that people can live in harmony. • It is an enforcing change agent that makes all citizens to adhere to the expected changing scenario of prevailing social values in an area. • It is usually law that catches up with prevalent social ills to be remedied.

CONSENT

Consent refers to the HCP agreeing to give information or advice or a warning to an adolescent, his/he natural parents, guardians and/or court who in turn agree with HCP. Such an agreement in legal parlance is 'consent' or 'risk bond'.

The importance of getting consent from the patient for delivering medical services by the HCP is a relatively new phenomenon of the 20th century (see Appendix 1-Table 1 and Table 2).

Appendix 1 - Table 1: Historical aspects of consent by patients
• The father of Western Medicine, Hippocrates (460 BC to 370 BC) provided a "paternalistic" concept that the physician would always provide what was in the best interest of the patient. Thus, the patient simply agreed to whatever the clinician suggested. • The revolutionary idea that patients had rights to agree or disagree with these recommendations was not considered in the United States until the 20th century. • Testimonies at the Post-World War II Nuremberg Trials (1945 and 1946) after atrocities committed by Nazi doctors established that doctors may not always have their patients' best interests in mind. • Legal cases and the Civil Rights Movement in the 20th century United States gradually established the rights of patients to consent (agree or disagree) with doctors' advice. • This pendulum of patients' rights has gradually swung to include that of adolescents as well in various situations.

HISTORY TAKING AND CLINICAL EXAMINATION

Before you begin taking history and doing a medical examination of an adolescent, it is important to take

Appendix 1-Table 2: Different nomenclatures of consent
Informed consent is also known as: • Risk bond • Assent • Dissent • Forewarning • Refusal to follow health care provider's (HCP's) advice
Consent for Adolescents Without Known Guardians • **Court Permission:** Adolescents whose parents/guardians are not known, e.g. street adolescent/child is brought sick needing medical/surgical attention, then HCP needs legal permission from court for medical interventions. The legal rule is that law court of appropriate jurisdiction is the designated guardian of such children under Guardians and Wards Act, 1890. Police or HCP needs to apply permission to court as per prescribed procedure. Usually court gives very specific permission and not a blanket permission for medical interventions for such adolescent.
Parental and Police Autonomy • Indian cultural history is very much endorsed by legal philosophy that parents essentially had complete autonomy over their children. Even today we are in "era of parental autonomy" where children are expected to obey parents and are punished by parents or other law enforcers such as the police if disobedience occurred.
Prevention of Litigation • In most of the cases filed against the medical professional it is alleged that no consent was obtained. • Obtaining of consent will thus be a cornerstone of protection against litigation.
Types of Consent Depending upon the circumstances in each case consent may be implied, express or informed. • **Implied Consent (Tacit Consent):** This is by far the most common variety of consent in both general practice and hospital practice. The fact that a patient comes to a medical professional for an ailment implies that he/she is agreeable to medical examination in the general sense. This, however, does not imply consent to procedures more complex than inspection, palpation, percussion, auscultation and routine sonography. For other examinations, notably rectal and vaginal and withdrawal of blood for diagnostic purpose, express consent (oral or written) should be obtained. For more complicated diagnostic procedures, e.g., lumbar puncture, radiology, endoscopy, CT scan, etc. express written consent should be obtained. • **Express Consent:** Anything other than the implied consent is express consent. This may be either oral or written. Express oral consent is obtained for relatively minor examinations or therapeutic procedures, preferably in the presence of a disinterested third party. Express written consent is to be obtained for: (i) all major diagnostic procedures, (ii) general anesthesia, (iii) for surgical operations, (iv) intimate examinations, (v) examination for determining age, potency and virginity, and in medico-legal cases. • **Informed Consent:** The concept of informed consent has come to the fore in recent years and many actions have been brought by patients who alleged that they did not understand the nature of the medical procedure to which they gave consent. All information must be explained in comprehensible non-medical terms preferably in local language about the (a) diagnosis, (b) nature of treatment, (c) risks involved, (d) prospects of success, (e) prognosis if the procedure is not performed, and (f) alternative methods of treatment. The physician's duty to disclosure is subject to the exceptions: (a) if the patient prefers not be informed and (b) if the medical professional believes in the exercise of coming to a sound medical judgement, that the patient is so disturbed or anxious that the information provided would not be processed rationally or that it would probably cause significant psychological harm. This is known as *Therapeutic Privilege*. In such a case it is advisable that the medical professional should consult the patient's family physician. Revelation of risk is always a compromise between reasonable information and the danger of frightening off the patient from beneficial treatment. The three important components of such consent are information, voluntariness and capacity. • **Proxy Consent (Substitute Consent):** All the above types of consent can take the shape of Proxy Consent e.g. parents for child, close relative for mentally unsound/unconscious patient, etc.

permission from both the parents/guardians and the adolescents themselves, in order to be safe and to prevent medico-legal problems.

The Adolescent Mind and Maturity

As youth traverses from childhood to adulthood, they reach a stage at which they can be considered competent enough to understand and agree to various treatment options. For the adolescent, this is a period of an intriguing mixture of vulnerability for many reasons. There are changes in the adolescent body that make the adolescent respond, behave and think like an 'adult'. Yet the 'mind' and the 'heart' are sensitive like that of a 'child'. For an Indian adolescent, this is a situation with conflict, since words such as 'child' as well 'adult' have strong roots in cultural connotations. It is believed that the body of adolescent has a 'child' inside.

The family sees the adolescent person as a prospective family member who will earn greater wealth, give better security and bring honor to family in future. The child is seen as a gift of God, but in Indian hierarchical fabric of society, adolescent's place is probably at its bottom. Advancing age in India is believed to be associated with increase in wisdom and power that befits respect as needed to be given to adolescent. Biological changes are markers and predictors of future human behavior; e.g. puberty means that the age for marriage is not very far away especially for a young pubescent girl in India.

The HCP must be aware of the various definitions of the law of the land regarding consent and confidentiality. It is good to be aware of the various forms of consents (see Box 1.5.3).

Consent or series of consents are required for treating sick and serious adolescents which is a continuous process as described below:

- HCP daily takes stock of medical situation/information on a continuous basis from adolescent patients guiding HCP to do relevant physical examination and if needed appropriate investigations.
- Based on a working diagnosis, HCP advices single or

Box 1.5.3: Various aspects of consent in adolescents
Medical informed consent Informed consent law developed from the intentional tort of battery, which protects the individual from an unwanted physical touching of the body by one having neither express nor implied consent of the person touched nor a privilege to do so.
Proxy consent To treat a minor without appropriate parental consent, usually shall be construed "assault and battery" as per prevailing • Legal philosophy. • Customs and usage of common law and tradition.
Informed Consent (for minors and parents) in India Any person who has completed 18 years of age as per Indian Majority Act–1975 is considered an adult. All adolescents on completion of 18 years are capable of giving consent, if otherwise there are no legal impediments.
Invalid consent • Consent is invalid if the adolescent is less than 18 years. • The adolescent below 18 years needs parental consent for medical treatment even at the cost of jeopardizing confidentiality. • Consent is given under fear, fraud or misrepresentation of facts, or by a person who is ignorant of the implications of the consent even if the person is above 18 years.
Consent of adolescent usually arrogates with confidentiality • Consent and confidentiality of medical treatment is a legally far-fetched dream in India. But at the same time parents and authorized adult relatives cannot arrogate with adolescent rights. • Legally, emancipated adolescent is given preference over parental wish in seeking medical treatment depending upon the facts and circumstances of the case brought before judiciary for interpretation and discretion; but are full of hassles.
Parental wishes over adolescent's consent • In general, in India parents pay for medical bills; hence the wishes of parents prevail over adolescent. • If adolescent is insured for medical treatment, an emancipated or liberated adolescent's wish may have a say over parental say in medical treatment.
Warning to HCP for overstepping authority of consent • Since all these fall in the grey area of interpretation and the use of their discretion, HCPs are warned that they are undertaking legal risks if the situation is not life-saving if they do not obtain consent. • Usually in emergency life-saving situations, HCP is at liberty to go ahead with medical treatment to save life and limb of a patient without consent.

multiple surgeries, drugs and/or non-drug treatment as per the situation for betterment.

- Each further evaluation of provisional diagnosis and/or monitoring of disease may need separate fresh consent.
- While this is being done medical professionals in tandem advise investigations to evaluate recovery or worsening of disease, to warn about side effects, adverse effects and complications of drug and/or non-drug and/or surgical treatment.

All these algorithmic exercises of monitoring are done by medical professionals to reduce health risks from disease/drugs and surgery continuously; thus consent is not one point activity; it could be a continuous process requiring oral, written, proxy consent or court order depending on facts and circumstances.

In a sick and serious adolescent, a number of times consent, re-consent, fresh consent and high risk consent are required. In other patients, permission to do medical termination of pregnancy (MTP)/abortion, to continue sequential multi-stage surgical treatment and to continue or discontinue life support as well as permission for research is required.

The HCP also needs to be aware of these issues when ordering investigations and giving treatment and also about issues of consent in special situations (see Box 1.5.4).

Box 1.5.4: Consent in special situations

Situations where consent may not be obtained:

- In medical life-saving emergencies, the well-being of the patient is of paramount importance; hence medical treatment precedes legal considerations.

Situations requiring extra caution:

- Medical professional should keep in mind certain high-risk situations, which are common causes for medical negligence actions.
- Situations that require extra caution are surgical treatment related to eye, ear spinal cord and brain.

CONFIDENTIALITY

Confidentiality takes patient's rights in a further direction and forces the clinician to consider the potential need of patients to provide information about their condition and consent for their treatment without others being involved.

Issues of Confidentiality in Adolescents

- Can HCPs give assurance to the adolescent that without his/her permission they will not divulge to their parent/s, certain issues of their health that involve them, their actions and their behaviors?
- Who is the patient—the adolescent? The parent? Whose rights does the clinician follow in this delicate clinical dance?
- Do the parents have the right to know whether their adolescent is homosexual, has a sexually transmitted disease, is suicidal or homicidal, has a substance use disorder, is receiving an abortion, or other issues considered by the patient to be so private that s/he does not want the parent to know these issues?
- Does the clinician not tell the parents and find out any important clinical information or inform parents with the risk of teen refusal to provide clinical data or failure to accept needed treatment?

It may be easier as well as more profitable for some clinicians to simply work with the parents and deal with the adolescent in a secondary manner. However, this increases morbidity and mortality for many youth.

The parents may win this battle, but adolescent may lose valuable health. Ideally parents can trust another adult (i.e. a clinician who provides confidentiality) to provide the best health care for their adolescent who demands confidentiality.

If the clinician tells parents about such sensitive concerns, the youth may lose confidence in this clinician and not tell him/her vital health information in the future, even if it results in complications, such as unwanted pregnancy from being sexually active without use of contraception or pelvic inflammatory disease from failure to screen for and find cervical *Chlamydia trachomatis*.

Like any adolescent in the world, the Indian adolescent also wants to be assured of confidentiality (see Box 1.5.5).

Box 1.5.5: What Indian adolescents may want to keep secret?

- Adolescents in India want to keep secret about sexual activity, venereal diseases, pregnancy, abortion and contraception.
- Adolescents do not want these matters to be disclosed to parents and family members.
- The disclosure of such personal health information by doctor in the above matters has the potential to be embarrassing, stigmatizing or discriminatory to adolescent.
- Hence many adolescents may prefer going to a quack who can assure them of confidentiality without disclosing to their parents, which results in adverse effects on their health with substandard medical care.

APPROACH FOR APPROPRIATE USE OF CONSENT AND CONFIDENTIALITY

History Taking

Legal aspects and the protocols for consent and confidentiality for adolescents vary from country to country and a clinician needs to be well versed with them. In adolescent clinical practice the approach will also be different depending upon the age of the adolescent: early middle or late adolescence. The changes in adolescence can result in a number of complexities in adolescent health care depending on their age, maturity, thinking skills, circumstances in life, local or national laws, and other factors.

- *Young or early adolescents (10-13 years of age)* are leaving childhood, entering puberty with preoccupation for body changes, and continuing sexuality processes. They typically are still dependent on parents for medical information and consent for care.
- **Middle adolescents (14-16 years of age),* usually accept their more adult-like secondary sexual characteristics, with more advance thinking skills (i.e. more formal versus concrete thinking), choosing peers over parents, engaging in sexual activity of various types, and typically want health care provided in a confidential manner that involves their (not their parents) consent in such issues as sexuality and mental health.
- *Late adolescents (17-19 years of age)* are physically mature, have more adult-like thinking skills, are more able to make decisions as adults, and demand confidentiality from providers. Their journey, however, is not complete, as their adult brains are established with development of a mature prefrontal cortex at some point in their 20s.

(*Most states in the USA note a minor is someone under 18 years of age while a few states list 19 as the age of majority. In India when one has completed 18 years age, s/he is considered as a major legally, except when court appoints a guardian, in which case age for majority shifts to 21 as per the Guardians and Wards Act, 1890.)

If an adolescent is seen and treated without the parent's knowledge, it can place the HCP in a delicate balance between dealing with the needs/wishes of adolescents versus the needs/wishes of their parents (guardians). Treatment of a minor without parent's consent may lead to a legal charge of 'assault and battery'.

In the USA, age of legal consent is defined by state law which can vary from state to state. This can complicate a variety of health care dilemmas such as ethical and policy issues seen in genetic testing of adolescents or over-riding an adolescent's decision against treatment of a medical condition (Health Record Privacy; US Health Insurance Portability and Accountability Act, HIPAA—see Appendix 1-Table 3).

The various laws in India and medicolegal aspects while doing general or medical super-specialty practice which also encompasses adolescent clinical practice should be read by every clinician (see Appendix 1-Tables 4A to 4I).

Appendix 1 - Table 3: Health record privacy (US Health Insurance Portability and Accountability Act (HIPAA))

- Concern with privacy of medical records in the US lead to the 1996 passage of The Health Insurance Portability and Accountability Act (HIPAA) which established Federal rules both securing patient access to protected medical data as well as patient control on the disclosure of this medical information.
- It deals with competent adults and defers to state law with regard to securing privacy of medical records of adolescents. Some confidentiality protections are found in the HIPAA law and are called the "HIPAA Privacy Rule".
- If a state law allows teenagers to consent to confidential health care, then this is secure from parents and requires authorization of written as well as verbal information by the youth for release.
- State laws can over-ride this Federal mandate and thus details of confidential data release are dependent on where this adolescent lives.
- Minors' rights for confidentiality in the US have also received some protection from the 1974 Federal FERPA (Family Educational Rights and Privacy Act) which was amended in 1994 in the Improving America's School Act (IASA).

Appendix 1 - Table 4A: Informed consent means reasonable information be given

- Informed consent is the legal embodiment of the concept that each individual has the right to make decisions affecting his or her well-being.
- It is generally accepted that individuals should consider– that is, trade-off–the risks and potential benefits flowing from their decisions. To do so, decision-makers must have knowledge of those risks and potential benefits.
- The law protects the individual's right to give informed consent by requiring the disclosure of information by the party to whom consent is given.

Appendix 1 - Table 4B: Risks involved in treatment, surgery and natural course of disease if no treatment is undertaken

Risk may be defined as "exposure to a chance of an injury or loss". It embodies two distinct factors:

- Chance relates to uncertain events–those that are not predictable in any single case, but for which a probability that an event will occur in any one case may be estimated.
- Medical informed consent law requires the disclosure of the risks of and alternatives to suggested medical procedures to enable patients to make knowledgeable decisions about the course of their medical care.

Appendix 1 - Table 4C: Information about materiality of risk undertaken while handling disease of a patient

- The "materiality" says that the physician's duty to disclose risk information increases as the magnitude of the risk increases. Further, if risks are of severe consequences, e.g. of death or serious disability, is material and should be disclosed independent of the frequency.
- "Severe risks (e.g. death, paralysis, loss of eye sight, hearing and any other sense organ damage) should always be disclosed, even when the probability of occurrence is almost negligible.
- Less severe risks, which have a high incidence of occurrence, likewise should always be disclosed.
- Nominal risks with little likelihood of occurrence need not be disclosed.

  Last but not the least is:
- Though everyone recognizes that frequency of occurrence, as an important component of risk, yet severity of risk though rare cannot be ignored while disclosure to patient like loss of vision, hearing, sensation, limb, ovary, testes, motor function and similar loss.

Appendix 1 - Table 4D: Legal implications of risk disclosure and informed consent

- The obligation to disclose risk information increases with increasing severity of the potential consequences of complications of disease, drug or surgery.
- Consent cannot be substituted for carelessness or unskillfulness or rash action of medical professional legally speaking for any action for negligence. Consent is the basic document that speaks about medical professional's explanation of disease, procedure and risk told to patient. Of course one cannot impose acceptance of unskillfulness and carelessness and risks arising out of non-availability of prescribed standards for carrying out treatment or procedure or surgery.
- Low risks with trivial complications of disease, drug or operation needs no disclosure.
- Thus informed consent is becoming a recognized basis for physician liability; the courts reasoned that any consent based on inadequate information was vitiated by the failure of the physician to disclose.
- Lack of informed consent is considered a matter of negligence of the physician to disclose necessary information to patients rather than battery.

Appendix 1 - Table 4E: Consent should address four elements of negligence to clear HCP from liability as below

Negligence requires that four elements be established for liability of the defendant:

1. A duty of defendant to meet a particular standard of care be explained in consent;
2. Chances anticipated failures to perform that duty be explained in consent;
3. Consent should remove possibility of causal connection between defendant's failure and plaintiff's injury; and
4. Consent should explain injury in fact is due to complication of disease or surgery and not because of failure to act as per standard medical care.

Appendix 1 - Table 4F: Onus of proof of information in consent

In order to recover damages for that outcome, the plaintiff must establish the elements of negligence, that:

- The physician had a duty to disclose particular information to the patient; disclosure did not occur;
- But for the non-disclosure, the tendered procedure would have been refused, and that the tendered procedure was the cause in fact of plaintiff's injury; and
- The plaintiff suffered an injury which can be compensated in terms of money.

Appendix 1 - Table 4G: Disclosure of information to TPA and mediclaim

In India for mediclaim, patient party receives personally, all information from doctor and submits to insurer or "under third party administrator [TPA] contracts" of insurer. Under cashless schemes doctor obtains specific prior consent to medical disclose information to TPA/insurer for clearing cashless claims.

Appendix 1 - Table 4H: Standards of disclosure in consent

There are two dominant approaches to defining the standard of disclosure of information by which the physician's duty to their patients is measured.

- One is to follow the "professional standard", or peer "accepted risks" requiring a physician to disclose information that other physicians possessed of the same skills and practising in the same or a similar community would disclose in the same situation.
- Second is to follow "materiality" or "prudent patient" approach.

Appendix 1 - Table 4I: When non-disclosure is excused in consent

- The courts recognize situations where a physician's nondisclosure will be excused.
- When, if a patient is incompetent to make a reasoned decision, then disclosure to the patient may not be required.
- Under the therapeutic privilege, the physician may withhold information if disclosure would be upsetting or otherwise would interfere with treatment or adversely affect the condition or recovery of the patient.
- Finally, the emergency exception applies in situations where attempting to secure consent could detrimentally delay proper treatment.
- Generally, physicians need not disclose risks of which the patient is already aware or risks that are commonly known.

Research suggests that different brain circuitry is involved when youth are involved in emotional, high risk behavior ('hot cognition') versus cognition in low emotional issues ('cold cognition').

- Does the adolescent have the mental capacity to consider effects of alternative treatments?
- Is s/he free of coercions?

In health care one seeks to identify which youth are legally able to function as adults in health care settings and which ones are not. Hence it is important to understand the concept of emancipated and mature minor (see Table 1.5.1 and Box 1.5.6).

Table 1.5.1: USA scenario–The emancipated vs. Mature minor

Term	*Comments*
Competence	It is a legal term in US law and is set at the age of majority which is 18 years in most states.
Capacity	General term: Ability of a person to make various decisions.
Emancipated youth	Emancipated youth is generally regarded as one who is married, is a parent, in the military, or living independently away from home and with his/her own income. S/he may be allowed to provide consent to treatment as well as be given confidential treatment that does not involve parent's knowledge without the permission of the youth.
'Mature minor'	This is a doctrine developed in the late 20th century. It notes that a youth is at or over 14 years of age, is capable of informed consent, and receives treatment that is for the minor's benefit and receives what is regarded as 'standard' care. Though this is not a legal term in the USA law, the medical term would allow the clinician to assess and treat some youth in a confidential manner if the clinician felt this was in the best interest of the competent adolescent patient. The clinician assesses the maturity of this patient and if s/he understands the clinician's explanations.
Judicial bypass—'mature minor'	Minors may utilize a process called obtaining a judicial bypass which involves getting a judge's permission for seeking confidential care apart from the parents if the youth ruled as a 'mature minor'. The level of developmental maturity has become the cornerstone of this mature minor doctrine that has withstood a number of court challenges in the USA. The US Supreme Court ruled in 1990 that a judicial bypass is needed for states where parental notification or consent is needed.
Services that can be utilized by a minor	A youth ('minor') may be treated for emergency care if either the parents are not available to provide consent or the clinician feels that confidential care is best as s/he evaluates/treats a youth for sexually transmitted infections (STIs), diagnoses pregnancy, or treats a youth for a substance use disorder. Laws vary from state to state in such issues as dealing with contraception, HIV testing/care, contraception and abortion.

Box 1.5.6: Evolving mature–minor concept in India: Circumscribed to sexual acts

- The age of consent is the age at which a person is considered to be legally competent to consent to sexual acts, and is thus the minimum age of a person with whom another person is legally permitted to engage in sexual activity. Legally, per se, person below the minimum age engaged in sexual activity is regarded as the victim, and older sex partner as the offender. But time and again this legal assumption is proven wrong. Age controversy was at zenith when in Delhi gang rape case of December 2012, one of the offenders was a minor.
- It was debated that real test of age in any crime should not depend on some arbitrary age limit set by Juvenile Justice Act. Real test of age depends upon mental maturity—whether the offender is mentally mature to understand the heinousness of the crime (irrespective of age).
- In India mature minor concept was invoked in cases of rape, but was declined by Supreme Court. Hence the Juvenile Justice (Care and Protection of Children) Bill, 2014 was amended to give powers to the Juvenile Justice Board to decide if a juvenile above 16 years, involved in heinous crimes like rape, would be tried in an adult court.

REPRODUCTIVE AND SEXUAL HEALTH ISSUES: PROVIDING SERVICES FOR ADOLESCENT SEXUAL AND REPRODUCTIVE HEALTH (ARSH)

1. Contraception

Issues of adolescent sexuality have created legal and ethical complexities for clinicians in all countries. The right to fertility and when to have children without the intrusion of members of society has been debated for years (see Box 1.5.7).

2. Rape, Incest, Sexual Abuse

In USA, adolescents may consent to treatment for rape, incest, and sexual abuse; in acute situations, additional rules apply to the emergency care of patients. Physicians may be required to notify parents in such cases unless the parent is considered as the perpetrator. The minor should agree to be examined as well as treated and informed of available services such as management of STDs, pregnancy, or psychiatric care. Some states insist that the youth be of a certain age or be classified as a mature minor.

Box 1.5.7: Contraception

Indian Scenario

- There is no law to enforce the HCP to inform or seek parental consent for prescribing contraceptives to adolescent.
- Generally adolescents are hesitant in seeking contraceptives from HCP known to family. This sometimes forces them to seek advice of quacks.
- India has no specific statute governing or controlling the manufacture, advertisement and sale of contraceptives in an exclusive manner. A comprehensive legislation in the field of contraceptives is the need of the hour.
- As per government policy all contraceptive services are also provided through medical and paramedical staff free of charge in all government primary health centers (PHC), community health centers (CHC), rural family welfare centers and district hospitals throughout the country.
- Under the free distribution scheme, condoms under the brand name 'Nirodh' are made available. This scheme also meets the requirements of condoms by states/union territories under the STD/AIDS control program. The scheme of social marketing of oral pills was launched in 1987. The brand name 'Mala D' is given to the product under social marketing program.

USA Scenario

- In 1970 the US Congress passed Title X of the Public Health Service Act which provided for national family planning services. The right of minors to seek sexuality-related health care has been acknowledged.
- Various challenges have arisen, but in general, sexually active adolescents have access to contraceptive services without the need to either notify parents or get parent's permission to obtain contraception.
- Many adolescents will not accept contraception if parental notification/consent is part of the prescription process.
- In some states physicians who find emergency contraception (EC) morally objectionable, may opt to refuse to inform about as well as provide ECs to adolescents and also refuse to refer the patient to other willing health care providers.
- Adolescent health care can provide conflicts in ethics, morality, duties as a physician, and the law for providers.
- Preservation of adolescent fertility has become complicated by technical advances of medicine in the 20th and 21st century.

Box 1.5.8: Adolescent and criminal liability

According to criminal law under Indian Penal Code, Section 82 considers that the child up to 12 years is not capable of committing an offence.

Section 83 says nothing is an offence which is done by a child who has not attained sufficient maturity of understanding to judge the nature and consequence of his/her conduct on that occasion.

Thus there is total immunity from criminal responsibility up to the age of 7 years.

From 7 to 12 years, the liability depends upon the capacity of understanding of the child.

From 12 to 18 years, though the liability is not conditional, the Juvenile Justice Act provides for care and protection of the rights of child in conflict with law, and certain special procedure and forum was created to judge the criminality with concern for all social circumstances which might have compelled or influenced to commit crime.

Rape by Adolescent

Age of consent for sexual acts: Section 375 Indian Penal Code, 1860 considers age of 16 years as the right age of consent to decide the criminality of the offence of rape.

In the case of marriage, sex with a female of 16 years or younger is considered rape under Section 375 except in the State of Manipur where this age is 14 years.

In India rape has defined in Indian Penal Code (IPC),1860. Section 375 of IPC considers age of 16 years as the right age of consent to decide the criminality of the offence of rape. In the case of marriage, sex with a female of 16 years or younger is considered rape under Section 375 except in the state of Manipur where this age is 14. Rape is an offence under Sections 375 and 376 of IPC, 1860 (see Box 1.5.8).

If an adolescent comes to HCP telling s/he was raped or sexual molestation has occurred, the HCP should inform the police. Only the medical report in 'SAFE' format and the treatment report should be submitted to the police. Failure to report may lead to the HCP being hauled up for keeping confidentiality as hiding the crime of rape or sexual molestation under POCSO (please see Chapters 4.6 and 4.7) and also under Sections 120A, 201, 212, 375, 376 of IPC, 1860 and if pregnant and secured abortion under Sections 312 to 315 of IPC and Section 156 of Criminal Procedure Code by the police.

3. Pregnancy and Abortion

USA Scenario

A minor may seek pregnancy diagnosis without parent's consent and then chooses to keep the baby, give the baby up for adoption, or get an abortion. Federal law has supported the confidentiality and consent questions for pregnancy-related care for minors. Once this minor becomes a parent, she is in charge of all decisions for her child. Placing the consent for procedures and other decisions for babies in the neonatal intensive care unit (NICU) in the hands of a young teen mother can be troubling to many in society.

The rights of a minor to seek an abortion without parental notification or consent remains a focal point of bitter controversy in the USA, as does the right of any female to seek an abortion. The landmark case, Roe v Wade in 1972, noted that seeking an abortion was between the physician and the female and not subject to government intervention. The USA Supreme Court has also allowed a minor to seek an abortion without parental notification or consent. However, it remains under intense argument in various states and no let-up in this battle is likely in American politics. Most states now require notification of at least one parent with two-thirds requiring parental consent and one-third notification, but not consent. A minor may be able to obtain a judge's order (judicial bypass) to avoid parental involvement. A minor can also refuse an abortion that is wanted by her parents.

Indian Scenario

If an adolescent girl becomes pregnant and seeks advice of HCP for termination of pregnancy, it is allowed under the MTP Act, 1971 which allows termination of pregnancy in adolescent. However consent in Form 'C' of MTP requires that the adolescent has to be a major person i.e. 18 years or above, otherwise the consent is invalid. As a minor she must take father/mother for MTP for consent to be legally valid. Though marriage under the age of 18 years is prohibited by law, in the rural India child marriages still take place and when an adolescent pregnancy occurs in wedlock the husband can give permission for MTP for his wife.

Social Scenario of Pregnancy in Unmarried Adolescent Girls in India

Being an unwed mother is still a social taboo especially in rural India. In India due to the fear of society and parents, an unmarried pregnant adolescent does not disclose to anyone about the pregnancy till the abdominal bulge become obvious which is often beyond 20 weeks which is the upper limit of the MTP Act. Unwed pregnant adolescent may also commit suicide to save family honor or sometimes they can be murdered by the family as 'honor killing'.

If delivery is conducted, there can be infanticide or dumping of the baby by roadside or in a temple, church or outside an orphanage. Though there are provisions for foster care and adoption, for fear of societal image babies are often abandoned. If the delivery is conducted in the hospital, the baby may be given for adoption on condition of anonymity or abandoned and mother runs away without formal discharge.

Risks for HCP When a Patient Lies About Her Age and Gets MTP Done in India

A pregnant unmarried adolescent minor often resorts to various measures to get an MTP done as an adult. She feigns to be married wearing *mangal sutra* (an auspicious and visible neck wear signaling that the woman is married) and indirectly declares that she is major. Many a time adolescent comes to HCP with an assumed name and boyfriend pretends to be her husband. For MTP, medical professional cannot insist upon proof of date of birth and marriage certificate to pin the lie told by the adolescent. At a later time, after lapse of months and years, say if parents or she herself wants to file a case FIR for rape (since as per legal definition of rape under Section 375 of IPC, 1860, this is a fit case to be registered with police station for rape) against boyfriend, the police will try to contact the HCP for finding out who signed the consent and if the girl has signed then whether the consent is automatically invalid (e.g. girl being minor or less than 18 years as per Indian law). The medical professional will be in trouble for hiding the criminal act of rape and performing abortion without a legally valid consent. The medical professional has to defend till the case goes on in an Indian court. Hence an obstetrician has to be extremely careful while performing MTP in unmarried minor adolescents. Unfortunately this legal situation leads to adolescents seeking the services of quacks who do not follow the law.

4. Sterilization

USA Scenario

In USA, sterilization is permitted only with the person's fully informed and voluntary consent. Considerable controversy exists with the sterilization of a minor who has intellectual disability and parents would need to obtain a court order for such a procedure. Most states allow a female 18 years or older to undergo voluntary sterilization.

Indian Scenario

In India, there is no clear law on sterilization. Government guidelines state that 'no person is to be sterilized unless: she/he has attained the age of 35 years, is married and the consent of both the partners has been obtained for such operation'. The operating doctor is further obliged to explain the nature of operation for sterilization which gives permanent sterility.

Adolescents do not come forward for sterilization operations in India. In a mentally challenged female adolescent, both parents should sign consent for sterilization. If either of parents disagrees then court order is required. Parents of mentally challenged male adolescent rarely opt for sterilization in India.

5. Sexually Transmitted Diseases (including HIV)

USA Scenario

Currently it is legal in all 50 states in USA for a minor to seek treatment for a sexually transmitted disease (sexually transmitted infection) without parental consent; some states require that the minor must be at least 12 or 14 years of age for privileges of consent. In some states, the treating physician can contact the parents if s/he feels this is necessary. Laws regarding HIV/AIDS remain under review and minors not given guarantees of confidentiality may not seek care for this condition. One state requires parental notification for a positive HIV test.

Indian Scenario

HIV/AIDS is not a notifiable disease in India. STD and HIV are associated with a lot of social stigmatization in India. Pre- and post-counseling for HIV test is mandatory in India. A positive test result can lead to immense psychosocial trauma to the extent of suicide. HIV testing in an adolescent <18 years cannot be done without the written consent of parents or guardians.

EMERGENCY TREATMENT

Physicians can evaluate and treat minors of all ages without parental consent if necessary when an emergency has been declared because of endangerment 'to life or limb', and delaying treatment (i.e., to find and/or notify parents) would be harmful to the minor. Some treatment facilities may require another person to act in *loco parentis* and provide consent for the treatment. Careful documentation of the emergency situation is necessary and the parents (guardians) notified as soon as possible. Mature minors may seek confidential emergency treatment, in general, for mental health conditions, drug and alcohol addiction, pregnancy-related conditions, contraception and STDs.

India does not have 'Good Samaritan' doctor (emergency treatment) legislation. Supreme Court of India said all medical emergencies be attended to save life of patients. Hospitals can be now punished for turning away patients of medico-legal aspects and insisting on deposit of money or first registering complaint with the police.

LESBIAN, GAY, BISEXUAL AND TRANSGENDER (LGBT) ISSUES

For more details please see Chapter 4.2. Legal aspects related to LGBT in India are highlighted in Box 1.5.9.

Box 1.5.9: Legal and social situation for lesbian, gay, bisexual and transgender (LGBT) people in India

Hijras (Transgender)

- Legal recognition for Hijras (transgender) as a gender separate from men or women, making the country one of the few in the world to legally recognize a third gender.
- Hijras were legally granted voting rights as a third sex in 1994.
- Due to alleged legal ambiguity of the procedure, Indian transgender individuals do not have access to safe medical facilities.
- On 15 April 2014, Supreme Court of India declared transgender people as a socially and economically backward class entitled to reservations in education and jobs, and also directed Union and State governments to frame welfare schemes for them.
- On 24 April 2015, the Rajya Sabha passed The Rights of Transgender Persons Bill, 2014 guaranteeing rights and entitlements, reservations in education and jobs (2% reservation in government jobs), legal aid, pensions, unemployment allowances and skill development for transgender people.

Indian Law Regarding Same Sex Sexual Activity

- Homosexual intercourse was made a criminal offence under Section 377 of the Indian Penal Code, 1860. Sexual activity between two persons of the same sex is criminalized and is punishable by incarceration (jail).
- On January 28, 2014 Supreme Court dismissed the review petition filed by Central Government, the NGO Naz Foundation and several others, against its December 11 verdict on Section 377 of IPC.
- In explaining the ruling the bench said: "While reading down Section 377, the High Court overlooked that a minuscule fraction of the country's population constitutes lesbians, gays, bisexuals or transgender people, and in the more than 150 years past, less than 200 persons have been prosecuted for committing offence under Section 377, and this cannot be made a sound basis for declaring that Section ultra vires Articles 14, 15 and 21."

MENTAL HEALTH

Laws vary from country to country with regard to mental health services for adolescents. Some countries may allow youth to voluntarily commit themselves to a mental hospital; others only allow outpatient treatment and/or require parental consent. In many countries a parent may voluntarily commit their minor with or without the minor's consent, if such management is considered necessary. A competent adolescent may refuse treatment unless the physician concludes that an emergency condition exists.

If an adolescent expresses or confesses to HCP about suicidal ideation/tendency, then one must treat this as an emergency and counsel and refer to a psychiatrist. If the adolescent has attempted suicide, HCP must inform the police. *We are not law enforcers.* In India, an HCP may be hauled up for hiding crime of attempt of suicide or suicide under Sections 120A, 201, 212 and 306 of IPC and Section 156 of Criminal Procedure Code by the police.

SUBSTANCE ABUSE

Adolescents may consent to treatment for substance abuse assessment and management and in general, must consent to disclosure to parents. Drug testing of a youth at parent's request and without the knowledge of the youth places the clinician in a complex dilemma (see Appendix 1-Table 5).

For laws in USA and for the Narcotic Drugs and Psychotropic Substances (NDPS) Act in India (see Appendix 1-Table 6).

END-OF-LIFE DECISIONS

Rights of parents, physicians, and adolescents can clash in emotional ways when confronted with a dying young patient. The physician must walk a delicate balance between wishes of parents, the adolescent, and even the clinician him/herself! Advanced directives can be helpful in this manner as well as determining the developmental state of the patient. Parents can be assured that they remain loving parents even with the death of their beloved child and even when they allow increasing decision-making on the part of their child. Youth dying in a hospital setting may benefit from hospital committees that deal with ethical issues of end-of-life decisions. Youth do best with the support of strong family ties, active involvement in decision making, palliative care, and good communication with the involved health care professionals.

Can the youth refuse treatment? The not-yet an adult and not a child status of this adolescent can stress everyone involved as this complex dilemma unfolds. Meetings to allow ventilation of the hospital or clinic staff are also helpful. Refusal for treatment on the part of the youth and/ or parent(s) may require legal intervention to resolve. The refusal of a patient for treatment in end-of-life issues or other

Appendix 1 - Table 5: Legal aspects of substance abuse in adolescents in USA
• In USA the 1944 Federal Public Health Service Act mandated that drug and alcohol treatment records were confidential.
• Even if a state law allows disclosure of a minor's record to the parents, Federal law, in general, prevents this unless the minor's situation poses a threat to the minor or someone else, the threat is reduced by such disclosure, and/or the minor is unable to provide consent. However, the laws are complex and the physician may act according to specific interpretation of one's state law versus the Federal law.
• It remains an area in flux in American law and health care for minors. Many states currently permit but do not require parental notification.
• If the youth and parents disagree about treatment, some states seem to side with the youth and others with the parents.

Appendix 1 - Table 6: NDPS (Narcotic Drugs and Psychotropic Substances) Act in India
• Article 47 of the Constitution of India which mandates that the 'State shall endeavor to bring about prohibition of the consumption except for medicinal purposes of intoxicating drinks and of drugs which are injurious to health'. Thus the same principle of preventing use of drugs except for medicinal use was also adopted in framing The Narcotic Drugs and Psychotropic Substances (NDPS) Act, 1985 (NDPS Act).
• The Governments' policy has thus been to promote their use for medical and scientific purposes while preventing their diversion from licit sources, and prohibiting illicit traffic and abuse. Unlike the earlier Opium Act and the Dangerous Drugs Act which it replaced, the NDPS Act has given the power of enforcement to various central and state law enforcement agencies. Not only consumption, but also possession and sale is non-bailable cognizable and non-compoundable offence under NDPS. If HCP has knowledge, should report otherwise under sections 201 and 202 of Indian Penal Code may be hauled up by NDPS authorities and police.
• Alcohol abuse producing alcohol dependence and it is not under NDPS. But the fact is in spite of NDPS Act, India's location close to the major poppy growing areas of the world, in "Golden Crescent" on the Northwest and "Golden Triangle" on the North-East makes it vulnerable to substance abuse. Different kinds of drug abusage apart from opium products are prevalent like abuse of cannabis and its products, ephedra plant and its products–'Ecstasy' and 'Ice'. The substance abuse is seen in adolescents coming from diverse socio-economic, cultural, religious and linguistic backgrounds not restricted to any geographical area.
• Indian college students, disheartened by the cost ineffective Heroin and Ecstasy have chosen to switch over to crystal Meth (Methamphetamine), which can be easily manufactured from Ephedrine and Pseudoephedrine. Methamphetamine is the father of all substances of all drugs in the market.
• Now even latest substance abuse is seen of anesthetic agent Ketamine, which is not a banned drug but illegally abused as 'date-rape drug'.
• With all legal provisions in place still adolescent/teenagers and young adults must be counseled and taught the ill-effects of drugs by HCP because it is observed that such drug abuse topics are avoided in Indian households, either due to the unwillingness of parents to discuss such issues, or due to ignorance. In most cases, parents live in denial, in spite of knowing that their adolescent/ teenagers are in fully exposed to substance abuse culture existing in India.

aspects of health care must be placed into the context of this specific situation, the developmental status of the minor, and the nuances of the specific state law(s) that are involved.

For Indian laws for end of life decision please refer to Appendix1-Table 7. For more details on palliative care, see Chapter 7.5.

Appendix 1 - Table 7: End-of-life decision–Legal aspects in India

- In India active or passive euthanasia is illegal. In India end-of-life decision/situation [EOLD] are wrongly equated with active or passive euthanasia.
- In India there is no formal process of discussion and documentation of 'not for resuscitation'/donot resuscitate [DNR].
- The doctors are morally and ethically obliged to provide good prognostication and initiate discussions around treatment options, benefits of life prolonging treatment, and resuscitation as per the Indian Medical Council (Professional Conduct, Etiquette and Ethics) Regulations, 2002. Left against medical advice (LAMA) is a common situation seen in Indian setting where family unilaterally withdraws treatment due to social or financial constraints. The interpretation of Gian Kaur case disallows the concept of Euthanasia as it violates Article 21 of the Indian Constitution. Withholding and withdrawing life support amounts to abetment of suicide and abetment of suicide is a punishable offence according to Indian Penal Code.
- Self-determination of patients relating to medical decisions is not well articulated in Indian Constitution and often legal eagles hedge behind Article 21. Indeed the position of the law with respect to death in dignity is unclear, as Indian courts have only addressed appeals for Euthanasia.

RESEARCH AND ADOLESCENTS

Research is an important component to academic work and the field of adolescent medicine will benefit by continued research on youth. Youth are often been excluded from research trials in favor of adults for reasons of greater profit and to avoid sensitive areas implicated in research on adolescents. A balance is required between the need to protect the adolescent from harm done from research and the need for more knowledge in adolescent medicine. Many academic institutions have special Institutional Review Boards (IRBs) and Ethics Committees to establish guidelines for and monitor research on adolescents. Waiving of parental permission for research on their adolescent should be done only under special situations:

- When parental involvement would significantly interfere with the study's results.
- In pharmaceutical research trials when the trials are deemed as low risk and enhanced recruitment for the study is needed.

India has the potential to be the prospective place for trials for many large multinational pharmaceutical agencies for low-cost drug innovations along with economical skill base. There is a potential for providing simultaneous benefits of newly developed drugs to Indians as well. However the involvement of adolescents in these trials needs to be critically evaluated (see Appendix 1-Table 8).

Appendix 1 - Table 8: Research and adolescents in India

India was failing to implement a rigid and stricter vigilance mechanism on the Pharmaceutical Companies who conduct such clinical trial at the cost of the lives of some vulnerable and poor individuals who are not even aware that in our country there is existence of "right" to lead a safe and healthy life.

- The Drugs and Cosmetic Rules 1940 read with the rule122 and its subsections as amended up to 2013 guiding Schedule Y of the Drugs and Cosmetic Rules 1945 contains requirement and guidelines for clinical trials. This also provides for institutional ethics committee [IEC] clearance for each and every clinical medical research stressing on consent, confidentiality and safety. The research in India has to follow following:
  - Firstly legal document to follow research is, "an application for registration of clinical research organization shall be made to the said authority accompanied by the information as required under Schedule Y-1. The New Drug Regulatory Process and Schedule Y comes under the purview of the Drugs Controller General of India (DCGI), who is the head of the Central Drugs Standard Control Organization (CDSCO), located in New Delhi. DCGI and IEC approvals for initiating trial, investigator qualifications and site details, central laboratory details, protocol amendments. 2. Responsibilities of sponsors. 3. Responsibilities of investigators. 4. Informed consent process. 5. Responsibilities of Ethics Committee. 6. Definitions and objectives of different phases of trials (I, II, III and IV). Human pharmacology (Phase I), Therapeutic exploratory trial (Phase II), Therapeutic confirmatory trial (Phase III), Post-marketing trials (Phase IV). Hence to maintain uniformity in trial processes, Schedule Y provides formats of critical documents, e.g., informed consent documents, study reports, EC approvals, reporting of serious adverse events.
  - Second legal document to follow is, ICMR has published detailed "Ethical Guidelines for Biomedical Research on Human Subjects" in the year 2006.
  - Third legal document to be followed is, the Indian Medical Council (Professional Conduct, Etiquette and Ethics) Regulations, 2002 in para 7.22 Research: Clinical drug trials or other research involving patients or volunteers as per the guidelines of ICMR can be undertaken, provided ethical considerations are borne in mind. Violation of existing ICMR guidelines in this regard shall constitute misconduct. Consent taken from the patient for trial of drug or therapy which is not as per the guidelines shall also be construed as misconduct.

LEARNING POINTS

- A clinician working with adolescents will face some ethical dilemmas that can be complicated by legal standards.
- Confidentiality should be ethically considered and utilized as possible when providing health care services to adolescents as well as when conducting research on adolescents.
- Some youth can be identified as emancipated allowing them to make health care decisions on their own while keeping parents appropriately informed.
- Older adolescents may demand clear confidentiality or they may not provide critical information regarding their health care.
- Clinicians may be in a delicate balance or clinical dance between adolescents and parents (guardians). Indeed shared decision making is ideal in a triad between the adolescent patient, parent (guardian) and clinicians. However, complications arise based on the developmental changing process of adolescence as this person transitions from childhood to adulthood.
- Middle and late adolescents typically demand and need more autonomy from parents. This is especially the case for those youth who may be called 'emancipated'.
- As the adolescent becomes more mature, the shift of clinical focus and consent needs to be with the teen patient and not the parent.
- Limits can be set by law such as getting others involved for suicidal youth, homicidal youth, psychotic youth, sexually abused youth, and other dilemmas.
- Clinical judgment is needed along with respect for adolescent needs for autonomy, parents' rights, and the laws where one is practicing. This same respect is needed when involving youth in research protocols or end-of-life decisions.

SUGGESTED READING

1. American Academy of Family Physicians, American Academy of Pediatrics, American College of Obstetricians and Gynecologists, and Society for Adolescent Medicine. Protecting adolescents: Ensuring access to care and reporting sexual activity and abuse. J Adolesc Health 2004;35:420-23.
2. Baldwa M. Consent and confidentiality. In: Bhave SY, Parthasarathy A, Nair MKC, Menon PSN, editors. Bhave's Textbook of Adolescent Medicine, 1st Edition. New Delhi: Jaypee Brothers Medical Publishers (P) Ltd. 2006; 26-34.
3. Baldwa M. Consent and confidentiality in legal scenario of adolescence in India. In: Bhave SY (Ed.) Adolescent Practice: Case Scenarios and FAQs; 1st Edition. New Delhi: Byword Books Pvt Ltd 2011;1-11.
4. Baldwa M, Tiwari S, Tiwari M, Shah N (Eds.). Legal Problems in Day-to-Day Pediatric Practice; 2nd Edition. Hyderabad: Paras Medical Publishers; 2010.
5. Campbell AT. Consent, competence and confidentiality related to psychiatric conditions in adolescent medicine practice. Adolesc Med Clin 2006;17(1):25-47.
6. Campbell AT, English JD. Law, ethics and clinical discretion: Recurring and emerging issues in adolescent health care. Adolesc Med. 2011;22(2):321-34.
7. Committee on Pediatric Emergency Medicine and Committee on Bioethics. Consent for emergency medical services for children and adolescents. Pediatrics 2011;128(2):427-33.
8. Daley AM, Sadler LS, Reynolds HD. Tailoring clinical services to address the unique needs of adolescents from pregnancy test to parenthood. Curr Probl Pediatr Adolesc Health Care 2013;43(4):71-95.
9. Diekema DS. Adolescent refusal of lifesaving treatment: Are we asking the right questions? Adolesc Med 2011;22(2):213-28.
10. Jones RK, Purcell A, Singh S, Finer LB. Adolescents' report of parental knowledge of adolescents' use of sexual services and their reactions to mandated parental notification for prescription contraception. JAMA 2005;293:340-45.
11. Lyren A, Silber TJ. Consent, confidentiality, and other related issues in the care of adolescents: Medical, legal, ethical, and practical considerations. In: Greydanus DE, Patel DR, Pratt HD (Eds.). Essential Adolescent Medicine. New York: McGraw-Hill Medical Publishing Div 2005; 29-42.
12. Padvi N, Padvi A, Gupta V, Baldwa M (Eds.). Textbook of Paediatric Anaesthesia. New Delhi: CBS Publishers and Distributors Pvt Ltd. 2015; Chapters 42 & 43; 546-56.
13. Plantz D, Lantos JD. Conscience, clinical ethics, and emergency contraception. Adolesc Med 2011;22(2):175-82.
14. Tiwari S, Baldwa M,Tiwari M, Kuthe A (Eds.). Textbook on Medicolegal Issues – Related to Various Medical Specialties; 1st Edition. New Delhi: Jaypee Brothers Medical Publishers (P) Ltd; 2012.
15. Welisch E, Altamirano-Diaz LA. Ethics of pharmacological research involving adolescents. Paediatr Drugs 2015;17(1): 55-59.

1.6

Handling Parents

Pramod Jog, Swati Y Bhave

INTRODUCTION

It is important while dealing with adolescent clients to ensure that they are assured of confidentiality and privacy. When the adolescents are legally minors and the parents are paying for the consultation they will insist on knowing everything about what you are discussing with the adolescents. The adolescent pediatrician has to strike a balance between taking care of the adolescent rights vs the rights of the parents to know all about their minor adolescents. It is very important to be aware of the legal and ethical issues while taking care of adolescent patients for legal and ethical issues (see Chapter 1.5).

There are many reasons why parents would bring their teen to the adolescent clinic (Box 1.6.1).

Bringing up an adolescent is quite a stress for parents. One can visualize a hormonal storm. The adolescent's hormones are surging up and the parents' hormones are going down due to menopause and andropause. This leads to mood swings in parents too. The parents are also going through midlife crisis on different fronts such as health, career, relationships etc. Their physical stamina as well as mental tolerance are reduced. Admonishing the parents and putting all the blame on them will only make them feel very guilty. At the same time, parents have to be told firmly to disregard some of the harmless issues of their children and pick their battles carefully. Otherwise, it is a perpetual war between them.

Pediatricians are used to dealing with parents when they are dealing with young children and hence trained to deal with parents. Clinicians from other specialties have to learn how to handle parents of teens (Box 1.6.2). Even for an experienced pediatrician managing parents of teens is not easy. Clinicians have to be ready with various different reactions and attitudes of parents.

- Some parents are very fed up of what they feel is "abnormal behavior" of the teen and expect you to accept that they are doing everything right, it is their teen who is very problematic and he or she should be changed. They expect you to "side" with them and improve their teen. Such parents react with hostility to any suggestion that their parenting may be the cause of the problem and needs to be changed.
- Some parents who have been either very strict or very indulgent with their teens, blame each other or themselves for the teen behavior. They are in remorse and already burdened with guilt that they have been bad parents. Such parents need reassurance that all they need to do is understand the adolescent behavior and change their pattern without feeling bad about what has happened in the past.

Box 1.6.1: Reasons for parents of adolescents visiting a clinic for help
1. Awareness of adolescent clinics and availability of adolescent physicians.
2. Modern adolescence is more stormy, fast and difficult to handle.
3. Newer issues have emerged which parents never faced in their own teenage.
4. Increasing number of nuclear families: so advice and support from elders is missing.
5. Since there are only one or two children in the family, parents are more focussed on them. They keep an eye on them and want to direct them in every sphere of life.
6. Often school authorities refer them for low academic performance or disruptive behavior in school.
7. Other physicians refer them.
The adolescent consultant should be aware of the fact that the presenting complaint may not be the main issue; it may just be the tip of the iceberg. It could be any of the following:
1. The parents' perception and interpretation of the issue.
2. A physical manifestation of underlying psychological problem.
3. Adolescent's cry for help as they cannot express some of their problems with the parents and need some outside help.

Box 1.6.2: Essential prerequisites of an adolescent pediatrician
An adolescent physician has to work not only as a medical expert but also as a well-wisher and confidant for the family.
Non-judgmental attitude: Reacting instead of responding, giving instant opinions should be avoided. Our own previous experiences and value systems sometimes prompt us to do this.
Knowledge about current local and global adolescent scenario: Globalization is changing the norms for adolescents very fast. If the physician has adequate knowledge, it will help her/him to educate the parents regarding acceptable and unacceptable behavior, as well as reasonable and unreasonable expectations of parents.
Empathetic yet assertive attitude: Have empathy for both parents and adolescents and make them understand each other.

- Some parents are very perplexed about what is happening to their teen and genuinely not able to comprehend what is going wrong and want to understand how to deal with the situation. Such parents respond well to the clinician explaining to them the normal psychosocial changes in adolescence and more amenable to tips on parenting.

HISTORY TAKING

The first session with parents can last for 40 to 45 minutes. An anxious adolescent in the waiting room can become bored or agitated and restless in the meantime. So, the first session should preferably be only with the parents. But if the adolescent has accompanied the parents it is a good idea to give the adolescent the HEEADSSS questionnaire to fill up which can take 30-45 minutes (see Chapter 1.3).

The first questions to the parents:

1. What is the main concern that has brought them to the clinic?
2. What are their expectations from the clinician?
3. What have they done till now to address the problems?

The HEEADSSS format of history taking can also be used with the parents as well as adolescents.

Most parents when they come to the clinic are quite distraught about the "problematic behavior" of their teen. Most often it is not the "problematic behavior" of the adolescent but their inability to understand the normal developmental milestones of early middle and late adolescence.

The first job after a good history taking is to analyze which behavior is within the normal range and which is definitely abnormal and needs analysis and management.

If the behavior is within the range of "normalcy" the parents need to be educated about the normal milestones and reassured that the problem is not serious and they should be given guidance and tips of parenting to handle the situation.

The adolescent should also be explained how his or her behavior though in the range of normalcy is leading to problems and counseling done to improve their communication with parents and make efforts to resolve the issue with negotiation. One major role which we have to play is to improve the understanding and communication between our adolescent clients and their parents.

MANAGEMENT

Though majority of the problems of the teens are due to problems of parenting, the physician has to be very careful not to appear accusing or blaming the parents as this will make them defensive as they will look at it as failure of their parenting and no one likes to be blamed. Hence one has to be very diplomatic in handling the situation and giving tips for parenting.

Education, Awareness, Preventive Counseling and Anticipatory Guidance

Generally, parents wake up only when a problem such as academic failure, falling in love or addiction occurs. This can be prevented by creating awareness among all stake holders such as adolescents, parents, school authorities and society in general about important adolescent issues. We will consider only the parents here. School parent-teacher meeting is a chance to interact with a large number of parents with similar concerns.

The following important points for wellbeing of an adolescent should be emphasized to all parents:

1. *Importance of good diet, adequate sleep and exercise:* Parents need to be educated about the importance of healthy diet and exercise. If adequate calories, proteins and vitamins are not given it will have a long term adverse effect on health. Whatever the academic pressure adequate physical exercise must be given priority. The effect of lack of exercise and sedentary lifestyle and onset of lifestyle disorders like obesity, diabetes type 2 and hypertension must be adequately explained. They should monitor the sleep pattern and look for signs of sleep deprivation.
2. *Flag signs of serious problems in adolescence:* Parents should be educated and warned about serious mental

issues like substance abuse, depression and suicide ideation. Timely medical help will prevent from the problem escalating. They also should be able to detect problems that can get their adolescent in conflict with law, e.g., underage and driving after drinking, using narcotics, conduct disorders and juvenile delinquency and not be in denial but get timely help.

3. *Communication:* Though quite difficult, communication with the adolescents must be maintained. Most of the times, parents are either scolding them or advising them or asking them questions. Normal small talk, eye contact, listening when they talk, are all signs of good communication. Understanding their point of view, respecting them and accepting their opinions will encourage them to confide, discuss and take advice on problems troubling them.
4. *Don't compare your adolescence:* Most parents give examples and compare their own adolescence with their children. Actually, this is not fair in many aspects, as the world has changed since then. Computer, mobile phone and internet have made today's adolescent's life totally different. This has to be brought to parent's notice. Though ethics remain same in all generations, the moral values change in each generation and that has to be accepted.
5. *Do not compare your adolescent to any one:* Each adolescent is a unique individual. Constant comparis on with siblings, cousins, children of friends and neighbours has a negative impact on the emotions and they will become rebellious.
6. *Educate about neurodevelopment:* Parents also need to be made aware that just as their teen's body is changing, the brain is changing too. Educate parents about the various aspects of the developing brain in adolescents. Rebelliousness, abstract thinking, experimentation and self-centeredness are manifestations of the changing brain.
7. *Become role models:* Parents should become role models for the qualities they want the teens to learn and adapt. Parents need to be fit and happy themselves. They have to learn to enjoy their hobbies, friends and exercise.
8. *Sexuality education* is still a taboo in our society. The correct word to use is 'Family life education' (FLE). Adolescent pediatrician can create awareness among parents regarding giving sexuality education to adolescents so that they are more open to their teens being exposed to these programs in their schools. This education also needs to be given to the parents so that they can accept some of the adolescent issues as natural. Parents also can be given guidance how to initiate and use opportunities to discuss sexuality issues that come in print and media. Grabbing opportunities to initiate discussions about taboo subjects like sex, pornography, romantic relationships, drug addiction etc. assures the adolescent that I can talk to my parents about anything.

Guidance Should also be Given on Some Common Issues that Cause Conflict

1. Academic Issues

Not doing well in academics is one of the most common reasons of a teen being brought to an adoelscent clinic. As a result of their natural rebelliousness, adolescents may start lagging behind in studies. The fact is, even though academics are the top priority for parents, children have other important issues uppermost in their minds. Some learning disabilities, too, emerge during adolescence.

It is important to remember that, academic failure is often the tip of the iceberg and a combined result of many factors like falling in love, depression, drug addiction, net addiction etc. A detailed discussion with parents may be able to point to one of these issues.

2. Relationships

- *Parent-teen relationships* undergo a major change during this period. Parents may feel alarmed that their teen is drifting away from them. You can explain to them that the ties with parents and family are restructured and new relationships are formed as a natural process of independent socialization.
- *Romantic relationships* of adolescents are a major concern for parents. It is understandable that it is very difficult for the parents to accept their child as a sexual being. You can help parents to understand the nature of such love or attraction. Such situations should be handled with maturity and openness and without panic.
- *The hormonal changes* make teens crave for a special friend. Regular discussion about various types of relationships, understanding healthy boy and girl relationships, choosing the right partner, understanding effect of media, parental concerns about the wellbeing of the teen etc. help the adolescent start a thought process in an objective sort of way.

3. Screen Time and Cyber Safety

- All electronic gadgets such as smart phones, tablets, computers and TV have to be considered under screen time. Usually, the 'screen time' issue results in 'scream time', with parents and children screaming at each other.

- Parents should be advised about the daily recommended limits, maximum 1 hour on week days and maximum 2 hours during holidays.
- Complete avoidance of media is not possible, hence you should tell parents to watch some programs along with the teens and utilize these opportunities to initiate a meaningful discussion in order to create media literacy.
- *Cyber safety:* Parents have to educate themselves about social networking and teach teens about the dangers of the net and how to protect themselves from becoming victims of cyberbullying, identity thefts, dangers of sexting, porn addiction etc.

4. Allowing Independence

Learning to "let go" and allow the teen to become independent: The way of nature is to make everyone independent. Teens are also becoming gradually independent. Therefore, they want to take their own decisions. Most of the time, parents do not let go. They interfere a lot. The results can be:

- Teens may become too dependent on parents and are unable to make their own decisions. This can be a great handicap in later life.
- On the other hand, some children may rebel and make some unwise moves.
- Or they may do things anyway but will make sure that the parents do not come to know about this. If caught will resort to lying.

At some stage, parents need to accept that the child is not their appendage but an independent human being.

LEARNING POINTS

1. To be able to successfully manage adolescent clients it is very important to take the parents on board. Without their active participation and support, adolescent issues will remain unresolved or only partially resolved.
2. The adolescent pediatrician has to strike a balance between taking care of the adolescent rights vs the rights of the parents to know all about their minor adolescents. It is very important to be aware of the legal and ethical issues while taking care of adolescent patients.
3. It is also important to be aware of all ethical issues and the laws of the land when dealing with adolescents.

Acknowledgements

Dr Vaishali Deshmukh, Adolescent Pediatrician, Dinanath Mangeshkar Hospital, Pune for her valuable suggestions.

SUGGESTED READING

1. Bhave SY, Pratt H, Kanikar A. Chapter 25.1 Adolescent Parenting: How and Why is it different? In: Bhave SY, Nair MKC, Parthasarathy A, Menon PSN (Eds). Bhave's Textbook of Adolescent Medicine, First edition. New Delhi: Jaypee Brothers Medical Publishers Pvt Ltd 2006; 875-87.
2. Tamboli S, Nimbalkar S. Parenting from Womb to Adolescent: IAP GDBP Academy, 2015 New Delhi; CBS Publishers and Distributors; 2015.

Pre-conception Care for Adolescents in Clinical Practice

1.7

Rajesh Mehta

INTRODUCTION

Adolescents (age 10-19 years) constitute over 20% (243 million) and young people (age 10-24 years) about 30% (358 million) of India's population. In absolute terms India has the largest population of adolescents in the world. Owing to population momentum, the adolescent population will continue to increase for next few decades to about 260 million in 2030 and 250 million by 2050. For the national development and economic growth, availability of large number of young people represents a huge demographic bonus for the country. However, this opportunity will only be realized through substantial investments in the education, health and development of adolescents. Many of the health conditions that adolescents face are related to underlying risk behaviors and have implications for immediate health, reproductive health outcomes as well as for health during adult life in the long-term, like the non-communicable diseases. Many of the health risk behaviors that are acquired during adolescence must be prevented before they begin. Pre-conception care package consists of interventions that effectively address these health risks.

PRE-CONCEPTION CARE: DEFINITION AND CONCEPT CLARIFICATION

Traditionally, pre-conception care has been at the risk of an assumption that it focuses at the event of conception thus possibly targeted at the women wanting to be pregnant. So the related services would fall in the domain of obstetricians and gynecologists. The new and broader concept of pre-conception care includes provision of the preventive care during adolescence that would prepare boys and girls for future life with wider health and social benefits. This new concept of pre-conception care has made it mandatory to involve all physicians dealing with adolescents to provide preventive care to both boys and girls.

Pre-conception care is defined as the provision of biomedical, behavioral and social health interventions to women and couples before conception occurs, aimed at improving their health status, and to reduce behaviors as well as mitigate individual and environmental factors that could contribute to poor maternal and child health outcomes.

In India and some other neighboring countries, early marriage followed by early pregnancy during adolescence is common and has adverse implications for both mother and their offspring. Health and social care provided before the conception can effectively improve health of adolescents in the immediate context as well as during later life in the long term. In this context, pre-conception care is especially important to delay first pregnancy (beyond adolescence) and too frequent pregnancies as well as preparing the young women to be healthy and ready for healthy pregnancy and healthy offspring and preparing young men to be partners in achieving these objectives. In addition to these immediate benefits, there are long-term benefits beyond reproductive health benefits.

As per the broader concept of the pre-conception care, reaching out to adolescent boys and girls will not only improve reproductive health but also ensure health during adulthood, in the long-term, by addressing the health risk behaviors–e.g. Non-communicable diseases (NCD) risk and other conditions.

Hence, pre-conception care package needs to be delivered across a life course beginning during adolescence (age 10-19 years), before pregnancy and between successive pregnancies for certain public health benefits (see Table 1.7.1).

EVIDENCE-BASED INTERVENTIONS FOR PRE-CONCEPTION CARE

Exhaustive reviews of the evidence of pre-conception care interventions in contributing to a range of health and development outcomes have been published by the Centers for Disease Control and Prevention, Erasmus University, the Health Council of the Netherlands and Aga Khan University. In addition, there are evidence-based WHO guidelines for several interventions that are

Table 1.7.1: Delivery of pre-conception care in life-course

Period in life-course	*Present status*	*Expected outcome*
Before pregnancy and between the successive pregnancies	From the perspective of RMNCAH (Reproductive-Maternal-Newborn-Child-Adolescent health) programs, these periods in life-course continuum of care have traditionally been weak	Preventive and management care in the immediate pre-pregnancy period and inter-pregnancy period could reduce maternal and childhood mortality. In the long term, pre-conception care could contribute to improving the health of babies and children as they grow into adolescence and adulthood
During adolescence (age 10-19 years)-extended period before the first pregnancy	These interventions could be provided during adolescence in an age-appropriate and contextual manner This is especially important for preparing the young women to be healthy and ready for healthy pregnancy and healthy offspring and preparing young men to be partners in achieving these objectives	This would keep the adolescents healthy, improve the reproductive health outcomes and in the long term ensure healthy adulthood (e.g. prevention of NCDs)

applicable to pre-conception care. There is a range of pre-conception care interventions that address priority health problems and have proven benefits for fetus, baby and the mother. Incorporating pre-conception health promotion into routine care is opportunistic because every clinical encounter before pregnancy offers an opening to explore and reinforce health promotion by addressing various issues (see Table 1.7.2).

BENEFITS OF PRE-CONCEPTION CARE

There is a range of benefits of the evidence-based interventions that positively affect the health and wellbeing of the mothers fetus/baby (see Table 1.7.3).

DELIVERING PRE-CONCEPTION CARE TO ADOLESCENTS IN CLINICAL PRACTICE

Adolescent health programs have evolved in several countries, including India, with the objectives of providing comprehensive and age-appropriate services to adolescent boys and girls. Indian adolescent health program envisages delivering holistic services with a multitude of interventions through clinics, field activities, school-based activities and communication activities. In addition Ministries of Women and Child Development, Education (Human Resource Development) and Youth and Sports, have programs targeting adolescent girls and boys. Elements of pre-conception care and promotion of health behaviors and healthy lifestyle could be integrated with the services delivered under these programs. Professional associations of Pediatrics and Gynecology in India have been supporting provision of adolescent health services. With their advocacy among private sector service providers pre-conception care services could also be delivered in private clinics. Adolescent clients (boys and girls) visit pediatricians, general physicians, family physicians and gynecologists for a variety of reasons like sickness, health concerns, immunization and health certification when joining higher education. These contacts could be effectively used to deliver the selected/prioritized pre-conception care interventions to adolescents (see Table 1.7.4).

In developed countries, a variety of preventive services guidelines for the adolescents have been proposed (see Table 1.7.5).

Federation of Obstetric and Gynecological Societies of India (FOGSI) has proposed an annual contact with adolescent clients to provide prioritized interventions (see Table 1.7.6).

LEARNING POINTS

- Pre-conception care is defined as the provision of a package of biomedical, behavioral and social health interventions to adolescent girls women and couples before conception occurs, aimed at improving their health status, and to reduce behaviors as well as individual and environmental factors that could contribute to poor maternal and child health outcomes.
- Such interventions could be delivered during two main periods: immediate pre-pregnancy period

Table 1.7.2: Effective interventions for pre-conception care		
	Fetus/Baby	*Maternal effect*
Folic acid insufficiency	Risk of neural tube defects in the fetus/baby	
Iron deficiency	Fetal growth restriction and low birth weight	Higher maternal morbidity and mortality
Undernutrition	Low BMI and short stature: Poor fetal development It also places the mother and child at risk of complications during pregnancy and childbirth	Short stature, maternal complications in pregnancy and delivery
Over-weight	Poor fetal health leading to preterm birth and stillbirth Complications: Macrosomia (large for gestational age), neural tube defects and other birth defects	Higher maternal morbidity and mortality: Hypertensive disease, gestational or pre-existing diabetes
Vaccine-preventable infections: Affect health and wellbeing of mother and fetus	Tetanus: Neonatal infection and death Rubella: Stillbirth, congenital rubella syndrome Hepatitis B: Neonatal hepatitis B infection	
Tobacco use	Preterm birth, low birth weight, birth defects (including oral cleft, limb-reduction defects, clubfoot, defects of eyes and gastrointestinal system, especially gastroschisis and abdominal hernias), sudden infant death syndrome (SIDS)	Infertility, spontaneous abortion, ectopic pregnancy, placenta previa, placental abruption, premature rupture of membranes
Environmental risks Exposure to ionizing radiation, pesticides, lead or mercury pollution, indoor air pollution	Poor fetal health	Poor maternal health
Genetic disorders	Single gene disorders (e.g. thalassemia, sickle cell disease) and chromosomal disorders (e.g. Down syndrome) that affect fetal and child health (some time) and life-long health problems	
Early pregnancies, unwanted pregnancies, and pregnancies in rapid succession	Higher morbidity and mortality for babies	Higher maternal morbidity and mortality for babies
Sexually transmitted infections (STIs), TORCH infections and human immunodeficiency virus (HIV)	Poor fetal and child health	Poor maternal health
Mental health disorders, including epilepsy: Perinatal stress and depression is associated	This leads to preterm birth; underweight and stunting medications for epilepsy are associated with birth defects and neurodevelopmental impairments	
Psychoactive substance use Abuse of alcohol and drugs before conception	Birth defects like fetal alcohol syndrome	Maternal morbidity

Table 1.7.3: Benefits of pre-conception care

Preventing too early pregnancies: Reduced risk for mother and baby in immediate and long-term	
Pregnancy <20 years risky for mother as well the fetus and newborn Pregnancy <15 years associated with higher reproductive morbidity and higher mortality	Delivery <19 years age: $\uparrow$preterm and LBW babies $\uparrow$ Adult coronary artery disease, hypertension and diabetes $\uparrow$ Chance of short stature $\downarrow$ School achievement $\uparrow$ Glucose intolerance during adulthood
Preventing too frequent and too close pregnancies: Prevent <Less 24 months interval Reduced risk of poor outcomes for the mother as well as the fetus and baby	
Preventing unplanned/unintended pregnancies Prevent serious psychological stress and social problems that can have long-term effects on health and wellbeing of girls and women	
Providing opportunity to screen and manage health risks	
Planned pregnancy has the benefit of screening and management of common conditions and unhealthy behaviors These are associated with poor outcome for mother and fetus	Prevents and treats anemia, STIs, TORCH infections, overweight-obesity, diabetes Prevents behavior like use of tobacco, alcohol, illicit drugs
Promoting healthy behaviors	
Health contacts before pregnancy occurs provide opportunities for the women and their partners to receive education and support for adopting healthy behaviors	Promotes balanced nutrition, micronutrient supplementation, physical activity, and immunization (e.g. rubella) for the benefit of the mother and the fetus
Providing opportunity to screen and prevent genetic disorders and environmental exposure	
Prevention from common genetic diseases (e.g. thalassemia) based on local factors and risk	Can educate to prevent exposure to environmental agents like second hand tobacco smoke, pesticides and agricultural chemicals that could affect the health of fetus

Table 1.7.4: Preconception care that can be provided to adolescents in routine clinical practice

Promoting balanced nutrition and micronutrient supplementation	Promoting adequate physical activity and preventing sedentary lifestyle
Prevention of injuries and accidents (the first killer of death among adolescents)	Prevention of violence including gender-based violence
Promoting safe sex behavior	Prevention of initiation and cessation of use of tobacco, alcohol and drugs
Immunization	

Table 1.7.5: Comparison among recommendations of adolescent preventive services in USA

Subject	*AAFP*	*AAP*	*AMA*	*BF*	*USPSTF*
Immunizations					
ACIP Recommendations	Yes	Yes	Yes	Yes	Yes
Health Guidance for Teens					
Normal Development	Yes	Yes	Yes	Yes	
Injury Prevention	Yes	Yes	Yes	Yes	Yes
Nutrition	Yes	Yes	Yes	Yes	Yes
Physical Activity	Yes	Yes	Yes	Yes	Yes
Dental Health	Yes	Yes	No	Yes	Yes
Breast/Testicular Self-examination	Yes	Yes	No	Yes	No
Skin Protection	Yes	Yes	Yes	Yes	Yes
Health Guidance for Parents					
Counseling for the Parents	No	Yes	Yes	Yes	No
Screening/Counseling					
Obesity	Yes	Yes	Yes	Yes	Yes
Contraception	Yes	Yes	Yes	Yes	Yes
Tobacco Use	Yes	Yes	Yes	Yes	Yes
Alcohol Use	Yes	Yes	Yes	Yes	Yes
Substance Abuse	Yes	Yes	Yes	Yes	Yes
Hypertension	No	Yes	Yes	Yes	Yes
Depression/Suicide	No	Yes	Yes	Yes	No
Eating Disorders	No	Yes	Yes	Yes	No
School Problems	No	Yes	Yes	Yes	No
Abuse	No	Yes	Yes	Yes	No
Hearing	Yes	Yes	No	Yes	No
Vision	No	Yes	No	Yes	No
Tests					
Tuberculosis	Yes	Yes	Yes	Yes	Yes
Papanicolau Smear	Yes	Yes	Yes	Yes	Yes
HIV	Yes	Yes	Yes	Yes	Yes
STD	Yes	Yes	Yes	Yes	Yes
Cholesterol	Yes	Yes	Yes	Yes	No
Urinalysis	No	Yes	No	No	No
Hematocrit	No	Yes	No	No	No
Periodicity of Visits	Tailored	Annual	Annual	Annual	Tailored
Target Age Range (Years)	13-18	11-21	11-21	11-21	11-24

AAFP: American Academy of Family Physicians; AAP: American Academy of Pediatrics; AMA: American Medical Association (GAPS); BF: Bright Futures; USPSTF: US Preventive Services Task Force; ACIP: Advisory Committee on Immunization Practices-CDC

Table 1.7.6: Health services adolescent girls annual visit at AFHS guidelines by FOGSI

Physical Check-up	*Development/Behavior Screening*	*Counseling/Anticipatory Guidance*	*Lab Tests (If indicated)*	*Life-skills*
Weight, height, BMI, SMR Systemic examination, BP Eye check up, visual acuity Hearing assessment Dental check up Breast/Testicular self-examination (older adolescents)	HEADSS screening	Normal development Nutrition Injury prevention Physical activity Safe sexual behavior Substance use–including tobacco and alcohol (older adolescents)	Hematocrit (if anemic) Cholesterol (if family history) STI/HIV (If sexually active)	Promote self-esteem, communication skills, coping with emotions and stress, negotiation and assertive skills, decision-making skills
Health Guidance for Parents Immunization–as recommended by FOGSI, IAP				

and inter-pregnancy period; and during adolescence. This approach strengthens the services across the reproductive-maternal-newborn-child-adolescent health continuum of care. To reach the target populations the evidence-based pre-conception care interventions can be integrated into existing health services.

- Pre-conception care can be delivered to adolescent girls and boys within the existing clinical practice.
- It contributes to health during adolescence, positive reproductive health outcomes and healthy adulthood, in the long-term.

Disclaimer: The author is a staff member of the World Health Organization. The author alone is responsible for the views expressed in this presentation and they do not necessarily represent the decisions, policy or views of the World Health Organization.

SUGGESTED READING

1. Dean SV, Imam AM, Lassi ZS, Bhutta ZA. Systematic review of preconception risks and interventions. Karachi, Aga Khan University, 2011.
2. Jack BW, Attrash H, Coonrod DV, *et al*. The clinical content of preconception care: An overview and preparation of this supplement. American Journal of Obstetrics and Gynecology, 2008,199 (Suppl. 2): S266-79.
3. Jackson CA, Henderson M, Frank JW, Haw SJ. An overview of prevention of multiple risk behaviour in adolescence and young adulthood. J Public Health (Oxf) 2012;34 (Suppl 1):i31-40.
4. Johnson K, Posner SF, Biermann J, *et al*. Recommendations to improve preconception health and health care–United States: A report of the CDC/ATSDR Preconception Care Work Group and the Select Panel on Preconception Care. Morbidity and Mortality Weekly Report 2006; 55:1-23.
5. Klein JD, Allan MJ, Elster AB, Stevens D, Cox C, Hedberg VA, Goodman RA. Improving adolescent preventive care in community health centers. Pediatrics 2001;107(2):318-27.
6. Report of a WHO technical consultation on birth spacing, Geneva, Switzerland, 13–15 June 2005. Geneva, World Health Organization, 2007 Available from: http://www.who.int/reproductivehealth/publications/family_planning/WHO_RHR_07_1/en/ Accessed on 26 July 2015.
7. Saraf DS, Nongkynrih B, Pandav CS, *et al*. A systematic review of school-based interventions to prevent risk factors associated with noncommunicable diseases. Asia Pac J Public Health 2012;24(5):733-52.
8. United Nations: World Population Prospects: 2012 Revision: Available from: http://esa.un.org/wpp/unpp/panel_population.htm; accessed on 26 July 2015.
9. World Health Organization Report 2012: Meeting to Develop a Global Consensus on Preconception Care to Reduce Maternal and Childhood Mortality and Morbidity World Health Organization Headquarters. Available from: http://www.who.int/maternal_child_adolescent/documents/concensus_preconception_care/en/ Accessed on 26 July 2015.
10. World Health Organization, 2011: Preventing early pregnancy and poor reproductive outcomes among adolescents in developing countries. Geneva. Available from: http://www.who.int/maternal_child_adolescent/documents/preventing_early_pregnancy/en/ Accessed on 26 July 2015.

Non-Communicable Diseases (NCDs)

1.8

Swati Y Bhave

INTRODUCTION

Non-communicable diseases (NCDs) are also known as lifestyle disorders, as they are caused by various factors in an unhealthy lifestyle such as (a) sedentary lifestyle and lack of exercise, (b) calorie dense food which is high in sugar, salt and trans fat, and (c) indulgence in tobacco and alcohol. Overweight and obesity are important determinants of health and lead to adverse metabolic changes, increase in blood pressure, unfavorable cholesterol levels and increased resistance to insulin. This leads to high risk of NCDs that include diabetes mellitus, coronary heart disease, stroke, and many forms of cancer. In 1990 only 40% of the NCD deaths were from developing countries but doubled to 80% in 2008. NCDs have globally increased the number of DALYs (i.e. Disability Adjusted Life Years).

For prevention of NCD it is extremely important to focus on adolescents, as many of the behaviors and the lifestyle pattern that adolescents adapt, form the nidus for the beginning of various pathophysiologies that lead to adverse life-long consequences (see Table 1.8.1). NCDs are a life course issue—most of the behaviors that cause NCDs generally begin in childhood—sedentary lifestyle and addiction of calorie-dense high sugar, salt and trans fat containing foods. These get well established in the adolescent or youth with the added component of tobacco

Table 1.8.1: Review of incidence of NCDs in adolescents
Obesity
75% of obese adolescents continue as obese adults
This increases their risk for development of metabolic syndrome
Eating pattern and parental and environmental factors are major contributors
Obesity, diabetes and cardiovascular diseases
By 15 years of age many adolescents who have obesity will have signs of diabetes and have high risk of developing atherosclerosis and cardiovascular disease
Teenage pregnancies have high risk of having low birth weight offsprings that have high risk of developing metabolic syndrome as adults
Cancer
Exposure to HPV virus in adolescence age group is a high risk for cervical cancer in adult women and head and neck cancers in both genders
Exposure to sun in adolescence can result in skin cancer in adulthood
Tobacco exposure
Teen smokers have high risk of asthma, chronic lung disease and cancer
Earlier the age of smoking higher the chance of chronic addiction in adulthood
Chronic alcohol dependence
Most alcohol-dependent adults begin experimentation and consumption as children or teens; and have high risk of addiction persisting in adulthood
Intentional and unintentional injuries
Violence leading to homicides or self harm and suicides; vehicle accidents specially under influence of alcohol are the highest cause of mortality in teens
Mental health disorders
75% of all mental illness have their onset in adolescence and youth
25% of youth have some mental illness before the age of 24 years
Violence
Aggression and violence is a major cause of morbidity and mortality in this age group

and alcohol and track into adulthood. Hence prevention of adult NCDs has to begin in childhood and adolescence.

The World Health Assembly in 2011, called upon member states to concentrate on youth in context of NCDs and made a resolution regarding the same. WHO recommends: Preventing and responding to NCDs must integrate a focus on adolescents. Every country needs to develop national programs on adolescent health to prevent NCDs and to have policies and legislation against the risk factors that lead to NCDs like banning of unhealthy processed and deeply fried food and sugary aerated drinks in school canteens, banning of tobacco and alcohol for youth etc.

Research has shown that the limbic system is predominant in adolescence and hence rewards seeking, experimentation and peer pressure leads to many of them indulging in use of tobacco and alcohol. The developing brain is more vulnerable to the adverse effects of substance abuse and the chance of addiction is much higher when use begins in the younger age. A majority of adults who have this faulty behavioral pattern have started this in the adolescent age.

The aim of this chapter is not to give a detailed overview of NCDs and their management, but to make clinicians dealing with adolescents aware that they have a very important role to play in prevention and screening for NCDs in their day to day practice of adolescent clients.

Regardless of the presenting symptoms and the problem as adolescent comes with, they should undergo a detailed history taking regarding his/her lifestyle and use of tobacco and alcohol. Preventive counseling and anticipatory guidance have to be given to every adolescent for physical activity, reducing screen time and sedentary lifestyle, healthy nutrition and prevention of gateway drugs of substance abuse namely tobacco and alcohol. It is also the need of the hour to screen adolescents for detecting early signs of metabolic syndrome specially in those who are overweight/obese and/or with a strong family history of risk factors.

HISTORY TAKING

Every adolescent regardless of what the presenting complaints are, should be screened for risk factors for NCDs (see Table 1.8.2). The first step is to ask about the four main behavioral factors that contribute to NCD.

Table 1.8.2: History taking–Risk factors in adolescents for NCDs

Risky behavior	*Causes*	*Results*
Poor eating habits Unhealthy diets	• Marketing and advertising impacts food habits adversely • Most are attracted to the very tasty, energy dense, 'High Sugar, High Salt' (HSHS) food with high levels of saturated fats and trans fats • Since these are very addicting they lead to sugar, salt and fat craving	• Overweight and obesity lead to high incidence of metabolic syndrome • Associated risk of type 2 diabetes, hypertension and cardiovascular risk factors • Nutritional deficiencies
Physical inactivity Lack of exercise	• Physical inactivity is on the rise due to many factors: Rapid urbanization, unsafe playgrounds, use of motorized transport, lifts for climbing stairs etc. that lead to a "obesogenic environment" • Addiction to electronic gadgets and spending many hours of "screen time"	• Insufficient physical activity and unhealthy diet can lead to many negative physical changes in adolescence • Type 2 diabetes, hypertension and cancers can be triggered by obesity
Tobacco use	• Majority of adult smokers begin in teenage • 25% teens begin smoking at less than 10 years of age	• Tobacco exposure increases risk for asthma and lung infections • Smoking by teen girls has adverse effects on fertility as well as morbidity and mortality in the fetus, newborn, infant and toddlers
Alcohol consumption	• Due to peer pressure and changing socio-cultural milieu, many adolescents have started alcohol consumption from school age also • Drinking from teenage has high risk of leading to addiction lasting into adult life	• Major risk factor for premature death and disability • High level of alcohol can lead to cancer and cardiac disease • Drinking and driving by underage teenagers cause many fatal road traffic accidents • Alcohol also increases other high risk behaviors: unprotected sex, intentional and unintentional injuries, and gender-based violence, mental illnesses and poor mental health

1. Poor eating habits/unhealthy diets (Foods containing high levels of sugar, salt, saturated fats and trans fats)
   - Ask for history weekly consumption of unhealthy food e.g. sugary aerated drinks, processed food, packaged food, etc.
   - Ask for weekly consumption of healthy foods e.g. salads, greens, fruits, vegetables, complex carbohydrates etc.

   For more details please see Section 4.
2. Physical inactivity and /or lack of exercise (see Boxes 1.8.1 and 1.8.2)
   - Ask for number of hours spent in sedentary activities per day.
   - Ask for the type of physical activities they do daily which include walking, climbing stairs, cycling etc. and the sports they participate in.
3. Tobacco use: This needs to be asked as direct questioning.
   - Have they tried tobacco products?
   - If yes, have they stopped at experimentation–just tried once to see how it feels or are they having regular consumption?
   - Assess at what level they are (see Box 1.8.3).

Box 1.8.1: Physical activity is an important correlate of health across the life course
The patterns of physical activity established in adolescence persist to adulthood.
The World Health Organization defines physical activity as any bodily movement produced by skeletal muscles that requires energy expenditure, including activities undertaken during one's daily life: working, traveling, house work, and engaging in recreational pursuits.
The term physical activity should not be confused with exercise, which is a subcategory of physical activity that is planned, structured, repetitive, and aims to improve or maintain one or more components of physical fitness.
Physical inactivity is on the rise in many countries, adding to the burden of non-communicable diseases in adults.
In 2013 WHO member states agreed to reduce physical inactivity by 10% in the framework of the global action plan for the prevention and control of non-communicable diseases. Policies and plans to address physical inactivity had been developed in about 80% of WHO member states. WHO recommends that adults have 150 minutes of moderate intensity activity per week.
There are major health risks of physical inactivity: • With it being identified as the fourth leading risk factor for global mortality, causing an estimated 3.2 million deaths each year. • As a risk factor in 6% of all deaths, physical inactivity is only outstripped by high blood pressure and tobacco use. • It carries the same level of risk of mortality as high blood glucose.

Box 1.8.2: Physical activity in adolescence
World Health Organization recommends that children and adolescents spend 60 minutes each day participating in moderate to vigorous intensity physical activity. Obesity prevention can be achieved by physical activity. At the time of puberty, adolescents are more vulnerable to obesity. During this time most teens also have reduced physical activity which is added risk factor. Prior to adolescence, the amount of time that boys and girls spend being physically active is pretty similar. Due to many factors like socio-cultural taboos, gender discrimination, lack of safe playgrounds etc., the physical activities of girls is markedly reduced after puberty. The affluent section of society in India is becoming extremely westernized and following the same sedentary lifestyle and unhealthy eating pattern. Many adolescents today have reduced energy expenditure, as their activites are sedentary with electronic gadgets. Unless this life pattern is changed, today's adolescents will have a unhealthy adulthood as compared to their parents.

Box 1.8.3: History taking for tobacco consumption
Stage 1: "Wanting" is the first symptom of nicotine addiction. It is mild transient desire to smoke that is easily ignored. A person can remain without tobacco without withdrawal symptoms.
Stage 2: Craving is more intense than wanting and intrudes upon the person's thoughts. It is more persistent and difficult to ignore.
Stage 3: Needing is an intense and urgent desire to smoke that is impossible to ignore. The individual must smoke to restore a normal mental or physical state.
Stage 4: Withdrawal symptoms of nicotine. Restlessness, anxiety, irritability, anger, difficulty in concentrating and disturbed sleep.

   - Ask for all tobacco products, smokeless or chewable e.g. gutka and smoking–including cigarettes, beedis and hookahs.
4. Harmful use of alcohol.
   - Alcohol is the second gateway drug of adolescence that can lead to hard core substance abuse. Hence direct questioning is extremely important.
   - Like tobacco, the level of alcohol craving and dependence has to be ascertained.
   - Driving under influence or drunken driving is a major cause of traffic-related accidents and morbidity and mortality in adolescents and young people.
   - A good tool to use in clinical practice is CRAFFT questionnaire for screening for alcohol and other substance abuse (see Box 1.8.4).

Box 1.8.4: The CRAFFT screening tool
The CRAFFT is a behavioral health screening tool for use with children under the age of 21 and is recommended by the American Academy of Pediatrics Committee on Substance Abuse for use with adolescents.
It consists of a series of 6 questions developed to screen adolescents for high risk alcohol and other drug use disorders simultaneously.
It is a short, effective screening tool meant to assess whether a longer conversation about the context of use, frequency, and other risks and consequences of alcohol and other drug use is warranted.
Screening using the CRAFFT begins by asking the adolescent to "I'm going to ask you a few questions that I ask all my patients. Please be honest. I will keep your answers confidential"; and then asking three opening questions.
The 3 opening questions are: **Part A During the PAST 12 MONTHS did you:** 1. **Drink** any alcohol (more than a few sips)? (Do not count a few sips of alcohol taken during family or religious events) 2. **Smoke** any marijuana or hashish? 3. **Use** anything else to get high? ("anything else" includes illegal drugs, synthetic marijuana, over-the-counter and prescription drugs, or things that people sniff or "huff")
If the adolescent answers **"No"** to all questions in Part A, the provider only needs to ask the adolescent the first question - **the CAR question only, then stop**. If the adolescent answers **"Yes"** to any question in Part A, the provider will ask **all 6 CRAFFT** questions.
CRAFFT is a mnemonic acronym of first letters of key words in the six screening questions. The questions should be asked exactly as written. **Part B** C–Have you ever ridden in a **CAR** driven by someone (including yourself) who was "high" or had been using alcohol or drugs? R–Do you ever use alcohol or drugs to **RELAX**, feel better about yourself, or fit in? A–Do you ever use alcohol or drugs while you are by yourself, **ALONE**? F–Do you ever **FORGET** things you did while using alcohol or drugs? F–Do your **FAMILY** or **FRIENDS** ever tell you that you should cut down on your drinking or drug use? T–Have you gotten into **TROUBLE** while you were using alcohol or drugs?
*Two or more YES answers on the CRAFFT suggest a serious problem and need for further assessment. © John R. Knight, MD, Boston Children's Hospital, 2015. All rights reserved. Reproduced with permission. For more information, contact ceasar@childrens.harvard.edu

- Anticipatory guidance and preventive counseling have to be given to all adolescents regarding adverse effects of alcohol as teens today are experimenting in school age; and going to pubs is considered to be 'modern and cool' behavior in college.
- Most adolescents are not aware of the adverse impact of alcohol on the developing brain and long term health (see Box 1.8.5).
- The alcohol content of commonly used alcoholic beverages are provided in Table 1.8.3.

Family history: Family history especially adults in the family having obesity, type 2 diabetes, hypertension, cardiovascular diseases, cancer, mental illness etc. is very important as this makes the adolescent at high risk for NCDs especially if s/he is overweight and obese.

PHYSICAL EXAMINATION

Important aspects in the physical examination related to NCD are:

- Height, weight and calculation of BMI, abdominal girth and waist hip ratio. This gives an idea about overweight and obesity (see Chapters 3.3 and 3.4 for more details).
- Measurement of blood pressure to check for hypertension (Chapter 5.3).
- Nicotine stains on fingers and teeth are important indicators for tobacco use.
- Signs and symptoms for substance abuse like unkept look, poor personal hygine, sniffing , tremors etc. For more details see Chapter 8.3.

INVESTIGATIONS

All overweight and obese adolescents and/or those with a family history of metabolic syndrome (Chapter 3.4) and other NCDs need appropriate investigations.

MANAGEMENT

1. If there is no evidence of any NCD related symptoms and signs, the adolescent should be congratulated and encouraged to follow the healthy lifestyle. Anticipatory guidance and preventive counseling can be given for tobacco and alcohol and their adverse effects on health.

Box 1.8.5: Facts about alcohol for anticipatory guidance and preventive counseling

Alcoholism, or alcohol dependence, is a disease that causes

- Craving - a strong need to drink.
- Loss of control - not being able to stop drinking once you've started.
- Physical dependence - withdrawal symptoms.
- Tolerance - the need to drink more alcohol to feel the same effect.

Alcohol abuse

You are not physically dependent, but your drinking can cause problems at home, work, or school.

It may cause you to put yourself in dangerous situations, or lead to legal or social problems.

It can cause damage to the liver brain, and other organs.

It can cause cancer of mouth throat esophagus, liver and breast.

Binge drinking is defined as consumption of alcoholic drinks in 2 hours or less

(a) 4 or more drinks for women

(b) 5 or more drinks for men

Binge drinking increases the chances of breast cancer, sexually transmitted diseases, heart disease, unintended pregnancy, and many other health problems.

Alcohol poisoning is caused by drinking large quantities of alcohol in a short period of time.

Very high levels of alcohol in the body can shut down critical areas of the brain that control breathing, heart rate, and body temperature, resulting in death.

Women's and girls' bodies respond to alcohol differently than men.

It takes less alcohol for women to get intoxicated because of their size and how they process alcohol.

There is no safe level of alcohol during pregnancy.

Alcohol can disrupt fetal development at any stage including the earliest stage when a woman is not even aware that she is pregnant.

Exposing their developing baby to high levels of alcohol, especially by binge drinking can lead to Fetal Alcohol Spectrum Disorders (FASD).

This is the umbrella term for the different diagnoses, which include fetal alcohol syndrome, partial fetal alcohol syndrome, partial fetal alcohol syndrome, alcohol-related neurodevelopmental disorder, and alcohol-related birth defects.

Drinking during pregnancy can also lead to sudden infant death syndrome.

Alcohol consumption also increases the risk of death from injuries, homicide, and suicide.

Drinking and driving lead to car accidents leading to your killing yourself and/or others.

The younger the age at which you start drinking higher the chance of your being chronic addict as an adult.

MRI imaging has shown that the effect of alcohol on a developing teen brain is loss of memory and reduction in the size of the hippocampus.

Source:

http://www.niaaa.nih.gov/alcohol-health/alcohols-effects-body

http://www.cdc.gov/vitalsigns/alcohol-screening-counseling/index.html

https://www.nlm.nih.gov/medlineplus/alcoholismandalcoholabuse.html

2. If there is no evidence of NCD but there is high risk family history, they should be advised to undergo routine screening and given guidance for prevention.
3. Appropriate treatment and management will be needed if there is evidence of any NCD like obesity, type 2 diabetes, hypertension etc.

Table 1.8.3: Alcohol content of commonly used alcoholic beverages

Type of alcohol	*Amount*	*Alcohol %*
Beer	12 oz	5
Wine	5 oz	12
Malt liquor	8-9 oz	7
Whiskey, Vodka, Gin, Rum, Tequila	1-1.5 oz	40-80
1 US oz = 30 ml		

LEARNING POINTS

1. All physicians need to be aware that prevention for NCD begins in the pediatric and adolescent age group.
2. It is very important to make adolescents, teachers and parents aware about NCDs and the risky behavior that leads to NCDs. Schools and parents have to make special efforts to protect adolescents from harmful substances such as tobacco, alcohol and foods containing high levels of saturated fats, trans fats, sugar and salt.
3. Exercise for 60 minutes daily has to be instituted in every adolescent's life.
4. Sedentary lifestyle and screen time addiction due to various electronic gadgets has to be drastically reduced both at home and school.
5. Every adolescent needs to be screened for both detection and prevention of NCDs. Those with risk factors need to be put on long-term follow-up.
6. Overweight and obese adolescents need to be completely investigated for metabolic syndrome and treatment instituted immediately to prevent further complications.
7. Preventive counseling and anticipatory guidance should be given to every adolescent against the use of tobacco and alcohol.

SUGGESTED READING

1. Blum R, Gates WH. Non-Communicable Diseases and Adolescents – An Opportunity for Action. AstraZeneca Young Health Programme, 2011. Available at www. astrazeneca.com; www.jhsph.edu; and www.plan-international.org
2. Dewitt DJ, Alfa EM, Offord DR, Osborne AC. Age at first alcohol use: A risk factor for the development of alcohol disorders. Am J Psychiatry 2000;157:745-50.
3. Freedman, DS, Zulu, M, Srinivasan, SR, Berenson, GS, and Dietz WH. Cardiovascular risk factors and excess adiposity among overweight children and adolescents: The Bogalusa Heart Study. Pediatrics 2007;150(1):12-17.
4. Gaffer A, Reddy KS, Singh M. Burden of non-communicable diseases in south Asia. BMJ 2004;328:807-10.
5. Gore F, Bloem P, Patton G, Ferguson J, Joseph V, Coffey C, Sawyer S, Mathers C. Global burden of disease in young people aged 10-24 years: A systematic analysis. Lancet 2011;377:2093-102.
6. Greydanus DE, Bhave SY. Editorial Obesity and Adolescents Time for increased physical activity: Indian Pediatrics 2004;41:545-50.
7. Patton GC, Coffey C, Cappa C, *et al.* Health of the World's Adolescents: A Synthesis of International Comparable Data. Lancet 2012;79(9286):1665-75.
8. Shah B, Kumar N, Menon GR, Khurana S, Kumar H. Assessment of burden of non-communicable diseases. Indian Council of Medical Research, New Delhi; 2004.
9. World Health Assembly. Youth and Health Risks. World Health Organization 2011; A64/28, 1-4.
10. World Health Organization. Global status report on non-communicable diseases 2010. Geneva: World Health Organization; 2011. Accessed at: http://www.who.int/nmh/publications/ncd_report2010/en/. Retrieved on: 14th October 2013.

Normal Growth and Physical Development in Adolescence

2.1

Vaman Khadilkar, Supriya Phanse Gupte

INTRODUCTION

During adolescence, changes in the physical characteristics and development of internal and external genitalia result in the maturation of a child to an adult capable of reproduction. Most issues of adolescence revolve around puberty and related emotional and psychosexual issues. Detailed understanding of puberty helps in the management of these health issues. Physical changes of puberty occur about two years earlier in girls as estrogen is a more potent hormone as compared to testosterone.

FACTORS INFLUENCING ONSET AND PROGRESSION OF PUBERTY

- The onset and progression of puberty is finely tuned by the hypothalamic-pituitary-gonadal (HPG) axis.
- At the time of puberty, the hypothalamus starts generating gonadotropin-releasing hormone (GnRH) pulses which stimulate the pituitary to secrete LH (luteinizing hormone) and FSH (follicle stimulating hormone) in a pulsatile manner.
- This in turn stimulates the ovaries in girls, and testes in boys to secrete estrogen and testosterone respectively.
- Several factors such as kisspeptin, control the onset of puberty.
- Energy availability markers such as leptin and insulin-like growth factor-1 (IGF-1) play a permissive role in onset of puberty.
- This explains the need of a critical body mass index (BMI) for onset of puberty and influence of chronic illness on onset and progression of puberty. Similarly genetic factors play a role in timing of onset of puberty.

Details of pubertal development in boys and girls is outlined in Table 2.1.1.

Table 2.1.1: Pubertal development

Adrenarche	Adrenarche is the maturation of the hypothalamic-pituitary-adrenal (HPA) axis leading to increased synthesis of androgens—DHEAS (dehydroepiandrosterone sulphate) and androstenedione. The secretion of these androgens leads to development of axillary and pubic hair and adult type body odor in both boys and girls. Though its timing is closely associated with the other pubertal changes, it may not always occur in concordance with pubertal development, and may occur earlier or later.
Gonadarche in girls	The primordial follicles undergo recruitment and maturation resulting in estrogen production and ovulation, with subsequent formation of corpus luteum and progesterone secretion. However menstrual cycles can be anovulatory for the first few months until ovulation is established. The ovaries slowly increase in size from the prepubertal volume of approximately 0.5 ml to >1 ml in puberty and finally achieve a post-pubertal volume (4-15 ml). The uterus grows from the small tubular structure in prepubertal period to the pear shaped and larger adult structure with endometrial lining formation. Uterine length >3.5 cm, a pear shaped contour and presence of endometrial echo herald the onset of puberty. Menstruation occurs at endometrial thickness of approximately 7-16 mm. Estrogen leads to development of the breasts with formation of glandular tissue as well as female distribution of fat, increase in bone mass and epiphyseal fusion of bones. Changes in physical appearance and internal hormonal milieu result in behavioral changes, mood swings and emotional lability.

Contd.

Contd.

Gonadarche in boys	Under the influence of LH, the Leydig cells in the testes secrete testosterone. FSH stimulates the development of Sertoli cells and formation of spermatids with subsequent spermatogenesis. The testes grow in size from a prepubertal volume of approximately 1-2 ml to 4 ml indicating onset of puberty and finally to adult size of approximately 12-25 ml. High circulating and local testosterone levels result in development of internal genitalia, beard growth, growth spurt, increased muscle mass, loss of fat mass, and adult physique. Dihydrotestosterone formed by conversion of testosterone is responsible for maturation of the external genitalia, prostate, and male pattern of baldness.
Growth spurt	Sex steroids are responsible for the growth spurt in both genders by increasing the pulsatility and amplitude of growth hormone (GH) pulses as well as direct effect on growth plate. In both girls and boys estrogen (due to peripheral aromatization of testosterone) leads to maturation of bones and final closure of growth plates and achievement of final height

Puberty is a physiological process and seldom needs medical intervention unless there is a pathological variation or psychological distress. The role of medical professional is mainly to ensure that things are progressing within the normal range and providing support to the adolescent and parents during this stage. It also involves managing the common issues of puberty and addressing issues of adaptation in adolescents with chronic diseases.

Common problems and issues of puberty have been enlisted in Tables 2.1.2 and 2.1.3 below and have been discussed in relevant parts of the chapter.

Table 2.1.2: Problems of puberty

In girls	*In boys*
Early puberty	Delayed puberty
Delayed puberty	Early puberty
Acne	Acne
Body odour	Body odour
Asymmetrical breast development	Gynecomastia
Leucorrhea	Buried penis
Dysmenorrhea and menorrhagia	Phimosis and paraphimosis
Pubertal goiter	Frequent erections
Hirsutism	Ejaculations and nocturnal emissions

Table 2.1.3: Issues related to puberty

Issues	*Comments*
Concerns of height	The timing of puberty is extremely variable in boys, with some starting and progressing much later than their peers. This needs reassurance and monitoring of puberty as it usually kick-starts spontaneously at a later stage. Constitutional delay of growth and puberty is common in boys; however it may need endocrine evaluation if causing too much psychological distress or if unduly delayed.
Change in voice	Boys may wake up one day to find their voice croaky and broken, causing distress. They need reassurance that it is a normal part of puberty and will settle down with time.
Involuntary erections and nocturnal emissions	May cause embarrassment need psychological support and reassurance.
Gynecomastia	Is a common occurrence needing reassurance, close monitoring and weight loss in obese boys.
Unequal testicles	Cause concern amongst boys. They are a normal occurrence and need reassurance.
Phimosis, paraphimosis and hypospadias	Are problems needing attention and appropriate referral.

APPROACH TO ASSESSMENT OF GROWTH AND PUBERTY

While assessing puberty in an adolescent, it is important to respect their privacy and individuality. Adolescents are neither old children nor young adults; their needs are different from either and a sensitive and individual approach is the key to a successful consultation. Maintaining eye contact with them during the consultation and valuing their opinion is of paramount importance.

HISTORY TAKING

- Puberty being an important part of adolescence, it is necessary to have an idea of the onset and progression of puberty in all adolescents.
- Most will progress normally through puberty with a range of variation in onset and progression which is in concordance with the variation seen in the population.
- Various issues of adolescence are associated with the pubertal stage (see Tables 2.1.2 and 2.1.3) and a broad idea of pubertal staging helps in addressing these issues.
- In scenarios wherein adolescents may be shy to allow examination, especially when there are no concerns of early or delayed onset of puberty, a brief history will suffice and uncomfortable examination can be avoided.
- Onset of pubertal changes before 8 years in girls and 9 years in boys is precocious puberty. Similarly absence of pubertal changes beyond 13 years in girls and 14

years in boys is suggestive of delayed puberty. Both are abnormal and need a proper examination followed by appropriate investigations.

History Taking in Girls

- It is a good idea to have a female chaperone while examining an adolescent girl.
- Some girls might find it uncomfortable to answer questions on such sensitive issues.
- Ensuring the comfort of both patients and parents while handling such issues is important.
- History of menarche and detailed history of the menstrual periods is very important. One must ask for the interval between periods, regularity, duration, whether they are heavy or light and dysmenorrhea should be enquired. Any abnormality warrants a referral to a gynecologist for investigations.
- Girls with menorrhagia need to be investigated and may require iron supplements.

The various stages of puberty are well depicted in the pictorial representation of Tanner staging of puberty in Figure 2.1.1 and Table 2.1.4. The duration of each stage is extremely variable. Often a pictorial representation of the Tanner staging of puberty helps in self-assessment of pubertal stage, if the examiner is not worried of a pathology or the adolescent is shy and does not comply with a formal examination.

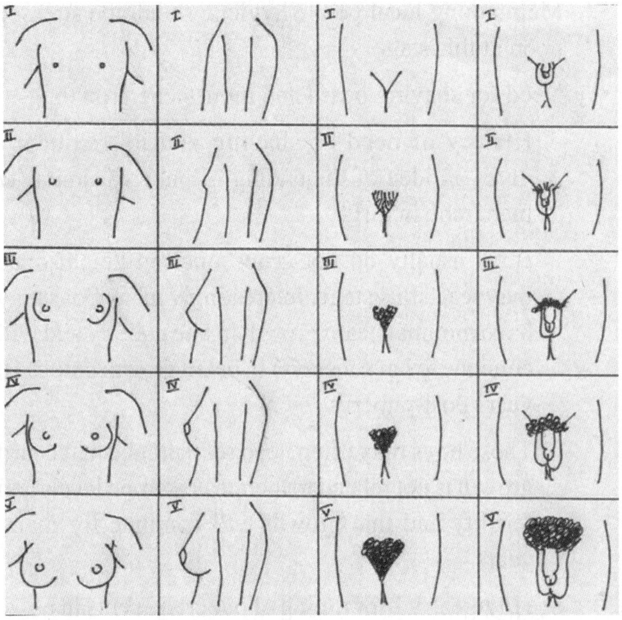

Figure 2.1.1: Tanner staging of puberty

History Taking in Boys

- As in girls, it is equally important to respect privacy and ask questions regarding puberty with an element of sensitivity.
- About 50% of boys are able to retract foreskin by midpuberty and almost 90% by end of puberty. Those unable to retract are more likely to develop phimosis and need monitoring.

Table 2.1.4: Tanner stages of puberty for girls and boys

Tanner Stage	*Girls*		*Boys*	
	Breast	*Pubic Hair*	*Genitalia*	*Pubic Hair*
I	Prepubertal	No hair/fine vellus hair	Prepubertal Testes < 2.5 cm in length (volume 1 to 3 ml)	No hair/fine vellus hair
II	Breast bud appears	Few pigmented hair around labia	Thinning and reddening of scrotum Testes >2.5 cm in length (volume 4-8 ml)	Few pigmented hair at base of penis
III	Areola and breast enlarge Primary mound is formed	Hair is coarser, darker, curly, and spreads over pubis	Increase in length of penis Testes: 3.3-4 cm in length (volume 10-15 ml)	Hair is coarser, darker, curly and spreads till mons pubis
IV	Areola and papilla project to form secondary mound	Adult type hair but not spread over medial aspect of thigh	Increase in length and breadth of penis, enlargement of glans, scrotal skin darkens Testes: 4.1-4.5 cm in length (volume 15-20 ml)	Adult type hair but does not extend over medial aspect of thigh
V	Adult breast contour, papilla projects, similar to stage III, larger areolae and size of breast tissue	Hair spreads to medial aspect of thigh	Adult type genitalia Testes: >4.5 cm in length (volume 25 ml)	Adult type hair; extends to medial aspect of thigh

- Maintaining local penile hygiene should be stressed upon at this stage.
- Need for shaving/beard and moustache growth
  - History of need of shaving and its frequency gives an idea of the ending of puberty similar to menarche in girls.
  - Boys usually do not grow much in height once they reach this stage. Interestingly many boys may have minimal beard growth in late puberty and will continue to have increase in beard growth upto 5-10 years post-puberty.
  - These boys may often need reassurance that beard growth is not related to their testosterone levels and fertility and that growth will continue for many years.

See Figure 2.1.1 for timing of pubertal events in boys.

Birth History

- History of birth weight and gestational age at time of birth may be enquired.
- Those born small for gestational age (SGA) have higher predisposition for early onset of puberty, rapid progression and should be monitored for the same.

Family History

- History of timing of menarche and age at shaving in parents and elder siblings gives a rough guideline of what should be expected in the adolescent being examined.
- History of delayed or early puberty in either parent and/or sibling may suggest a similar trend in the adolescent.
- Family history of thyroid illness, autoimmune disorders like psoriasis, connective tissue disorders and celiac disease should be asked, as a positive history increases risk of autoimmune illnesses in adolescence.

History of Intercurrent Illness

- Children with chronic illnesses such as cardiac conditions, asthma, chronic respiratory disease (e.g. Cystic fibrosis), liver diseases, malabsorption syndromes, type1 diabetes, renal disorders and those on long-term steroid therapy, may not naturally progress into puberty.
- It is important to keep an eye on puberty in children with these conditions.

Diet History

Adequate Intake of Calories, Nutrients and Micronutrients

- This is a stage of increased need for calories and protein intake.
- Girls especially are predisposed to anorexia nervosa at this stage.
- This can delay the pubertal onset and progression.

Intake of Calcium and Exposure to the Sun (Vitamin D)

- Maximum accruement of bone mass occurs in the critical pubertal years, which lasts for life.
- It is important to ensure adequate calcium intake and vitamin D levels in this age to reduce chances of fractures in adolescence and osteoporosis in adulthood.
- Prevention and treatment of vitamin D deficiency is important to ensure adequate bone accrual.

History of Physical Activity

- Physical activity strengthens muscles and bones and plays an important role in bone accruement as well.
- With the rising incidence of obesity amongst adolescence, healthy practices should be encouraged in all.
- The Center for Disease Control (CDC), USA recommends 60 minutes of physical activity daily with aerobic activity being the major component and stress on muscle strengthening and bone strengthening activities at least thrice a week.
- However excessive physical activity, as seen in boys and girls training for competitive sports can hamper puberty.
- History of details and duration of physical activity is helpful to have an overall overview of the situation.

PHYSICAL EXAMINATION

Anthropometry is a very important part of physical examination.

Height

- Measurement of height at routine visits every 6 monthly/yearly and plotting it on growth charts is extremely useful.
- It gives the examiner an idea of growth trend, growth spurt and achievement of final adult height. Caution should be exercised while giving adult height

predictions based on trends on growth charts because, skeletal maturity progresses rapidly with puberty.

- Thus an adolescent may suddenly stop growing in spite of following a trajectory, if puberty is nearing completion.

Method of Height Measurement

- The subject stands straight against a stadiometer. Footwear should be removed. The back of the heels, buttocks, scapulae and occiput should be touching the vertical board behind.
- The eyes should be facing forwards with the line drawn from outer canthus of eye to tragus, parallel to the horizontal plane.
- The examiner must then apply gentle pressure over the mastoids to assess the actual height, and measure till the last mm at the level of the measuring board.
- See Figure 2.1.2 for method of height measurement.

Weight

- Weight is usually measured at clinic visits.
- It should also be plotted on growth chart and interpreted in relation to the height.

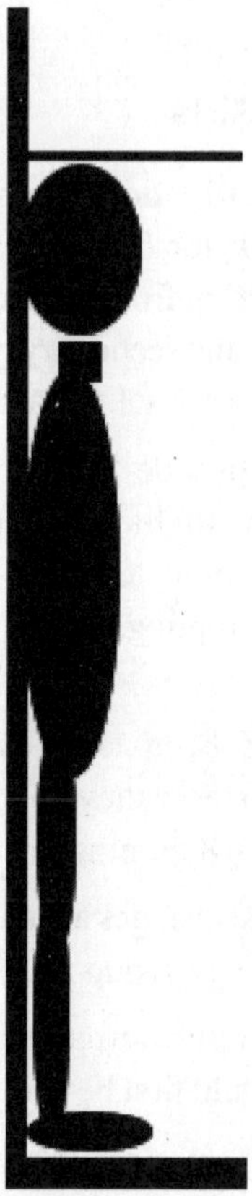

Figure 2.1.2: Measurement of height using stadiometer

- An upward trajectory of weight is a warning bell for active efforts to be taken to control weight.
- Similarly a downward trajectory from the normal may be a sign of an underlying illness like anorexia nervosa, hyperthyroidism, diabetes or systemic illness.

BMI (Body Mass Index)

- Body mass index = weight (kg)/height $(m)^2$.
- It is a better indicator of overweight and obesity than weight alone as it takes into account, weight in relation to height.
- Critical BMI is necessary for normal puberty, due to permissive role of Leptin and other energy availability markers at the level of hypothalamus to generate GnRH pulses to start puberty.
- Thus girls with anorexia nervosa or low BMI may face problems in pubertal progression. Similarly young obese girls may go early into puberty.
- To assess physical growth in childhood and puberty, age and community appropriate percentile charts are of paramount importance. Indian children's growth spurt during pubertal years appears relatively less pronounced as compared to their Caucasian counterparts. The Indian Academy of Pediatrics in 2015 have revised growth references to assess modern Indian children's growth parameters (Refer to Chapter 11.1 to 11.4 (Annexure) for growth charts).

General Examination

Scalp

Increased sebaceous secretion may lead to oily scalp, hair fall and seborrheic dermatitis.

Face

- Acne over forehead and cheeks is a common occurrence.
- Appearance of dark, coarse hair over face in boys indicates final stage of beard growth. There is a wide inter-individual variability in terms of hair distribution, density of hair and frequency of shaving amongst boys and all are usually within the normal population limits.

Hirsutism

- Male pattern of hair growth in a female is hirsutism which is usually caused by androgen excess in a girl.

- Hirsutism specially in obese adolescent girls should be monitored and investigated for an element of polycystic ovarian disease or non-classical CAH in light of history of irregularity of menstrual periods.

Neck

- Pubertal goiter is commonly seen in girls of pubertal age.
- This is due to overactivity of the thyroid gland to meet the increased requirements of pubertal years.
- However in the presence of goiter, assessment of thyroid function and antibody measurement is necessary to rule out autoimmune hypothyroidism, a common entity at this age.

Trunk

Gynecomastia in Boys

- Pubertal gynecomastia is commonly seen in boys in mid-late puberty.
- It may be unilateral or bilateral and usually less than 3-4 cm. This occurs due to peripheral conversion of testosterone to estrogen which acts on the glandular tissue leading to gynecomastia.
- An element of lipomastia often coexists in obese boys.
- Rarely, it may be an indicator of an underlying testicular neoplasm, Klinefelter syndrome or concomitant medication use.
- Most boys need reassurance and periodic reevaluation.
- Those with gynecomastia > 5 cm, or persisting for > 18 months and causing significant psychological trauma, will need careful evaluation, trial of medical treatment or cosmetic surgery.

Horizontal and Vertical Striae

- Horizontal pale to pink scars (stretch marks) are often seen over the lower back and shoulder in boys who have had a rapid and large growth spurt due to rapid growth of trunk.
- Rapid gain of weight leads to appearance of striae over lower abdomen, hips and thighs, commonly seen in obese adolescents.

Stigmata of Syndromes and/or Systemic Illness

Turner Syndrome

Short stature and failure of onset or progression of puberty may be the only apparent signs of Turner syndrome in girls. If these are present, examine for other signs such as antimongoloid slant of eyes, ptosis, nevi, webbing of neck, low posterior hair line, heart murmur, difference in upper limb-lower limb blood pressures, wide carrying angle, Madelung deformity and hyperconvex nails.

Chronic Systemic Illness

Jaundice, organomegaly, signs of vitamin deficiencies in malabsorption syndromes, signs of cardiac failure, knock knees seen in chronic renal failure and hypophosphatemic rickets etc. should be looked for.

EXAMINATION OF PUBERTY

- Before starting examination, it is a good idea to ask the adolescent especially if older, if he/she would like a parent accompanied during examination.
- Ideally a chaperone should be present during examination.
- A quick and informal examination is easier and less traumatic for the adolescent, as long as it provides all the necessary information to the examiner.
- For examination of axillary hair, ask the adolescent to place both hands over the head, this enables a quick examination of the presence and coarseness of axillary hair.

Examination in Girls

- Examination can be done in sitting or lying down position, to look for breast development, with the examiner inspecting from the front and side profile to identify primary and secondary mound and contour of breasts. See Figure 2.1.1 for assessing Tanner stage.
- Using the stethoscope to listen to the chest gives an opportunity to have a quick look as well. During examination, look for breast staging, skin discoloration, dimpling, lumps and discharge from nipples.
- Asymmetry of breasts is common and needs reassurance as usually they will become symmetrical over a period of 18 months to 2 years.
- Fibrocystic breast changes are the most common cause of lumps in this age group and are usually benign.
- For examination of external genitalia in girls, breast examination should first be completed, with the chest covered.
- Distribution of pubic hair is looked at to define stage of pubarche.

- If there are concerns of androgenization, clitoromegaly should be looked for.
- Ask for mother's help with undressing and assistance to look for clitoromegaly.
- No other examination is usually needed for adolescent girls if there are no concerns.
- Leucorrhea, a whitish watery vaginal discharge may be seen in girls before their first period and is physiological.
- In older girls, presence of vaginal discharge may need gynecological referral to rule out vaginitis.

Examination in Boys

- Examination of external genitalia in boys can be done in standing or lying down position.
- A prior discussion of the examination procedure with the adolescent helps in allaying anxiety and resulting cooperation during examination.
- It may be difficult to examine the testes in an anxious adolescent, wherein both testes might retract on attempt to palpation.
- The development of penis and scrotum is assigned a pubertal stage. See Figure 2.1.1 for Tanner staging.
- Young boys may have concerns regarding size and shape of their penis (average length 5-15 cm), which may need reassurance by the examiner.
- Those with hypospadias should be asked regarding curvature (chordee) which may need surgical intervention.
- Varicoceles may be present, usually unilateral and need no intervention unless large as they may affect spermatogenesis.
- Presence of hydrocele needs examination of inguinal hernia and appropriate referral.
- Persistence of phimosis (inability to retract foreskin over glans) during puberty with complications like paraphimosis (wherein, the foreskin is retracted tightly around the glans causing edema and pain due to restriction of blood supply) will need surgical intervention.
- Testicular volume is measured by holding the testes between the index finger and thumb and comparing it with beads of Prader's orchidometer.
- Obese adolescents are often brought with suspected micropenis. A careful examination reveals a normal sized penis buried in subcutaneous fat. It usually needs reassurance and monitoring for pubertal progression.

Important points to remember in history taking and physical examination are summarized in Table 2.1.5 in girls and Table 2.1.6 in boys.

INVESTIGATIONS

Adolescents progressing normally through puberty do not need investigations. Only those who have some concerns either on history or examination need further investigations.

- *Hemoglobin:* Girls having menorrhagia are at risk of iron deficiency anemia. Routine hemoglobin estimation is helpful to guide treatment if needed.
- *Thyroid function tests with anti-thyroid peroxidase (TPO) antibodies:* If presence of goiter or positive history.
- *Celiac screen*: If anemic, having abdominal complaints, not gaining weight.
- Vitamin D may be measured if suspected deficiency, need to be supplemented with vitamin D during growth.
- Investigations to diagnose chronic illness, if positive findings on history and examination.

MONITORING AND MANAGING PUBERTY

An annual review during a clinic visit will suffice if no other concerns:

- Healthy eating and avoidance of high calorie junk food.
- Ensure adequate calcium and vitamin D intake.
- Encourage physical activity.
- Approach medical care if any concerns regarding physical changes or psychosexual issues.
- Ongoing support and monitoring of puberty.

Physicians dealing with pubertal issues need to do counseling to the parents and adolescents themselves.

Mothers of Adolescent Girls

- Mothers of girls should be encouraged to talk to their daughters at peripubertal age, regarding the changes of puberty, being experienced by them.
- Mothers may need support and information on these issues which can be provided by the practitioner.
- With breast development, girls may need supportive inner wear. This may bring mixed reactions amongst girls, with some excited towards change to womanhood while others embarrassed about it especially if

Table 2.1.5: Important points to remember: History taking and physical examination in girls

Physical signs	*Comments*
Onset of thelarche Puberty begins with the appearance of breast buds (B2). Girls often complain of soreness or tenderness on one or both sides. Time since when supportive inner wear is being used is also a useful history to judge the stage of breast development.	The breast bud stage is associated with growth spurt. This is followed by development of a primary mound (B3). Subsequent development of the areolae and nipples and formation of the secondary mound (B4). Finally the contour of the adult breast.
Onset of pubarche/adrenarche This is followed by appearance of pubic and axillary hair a few months later. Ask mother and adolescent–approximate time when they were first noticed.	Breast development and hair growth progress together. Ask for texture and density of hair—few or many, fine downy or coarse black and curly, and extension to pubic triangle.
Onset of menarche Menstruation ensues about 18 to 30 months later. The onset of menarche heralds the completion of puberty. It is important to note the date of first menstrual period.	It signifies the completion of growth spurt, and the height gain after this is usually minimal. The first menstrual bleed is variable from spotting to frank bleeding for few days. It may take 18 months to 2 years for the periods to regularize.
Body odor	History of an increased tendency to sweat and body odor is commonly seen as a marker of adrenarche. The spectrum may be variable, with some parents and children finding it distressing, while others hardly noticing it.
Acne	The occurrence of acne on face is commonly seen and causes a lot of distress amongst young adolescent girls. These may wax and wane with time. If absent at the time of consultation, history might be helpful.
Pubertal growth spurt It happens in the early pubertal stages (2-3) in girls.	This usually coincides with the growth spurt of puberty and often noticed by parents. Height gain is very slow in later stages of puberty in girls and minimal after onset of menarche. Thus it is an important piece of information that helps in assessing the growth already done and the remaining potential.
Psychosocial changes and emotional lability	Changes in external appearance and hormonal milieu lead to social and emotional changes. Mothers usually notice these changes in girls with estrogenization. Girls usually become more conscious of their self and surrounding with emphasis on specific dressing, grooming and behavioral changes. Mood swings and emotional lability is commonly seen.

younger. Mothers need to learn sensitive handling of the situation and support is important.

- An important aspect mothers need to discuss is menstruation. Many concerns in adolescent girls are related to menstruation. The first period can be a matter of distress and surprise to most girls. These discussions should begin once breast development has started as some girls may achieve menarche earlier than others. Information leaflets can be helpful. Some practitioners arrange special educational visits for the peripubertal age group to support their needs.
- ***For more about normal menstruation and menstrual hygiene please see Chapter 2.4.***
- With progression of hair growth to thick curly adult stage in pubic area, axillary regions and on legs. Due to effect of media most girls wish to remove body hair. Mothers need to help girls to make a choice about method of hair removal. If shaving is opted for advice regarding use of warm water, soap and a clean razor, avoid sharing with other members should be stressed. Care of personal hygiene in beauty parlors should be advised.

Table 2.1.6: Important points to remember: History taking and physical examination in boys	
Physical signs	***Comments***
Onset of puberty usually begins with testicular enlargement (testicular volume 4 ml) and enlargement of scrotal sac with thinning and reddening of scrotal skin.	This stage lasts for a few months.
Onset of pubarche/adrenarche Pubic hair usually appears at the base of the penis after the start of testicular and scrotal enlargement and spread over pubic triangle. Axillary hair growth also increases from fine downy hair to thick, coarse and curly hair.	There is gradual increase in length followed by increase in both length and breadth of the penis. Pubic hair increase in number, thickness, become curlier and spread over the pubic triangle, inner aspect of thigh and abdomen.
Changes in external genitalia An overall history of whether "there are changes down below" of an adult man gives an idea of onset and progression of puberty.	A pictorial representation of Tanner staging using charts may be helpful. However it is important to remember that boys usually over-rate their puberty while girls tend to under-rate their pubertal stage.
Ejaculations Often nocturnal, they begin at around 13 years of age (SMR stage 3).	Onset of involuntary erections in sleep at night and early morning is normal.
Breast Boys may also develop soreness of their nipples and some breast development. This may be pubertal gynecomastia, a common occurrence during SMR stage 3-4, or lipomastia secondary to obesity.	The condition needs close monitoring and may need referral to a pediatric endocrinologist.
Voice change and Adam's apple prominence	With the increasing size of larynx and vocal cord thickening, breaking of voice begins in mid-late puberty and results in final deepening of voice and prominence of Adam's apple. It may be difficult for the examiner to notice this if the boy is seen for the first time. Asking parents if they have noticed a change in voice is helpful. This stage usually occurs late in puberty and suggests it is nearing completion.
Body odor	The rise in androgen levels changes the fatty acid composition of sweat resulting in an adult body odor which can be a problem in young boys. Use of deodorants and maintenance of personal hygiene is important.
Acne	Acne commonly occurs during all stages of puberty. Sebum secretion increases under influence of androgen. This along with blockage of sebaceous glands, results in blackheads, whiteheads and acne. Frequent washing of face and hygiene is useful.
Pubertal growth spurt Unlike girls, growth spurt in boys occurs at later stages (stage 3 and 4) of puberty.	They grow with a greater spurt (10-12 cm/year) as compared to girls to achieve an adult height. History of perception of one's height as compared to peers in class, rapid change in shoe size and outgrowing clothes are suggestive of growth spurt.
Psychosocial changes and emotional lability	As in girls, changes in external and internal milieu lead to behavioral changes in boys as well. A major contributor to many social issues is lack of cognitive and emotional maturity. Cognitive immaturity results in poor judgement, hasty and impulsive decisions. Emotional immaturity leads to poor control of emotions and emotional outbursts. These are a part of puberty and need a sensitive approach.

Counseling of Fathers of Boys

- Fathers may need to help their boys understand changes of puberty with appropriate help from health care providers.
- Some boys may be more comfortable talking to the father while some with the mother.
- With the onset of pubertal changes, pre-adolescent and adolescent boys tend to become more conscious about themselves and modest while bathing or changing clothes.
- Respecting their privacy becomes important.
- While maintaining privacy, it is important to monitor the pubertal changes, keeping in mind the wide variation in onset and progression of puberty amongst boys.
- Conversations become more of discussions rather than unilateral talks.
- Good natured teasing should be avoided as it can embarrass boys easily at this age.

Counseling Adolescent Girls and Boys

- It is important for adolescents to understand these physical, sexual and emotional changes.
- Emphasize that these changes are normal and occur due to hormones produced in their bodies.
- Reassuring that while they may start at a different time as compared to peers, all will finally reach the adult stage and these variations are normal.
- Adolescents are extremely self-conscious at this stage and understanding this is important.

LEARNING POINTS

- Puberty is a tumultuous phase in the life of an individual.
- A close watch on its progression and adequate support during this phase is of paramount importance for the physical and mental health of these young adults.
- Assessment of puberty encompasses history of changes noticed by self or parents, presence of chronic illness, family history of timing of puberty and any abnormality of tempo of puberty noticed.
- Early or delayed puberty needs referral to an endocrine expert.
- Examination involves a thorough general examination as well as sexual maturity rating to assess stage of puberty.
- For those children who do not have any concerns of puberty and are hesitant to have a formal clinical examination a self assessment of pubertal staging using pictorial chart is helpful.
- Awareness among medical professionals regarding pubertal issues faced by adolescents and ways of dealing with them is important.
- Common pubertal problems include acne, excessive body odour, hirsutism, pubertal gynecomastia, asymmetrical breast development and menstrual irregularity.
- Sensitive approach with due respect to their privacy and opinions is key to effective management of various issues at this stage.

SUGGESTED READING

1. Blakemore SJ, Burnett S, Dahl RE. The role of puberty in the developing adolescent brain. Hum Brain Mapp 2010;31(6):926-33.
2. Bridges NA, Cooke A, Healy MJ, Hindmarsh PC, Brook CG. Growth of the uterus. Arch Dis Child 1996;75:330-31.
3. Kaplowitz PB, Slora EJ, Wasserman RC, Pedlow SE, Herman-Giddens ME. Earlier onset of puberty in girls: Relation to increased body mass index and race. Pediatrics. 2001;108(2):347-53.
4. Marshall WA, Tanner JM. Variations in pattern of pubertal changes in girls. Arch Dis Child 1969;44(235):291-303.
5. Menon PSN, Ammini A. Normal puberty. In: Pediatric Endocrine Disorders. Eds. Desai M, Bhatia V, Menon PSN. Chennai; Orient Longman; 2001.
6. Rathi N, Rathi A. Vitamin D and Child Health in the 21st Century. Indian Pediatr 2011;48(8):619-25.
7. Rogol AD, Roemmich JN, Clark PA. Growth at puberty. J Adolesc Health 2002;31(6 Suppl):192-200.
8. Tanner JM, Whitehouse RH. Clinical longitudinal standards for height, weight, height velocity, weight velocity, and stages of puberty. Arch Dis Child 1976;51:170-79.
9. Terasawa E, Guerriero KA, Plant TM. Kisspeptin and puberty in mammals. Adv Exp Med Biol 2013;784:253-73.
10. Westwood M, Pinzon J. Adolescent male health. Paediatr Child Health 2008;13(1):31-36.

Issues in Growth

2.2.1

PSN Menon, M Vijayakumar

INTRODUCTION

Our young generation is increasingly concerned about the physical appearance, thanks to media, sports, cinema, modeling, fashion shows and beauty contests. It is not uncommon for parents and/or adolescents to seek medical consultation regarding stature and pubertal development. According to the recent Indian standards based on multicentric studies, the Indian adolescents still lag behind their western counterparts in stature (see Chapter 2.1 and Annexures 11.1 to 11.4). Adult stature is around the 10–20th percentile of Center for Disease Control (CDC-USA) growth charts. It is possible that the secular trend for growth for our population is still unfinished. Or this may be the true ethnic difference of Indians from Western adolescents. The physician caring for adolescents should be conversant about the growth charts that he/she is following.

SHORT STATURE

Short stature is defined as height below 2 standard deviations or below 3rd percentile of the mean of national standards for age and sex. Growth velocity below 25th percentile is also considered as short stature. Many disease processes, both endocrine and non-endocrine, may affect the growth of the adolescent adversely. Most chronic systemic diseases result in short stature. Accurate and serial measurement of growth parameters is of paramount importance to assess the growth status during this period (see Chapter 2.1 for details).

The various causes of short stature are listed in Table 2.2.1.1. Which adolescents require evaluation is listed in Box 2.2.1.1.

HISTORY TAKING

History should start from antenatal period, since growth faltering starts in utero in majority of cases.

- Birth weight and length are important.
- If the adolescent was born small for gestation (SGA), the underlying cause can be traced in intrauterine period (may be a genetic syndrome or intrauterine infection).

Table 2.2.1.1: Causes of short stature in adolescents
1. Physiological short stature
• Genetic or familial short stature (FSS) • Constitutional delay in growth and puberty (CDGP)
2. Disorders with underlying pathology/etiology
• *Malnutrition:* Inadequate intake, malabsorption (Celiac disease, Crohn's disease), vitamin D or mineral (iron, calcium, zinc) deficiencies • *Children born small for gestational age (SGA):* Intrauterine growth retardation, Russell-Silver syndrome, 3M syndrome
Chronic systemic diseases
• Gastrointestinal and hepatobiliary: Chronic hepatic disorders, chronic inflammatory bowel disease • Renal: Chronic renal failure, renal tubular acidosis • Cardiovascular: Congenital cardiac diseases • Pulmonary: Cystic fibrosis, infections, bronchial asthma • Hematology: Hemolytic anemia, nutritional anemia
Chronic infections: Malaria, HIV, tuberculosis, parasitic disorders
Endocrine disorders
• Disorders of the hypothalamic–pituitary-GH-IGF-1 axis leading to growth hormone (GH) deficiency or hypopituitarism or panhypopituitarism: ♦ Congenital GH deficiency ♦ Acquired GH deficiency due to post-radiation or chemotherapy, post-neurosurgery, trauma, infections ♦ IGF-1 deficiency ♦ GH insensitivity
• *Hypothyroidism:* Late onset congenital forms, chronic lymphocytic thyroiditis • Adrenal: Cushing syndrome • Disorders of puberty • Hypoparathyroidism and pseudohypoparathyroidism • Disorders of vitamin D metabolism
Genetic/Syndromic disorders: Turner syndrome, Down syndrome, Noonan syndrome, Prader-Willi syndrome, Aarskog syndrome, Neurofibromatosis, DiGeorge syndrome, Neural tube defects
Metabolic disorders and skeletal dysplasia
Malignancies (Hematologic): Post-therapy
Psychosocial/Stress factors
Chronic medications: Glucocorticoids, High dose androgens/estrogens, Medications used for ADHD
3. Idiopathic short stature

Box 2.2.1.1: Who needs evaluation?

- An adolescent needs evaluation for short stature if his/her height is below the 3rd percentile or below 2 SD of the mean of the growth standards.
- Adolescents who are significantly short for their midparental height (MPH) or target height (TH) even if they are within the normal percentiles should also be evaluated on the same lines.
- Adolescents within normal height percentiles but with a height velocity less than 25th percentile over a period of observation for 6 to 12 months or crossing down two major percentiles also merit evaluation.

- History of neonatal hypoglycemia or hyperbilirubinemia is a clue for hypopituitarism.
- History of developmental delay or learning disabilities should be sought for (e.g. hypothyroidism, Down syndrome).
- Detailed nutritional history for finding out evidence of macro- and micronutrient deficiencies should be recorded.
- An account of pubertal pattern of both the parents is essential.
- Various clues to rule out any systemic disease will also be obtained from a careful history (e.g. chronic or recurrent cough, persistent diarrhea, jaundice, polyuria, breathlessness and bluish discoloration of tongue).

Psychosocial Short Stature

It is important to remember that emotional factors also affect growth and hence psychosocial history taking is important, to rule out psychosocial short stature.

- Growth is adversely affected by hostile social or environmental conditions like parental disharmony, divorce and, lack of affection from the care givers.
- Growth can resume once these adverse conditions are removed.

These are discussed elsewhere in the book (see Sections 3, 5 and 8).

PHYSICAL EXAMINATION

Careful clinical examination is necessary to rule out clinical conditions:

- Physical signs for chronic systemic diseases: pallor, cyanosis, clubbing, hypertension, heart murmur or hepatosplenomegaly.
- Macro- or micronutrient deficiency: wasting, bow legs and Bitot's spots.
- Endocrine disorders:
  - Hypopituitarism: Doll like face, single central incisor tooth and micropenis
  - Hypothyroidism: Coarse facial features, abdominal distension, dry skin and goiter
- Genetic syndromes: Webbing, shield like chest, wide carrying angle and simian crease.

Anthropometric Parameters and Puberty

Height, weight, body mass index, arm span, upper segment to lower segment ratio and plotting a growth chart are essential. This has to be compared with midparental height (MPH). These are detailed in Chapter 2.1.

During pubertal age the following is very important:

- Measurement of testicular volume (< 4 ml is prepubertal).
- Stretched penile length.
- Staging of puberty by Tanner charts (pubic hair and breast development); see Chapter 2.1 for details.

The major clinical features of physiological and idiopathic short stature are provided in Box 2.2.1.2 and pathological forms in Boxes 2.2.1.3 and 2.2.1.4.

INVESTIGATIONS

The number of tests the adolescent undergoes for evaluation of short stature differs from center to center. The cost economics of these tests makes it imperative that careful anthropometry is the ultimate decider as to who needs detailed evaluation and management. A panel of screening tests is suggested only when no clinical pointer to the diagnosis exists. Investigations should be tailor made based on history and clinical examination findings.

Table 2.2.1.2 lists the screening or level 1 investigations frequently performed.

Box 2.2.1.2: Physiological and idiopathic forms of short stature

Constitutional Delay in Growth and Puberty (CDGP)

- CDGP is probably the most common cause of short stature and pubertal delay.
- History of retarded linear growth in the first 2-3 years of life; but resume normal growth thereafter.
- Review of the growth records shows a growth pattern below the 3rd centile of standard growth curves.
- Typically they have delay in the onset of pubertal growth spurt *(late bloomers).*
- They continue their linear growth till puberty is completed, getting more time for their growth.
- Final adult height is within normal ranges; but remains relatively short.
- Usually either of the parents might have had a similar growth pattern in childhood.
- The bone age is delayed, usually corresponding to the height age.

Familial Genetic Short Stature (FGSS)

- These adolescents have short stature with normal birth weight, normal growth velocity,
- Bone age corresponds to chronological age, predicted final adult height within the range of midparental height (MPH).
- Family history of short stature is often present; at least one of the parents is short. Extended family history is of great help.
- Growth pattern is below 3rd centile but parallel to the standard lines in the growth charts.
- Puberty is attained at an appropriate age.
- They finally land up as short adults.

Idiopathic Short Stature (ISS)

- A small group of adolescents remain short despite all interventions with no clear etiology evident on clinical evaluation and usual investigations.
- Their growth potential falls below the national standards.
- The height is below 2 standard deviations below the mean for the age, sex and population.

Box 2.2.1.3: Systemic forms of short stature in adolescents

Undernutrition

- This is one of the most important causes, especially in developing countries.
- Even if the patient has a primary hormonal/systemic disease, undernutrition may be a compounding factor, making the diagnosis more complicated.
- The weight age is more affected than height age and the adolescent has clinical features of *wasting.*
- They may also have features of associated *micronutrient deficiencies* like iron, calcium, zinc, and vitamin D, all contributing to slow linear growth (Refer to Section 3 for more details).

Chronic Systemic Illnesses

In any case of short stature, clinical features of an underlying systemic illness should be carefully looked for. Often the characteristic features may not be evident and short stature may be the only clinical manifestation. The most common among these conditions are:

- Malabsorption (celiac disease)
- Chronic anemia (hemolytic anemia or nutritional anemia)
- Congenital heart diseases (cyanotic and obstructive)
- Chronic lung diseases (asthma and cystic fibrosis)
- Chronic renal disease (chronic renal failure and renal tubular acidosis)
- Chronic liver diseases
- Chronic or recurrent infections (tuberculosis, HIV/AIDS infection, infestations (giardiasis)

In almost all of these conditions, *weight will be more affected than height,* manifesting as wasting. *Bone age shows a mild delay (1-2 years).*

Adolescents Born as Small for Gestational Age (SGA)

- Babies born with a birth weight or length below 2 standard deviations from the mean for gestational age are considered as SGA.
- Most of the SGA babies catch up their growth potentials by about 2 years, but at least 10% of them remain short.
- Russel-Silver syndrome is a prototype of SGA.

Many of them seek advice around adolescence about the possibility of gaining further height and possible growth hormone (GH) therapy.

Box 2.2.1.4: Endocrine and genetic forms of short stature in adolescents
Endocrine Disorders • Most congenital endocrine deficiencies manifest at an early age and newborn screening helps to pick up some at an early age. • It is not uncommon to diagnose an endocrine disorder manifesting at around puberty, often due to an acquired insult or as a late manifestation of an evolving congenital disorder. • Common among this group is *hypothyroidism* (due to chronic autoimmune thyroiditis or following ectopic thyroid) and rarely *hypopituitarism* (autoimmune disease, post-chemotherapy and radiation), or *Cushing syndrome*. • Here *linear growth is more affected than weight.* • *Bone age is markedly delayed* in hypopituitarism and hypothyroidism. • Careful clinical evaluation would show some of the characteristics of the hormone deficiency.
Genetic Syndromes and Skeletal Dysplasia • Most manifest in infancy and childhood; and many seek consultation again during adolescence. • A few genetic syndromes are associated with late onset growth retardation and the characteristic physical features and associated co-morbidities may not be evident e.g. Turner, Noonan, Down, Prader-Willi and Williams syndromes.

Table 2.2.1.2: Level 1 screening investigations for short stature

Tests	***Reasons***
Complete blood counts	To rule out anemia, infections and malignancy
ESR	To rule out chronic inflammatory and collagen vascular disorders
Protein, albumin: globulin ratio, transaminases	Index of nutrition and hepatic function
Blood urea, creatinine, venous blood gasses	To determine renal function and to detect renal tubular disorders
Calcium, phosphate, alkaline phosphatase	Hepatic and renal functions and rickets
Urine tests	Fresh urine for pH, osmolality, specific gravity: Renal tubular disorder, diabetes insipidus Sugar, protein and casts: Diabetes mellitus and urinary tract infections
Fasting blood sugar	To rule out diabetes mellitus and hypoglycemia
Stool tests	Fresh stool for parasites (giardiasis)
Imaging	• *X-ray of hands for bone age* preferably by Greulich and Pyle or Tanner Whitehouse method • *X-ray of skull for sella* (pituitary tumor) and suprasellar calcification (craniopharyngioma) • Other X-rays as required based on clinical evaluation

Table 2.2.1.3 lists the level 2 investigations further detection of a specific etiology. Adolescents with failure to thrive or poor weight for height should undergo studies for renal tubular acidosis and malabsorption (Table 2.2.1.3).

Table 2.2.1.3: Level 2 investigations for short stature

Tests	***Reasons***
Thyroid function tests	Total or free thyroxine (T4) and thyroid stimulating hormone (TSH): Hypothyroidism Anti-thyroid antibodies: Chronic autoimmune thyroiditis
Karyotyping	In girls with unexplained short stature to exclude Turner syndrome
Genetic studies	To detect Down or Prader-Willi syndromes
Morning cortisol	Suspected adrenal pathology
Provocative GH testing	To confirm GH deficiency
Cardiac evaluation	Echocardiography in Turner and Down syndromes
Ultrasound of abdomen	Detect renal malformations
Studies for renal tubular acidosis	Venous pH and bicarbonate, ammonium chloride or bicarbonate loading test
Studies for malabsorption	Celiac disease (D-xylose test, jejunal biopsy, anti-tissue transglutaminase [TTG] antibodies)
Brain imaging	Hypothalamus and pituitary in confirmed GH deficiency

In adolescents suspected with GH deficiency, GH stimulation testing should be done after sex steroid priming. Insulin-like growth factor-1 (IGF-1) and/or its binding protein-3 (IGFBP3) levels are often used as a screening test for GH deficiency. Details of GH testing are given in Box 2.2.1.5.

Box 2.2.1.5: Growth hormone stimulation test

- Priming with sex steroids is done in all children with bone age > 10 years
  - ♦ ***Boys:*** Depot testosterone 100 mg IM 3-5 days before the test
  - ♦ ***Girls:*** Ethinyl estradiol 50-100 µg/day (oral) for 3 consecutive days OR Premarin 5 mg (oral), the night before and morning of the test
- Thyroid function tests should be normal before the test
- All tests are done after an overnight fasting
- 2 standard provocative tests are recommended
- Stimulants used:
  - ♦ Insulin (0.05-0.1 IU/kg IV)
  - ♦ Clonidine (0.15 mg/m^2 PO)
  - ♦ Arginine (0.5 g/kg; maximum 30 g; in normal saline IV)
  - ♦ L-Dopa (250 mg in < 35 kg, 500 mg in > 35 kg; PO)
  - ♦ Glucagon (0.1 mg/kg IM)
- Sampling done at 0, 30, 60, 90 and 120 minutes
- Interpretation: Peak GH level following stimulation
  - ♦ < 5 ng/ml – Severe deficiency
  - ♦ 5-10 ng/ml – Mild to moderate deficiency
  - ♦ > 10 ng/ml – No deficiency

MANAGEMENT

- Specific therapy for short stature should be directed against its etiology especially if a treatable cause has been found.
- FGSS and CDGP: Adolescents and their families should be reassured about the absence of a disease. GH is not usually indicated in their management.
- Irrespective of the etiology, the importance of a balanced diet and healthy lifestyle with exercises should be advocated.
- Pediatricians have a great supportive role to play in the management of these adolescents.
- The pressure from the peers especially opposite gender and the family can often be very demanding and the teens may need the support of a professionally trained clinical psychologist.

The pros and cons of using growth hormone are discussed in Box 2.2.1.6.

Box 2.2.1.6: Growth hormone (GH) therapy

With the easy availability of GH and the claims about the benefits of GH therapy in various forms of short stature available through net, it is common to see adolescents (and their parents) seeking advice regarding GH therapy for short stature.

Indications: Apart from GH deficiency, recombinant human GH is indicated in:

- Turner syndrome
- Adolescents with SGA
- Prader-Willi syndrome (PWS)
- Idiopathic short stature (ISS)
- Noonan syndrome
- Chronic renal failure (CRF)

All other indications are considered experimental now according to EMA (European Medicines Agency) and FDA (USA).

Administration:

GH is given as daily subcutaneous injections at night.

The dose ranges from 25-50 µg/kg/day.

- The dose should be increased during puberty since physiological requirement of GH is more during this period.
- Treatment is continued till final height has been achieved.

Stopping therapy:

- Poor growth velocity—height gain < 2 cm per year and attainment of bone age of 14 years in girls and 16 years in boys—is usually considered as indications for stopping the treatment.

Adverse effects:

Usually GH is a well tolerated drug. Adverse effects are uncommon and include:

- Carpal tunnel syndrome
- Pseudotumor cerebri
- Slipped capital femoral epiphyses
- Glucose intolerance

Should GH Therapy be Given in Idiopathic Short Stature?

In practice affording parents are likely to ask for GH therapy. Surveys in USA and Europe have shown that many pediatric endocrinologists prescribe GH for short normal children.

The individual physician's decision is based on degree of short stature, growth rate, and degree of maturation in terms of bone age.

Other factors affecting such a decision was cost of therapy, family's expressed wishes, physician's belief about effect of short stature on child's well-being and potential benefit of such therapy.

The likelihood of prescription is high if the child's height was below 3rd percentile, bone age is normal and the child was male.

- The American Academy of Pediatrics (AAP) Committee on Drugs and Committee on Bioethics recommends GH for very short children whose ability to participate in basic activities of daily living is limited as a result of their short stature and who have a condition for which GH is effective.
- The follow-up studies showed that boys gain about 5 cm and girls about 6 cm by such long-term treatment.
- There is no relation between the increase in adult height with any anthropometric or biochemical markers.
- This means that we cannot at the moment predict which child will benefit with an increase in height and how much will be the gain following GH therapy.
- Prescription of GH should remain with a specialist who has experience in monitoring such therapy.

Box 2.2.1.7 details the use of other drugs in the management of short stature.

Box 2.2.1.7: Other drugs used for short stature

Testosterone/Estrogen:

- It is used in CDGP to increase height velocity and generate secondary sexual characters.
- It is usually administered as intramuscular (IM) injections, once a month in a dose of 50-100 mg for 3-6 months.
- Oral preparations are also available.
- Girls may be given ethinyl estradiol 5 microgram or conjugated estrogen (Premarin) 0.3 mg daily for 4 to 6 months.

Oxandrolone:

- It is an anabolic steroid is often prescribed for ISS and Turner syndrome.
- Usual dosage is 0.03-0.05 mg/kg/day from the age of 8-10 years onwards.

Low Dose Estrogen:

- Started early, has positive effects on growth.
- Pubertal induction is started at the age of 12 years, gradually increasing to adult dose within 4 years.

Gonadotropin Releasing Hormone (GnRH) Analogs:

- GnRH analogs block sex steroid production and thus delaying pubertal onset.
- It can result in an increase in adult height.
- In practice this has relatively a modest efficacy needing long term therapy.
- More height gain is seen in younger children with longer duration of treatment.
- Giving GnRH analog along with GH results in better final height.

Aromatase Inhibitors (Testolactone, Anastrozole or Letrozole):

- Probably more effective than GnRH analogs as they do not delay puberty in boys.
- However the safety data is scarce and therapy is considered experimental.

TALL STATURE

Tall stature is defined as height more than 2 standard deviations (97th percentile) above the mean for age, gender and population. Even though most cases are normal variants such as familial and constitutional, tall stature and height acceleration may be a clinical manifestation of underlying serious diseases such as Marfan syndrome or GH excess.

Most adolescents seeking advice for tall stature do not have any abnormality on evaluation. Common causes of tall stature are given in Box 2.2.1.8.

Box 2.2.1.8: Common causes of tall stature

- Familial (constitutional) tall stature
- Exogenous obesity
- Marfan syndrome
- Klinefelter syndrome
- Homocystinuria
- Hyperthyroidism
- Excess growth hormone (GH) secretion
- Beckwith-Wiedemann syndrome
- Androgen insensitivity syndrome (AIS)
- Androgen/estrogen deficiency

History Taking

History should include a detailed family history of tall stature.

- In familial tall stature, there are no abnormalities detected during physical examination and the bone age corresponds to chronologic age. Height of the subject is consistent with midparental height, whereas in pathologic tall stature, the adolescent's projected height greatly exceeds MPH.
- Evaluation of body proportions is very essential in the differential diagnosis. Those with Klinefelter syndrome and Marfan syndrome have decreased upper-to-lower segment ratio and their arm span is at least 5 cm more than height.
- Measurements of BMI and plotting on a BMI chart help to detect exogenous obesity associated with tall stature during pubertal period with mild bone age acceleration. But final adult height is not much affected because of early epiphyseal fusion.
- Several conditions have their own distinct clinical features.
  - Patients with Klinefelter syndrome have mental retardation, gynecomastia and small testes.
  - Marfan syndrome has arachnodactyly, ocular abnormalities (superotemporal lens subluxation) and cardiac anomalies.

- Homocystinuria shares many of the clinical features of Marfan syndrome, but lens subluxation is inferonasal.
- Beckwith-Wiedemann syndrome is associated with overgrowth, advanced bone age, macroglossia, omphalocele and hypoglycemia.
- Sotos syndrome (cerebral gigantism) is associated with excessive physical growth, large head size, and advanced bone age.

- Assessment of sexual maturity helps to differentiate tall stature caused by precocious or delayed puberty.
  - Precocious puberty is characterized by accelerated linear growth during childhood. But if untreated, because of accelerated skeletal maturation and early fusion of epiphyses, final adult height is compromised.
  - In contrast, delayed puberty will have short stature during childhood, but they attain final height later, continuing to grow even after pubertal age.

Investigations

- If history is suggestive of familial tall stature and physical examination is normal, investigations are not needed. Bone age evaluation is all that is needed in such cases.
- Chromosomal analysis is indicated if the clinical picture is suggestive of Klinefelter syndrome.
- Thyroid function tests are indicated in suspected hyperthyroidism.
- IGF-1 and IGFBP3 levels should be measured if clinical suspicion of GH excess is entertained.
- In such cases, an MRI of brain is essential to find out the status of pituitary gland.

Management

- Parents and the adolescent should be reassured in familial tall stature.
- In severe cases of tall stature (e.g. Marfan syndrome), a trial of sex steroids is tried in early puberty, to accelerate puberty and cause early epiphyseal fusion.
- In conditions such as GH excess, surgical removal of the causative lesion may be the only option.
- Somatostatin analogs (e.g. octreotide) or dopamine agonists (e.g. bromocriptine) are tried to suppress GH levels.

LEARNING POINTS

- Short stature is diagnosed when the height is below 2 standard deviations or below 3rd percentile of the mean of the growth standards for age and sex and/or height velocity below 25th percentile.
- CDGP is probably the most common cause of short stature and pubertal delay.
- It is important to remember that emotional factors also affect growth and hence psychosocial history taking is important, to rule out psychosocial short stature.
- In adolescents suspected with GH deficiency, GH stimulation test should be done after sex steroid priming. Insulin-like growth factor-1 (IGF-1) and/or its binding protein-3 (IGFBP3) levels are often used as a screening test for GH deficiency.
- The American Academy of Pediatrics (AAP) Committee on Drugs and Committee on Bioethics recommends GH for very short children whose ability to participate in basic activities of daily living is limited as a result of their short stature and who have a condition for which GH is effective.
- Tall stature is defined as height 2 standard deviation (97th percentile) above the mean for age, gender and population.
- Most adolescents seeking advice for tall stature do not have any abnormality on evaluation.
- In severe cases of tall stature (e.g. Marfan syndrome), a trial of sex steroids is tried in early puberty, to accelerate puberty and cause early epiphyseal fusion.

SUGGESTED READING

1. Backeljauw PF, Dattani MT, Cohen P, Rosenfeld RG. Disorders of growth hormone/insulin-like growth factor secretion and action. In: Sperling MA. Pediatric Endocrinology, 4th ed. Philadelphia: Elsevier/Saunders 2014; 291-404.
2. Bajpai A, Menon PS. Growth hormone therapy. Indian J Pediatr 2005;72;139-44.
3. Bajpai A, Kabra M, Gupta AK, Menon PS. Growth pattern and skeletal maturation following growth hormone therapy in growth hormone deficiency: Factors influencing outcome. Indian Pediatr 2006;43(7):593-99.
4. Bajpai A, Menon PS. Insulin like growth factors axis and growth disorders Indian J Pediatr 2006;73(1):67-71.
5. Cuttler L, Silvers JB, Singh J, *et al.* Short stature and growth hormone therapy: A national study of physician recommendation patterns. JAMA 1996;276:531-37.

6. Downie AB, Mulligan J, McCaughey ES, Straford RJ, Betts PR, Voss LD. Psychological response to growth hormone treatment in short normal children. Arch Dis Child 1996;75:32-35.
7. Editorial: On adult height of children with idiopathic short stature. N Engl J Med 1999;340:502-07.
8. Growth Hormone Research Society Consensus guidelines for the diagnosis and treatment of growth hormone (GH) deficiency in childhood and adolescence: Summary statement of the GH Research Society. GH Research Society. J Clin Endocrinol Metab 2000;85;3990-93.
9. Oberfiled SE, Growth hormone use in normal short children– A plea for reason. N Engl J Med 1999;340:557-59.
10. Rosenbloom AL, Connor EL. Hypopituitarism and other disorders of the growth hormone-insulin-like growth factor-1 axis. In: Lifshitz F. Pediatric Endocrinology; 5th ed. New York: Taylor and Francis Inc 2006; 65-99.

Issues in Pubertal Development

2.2.2

PSN Menon, M Vijayakumar

INTRODUCTION

Puberty is a critical period of development in an adolescent's life. The changes occurring in the hormonal milieu ensure not only acceleration in growth and gain in sexual maturity, but also the capacity for reproduction along with acquisition of peak bone mineral mass. Thus any delay or arrest in pubertal development would be harmful for health and well-being of an adolescent.

DELAYED PUBERTY

Late appearance of secondary sex characteristics is a major concern for most adolescents and is one of the common reasons for seeking medical attention.

- Often this leads to a sense of inferiority and associated psychological concerns.
- Adolescents with delayed puberty are often victims of harassment and bullying at school, play and sports activities.
- Constitutional delay in growth and puberty (CDGP) can affect academic performance and cause social problems in adolescents.
- The concern and fear of being left behind by their peers make them shy and withdrawn to the extent that some might not even seek professional help.

Age at onset of puberty varies in boys and girls and is influenced by genetic factors and ethnicity as well as environmental factors including nutrition, physical activity, and presence of illnesses especially endocrine disorders. In general, delayed puberty is defined as:

- Absence of enlargement of testes in boys (> 4 ml) by the age of 14 years or breast budding in girls by the age 13 years.
- Absence of menarche by the age of 16 years in girls.
- The term *'pubertal arrest'* is used to indicate lack of progress of puberty over two years or failure to complete the puberty (menarche in girls and complete genital development in boys) within 5 years after the onset of puberty.

Majority of cases are physiological and boys outnumber girls. Major causes of delayed puberty are listed in Table 2.2.2.1.

Table 2.2.2.1: Etiology of delayed puberty
A. Hypogonadotropic Hypogonadism (Low LH and FSH)
• Constitutional delay in growth and puberty (CDGP)
• *Genetic and syndromic causes:*
♦ Kallmann syndrome
♦ Multiple pituitary hormone deficiencies
♦ Prader-Willi syndrome
♦ Biedl-Bardet and Laurence-Moon syndromes
♦ CHARGE association
• *CNS tumors:* Craniopharyngioma, optic nerve glioma, pituitary tumors, Langerhans histiocytosis
• Post-infections: Meningitis, encephalitis
• Trauma, pituitary stalk transection
• *Malignancy:* Cranial irradiation, chemotherapy
• *Chronic systemic diseases:* Asthma, cystic fibrosis, inflammatory bowel disease, thalassemia, chronic renal diseases, diabetes mellitus
• *Endocrine:* Hypothyroidism, Cushing disease
• Malnutrition, anorexia nervosa
• Psychogenic, chronic stress
• Exercise
• *Drugs:* Corticosteroids
B. Hypergonadotropic hypogonadism (High LH and FSH)
• *Turner syndrome and its variants (in girls):* 45,X; 46,XX/45 X; 46,XY/45,X
• *Klinefelter syndrome and variants (in boys):* 47,XXY, 46,XY/47,XXY
• Ovarian dysgenesis
• *Primary ovarian failure:* Autoimmune, metabolic (galactosemia)
• Testicular dysgenesis
• *Genetic:* Noonan syndrome, Robinow syndrome
• Anorchia, cryptorchidism
• Defective testicular synthesis and action
• *Infections:* Mumps, orchitis
• Testicular irradiation, drugs

History Taking

The following points should be noted during the interview:

- Delayed puberty is often associated with short stature. A detailed history regarding the growth pattern of the adolescent since birth and pubertal development should be taken.
- It is important to know whether puberty failed to occur, or it began but failed to progress or even regressed.
- Detailed history to rule out any chronic or intermittent systemic illnesses that may delay the onset of puberty (functional hypogonadotropic hypogonadism), as well as use of medications, nutritional status, and psychosocial functioning.
- Excessive exercise (those participating in athletics and gymnastics).
- A family history, including childhood growth patterns and age at pubertal onset of the parents and siblings.
- Specific symptoms like sensation of smell (anosmia or hyposmia) and galactorrhea (e.g. Kallmann syndrome).
- Delayed cognitive development associated with obesity or dysmorphic features suggest an underlying genetic syndrome.
- Weight gain, slow growth and poor scholastic performance (e.g. hypothyroidism).
- Collecting previous and present anthropometric measurements (height and weight) and plotting in a growth chart will help in assessing the growth pattern.

Physical Examination

- Recording of the sexual maturity rating (SMR, see Chapter 2.1) according to Tanner staging along with measurement of testicular volume and stretched penile length in boys may help to confirm whether the pubertal changes have already taken place, thus re-assuring the adolescent and parents.
- Measurements of upper and lower segment may be helpful in excluding some genetic conditions (Klinefelter syndrome).
- Eunuchoid proportions strongly suggest hypo-gonadism.
- Look for any stigmata of a genetic syndrome (webbing of the neck, broad chest and wide carrying angle as in Turner syndrome; almond shaped eyes, obesity and clinodactyly in Prader-Willi syndrome).

Box 2.2.2.1: Major forms of delayed puberty

Constitutional delay in Growth and Puberty (CDGP, see Chapter 2.2.1)

- This is the most common cause of delayed puberty; it accounts for ~70% boys and ~30% girls with delayed puberty.
- We do not know what exactly causes CDGP; but it has a strong genetic basis.
- The normal pre-pubertal growth deceleration is prolonged and is believed to be due to slow development of GnRH pulse secretion.
- They will lag behind their peers in attaining secondary sexual characters and growth velocity (late bloomers).
- Affected boys are often more distressed by short stature than by delay in puberty.
- Major diagnostic features include:
  - Similar history of delayed puberty in parents or siblings.
  - Physical examination is unremarkable.
  - Bone age is slightly delayed, consistent with the extent of pubertal development.
  - Usually final height and pubertal development will be normal (at par with his/her peers).

Chronic Systemic Illness

- Chronic systemic illnesses affect pubertal growth spurt and final maturation by disturbing the physiologic function of growth and puberty.
- Medications used in these conditions (e.g. glucocorticoids, chemotherapy and radiation therapy) adversely affect the pubertal development and maturity.
- Associated nutritional deficiency also delays pubertal development.
- Examples include inflammatory bowel disorders, cystic fibrosis, diabetes mellitus, rheumatoid arthritis, thalassemia and leukemia (both during active disease and after completion of therapy) etc.

The major forms of delayed puberty encountered in common clinical practice include CDGP and those secondary to chronic systemic illnesses (Box 2.2.2.1).

It is not uncommon to see adolescents seeking advice with an endocrine or genetic disorder (Table 2.2.2.2). Classifying them on the basis of serum levels of sex hormones and gonadotropins would help to identify the etiology, advise appropriate management and for appropriate counseling. Girls with Turner syndrome may present with a history of amenorrhea without the characteristic physical findings (Box 2.2.2.2).

- While constitutional delay is more commonly seen in adolescent boys, gonadal pathology is more often detected in adolescent girls (around 40% compared to 10% in adolescent boys).
- Hypothalamic-pituitary defects account for nearly 30% and chronic systemic illnesses in about 10% of those presenting with pubertal delay in both groups.

Table 2.2.2.2: Endocrine and genetic causes of delayed puberty

Hypogonadotropic hypogonadism (Low LH and FSH)

- Pubertal delay is due to reduction or absent production of gonadotropins (LH and FSH) or its action.
- Isolated gonadotropin deficiency occurs as a feature of Kallmann syndrome associated with anosmia. Thus testing of smell is important in pubertal delay.
- It may be a part of syndromes like Bardet-Biedl, Laurence-Moon or CHARGE syndrome. Thus examination of all systems for possible abnormalities and dysmorphic features will help to make a diagnosis.
- Several genes, including *KAL1, FGF8 and FGFR1* are shown to be linked to this condition. Some are associated with other anterior pituitary hormone deficiencies.
- It may also be acquired, secondary to tumors, surgery, trauma or radiation involving brain or hypothalamic-pituitary region.

Hypergonadotropic hypogonadism (High LH and FSH)

- Delayed puberty associated with elevated serum LH and FSH is due to diseases causing gonadal insufficiency.
- Turner syndrome is the prototype in girls.
- They will have elevated FSH as early as 9-10 years of age.
- In boys, Klinefelter syndrome is the most common cause of this condition.
- In addition local radiotherapy, chemotherapy, or surgery can also lead to hypergonadotropic hypogonadism.

- Idiopathic hypogonadotropic hypogonadism (IHH) is characterized by low gonadotropin levels probably from GnRH deficiency.
- Kallmann syndrome is an example of IHH with absent or diminished sensation of smell (anosmia/hyposmia) and is an X-linked disorder.
- Prader-Willi syndrome is also a form of IHH caused by a deletion on the short arm of paternal chromosome 15 associated with mental subnormality and hyperphagia often with diabetes mellitus.
- Hypergonadotropic hypogonadism in adolescent girls may be due to Turner syndrome characterized by ovarian dysgenesis.
- The term pseudo-Turner syndrome or Noonan syndrome is used to describe those with features of Turner syndrome but with a normal karyotype, commonly seen in males.
- Klinefelter syndrome is characterized by an abnormal karyotype (47,XXY) with hypergonadotropic hypogonadism and testicular dysfunction in boys.

Box 2.2.2.2: Common genetic forms of delayed puberty

Klinefelter Syndrome (Figure 2.2.2.1)

- Klinefelter syndrome occurs in approximately 1 in 1000 males, and is the most common form of male hypogonadism.
- It is associated with the characteristic karyotype of 47,XXY.
- Children with Klinefelter syndrome often enter puberty normally but will have pubertal arrest.
- The clinical features include small, firm testes, impaired spermatogenesis, long legs but not long arms and gynecomastia.
- Prepubertally, patients can be detected by the disproportionate length of the extremities.
- Neurobehavioral abnormalities, primarily in language, speech, learning, and frontal executive functions, are common.
- Conditions associated with Klinefelter syndrome include aortic valvular disease, ruptured berry aneurysms, breast carcinoma and other malignancies such as acute leukemia, lymphoma, and germ cell tumors at any midline site; systemic lupus erythematosus; and osteoporosis.
- There is an increased risk of diabetes mellitus, thyroid disease, fatigue, varicose veins, and essential tremor.

Turner Syndrome (Figure 2.2.2.2)

- It is the most common form of hypergonadotropic hypogonadism in females.
- It is the syndrome of gonadal dysgenesis, a sporadic disorder with an incidence of 1 per 2500 live-born girls in which all or part of the second sex chromosome is absent.
- Turner syndrome may be recognized in the newborn period. Affected newborn infants may have cystic hygromas in the neck and lymphedema of the extremities.
- Other frequent features are short stature, distinct facies with micrognathia, a fish-mouth appearance, high-arched palate with dental abnormalities, epicanthic folds, ptosis, low-set or deformed ears, short neck with low hairline, webbed neck, and recurrent otitis media, often leading to impaired hearing.
- A broad, shield like chest leads to the appearance of widely spaced nipples, and the areolae are often hypoplastic.
- Skeletal defects include short fourth metacarpals and cubitus valgus (which may develop after birth), Madelung deformity of the wrist, genu valgum and scoliosis.
- There are extensive pigmented nevi, a tendency to keloid formation, and hypoplastic nails.
- Cardiovascular anomalies affect the left side of the heart and include coarctation of the aorta, aortic stenosis, and bicuspid aortic valves; the latter individuals are at risk for a dissecting aortic aneurysm.

Kallmann Syndrome

- The most common form of idiopathic hypogonadotropic hypogonadism (IHH) is characterized by anosmia or hyposmia resulting from agenesis or hypoplasia of the olfactory lobes or sulci in association with GnRH deficiency.
- Because affected individuals often do not notice impaired olfaction, testing with graded dilutions of pure scents is necessary.
- Mutations in *KAL1, FGFR1/FGF8, PROK2/PROKR2, NELF, CHD7, HS6ST1, WDR11 and SEMA3A* are associated with defects in neuronal migration, leading to Kallmann syndrome.
- Associated defects that may accompany Kallmann syndrome include cleft lip, cleft palate, imperfect facial fusion, seizure disorders, short metacarpals, pes cavus, neurosensory hearing loss, cerebellar ataxia and nystagmus, ocular motor abnormalities, unilateral or rarely bilateral renal aplasia or dysplasia, and bimanual synkinesia.

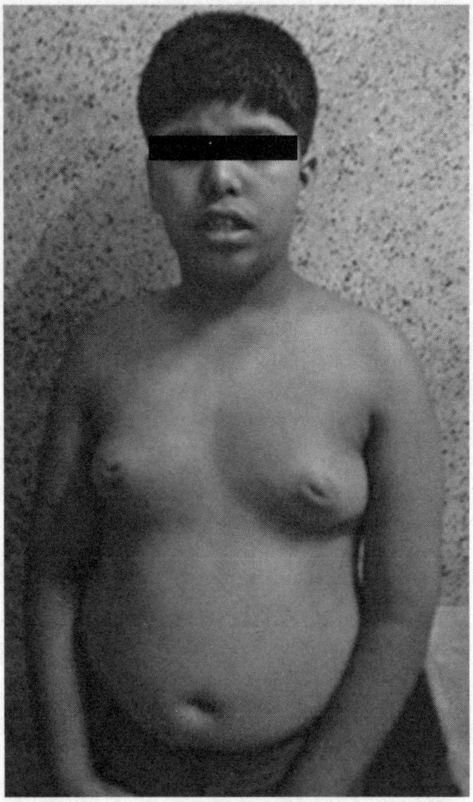

Figure 2.2.2.1: A 4-year-old boy with delayed puberty and gynecomastia. The karyotype was suggestive of Klinefelter syndrome (47,XXY)

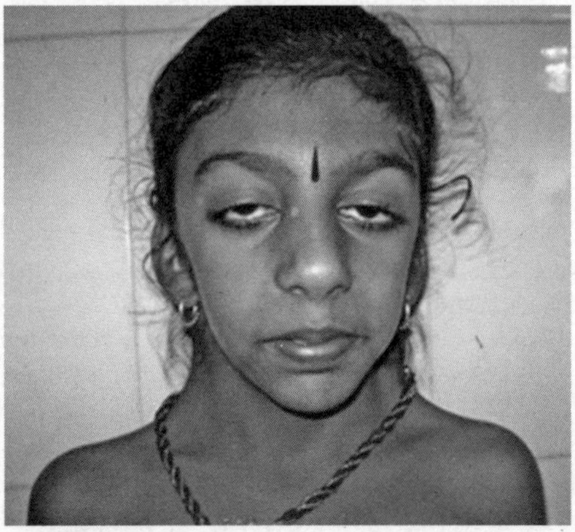

Figure 2.2.2.2: An adolescent girl with primary amenorrhea with hypergonadotropic hypogonadism. Note the features of Turner syndrome including webbing of neck, bilateral partial ptosis and low-set and abnormal ears

Investigations

- *Bone age:* Hormonal causes such as hypothyroidism and hypopituitarism produce marked delay in bone age. Constitutional delay in growth and puberty (CDGP) and chronic systemic diseases (see Chapter 2.2.1) produce slight delay in bone age.
- *Serum gonadotropins (LH and FSH) and sex hormones (testosterone in boys and estradiol in girls):* These tests help to differentiate the patients into hypogonadotropic (low LH and FSH and low sex hormones) and hypergonadotropic (high LH and/FSH with low sex hormones) hypogonadism.
- *Pelvic ultrasound:* This helps to visualize the internal genitalia especially in girls. In Turner syndrome streak ovaries are seen.
- *Genetic studies:* In Turner syndrome and Klinefelter syndrome, the karyotype is diagnostic. In Prader-Willi syndrome, methylation studies are helpful. Microarrays and next generation sequencing (NGS) help to detect many who cannot be clinically diagnosed.
- *MRI scan of brain* for pituitary gland is useful in many hypogonadotropic cases.
- *Thyroid hormone tests* (free or total thyroxine [T4] and TSH) should be performed in suspected cases of hypothyroidism.
- Serum IGF-1 levels may be done, especially if bone age is markedly delayed.
- The screening tests to rule out causes of functional hypogonadotropic hypogonadism should include the following: complete blood counts, ESR, kidney and liver function tests, serum electrolytes including bicarbonate, serum calcium, and phosphorus and screening for celiac disease in high risk groups.
- Differentiating CDGP from idiopathic hypogonadotropic hypogonadism (IHH) is often difficult. Serum total testosterone value > 50 ng/dL, GnRH agonist (triptorelin or luprolide) stimulated peak LH value > 14 IU/L and a hCG stimulated total testosterone increase of > 260 ng/dL suggest the diagnosis of CDGP. Serum inhibin B levels > 35 pg/ml is highly suggestive of CDGP. However, none of these tests are completely reliable for differentiating CDGP and IHH.

Management

- In case of chronic systemic illness, *management of the primary disorder* is of paramount importance. These include adequate treatment of bronchial asthma, transfusion with proper chelation in hemolytic anemia, surgical management of complex heart diseases, and nutritional support in undernutrition and anorexia nervosa.
- *Therapy with sex steroids* should be started if there are no signs of puberty by 14 years of age in boys and 13 years in girls. Treatment should be started at a low dose to begin with and then gradually increased over months to years.

- Many cases of *pubertal delay are secondary to CDGP.* In these cases, a small dose of *sex steroids* will act as a priming dose which will subsequently stimulate GnRH secretion. Treatment can be stopped in these children as soon as testicular volume is > 3 ml in boys or breast development has attained stage 3 in girls. In these children, further pubertal progress should be monitored closely.
- In boys, *testosterone preparations* (oral, injectable, and transdermal) are used as treatment. Testosterone injectable preparations are used in a dose of 25–50 mg once in 4 weeks. The dose can be gradually increased (if there is no response) by 25–50 mg at 6–12 month intervals over 3–4 years for full adult replacement (100 mg/week).
- In girls, treatment with *estrogen* produces development of secondary sexual characters and physical growth. Commonly used preparation is estradiol valerate. Conjugated estrogens (0.3 mg/day PO) or ethinyl estradiol (5 µg/day PO) can also be used. Transdermal preparations are also available. The dose can be gradually increased over months till breakthrough bleeding occurs. At this time cyclical progesterone (medroxyprogesterone) is added for 10–12 days in a month to the estrogen regime.
- *Girls with Turner syndrome* are managed with estrogen replacement and addition of cyclical progesterone at appropriate time. Addition of an anabolic steroid oxandrolone and growth hormone helps to improve short stature.
- *Boys with Klinefelter syndrome* require lifelong administration of testosterone, testicular prosthesis and in selected cases mastectomy for management of gynecomastia.

PRECOCIOUS PUBERTY

Precocious puberty is defined as appearance of secondary sexual characters before 8 years in girls and 9 years in boys. This condition is due to premature secretion of gonadal steroids. It can be central or gonadotropin-dependent precocious puberty, which is due to premature activation of hypothalamic-pituitary-gonadal (HPG) axis or be a peripheral or gonadotropin-independent type, as a result of gonadal steroid production from ovaries, adrenals or testes. It can also develop from excess steroids from exogenous sources. It may be a normal variant in some (premature thelarche and premature pubarche).

Gonadotropin-Dependent Precocious Puberty

- Majority of girls with this type of sexual precocity have no organic cause (90%).
- Younger the age, more the chance of underlying organic etiology.
- In boys, 90% will have an associated organic cause. Hence all boys with precocious puberty should undergo detailed investigation (Table 2.2.2.3).
- In older girls (> 6 years), chance of identifying an organic cause is very low even after extensive investigations.

Gonadotropin-Independent Precocious Puberty

- Here the secretion of sex steroids is independent of HPG axis.
- In males, familial testotoxicosis (male-limited gonadotropin-independent precocious puberty) is an autosomal dominant condition, due to premature Leydig cell and germ cell maturation.
- McCune-Albright syndrome (MAS) occurs in both sexes and is characterized by the triad of hyperpigmented macules with irregular edges, polyostotic fibrous dysplasia and endocrinopathies.
- Non-classic congenital adrenal hyperplasia (CAH) can present with precocious puberty.
- Adrenal and gonadal tumors can be virilizing or feminizing.
- Hypothyroidism can rarely present as precocious puberty.

Table 2.2.2.3: Causes of precocious puberty
A. Central (gonadotropin-dependent) precocious puberty
• Idiopathic
• *Congenital anomalies:* Septo-optic dysplasia, hydrocephalus
• *Brain tumors:* Hypothalamic hamartoma, optic nerve glioma
• *Post-infectious:* Meningitis, encephalitis
• Birth asphyxia
• Post-radiation, surgery, trauma
B. Gonadotropin-independent precocious puberty
• *Ovarian:* Cysts, tumors (virilizing/feminizing)
• McCune-Albright syndrome
• *Testes:* Testotoxicosis, testicular tumors
• *Adrenal:* Congenital adrenal hyperplasia, adrenal tumors (virilizing/feminizing), Cushing syndrome
C. Exogenous sex steroids administration
D. Hypothyroidism
E. Normal variants
• Premature thelarche
• Premature pubarche

Physical Examination

A carefully plotted growth chart is a must for evaluation.

- Tanner staging should be done separately for each parameter—Breast development and pubic hair development in girls and testicular and pubic hair development in boys.
- In boys testicular volume will be pubertal (> 3 ml) in gonadotropin-independent (peripheral) precocious puberty since HPG axis is not stimulated, testicular volume will remain pre-pubertal and corresponds to chronological age.
- Presence of neurocutaneous markers such as *café-au-lait* spots are seen in MAS or neurofibromatosis.
- Detailed neurological evaluation including fundus is a must in suspected intracranial pathology in young boys.
- Palpable abdominal mass may be an adrenal or ovarian tumor.

Investigations

- *Measurement of gonadotropins (LH and FSH) following GnRH stimulation:* A single IV bolus of GnRH is given and plasma LH and FSH are measured at 0, 20 and 60 minutes. Gonadotropin-dependent precocious puberty (central) is characterized by elevated LH (> 3-4 IU/L) and FSH (> 2-3 IU/L) with LH predominance. In premature thelarche, there is a predominance of FSH.
- *Neuroradiological imaging:* CT/MRI of brain is mandatory in all boys with precocious puberty and in girls > 6 years. In pre-adolescent girls, neuro-imaging is not a must.
- *ACTH stimulation test* is done in suspected non-classic CAH. Measurement of stimulated levels of 17α-hydroxyprogesterone is diagnostic of CAH.
- *Ultrasound abdomen:* Adrenal mass with < 5 cm size is usually benign. Autonomously functioning multiple leutinized follicular cysts of ovaries are seen in MAS.

Management

- Treatment is considered in children who show evidence of progression and the natural progress is leading to unwanted consequences.
- *Gonadotropin-dependent (central) precocious puberty:* Gonadotropin releasing hormone (GnRH) analog is the treatment of choice. Various preparations such as leuprolide acetate, triptorelin (monthly or 3-monthly), histrelin (implant) are being used for this purpose. Depot preparations are usually preferred.
- *Adrenal and gonadal tumors:* Surgical resection is the treatment of choice.
- *CAH:* Hydrocortisone and fludrocortisone should be administered in replacement doses.
- *Familial testotoxicosis:* Ketoconazole, aromatase inhibitors such as testolactone, anastrozole and spironolactone are used.

GYNECOMASTIA

- Gynecomastia is a benign enlargement of male breast as a result of proliferation of ductular elements.
- Breast enlargement due to excessive adipose tissue is called as lipomastia (pseudogynecomastia).
- Gynecomastia can be unilateral or bilateral and symmetric or asymmetric.
- About 50-60% of boys during puberty have some amount of breast enlargement.
- Usually it is physiological, but in rare occasion it may be a sign of an underlying endocrine or systemic disorder.
- Around 80% of physiological cases resolve within 1–2 years.

Pathophysiology

- Gynecomastia is characterized by proliferation of mammary ductules in a fibroconnective tissue stroma.
- Male breast tissue has androgen as well as estrogen receptors. Androgens inhibit and estrogen stimulates breast tissue proliferation.
- Gynecomastia results from either due to excess estrogen action or deficient androgen action (Table 2.2.2.4).
- During early pubertal period, there will be an initial rise in serum estrogen level compared to testosterone level, resulting in gynecomastia.
- During late puberty, adult androgen to estrogen ratio is established, leading to resolution of breast enlargement.
- During the early phase, ductal and epithelial proliferation occurs, with some inflammation and edema resulting in tenderness in some boys.

Table 2.2.2.4: Pathological causes of gynecomastia

A. Estrogen Excess	
Exogenous administration	• Dietary products–phytoestrogen, soy • Estrogen containing creams • Abused drugs–anabolic steroids (abuse for body building), marijuana, heroin, amphetamine
Endogenous production	• *Testes*–Leydig cell tumors, Sertoli cell tumors • *Adrenal gland*–Feminizing adrenal tumors
Increased aromatization	• Obesity • Hyperthyroidism • Liver diseases • Drugs
B. Androgen Deficiency	
Hypogonadism	• Klinefelter syndrome • Cancer chemotherapeutic drugs • Testicular radiation • Infection–Mumps orchitis • Drugs–Ketoconazole, spironolactone • Secondary hypogonadism –Pituitary or hypothalamic diseases
Decreased androgen action	• Drugs–Cimetidine, digoxin • Androgen insensitivity syndrome (AIS)

History Taking

- Many boys use anabolic steroids for body building. Some anabolic steroids are aromatized to estrogen resulting in breast enlargement.
- Illicit drugs like heroin or marijuana can also cause breast enlargement. Hence careful history of drug usage is a must.
- Take a detailed history and look for any signs of underlying chronic systemic diseases like liver disease or renal disease.

Physical Examination

- The first step is to differentiate true gynecomastia from lipomastia (pseudogynecomastia). Patient should be in lying position with his hands clasped beneath his head. Breast tissue is slowly compressed between the forefinger and thumb, beginning from the sides of the breast. In true gynecomastia, breast tissue can be palpated under the nipple areolar complex and it feels firm and rubbery (Box 2.2.2.3).
- Examination of both breasts is essential. Even though breast cancer is very rare in boys, it should be suspected when palpable masses are hard, fixed, associated with nipple discharge, skin changes or lymphadenopathy (Figure 2.2.2.3).
- Assessment of anthropometry including body mass index (BMI) is important. *Gynecomastia is a common finding in obese boys.* This is because of increased peripheral conversion of androgen to estrogen in the adipose tissue.
- Careful examination of the external genitalia should be done for documenting testicular size and detecting testicular masses.
- Degree of secondary sexual development should also be assessed.
- Partial (PAIS) and complete androgen insensitivity syndromes (CAIS) have varying degrees of genital underdevelopment.
- Palpable abdominal mass may be detected in adrenal tumors.
- On general examination, features of underlying chromosomal anomalies should be looked for.
- Tall eunuchoid habitus with small rubbery testicles is associated with Klinefelter syndrome.

Box 2.2.2.3: Clinical evaluation of gynecomastia–Essential steps
• Careful history to look for exogenous administration of drugs including anabolic steroids
• Careful palpation to rule out lipomastia
• Examination of both breasts
• Assessment of anthropometry, BMI and development
• Look for features of chromosomal anomalies and chronic systemic illness
• Examination of genitalia (Testicular size and consistency. Look for any ambiguity)

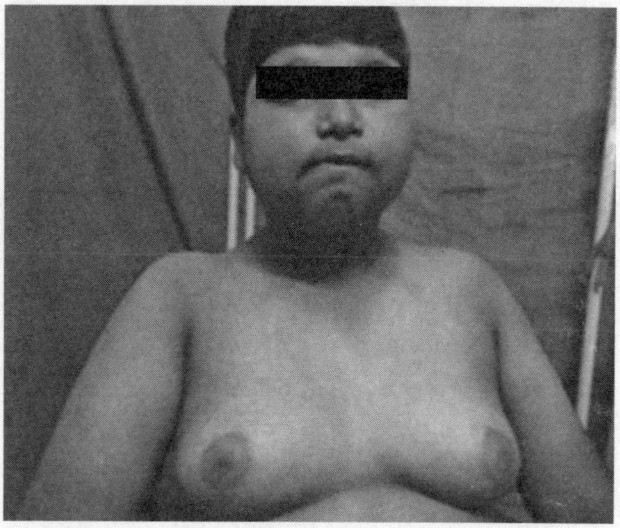

Figure 2.2.2.3: Adolescent idiopathic gynecomastia

Investigations

- If he has normal pubertal development and both history and physical examination do not reveal any abnormality, further investigations are not needed. He should be followed up regularly.

Management

- Pubertal gynecomastia does not require any treatment.
- Treatment of underlying disease and abstinence from the offending drug will result in reduction in breast size if a specific cause is detected.
- Clinical studies to evaluate the efficacy of certain drugs in decreasing the breast size in these children are ongoing.
- These include drugs which block estrogen effects in the breast tissue (anti-estrogens such as tamoxifen), decrease estrogen production (aromatase inhibitors such as testolactone and anastrozole) or androgens to suppress the effects of estrogen (non-aromatisable androgens like dihydrotestosterone, DHT). Till date, none of their effects are satisfactory.
- Various surgical options include liposuction or excision of glandular tissue by means of periareolar incision.

LEARNING POINTS

- Delayed puberty is more common in boys and majority have constitutional delay in growth and puberty.
- Delayed puberty in a girl requires more vigilant work-up since constitutional delay is uncommon. Genetic and chromosomal anomalies should be ruled out in them.
- Premature pubertal onset is much more common in girls than boys and majority is idiopathic.
- In boys, majority is associated with organic pathology and MRI of brain (pituitary and hypothalamus) is mandatory.
- The major clinical parameter used to differentiate central from peripheral precocious puberty is testicular volume.
- Treatment of precocious puberty is considered only when the early pubertal growth spurt affects the height and other characters of the patient.
- 50-60% boys will develop breast enlargement during pubertal growth spurt but many will get resolved within few years.
- Obese children will have lipomastia which should be differentiated from true gynecomastia by clinical examination.
- Careful history regarding the use of illicit drugs like anabolic steroids (for body building) is a must.
- General examination should include looking for any features of chromosomal disorders and chronic systemic illness.

SUGGESTED READING

1. Bajpai A, Menon PSN. Precocious puberty. In: Desai MP, Menon PSN, Bhatia V, eds. Pediatric Endocrine Disorders. 3rd edition. Hyderabad; Universities Press 2014;144-58.
2. Bajpai A, Menon PSN. Contemporary issues in precocious puberty. Indian J Endocrinol Metab 2011;15;172-79.
3. Colaco P. Precocious puberty. In: Gupta P, Menon PSN, Ramji S, Lodha R, eds. PG Textbook of Pediatrics, 1st edition. New Delhi; Jaypee Publishers 2015;2332-36.
4. Dickson G. Gynecomastia. American Family Physician 2012;85:716-22.
5. Johnson RE, Murad H. Gynecomastia: Pathophysiology, Evaluation and Management. Mayo Clin Proc 2009;84(11): 1010-15.
6. Laituri CA, Garey CL, Osttie DJ, St. Peter SD, Gittes GK, Snyder CL. Treatment of adolescent gynecomastia; J Pediatr Surg. 2010;45:650-54.
7. Menon PSN, Vijayakumar M. Precocious puberty–Perspectives on diagnosis and Management. Indian J Pediatr 2014;81(1): 76-83.
8. Narula HS, Carlson HE. Gynecomastia. Endocrinol Metab Clin N Am 2007;36:497-519.
9. Rosen DS. Delayed Puberty. Pediatrics in Review 2001; 22(9):309-15.
10. Sarathi V, Shah NS. Delayed puberty. In: Gupta P, Menon PSN, Ramji S, Lodha R, eds. PG Textbook of Pediatrics, 1st edition. New Delhi: Jaypee Publishers 2015;2328-31.
11. Virmani A. Gynecomastia. In: Gupta P, Menon PSN, Ramji S, Lodha R, eds. PG Textbook of Pediatrics; 1st edition. New Delhi; Jaypee Publishers 2015;2337-39.
12. Zacharin Z, Banerjee I. Delayed Puberty. In: Desai MP, Menon PSN, Bhatia V, eds. Pediatric Endocrine Disorders, 3rd edition. Hyderabad; Universities Press 2015;132-43.

Psycho-Social-Emotional Development

2.3

Sharad Agarkhedkar, Swati Y Bhave

INTRODUCTION

There is no standard definition of "adolescence". Chronological age is one way of defining adolescence. WHO defines adolescence to be between the ages of 10 and 19 years.

Adolescence is a very dynamic and important state of human development where a child has to transform into an adult. This leads to many changes happening at the same time in the physical, psychological, emotional and social environment. At physical level changes in puberty are often difficult to handle unless they are primed to understand the process. This leads to body image issues because they look gawky and awkward and have constant pressure of media to look cool and hep. Due to intense academic competition there is tremendous pressure in school and home for career choices and performance. Unless empowered with coping skills with programs like life skill education, it may become difficult for them to deal with various stresses and this increases the incidence of mental health issues like anxiety, depression and suicide. Adults tend to treat them as child or adult at varied times; this leads to confusion and identity crisis in the mind of the teens and leads to career pressures. The developing brain with its limbic preponderance leads to reward seeking and experimentation which results in high risk behavior compounded by peer pressure.

Most adults are not aware about the neuro-development and impact on adolescent behavior (see Chapter 1.8). They are also not aware about the psycho-emotional-social and sexual development of adolescence (see Chapter 4.1). Hence many parents and teachers have a lot of misunderstanding and misinterpretation of teen behavior, leading to conflicts at home and school. Clinicians need to educate teens themselves and parents and teachers through school and community programs (see Chapter 1.8).

Physical and hormonal changes during puberty also lead to psycho-social changes and directly affect not only the physical health parameters but also influence their final personality as an adult in the society. Biological and psychological changes of puberty are seen in all races and cultures, but psycho-social changes are culture specific and occur in the context of social environment. The tasks involved in social life move from dependence to independence, developing the adolescent's identity and maturation in the peer relationships. Some are very aggressive, others are very submissive.

Every adolescent goes through a confused state of mind:

- Who am I?
- What's the goal of my life?
- Am I capable enough?
- How will I sail through life? etc.

Their developing cognitive skills help to improve their abstract thinking and reasoning powers. Emotional development helps them to get a sense of personal identity. Social development helps them to relate to both peers and adults. They also develop greater sense of self awareness and their own set of moral values and ethics.

Adolescent development is divided into three phases: early (10-13 years), middle (14-16 years) and late (17-19 years) (Table 2.3.1).

PSYCHO-SOCIAL DEVELOPMENT

Most adolescents can go through these phases fairly smoothly, specially when they have a stable environment at home and school. If adults give them a positive psycho-social support, they also develop a positive self-esteem, which is a protective factor against risk-taking behavior. If an adolescent is different from peers by having early puberty (early bloomers) or late puberty (late bloomers), though they are still perfectly in the range of normalcy, it leads to lot of problems as he or she does not fit with peers. Unless educated about body changes that occur during puberty, many adolescents develop issues of body image which are more marked in girls and can also lead to eating disorders. Such adolescents need to receive timely counseling before it escalates into a mental illness. Boys who are early bloomers are at an advantage as they are bigger and stronger than peers. This can result in positive action–they assume and are being accepted as leaders. But it can also lead to aggression and bullying of others. An early bloomer girl has a "woman's mature body with a child's innocent mind". Such girls become targets of older

Table 2.3.1: Psycho-social changes in adolescence

Adolescence phase	*Psychological*	*Social*
Early (10-13 years)	Emotional lability, hot cognition. As they emotionally mature they want to become independent and this may lead to their being somewhat detached from the family. Body image issues may still be seen in some specially with late bloomers They are very conscious about self and feel. They are the focus of attention of everyone around Awareness of sexual identity Reward orientation	Peer identification begins, prefers peers Socially–Moves away from family Wants to avoid family get-togethers and outings Are curious about opposite sex but pretend to ignore opposite sex peers Their dressing sense, tattoos, hair styles, ear piercings etc. follow peer group pattern Sensation seeking exploratory behavior e.g. smoking Initiation of moral concepts
Mid (14-16 years)	Emotional separation continues. Wants to be left alone. Want privacy. Can put no-entry board on their doors Abstract thinking consider themselves invincible Verbal dexterity is increased Idolisation (Religious political) Period of heightened vulnerability to risk taking and problems in regulation of affect and behavior Rise late in the morning Untidiness issue of conflict with parents Rejection and Rebellion	Conflict over finances–feel parents are ATMs Attracted to opposite sex friends Transient phase–Same sex attraction can occur Experimentation starts (Need to talk about safe sex before this stage) Sex thoughts, self-stimulation is at peak Some girls may hate menstruation and require counseling for acceptance Fantasize about heroes and heroines Addiction to social networking Late night watching TV or internet Like to participate in lot of social and extracurricular activities Like to learn new languages Planning for vocation
Late (17-19 years)	Personal identity Complex abstract thinking *Neer, Kshir, Vivek* (Law and morality) Impulsiveness decreases Thoughts about future–Progress in education and employment career, what sort of person they want to be, religious and political views start getting get crystalized Want to start become financially independent	Period of terrible teens is over for most They come back to family structure and norms Their views are mature and outlooks are broader They do understand others' viewpoints and reason for the same They are aware of their rights and responsibilities Less of peer group more of intimate relations Can be aware that they have a different sexual orientation

boys and "sugar daddies" for sexual exploitation and abuse. She may also learn to use her body to her advantage, to get privileges. Girls with early puberty can also fall prey to unhealthy risk-taking behaviors like smoking, excessive dieting leading to eating disorders. Boys who are late bloomers are perceived as tiny and weak and can become victims of abuse especially by older homosexual boys or men. It can also lead to poor self-esteem due to negative body image, as girls do not think them sexually attractive. This also puts them at a higher risk of abuse of anabolic steroids, and harmful high protein supplements in order to do body building.

A late bloomer girl also develops poor body image and lowered self-esteem, as boys do not think them sexually attractive. This can lead to high risk sexual behavior like sexting etc. to attract attention.

COGNITIVE DEVELOPMENT

Cognitive competence includes the ability to reason effectively, solve problems, think abstractly, and plan for the future. Cognitive maturity enhances ability to do introspection and make mature decisions.

Early adolescence has "concrete thinking" which means understanding of immediate and short-term consequences. By middle adolescence "Abstract thinking" begins to emerge, which becomes more fine-tuned in late adolescence. Abstract thinking gives them reasoning skills which helps them to understand that there can be multiple outcomes of their action. In a calm state of mind, most middle and late stage adolescents will understand and accept adult advice. Though capable of abstract thinking, whenever they face with a stressful situation, their emotional storm can overwhelm them and they can revert to temporary concrete thinking and hence wrong decisions are often made in the heat of the moment.

Adolescent girls are better at reading and social skills and boys are better at their athletic (specially spatial orientation) and mathematical skills.

However there is a lot of debate of "nature vs nurture" in these gender related differences–whether these differences are due to gender stereotyping and upbringing or genetic in origin.

MORAL DEVELOPMENT

This refers to the development of a sense of values and ethical behavior, moral reasoning and pro-social behavior; and is very much dependent on the socio-cultural and religious milieu of his or her upbringing. Moral values shape up human personality and decide how a person will behave in society and with other human beings.

EMOTIONAL DEVELOPMENT

For a holistic personality development it is very important to have emotional skills necessary to manage stress and be sensitive and effective in relating to other people. These skills have been called "emotional intelligence" or EQ. This involves self-awareness, relationship skills—the ability to get along well with other people and to make friends. The most important skills that adolescents may develop as a part of their emotional development include recognizing and managing emotions, developing empathy, learning to resolve conflict constructively and developing a cooperative spirit.

It also includes development of the "positive self", that is *identity development* which is a very important aspect of adolescent development. This includes:

1. **Self concept:** Self-concept is our perception or image of our abilities and our uniqueness. This can be about personal qualities like looks, grooming, athletic capacity, professional goals, interests and personal values and opinions about religion, politics etc.
2. **Self-awareness:** Self-awareness is a psychological state in which people are aware of their traits, feelings and behavior. This refers to understanding oneself. Self-esteem is what one feels about oneself. It describes a person's overall sense of self-worth or personal value. Positive self-esteem nurtures a person to behave positively. Self-esteem can be as a whole or about different aspects–body image, intellect, social skills, etc. It is important for parents and teachers to help adolescents to develop positive self-esteem and a sense of identity. Because this is one of the important protective factors against high-risk behavior in adolescents like eating disorders, substance abuse, unsafe sexual experimentation etc.

Peer group is very important for developing a sense of identity and learning social skills specially during early adolescence. Being accepted and appreciated by peers is very rewarding for personality development. The influence of the peer group will depend on the stage of development.

Protective Factors for Prevention of High Risk Behavior by Adolescents

Stable, protective, nurturing environment at home, school and community fosters positive adolescent development and protects from high-risk behavior.

Family Relationships

A close bond between parents and teens is shown by many researchers to be a protective factor against high-risk teen behavior. Some amount of conflict between adolescents and parents appears to be a way of learning how to become independent from parents and at the same time also wanting to be close to them. Care should be taken to remain connected and assure them of unconditional love even during conflict situations.

School: Adolescents spend a large part of their life in school and learn to develop social and cognitive skills with peers. It also provides safety and stability. If teachers show partiality or favoritism to students, it will have an adverse effect on the self-esteem of the student concerned and emotions of the peers. Good teachers should act as ideal adult role models. Negative behavior by teachers can lead to negative behavior of students.

Community: The important supportive factors in a community include safe environment, safe schools, strong religious leaders with positive effect of religion; unsafe criminal neighborhoods foster school drop outs and juvenile delinquency.

LEARNING POINTS

1. Normal adolescence development is the foundation stone of healthy adulthood.
2. The three phases include early (10-13 years), mid (14-16 years) and late (17-19 years) adolescence, which have distinctive elements in physical, cognitive, emotional, psycho-social development.
3. Clinicians dealing with adolescents need to be well aware of these phases as this knowledge guides the approach to an adolescent patient.
4. Parents and teachers also need to be educated regarding these phases so that they do not misinterpret "normal adolescent behavior" as an abnormal wayward behavior.
5. Normal psycho-social development is affected by a variety of factors such as, personality of the adolescent, the parenting style, the atmosphere at home, school and community, peer influences, mentors and role models available. Timely interventions provided help in developing coping skills like WHO–LSE program etc.

SUGGESTED READING

1. American Psychological Association. Developing Adolescents: A Reference for Professionals. Washington, DC; American Psychological Association, 2002.
2. Bansal CP. Mission Kishore Uday: Getting IAP ready to meet the challenge of adolescent health. Indian Pediatr 2013;50: 831-32.
3. Bhave SY, Yadav S. Normal Adolescent Development. Indian J Pract Pediatr 2015;17(2):85-89.
4. Casey BJ, Getz S, Galvan A. The adolescent brain. Developmental Review 2008;28(1):62-77.
5. Erikson EH. Identity: Youth and Crisis, New York: Norton; 1968.
6. Kliegman R, Stanton B, Geme J St, Schor N, Eds.Nelson Textbook of Pediatrics, 20th edition, Chapter 110. Adolescence Development. Philadelphia; Elsevier 2015;926-36.
7. Santrock JW. Adolescence, 8th Ed. New York: McGraw-Hill; 2001.
8. Spear LP. The adolescent brain and age-related behavioral manifestations. Neuroscience and Biobehavioral Reviews 2000;24(4):417-63.
9. Steinberg L, Morris AS. Adolescent Development. Annual Rev Psychol 2001;52:83-110.
10. Zimmerman M, Copeland L, Shope J, Dielman T. A longitudinal study of self-esteem: Implications for adolescent development. J Youth Adolesc 1997;26:117-42.

Menstruation

2.4

Swati Y Bhave, Vasudha A Mashankar

INTRODUCTION

The onset of menstruation (also referred to as monthly period or menses) in adolescent girls is an important milestone in their development and puberty. This signals that the girl's body is now capable of procreation. In many cultures, this event is publicised and celebrated by the family. However in rural and conservative Indian families which still follow old traditions, this milestone leads to the imposition of a lot of social and cultural restrictions on the girl. How the family views her menstrual cycles has a great impact on her perception of pubertal changes. The menstrual cycle includes the period of time from the first day of menses and end with the first day of the next cycle. Monitoring that a young daughter in the family is having a regular monthly period is a great concern in many families, especially for the mother. Any disruption in this menstrual cycle can lead to significant concern and anxiety as the fear of pregnancy is paramount. It is important to remember that for the first 12-18 months after menarche, the periods may be irregular due to anovulatory cycles. Knowledge of normal ranges (Box 2.4.1) as well as an understanding of physiology (Table 2.4.1) are very important for young girls and their mothers.

It is also very important to educate the girls and their mothers about menstrual hygiene (Box 2.4.2) and hold school and community programs on this subject. This will help dispel the myriad of myths and taboos regarding this normal physiological process. Enhanced awareness about menstrual hygiene will also help reduce urinary and reproductive tract infections in young girls.

Box 2.4.1: Normal menstruation
Onset of menarche is at SMR (Sexual Maturity Rating) of 3–4.
The normal range for age at menarche is 9–14 years.
The normal menstrual cycle interval is average 28–30 days (range 21 to 36 days; may be longer [45 days] in teenagers).
The normal duration of bleeding is 2–8 days; normal flow as requiring 3 menstrual pads per day.
First 1–2 years after menarche many girls have anovulatory cycles.
Normal blood loss 13–80 ml.
Fully soaked pad or tampon will hold 5–15 ml blood.
Primary amenorrhea: No menarche by 15.5 years in the presence of other pubertal development.
Secondary amenorrhea: In the presence of menarche, absence of vaginal bleeding for > 3 months.

Although most adolescents will develop normal, regular menstrual cycles, a significant number may require gynecologic follow-up for persistent abnormal uterine bleeding.

MENSTRUAL ABNORMALITIES

Abnormal uterine bleeding is defined as menstrual cycles of less than 20 days or more than 40 days in duration, or a blood loss over 80 ml. *Menorrhagia* is defined as

Table 2.4.1: Phases of menstrual cycle

Follicular/Proliferative/Preovulatory Phase	*Ovulatory Phase*	*Luteal/Secretory/Postovulatory Phase*
Usually lasts from day 1 to day 14 (range 7-12 days). Important for recruitment and maturation of follicles. In early follicular phase: ↑FSH, ↑LH, in response to pulsatile secretion of GnRH. Granulosa cells of growing follicles secrete more estradiol.	LH surge occurs over 36-48 hours. It causes release of the mature ovum. LH surge is stimulated by high levels of estradiol, GnRH and increasing progesterone levels. Estradiol levels start dropping after LH surge; progesterone continues to rise.	Constant length of 14 days; progesterone levels peak 5-6 days after ovulation. Prepares the uterine bed for receiving the fertilized egg should pregnancy occur. If no pregnancy, the corpus luteum degenerates. Low estradiol and progesterone levels lead to sloughing of the endometrium and start of next menstrual cycle.

Box 2.4.2: Tips for menstrual hygiene
• Use clean undergarments and change them regularly.
• Avoid tight fitting synthetic material that does not breathe as it can lead to accumulation of sweat and secretions and lead to infection and rashes.
• Have a daily bath.
• Follow all instructions while using sanitary pads and tampons.
• Keep genital area clean–wash with plain water (no soap) after urination and each use of toilet to avoid infection.
• Always wash or clean the area in a motion that is from the front to back. Never wash in the opposite direction. Washing in the opposite direction can cause bacteria from the anus to lodge in the vagina and urethral opening, leading to infections. Keep area between legs dry to prevent chafing.
• Frequently change sanitary pads (ideally every six hours, earlier if flow is heavy) even if not fully soaked to prevent infection.
• Do not use soap or deodorant to clean the inside of the vaginal tract, as the vagina has its own self-cleaning mechanism.
• Clean the genital area before changing pads to prevent bad odor.
• Do not wear tampons for long hours to avoid the risk of TSS, i.e. Toxic Shock Syndrome.
• Dispose of sanitary pads by properly wrapping them in newspaper or any other paper and putting them in a waste basket. This will prevent the spread of infection and the emission of foul smell.
• It is important to wrap it well in newspaper or any other paper and put in waste basket. Avoid putting in a toilet as it will block the toilet.
• It is very important to wash your hands well after you discard your used napkin, as you are likely to touch the used portion of the pad or tampon while discarding.
• Take care to prevent pad rash by not using more than one pad at a time and cleaning well.

menstrual bleeding over 80 ml and bleeding lasting over 7 days. Menorrhagia at menarche is associated with anovulatory cycles. Menorrhagia at menarche needs to be evaluated to rule out hematological disorders such as von Willebrand's disease or other bleeding disorders or rarely a hepatic disorder or malignancy.

It is important to know the various other causes of abnormal uterine bleeding (Table 2.4.2) to be able to diagnose and manage them.

CLINICAL PRESENTATION

When the menarche is delayed, or there is amenorrhea, or any other problems in menstruation in an adolescent girl, it is more likely that an educated mother will consult a gynecologist first and not discuss the matter with the adolescent's clinician. However many mothers and adolescents are not aware of what are the characteristics of normal menstruation (Box 2.4.1), nor are they aware of the various manifestations that indicate that there is something wrong with the menstrual cycle (Tables 2.4.1 and 2.4.3). Hence, menstrual problems are often neglected.

Often if excessive loss of blood in a menstrual cycle is reported by the adolescent, it is assumed to be normal by the mother and no medical attention is sought. This compounds the iron deficiency anemia which already exists in adolescent girls due to inadequate nutrition and other factors (for more on this, please see Chapters 3.2 and 5.7).

HISTORY TAKING

A detailed history about menstruation should be taken in

Table 2.4.2: Causes of abnormal uterine bleeding

Physiological	Anovulatory cycles leading to dysfunctional uterine bleeding (DUB)
Coagulation disorders	Congenital and acquired bleeding disorders, von Willebrand disease
Blood dyscrasias	Idiopathic thrombocytopenic purpura
Trauma	Foreign body, intrauterine contraceptive device (IUCD)
Endometrial problems	Endometritis, endometrial polyps, fibroids, endometrial carcinoma
Ovarian problems	Polycystic ovarian disease
Endocrine problems	Hypothyroidism, hyperprolactinemia
Systemic illnesses	Chronic renal failure, severe liver disease, systemic lupus
Pregnancy and its complications	Ectopic pregnancy, threatened/incomplete abortion, spontaneous abortion
Psychiatric problems	Eating disorders–anorexia nervosa
Miscellaneous	Excessive exercise or dieting

Table 2.4.3: Abnormalities in menstruation			
Frequency:	*Polymenorrhea:* Frequent cycles of bleeding < 21 days. Cycles may be regular or irregular.	*Oligomenorrhea:* Infrequent cycles > 42 days interval.	*Irregular menses:* Bleeding frequency varies, but cycles are > 21 days, and <45 days interval.
Amount:	*Hypermenorrhea:* Profuse menstrual flow of normal duration and regular cycles.	*Hypomenorrhea:* Decreased menstrual flow of normal duration and regular cycles.	
Amount & duration:	*Menorrhagia:* Excessive and prolonged menstrual bleeding, defined as more than six "fully soaked pads" per day. Regular cycles.	*Metrorrhagia:* Intermenstrual irregular bleeding between regular periods.	*Dysfunctional uterine bleeding (DUB):* Prolonged excessive menstrual bleeding associated with irregular periods. The common etiology is absence of ovulation.

Box 2.4.3: Symptoms requiring evaluation

- No menstrual period 3 years after breast development
- No signs of pubertal development by 13 years of age
- No periods by 14 years with signs of hirsutism
- No periods by 14 years and history of eating disorder or excessive exercise
- Markedly irregular periods following regular periods
- Gap of more than 90 days between 2 periods
- Period lasting longer than 7 days
- Periods requiring frequent pad/tampon changes–soaked every 1-2 hours

every girl regardless of what presenting complaints she has been brought with (Table 2.4.2 and Box 2.4.3).

The questions asked should include:

- Onset of age of menarche?
- Frequency and duration of each cycle?
- Regularity of the cycle?
- Amount of blood loss (how many soaked pads per day?).
- If more than 3 soaked pads per day–whether symptoms suggestive of iron deficiency anemia present?
- Presence and severity of premenstrual syndrome (Box 2.4.4).
- Presence and severity of symptoms of dysmenorrhea (Box 2.4.5).
- Are there symptoms suggestive of secondary dysmenorrhea? (Box 2.4.5).
- If yes, whether there is a family history of endometriosis?
- History of medical conditions like Müllerian or renal anomalies?
- History for sexual activity for diagnosis of pelvic inflammatory disease.

History should also be taken to rule out various medical causes that can lead to abnormal uterine bleeding (Table 2.4.2).

CLINICAL EXAMINATION

A thorough clinical examination should be done to identify symptoms of anemia and to rule out medical conditions outlined in Table 2.4.3.

INVESTIGATIONS

Depending upon the clinical presentation, history and physical examination, the various investigations that need to be carried out to exclude the different causes of abnormal uterine bleeding (Table 2.4.2) include:

- Complete blood counts.
- Evaluation of bleeding profile (bleeding time, prothrombin time (PT) and partial thromboplastin time, PTT).
- Pregnancy test.
- Liver and kidney function tests and thyroid profile.
- Autoimmune disease screening.

Dysmenorrhea

- Pelvic ultrasound is indicated in the evaluation of pelvic pain, but is of not much use in non-ovarian endometriosis. It may reveal an obstructive anomaly or adnexal mass, which may have been difficult to feel in the physical examination.
- Diagnostic laparoscopy is indicated for endometriosis only if there is no relief in pain despite treatment, as most parents are concerned about subjecting their young daughters to laparoscopy.

Box 2.4.4: Premenstrual syndrome (PMS)
Adolescents can have menstrual dysfunction and associated symptoms, which can be a cause for anxiety.
Health care providers should be able to differentiate symptoms that accompany normal menstruation from those that represent significant pathology.
Most females experience pre-menstrual symptoms as a component of normal ovulatory menstrual cycles.
When these symptoms start to impact quality of life and cause functional impairment, for instance missing school days, then a diagnosis of PMS is made.
PMS is a broad spectrum of physical or emotional symptoms that occur cyclically before menses, and improve after the onset of menses.
The temporal relationship of symptoms with the menstrual cycle is important for diagnosis.
The onset of symptoms in the periovulatory period with continuation into the early phase of the next menstrual cycle, and absence of symptoms in the intervening period, is characteristic of PMS.
Physical symptoms include tenderness of breasts, edema of legs, abdomen or breasts, abdominal bloating and pain, weight gain, headache, acne, constipation, appetite changes and food cravings.
The emotional symptoms include mood swings, feeling of stress, nervousness, irritability, anxiety, anger, depression, lethargy, change in libido and fatigue.
The precise pathophysiology of PMS is not known. It is the result of complex interactions between the sex steroid levels around ovulation and neurotransmitters in the brain such as serotonin and GABA. There seems to be genetic predisposition and susceptibility.
Various proposed pathophysiological mechanisms are estrogen excess, progesterone deficiency, pyridoxine (B6) deficiency, vitamin A deficiency, increased melatonin and prostaglandin levels, alterations in insulin receptor binding and glucose metabolism, and allergic response to environmental agents and food.

Box 2.4.5: Dysmenorrhea
Mild dysmenorrhea or painful menses are seen in almost 50% girls. Generally this is relieved with simple measures like rest, a hot water bag, antispasmodics and/or paracetamol or non-steroidal anti-inflammatory drugs (NSAIDs). The symptoms are low back ache, cramps in the legs, nausea, vomiting and headache. These symptoms usually occur only in some cycles. Investigations to rule out pathological causes are needed when: (a) Severe pain not responsive to above measures (b) Symptoms last through the whole cycle and are present in every cycle (c) When such symptoms are associated with clots or excess bleeding.
Pathogenesis: The withdrawal of progesterone in the premenstrual period causes cell membranes to release phospholipids which get converted into prostaglandins and leukotrienes. The prostaglandins cause uterine ischemia and pain. Prostaglandin F2-alpha causes myometrial contractions, vasoconstriction, and ischemia, whereas prostaglandin E2 causes vasodilatation. Elevation of myometrial resting as well as contractile tone, increase in the frequency and irregularity of contractions–all contribute towards pain. The leukotrienes cause systemic symptoms like vomiting, headache etc. Other predisposing factors: BMI < 20, early menarche, menstrual irregularities, presence of premenstrual symptoms.
Types of Dysmenorrhea: 1. *Primary or physiological:* Due to changes during the menstrual cycle as described above. 2. *Secondary or pathological:* Endometriosis, structural anomalies, pelvic inflammatory diseases, ovarian cysts, benign uterine tumors, adhesions, pelvic inflammatory disease, cervical stenosis, and congenital anomalies such as genital atresia. In adolescents with chronic and severe intractable pelvic pain and dysmenorrhea, endometriosis is probably the most common cause. It can present with atypical symptoms such as dyschezia (difficulty in defecation) and dysuria (painful micturition).

Polycystic Ovarian Disease (PCOD) or Syndrome (PCOS)

This has emerged as a very common and important cause of menstrual irregularity in adolescent girls all over the world (Box 2.4.6).

Clinical features of PCOS include:

- Menstrual irregularity: Oligomenorrhea, amenorrhea, menorrhagia, metrorrhagia and dysmenorrhea.
- Truncal obesity.
- Signs of hyperandrogenism (hirsutism, acne)

Box 2.4.6: Polycystic ovarian disease (PCOD) or syndrome (PCOS)
PCOS is a syndrome of ovarian hyperandrogenism (causing hirsutism) and chronic anovulation in women without an underlying adrenal or pituitary cause. Most cases are obese but PCOS can also occur in lean girls.
Unless intervention is done early, there is high chance of reduced fertility which is the main presentation in young married women.
Menarche typically begins at a normal age but can be delayed. Ovarian androgen excess and relatively diminished levels of estrogen may impair follicular development, resulting in anovulation and/or oligo/amenorrhea. There is high risk of endometrial hyperplasia and cancer, breast cancer and ovarian tumor.
Hyperinsulinemia is a common mechanism: Insulin acts synergistically with luteinizing hormone (LH) to increase production of androgen by the ovarian theca cells while also decreasing the level of sex hormone-binding globulin. Clinical/biochemical evidence of hyperandrogenism.
Hyperinsulinemia and insulin resistance are associated with metabolic syndrome and increased incidence of type 2 diabetes mellitus, hypertension and cardiovascular disease.
Ultrasound may show polycystic appearing ovaries with a smooth pearly colored thickened cap; follicles >10 in number; each measuring 2-8 mm in diameter, located peripherally on the ovary.
There is evidence that the origin of PCOS may be in the prenatal period. Genetic studies also show an association of PCOS to type 2 diabetes and metabolic syndrome.

- Insulin resistance marker, acanthosis nigricans which is a raised, velvety, hyperpigmentation of the skin seen in the axilla, neck, and intertriginous areas.

Pelvic examination can be done in sexually active adolescents, whereas in others as per abdominal examination for palpable uterus, tenderness in pubic or pelvic area.

- In 2003 the Rotterdam criteria defined PCOS as being present when 2 out of 3 criteria are present i.e. clinical or biochemical hyperandrogenism, oligo/anovulation, and/or radiographic evidence of polycystic ovaries.
- A polycystic ovary is defined as one which contains at least 12 or more follicles (2-9 mm) in the periphery, or an ovarian volume > 10 ml.
- Goals in the diagnosis of PCOS are to confirm ovarian hyperandrogenism and menstrual dysfunction while excluding other causes of hyperandrogenism and menstrual dysfunction, such as adrenal/ovarian tumors, non-classical adrenal hyperplasia, thyroid disease, hyperprolactinemia and Cushing syndrome.
- Hormone assays for free and total testosterone and dehydroepiandrosterone (DHEA), prolactin and thyroid stimulating hormone. FSH levels may be required to exclude ovarian failure in girls without signs of hyperandrogenism.

MANAGEMENT

Acute Case Management

In case of life threatening bleeding (where the adolescent is hemodynamically unstable) immediate hospitalization, intravenous fluids and/or blood transfusion is required.

Intravenous conjugated estrogen may be needed if the bleeding does not stop in this situation.

Outpatient Clinic Management

Mild cases (hemoglobin >12 g/dl) can be managed with reassurance, menstrual calendar, prescription of multivitamins and iron, and re-evaluation in 3 months.

Moderate bleeding cases (hemoglobin 10-12 g/dl) are managed with oral contraceptives, iron supplementation, menstrual calendar and revaluation in 1-3 months.

High-dose oral medroxyprogesterone acetate therapy in the management of excessive DUB in adolescents has been found to be very effective.

Rapid saturation of the endometrium with progestogens also seems to be a highly effective method of treatment for excessive DUB in adolescents.

Premenstrual Syndrome

The goal is to improve quality of life in PMS. Accordingly, the treatment given in cases of PMS is symptom-centric.

An important aspect of such treatment is also to educating the patient about the normal menstrual cycle and associated symptoms, and teaching her self-care measures to alleviate the severity of symptoms.

- Milder forms of PMS may benefit from reassurance, healthy lifestyle and regular exercise (in the form of yoga and behavioral therapies).
- Other general measures include relaxation, low-fat/high-fibre diet and decreased consumption of salt, sugar, caffeine and alcohol.
- Various other treatments that have been tried with varied success include pyridoxine (vitamin B6), vitamin A, D and E; mefenemic acid, essential fatty

acids such as gamma linolenic acid (evening primrose oil), minerals (calcium, magnesium, iron, zinc and manganese), diuretics, natural progesterone, oral contraceptives, GnRH analogs and danazol.

- Fluoxetine (selective serotonin uptake inhibitor) may be used in premenstrual dysphoric disorder with severe affect symptoms.
- Severe cases warrant the use of combination oral contraceptive pills to suppress ovulation, and thus alleviate symptoms.

Dysmenorrhea

Even though it is a common problem, medical help is rarely sought for the same, and over-the-counter (OTC) drugs are often taken. However these result in the consumption of an inappropriate choice or dose of drugs.

- Pharmacotherapy remains the first line of treatment with non-steroidal anti-inflammatory drugs (NSAIDs). The commonly used drugs are ibuprofen (200-400 mg 4-8 hourly), and mefenemic acid (250 mg 6 hourly or 500 mg 8 hourly). Naproxen may also be used.
- Prostaglandin synthetase inhibitors have been found to relieve symptoms of primary dysmenorrhea.
- Hormonal contraceptives are used to suppress ovulation and subsequent progesterone production, when usual pharmacotherapy fails.
- Lifestyle changes such as dietary modification, yoga, exercises, and decrease in smoking have been proposed as treatment. However, there is lack of adequate evidence to support the effectiveness of these modalities.

Endometriosis

- Endometriosis presents with at least 6 months duration of noncyclical pain, which is non-responsive to oral contraceptive pills (OCP) and NSAIDs.
- Young patients with clinically suspected endometriosis may bypass the laparoscopy and instead are placed on 3 months of gonadotropin-releasing hormone agonist (GnRH-a). GnRH-a creates a hypoestrogenic and hypogonadal state which is not conducive to the growth of ectopic endometrium. Side effects of GnRH-a are mainly due to the hypoestrogenic state that it creates; a major side effect is the decrease in bone density.
- Danazol decreases the ectopic endometrial tissue volume by inducing a hyperandrogenic state. It cannot be recommended in adolescents with endometriosis because of its hyperandrogenic side effects.

Polycystic Ovarian Syndrome (PCOS)

A multi-specialty team approach is needed in the management of an adolescent with PCOS. Treatment is directed towards all aspects.

(a) *Normalization of menstruation:* Cyclic progestin and oral contraceptives (combined or progestin only) can be used to correct menstrual irregularity which also helps in reduction of acne.

(b) *Hirsutism and acne* (for treatment, refer to Chapter 6.4).

(c) *Counselling and psychotherapy:* Patients suffer from psychological disturbances and body image issues due to obesity, acne, hirsutism and acanthosis nigricans.

(d) *Treatment of obesity and insulin resistance (Chapters 1.8 and 3.3)*: Lifestyle modification by decreasing intake of calories and regular exercise helps to decrease weight, and reduce the waist circumference. This results in improving insulin sensitivity and fasting insulin levels. Good results are obtained by using insulin-sensitizing agent metformin (Chapter 3.4).

(e) *Metabolic syndrome and associated morbidity* (Chapter 3.4).

LEARNING POINTS

- Adolescent girls, mothers and teachers in schools need to be educated on normal menstruation and abnormalities in menstruation so that they will know when to get professional consultation.
- Knowledge about menstrual hygiene will prevent infections of the reproductive and urinary tracts in young girls, which is are presently very common.
- Lack of knowledge about what is excessive blood loss leads to many adolescent girls not receiving timely intervention. This eventually leads to the prevalence of a high incidence of iron deficiency anemia, which reduces a patient's cognitive ability, academic capability and causes them to suffer due to poor physical energy.
- The common menstrual disorders in adolescents are dysmenorrhea, premenstrual syndrome, abnormal uterine bleeding, amenorrhea, and polycystic ovarian syndrome.

- Polycystic ovarian syndrome is a combination of ovarian hyperandrogenism and chronic anovulation. As PCOS leads to long-term morbidity of low fertility and metabolic syndrome in the long-term, it needs to be detected and treated early.

SUGGESTED READING

1. American College of Obstetricians and Gynaecologists. Polycystic ovary syndrome. ACOG Practice Bulletin No. 108. Obstet Gynecol 2009;114(4):936-49.
2. American College of Obstetricians and Gynaecologists Committee opinion 2006, reaffirmed by American Academy of Pediatrics Committee on Adolescence 2009.
3. Bevan JA, Maloney KW, Hillery CA, Gill JC, Montgomery RR, Scott JP. Bleeding disorders: A common cause of menorrhagia in adolescents. J Pediatr 2001;138:856-61.
4. Grimes DA. Estimating vaginal blood loss. J Reprod Med 1979;22:190-92.
5. Menstrual Hygiene URL http://menstrupedia.com/articles/hygiene/necessary-hygiene accessed on 22nd Sep 2015.
6. Menstrual cycle URL http://www.acog.org/Resources-And-Publications/Committee-Opinions/Committee-on-Adolescent-Health-Care/Menstruation-in-Girls-and-Adolescents-Using-the-Menstrual-Cycle-as-a-Vital-Sign accessed on 22nd Sep 2015.
7. Polycystic Ovary Syndrome Writing Committee. American Association of Clinical Endocrinologists position statement on metabolic and cardiovascular consequences of polycystic ovary syndrome. Endocr Pract 2005;11(2):125-34.
8. Practice Committee of the American Society for Reproductive Medicine (2006). The evaluation and treatment of androgen excess. Fertility and Sterility, 86 (4, Suppl): S241-S247.
9. http://www.msdmanuals.com/professional/gynecology-and-obstetrics/female-reproductive-endocrinology/female-reproductive-endocrinology accessed on 26th September, 2015.

Overview of Nutrition 3.1

Elizabeth KE, Bindusha S

INTRODUCTION

Adolescence is the last chance for a child to attain his/her growth potential. Development of bone mass is essential during this period as this forms the ground for maintaining mineral integrity of the bone in later life. The pattern and proportion of various body components like body water, muscle mass, bone and fat increase during the entire childhood and adolescence to reach adult values by about 18 years. The nutritional needs of the adolescent girls are of particular importance as they have to prepare for motherhood. These rapid anabolic changes require more nutrients per unit body weight. Eating behavior of an adolescent depends on the knowledge about healthy diet, attitude of the adolescent and his/her family and behavioral and lifestyle factors in addition to food availability. Adolescence is the age in which the child attains nutritional independence. It is usually the adolescent who decides when to eat, what to eat and where to eat rather than the family. So, adolescence is the ideal age for nutrition education.

Prior to puberty the nutritional needs of boys and girls are same. But during adolescence there is change in the body composition and biological functions, which will result in gender specific requirement of nutrients. The requirement of nutrients will be more during the period of rapid growth, so that the requirements of specific nutrients vary during the different stages of adolescence (Tables 3.1.1 and 3.1.2). Box 3.1.1 provides some tips for making a healthy diet plan for adolescents.

Table 3.1.1: Daily nutrient requirement for adolescents–Indian Council of Medical Research (ICMR), 2011

Age group	*Energy (kcal)*	*Protein (g)*	*Fat (g)*	*Calcium (mg)*	*Iron (mg)*	*Zinc (mg)*
Boys 10-12 years	2190	39.9	35	800	21	9
Girls 10-12 years	2010	40.4	35	800	27	9
Boys 13-15 years	2750	54.3	45	800	32	11
Girls 13-15 years	2330	51.9	40	800	27	11
Boys 16-18 years	3020	61.5	50	800	28	12
Girls 16-18 years	2440	55.5	35	800	26	12

Table 3.1.2: Approximate recommended dietary allowances (RDA) of vitamins and minerals–ICMR, 2011

Age group	*Vit A μg/d*	*Thiamin mg/d*	*Riboflavin mg/d*	*Niacin mg/d*	*B6 mg/d*	*Vit C mg/d*	*Folate μg/d*	*B12 μg/d*	*Mg mg/d*
Boys 10-12 years	Retinol 600	1.1	1.3	15	1.6	40	140	0.2 -1	120
Girls 10-12 years		1.0	1.2	13	1.6				160
Boys 13-15 years		1.4	1.6	16	2.0	40	150	0.2-1	165
Girls 13-15 years		1.2	1.4	14	2.0				210
Boys 16-18 years		1.5	1.8	17	2.0	40	200	0.2-1	195
Girls 16-18 years		1.0	1.2	14	2.0				235

Box 3.1.1: Tips for making a healthy diet plan for adolescents

An adolescent boy is expected to take one unit of calories (2400 kcal) as equivalent to the requirement of an adult sedentary male.

Adolescent girl requires 2100 kcal/day, which is more than the requirement of her mother. Carbohydrates should make up 45–65% of energy intake; protein 10–30%; and fat 25–35%.

Dietary fat should come primarily from sources of polyunsaturated and monounsaturated fatty acids, such as fish, nuts, and vegetable oils.

Trans fats, found in hydrogenated oils used primarily in bakery products, should be avoided altogether because they increase serum levels of low density lipoprotein.

Dietary intake of total cholesterol, found in animal products, should be limited to 300 mg/day.

Box 3.1.2: Calcium and iron requirements in adolescence

Growing children and adolescents particularly require more calcium. Recommended dietary allowances for calcium are about 800 mg/d only. It is desirable to give higher quantities of calcium to achieve high peak bone mass. Due to inadequate exposure to sunlight adolescents are at risk of vitamin D deficiency also.

According to NFHS 3 survey over 55% of both adolescent girls and boys are anemic.

RDA of iron varies between 21–32 mg per day depending on the stage of adolescence.

Adequate intake of iron should be ensured as iron is needed:

- To build up the blood volume and muscle mass and myoglobin especially in boys.
- To prevent the development of anemia due to menstrual loss in girls.

Indian diet has the non-heme iron present in the grains and vegetables which has very low bioavailability and hence is poorly absorbed.

SPECIAL ISSUES OF ADOLESCENTS WITH RESPECT TO NUTRITION

Malnutrition among adolescents may be due to various reasons other than nonavailability of food. Box 3.1.2 provides some important information regarding calcium and iron requirements in adolescents.

- Many adolescents consume less food due to lack of time as they are engaged in a period of stressful studies.
- Breakfast is often missed or eaten hurriedly. Food fads and fast food culture also lead to malnutrition.
- Fast foods are high in calories, fat and sodium but fail to provide enough vitamins and minerals needed during this stage.
- Very little information is available about the nutrient composition of fast foods.
- Food additives like mono sodium glutamate (MSG, ajinomoto) and coloring agents used for preparation of fast foods are antinutrients.
- Soft drinks also provide only empty calories. They may contain antinutrients. Consumption of soft drinks will kill the appetite and promote skipping of meals.
- Junk food is defined as items with high fat, high sugar, high salt and also high preservatives/pesticides/additives (HFSS-P).

PSYCHOSOCIAL FACTORS AFFECTING FOOD INTAKE

- Peer pressure, media influence and rapid changes in the body size and shape may make them uncomfortable about their bodies.
- Some children especially girls eat less food as they want to remain slim. Box 3.1.3 details some relevant issues related to nutrition in adolescent girls.
- In some families, adolescent girls eat last and least due to ignorance and poverty.
- Psychological problems and eating disorders like anorexia nervosa and bulimia may also interfere with adequate nutrition.
- Adolescence is the period during which experimentation starts in all fields. Dietary experimentation in the form of strict vegetarianism without proper knowledge about the healthy meal plans may also lead to malnutrition. Box 3.1.4 discusses briefly some important aspects of vegetarianism in adolescents.
- It is the vulnerable stage for developing wrong food habits. Distinctive likes and dislikes for food may develop in this age. Developing unhealthy food habits may lead to nutrient deficiency. In addition to consumption of a nutritious well balanced diet, appropriate lifestyle practices and involvement in physical activity such as games/sports should be encouraged among children and adolescents.

Box 3.1.3: Special issues in adolescent girls

Adolescent girls have to be prepared for future motherhood.

But even those who do not wish to reproduce should have good nutrition to contribute to a healthy workforce of the nation.

Improving her nutritional status will contribute to the breaking of intergenerational malnutrition, poverty and chronic diseases.

It will also result in better pre-pregnancy weight and better body stores of nutrients.

Iron deficiency in adolescent girls may lead to preterm delivery and low birth weight of the offspring.

An adequately nourished mother will transfer adequate nutrients to the baby through placenta and breast milk without depleting her own stores.

Adequate folate sources in the mother will decrease the incidence of neural tube defects in the baby.

Adequate bone health will prevent cephalopelvic disproportion (CPD) and reduce the risk of obstructed labor.

Box 3.1.4: Vegetarianism

Vegetarianism is considered as a healthier option by some.

It may have low risk of obesity, hypertension, coronary arterial disease and colon cancer.

Vegans are at risk of calcium, iron and vitamin B12 deficiencies; hence need to take whole grains and germinated seeds.

Adolescents are easily carried away towards idealism.

Whether it is healthy or not will depend on the degree of vegetarianism.

Lacto-ovo-vegetarians have very little nutritional risk except iron deficiency due to lack of heme iron.

Fruitarians who eat only fruits are at the risk of protein, sodium, calcium and other mineral deficiencies.

MINERAL AND VITAMIN DEFICIENCIES PREVALENT IN ADOLESCENTS

History Taking

A very detailed dietetic history should be taken, especially if the adolescent is overweight or underweight. Table 3.1.3 provides the details about nutrients such as their requirement, sources and common micronutrient deficiencies during adolescence.

Iron Deficiency

- A detailed dietary evaluation regarding the frequency and type of iron rich food consumed will give a clue to iron deficiency.
- If the dietary intake of iron appears to be sufficient, history of chronic or acute blood loss should be sought.
- Menorrhagia is a common cause for iron deficiency in girls.
- Gastrointestinal tract is another common site of blood loss, which may be in the form of overt or occult bleeding.
- Worm infestations, especially hookworm infestation can also result in iron deficiency due to overt or occult bleeding.

Vitamin B12 Deficiency

- Vegans, who don't consume even milk or egg are at special risk.
- It is associated with atrophic gastritis, *Helicobacter pylori* infection and other gastrointestinal inflammations like celiac disease.
- Chronic use of proton pump inhibitors or H2 receptor blockers may lead to vitamin B12 deficiency.

Calcium Deficiency

- The amount of clothing worn and skin color will affect the vitamin D level of the children as cutaneous production is the major source of vitamin D.
- Enquire about intake of fish oil, fatty fish, egg yolk and vitamin D fortified food items.
- Milk and milk products are the major sources of dietary calcium. When consumption of milk is low, cereals become the major dietary source of calcium.
- Consumption of calcium rich food like raggi, rajkeera (amaranth), gingelly seeds, sea food, fish, mutton and green leafy vegetables should be noted.

Essential Fatty Acid Deficiency

- Essential fatty acid deficiency may be associated with malabsorption, restriction of dietary fat intake, or wrong choice of dietary fats.
- Enquire about intake of omega-3 fatty acids like legumes, fish and green leaves.
- Hydrogenated vegetable oils and animal fats are poor sources of EFA.

Iodine Deficiency

- The geographic area is the most important factor which determines the adequacy of iodine in the diet. In India, the endemic belt of iodine deficiency disorders (IDD) extends from the Jammu and Kashmir in the north, through parts of Punjab, Haryana, Himachal Pradesh, Uttar Pradesh, Northern part of Bihar, and West Bengal to North-Eastern states.
- IDD is reported in all states in India. They are known as extra-Himalayan foci of IDD. Even coastal areas have been found to be endemic for IDD.

Table 3.1.3: Common micronutrient deficiencies in adolescence

Nutrient	*Requirement*	*Sources*	*Features of deficiency*
Iron	21-32 mg/day	Meat, fish, liver	Microcytic hypochromic anemia, brittle nails, atrophic tongue, poor concentration, poor scholastic performance
Iodine	150 µg/day	Sea food, fish	Goiter, iodine deficiency disorders
Vitamin D	400 IU/day	Cutaneous synthesis, fish oil, fatty fish, egg yolk	Hypocalcemia, tetany, growth retardation, fractures, rachitic changes
Calcium	1200 mg/day	Milk and milk products, raggi, gingelly seeds, sea foods, fish, mutton	Tetany, growth retardation, failure of mineralization of bones, fractures, rachitic changes
Zinc	11-12 mg/day	Meat, liver, fish, milk, cereals, pulses, nuts	Growth failure, depressed immunity, anorexia, diarrhea, reproductive failure
B12	0.2-1 µg/day	Animal foods, meat, egg	Megaloblastic anemia, glossitis, neuropsychiatric symptoms, paresthesia
EFA	1-3% of total calories	Fish, vegetable oils like sunflower oil	Phrynoderma, follicular hyperkeratosis, learning disability, hyperactivity

- Enquire about intake of iodized salt. Daily intake of 10 grams of iodized salt will provide at least 150 µg of iodine per day. RDA of iodine is 150 µg/day for adolescents and adults.
- Presence of goitrogens in the diet which interfere with the production and utilization of thyroid hormone is another important cause. Foods like jowar, tapioca, cabbage, cauliflower, mustard seeds and groundnuts contain goitrogens in significant quantities.

Zinc Deficiency

- Zinc deficiency is rare in people who take nonvegetarian diet as meat, liver, fish and milk are very good sources of zinc.
- Though cereals, pulses and nuts are also rich sources of zinc, it will be lost on milling and processing of the grains.
- Intestinal absorption of zinc is markedly inhibited by the phytate and tannin content of the diet. Indian vegetarian diets are rich in phytate and thus bioavailability of zinc is poor in them.

CLINICAL EXAMINATION

Clinical Features of Iron Deficiency

- Iron deficiency affects the linear growth.
- Behavior changes: They lead to lack of concentration, poor scholastic performance, mood changes, and chronic headache.
- Iron deficiency predisposes to infections and lowers the physical fitness.
- In severe iron deficiency the nails will become flat and brittle or may even become spoon shaped.
- The tongue may become smooth due to atrophy of the papillae.

Clinical Features of Vitamin B12 Deficiency

- Neurological symptoms like paresthesia and peripheral neuritis, gastrointestinal symptoms like anorexia and glossitis may be present.
- Neuropsychiatric symptoms like depression, irritability, negativism, impaired concentration and attention and insomnia are common.

Clinical Features of Calcium and Vitamin D Deficiency

- Recent onset vitamin D and calcium deficiency during adolescence is unlikely to present with florid rickets.
- Deficiency of calcium and vitamin D during adolescence will result in failure to attain maximum muscle mass and height potential of that individual.
- There is also increased chance of fractures.
- Children may also present with muscle cramps due to hypocalcemia.

Clinical Features of EFA Deficiency

- EFA deficiency affects mainly skin, brain and retina.
- Skin changes include dry and scaly skin–phrynoderma, brittle nails, cracking of heels and follicular hyperkeratosis.
- Changes in visual acuity, attention deficit, hyperactivity, learning problems are also reported with EFA deficiency.

Clinical Features of Iodine Deficiency

- Iodine deficiency leads to endemic goiter.
- Iodine deficiency disorders (IDD) include abortion, stillbirths, low birth weight, cretinism, neonatal chemical hypothyroidism, psychomotor defects, impaired coordination, mental retardation and hypothyroidism.

Clinical Features of Zinc Deficiency

- Zinc deficiency can result in growth failure, depressed immunity, anorexia, diarrhea, altered skeletal function and reproductive failure.
- Zinc deficiency during adolescence will affect the final adult height.

INVESTIGATIONS

Iron Deficiency Anemia

- Hemoglobin and hematocrit will be reduced depending on the severity of anemia.
- MCV, MCH and MCHC will be low and RDW will be increased in iron deficiency anemia. Peripheral smear will show microcytic hypochromic anemia with anisopoikilocytosis.
- Serum iron, serum ferritin and transferrin saturation will decrease and the total iron binding capacity will increase.
- Serum free erythrocyte protoporphyrin will also increase in iron deficiency.

Vitamin B12 Deficiency

- Macrocytic anemia with hypersegmented neutrophils.

- Serum B12 level is usually < 1125 pmol/L.
- Schillings test can be done to demonstrate B12 malabsorption in indicated cases.

Calcium and Vitamin D Deficiency

- Biochemical changes include hypophosphatemia, hypocalcemia, and raised alkaline phosphatase levels.
- X-ray shows osteopenia and pathological fractures. There may be delayed maturation of the ossification centers. Rachitic changes are evident in severe and long-standing vitamin D deficiency.
- Serum 25 hydroxy-vitamin D level < 20 ng/ml indicates vitamin D deficiency. Levels >30 ng/ml are considered ideal in growing age in view of the added extra-skeletal effects.

EFA Deficiency

- EFA deficiency is confirmed by measuring the triene/tetraene ratio (T/T ratio).
- T/T ratio >0.4 in serum phospholipid indicates EFA deficiency.

Iodine Deficiency

- Urinary iodine excretion will be reduced in iodine deficiency. It can be tested by using dipstick.

Zinc Deficiency

- Serum zinc level < 60 μg/dl indicate zinc deficiency.

MANAGEMENT

Management of common nutritional deficiencies are summarized in Table 3.1.4.

LEARNING POINTS

1. Adolescence is the last chance for a child to attain his/her growth potential; educate parents about the amount of food that the adolescent should consume.
2. An adolescent boy should eat as much as his father eats (2400 cal) and the adolescent girl should eat a little more than what the mother eats (2100 cal).
3. Development of bone mass is essential during this period as this forms the ground for maintaining mineral integrity of the bone in later life.
4. Adolescence is the age in which the child attains nutritional independence. Eating behavior of an adolescent depends on the knowledge about healthy diet, attitude of the adolescent and his/her family and behavioral and lifestyle factors in addition to food availability. It is usually the adolescent who decides when to eat, what to eat and where to eat rather than the family. So, adolescence is the ideal age for nutrition education.
5. Ensure a balanced diet by including all food groups every day. Food pyramid will help in the choice of balanced diet (see Figure 3.1.1). Include cereal pulse combination, roots and tubers in adequate quantities, vegetables and fruits liberally, milk, milk products and meat in moderation and oils, fats and sugars sparingly.
6. Ensure variety within each food group. Food fads must be avoided as it may evolve as a social handicap.

Table 3.1.4: Management of various nutrient deficiencies in adolescence

Nutrient	*Treatment*	*Comments*
Iron	Therapeutic: Oral iron in dose 3-4 mg/kg/day. Prophylactic/preventive: Weekly iron folic acid supplementation programme (WIFS) of Government of India–Iron-folic acid supplements of 100 mg elemental iron with 500 μg folic acid using a fixed day approach.	Continue for 3 months after correction of anemia to replenish the body stores of iron. Biannual deworming with a broad spectrum antihelmenthic like albendazole and correct hand washing techniques will prevent worm infestation. Screening of target groups.
Vit B12	Daily dose of 1000 μg oral B12. Intramuscular 1000 μg once daily for 7 days; followed by 1000 μg once a week for one month; followed by 1000 μg/month.	For treatment of hematological manifestations only. Parenteral B12 is required for treatment of neurological disease.
EFA	Supplementation with omega-3 fatty acids.	10% of total energy should be from saturated fatty acids, 10% from monounsaturated fatty acids and 10% from polyunsaturated fatty acids. EFAs should provide 1-3% of total calories.
Vitamin D	Vitamin D 2000-5000 IU/day for 4-6 weeks followed by 800 IU/day. Calcium 1200-1500 mg/day.	High calcium intake should be ensured throughout the adolescence.
Zinc	20 mg/day for 14 days.	Giving zinc during diarrhea will prevent zinc deficiency.

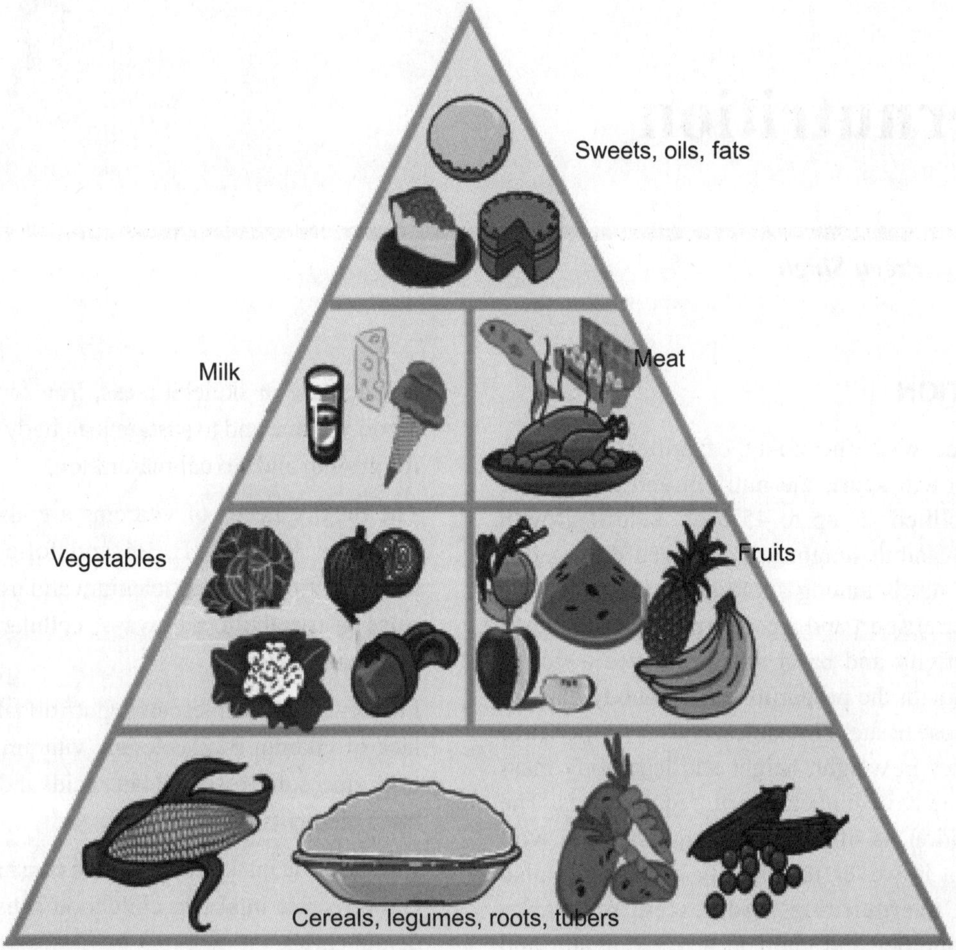

Figure 3.1.1: Food pyramid including all food groups and restricted use of oil, fat and sugars

7. Include micronutrients and antioxidants in the diet. Vitamin A, vitamin C, folic acid, iron, iodine and zinc are essential for the optimal growth of an adolescent.

SUGGESTED READING

1. Brown JE. Nutrition basics, Nutrition through life cycle, 4th ed. USA: Wadsworth 2011;2-44.
2. Elizabeth KE. Nutrition and Child Development, 5th ed. Hyderabad: Paras; 2015.
3. National Institute of Nutrition. Nutrient Requirements and Recommended Dietary Allowances for Indians – Report of the Expert Group of the Indian Council of Medical Research, Hyderabad; 2009.
4. National Institute of Nutrition. Dietary guidelines for Indians. A manual, 2nd ed. Hyderabad; 2010.

Undernutrition

3.2

Satinder Aneja, Preeti Singh

INTRODUCTION

In adolescence with the onset of puberty and the accelerated growth spurt, the nutrient and the caloric needs are amplified, as up to 45% of skeletal growth and 15–25% of adult height are achieved during this phase. Energy needs among adolescents vary with the timing of pubertal spurt and are determined by the level of physical activity and basal metabolic rate which is closely related with the proportion of lean body mass in relation to adipose tissue. The adolescent boys experience greater increases in weight, height and lean body mass than girls, hence have higher caloric requirements. The term 'malnutrition' is often used interchangeably with undernutrition, however technically speaking it also encompasses 'overnutrition'. Adolescent pregnancy exposes both mother and child to adverse health and socioeconomic consequences, particularly if the mother is undernourished or stunted. This further translates into a vicious cycle of intergenerational malnutrition, poverty and chronic disease.

DETERMINANTS OF UNDERNUTRITION IN ADOLESCENCE

- Severe malnutrition is not common except in presence of underlying chronic diseases such as tuberculosis (TB), human immunodeficiency virus (HIV) infections, parasitic infestations, chronic liver and renal diseases and celiac disease or in emergency situations such as famines.
- Either the dietary intake is inadequate in terms of energy and protein than recommended due to lack of awareness of increased nutrient needs, restrictive dieting, socioeconomic deprivation or impaired utilization secondary to chronic illness.
- Gender inequality gets widened during adolescence with girls predisposed to inadequate intakes because of social discrimination, dieting or lower energy intake and pregnancy.
- The need for minerals in adolescence increases with the accelerated muscular and skeletal growth–calcium for increase in skeletal mass, iron for expansion of blood volume and to sustain lean body mass and zinc for growth and sexual maturation.
- The dietary needs of vitamins are also augmented. Vitamins A, C, D, E, B6 and folic acid and the minerals zinc, copper, selenium and iron all play key roles in metabolic pathways, cellular function and immune function.
- For vegetarian adolescents, nutritional risks include lack of vitamin B12, calcium, vitamin D, riboflavin, iron, zinc, some essential fatty acids and perhaps some trace elements.
- Low fluoride intake coupled with consumption of high carbohydrate intake in childhood is associated with dental caries.
- Even in setting where food resources are adequate, the mean caloric intake of adolescents can be suboptimal due to poor and unhealthy food habits during this age.
- Anorexia nervosa and bulimia nervosa are nutritional and weight control practices often seen in adolescent females either to lose weight or to minimize weight gain.
- The nutritional status of adolescent girls is an index of their reproductive morbidity and mortality. Girls who become pregnant at an early age are at risk of depletion of their nutritional reserves.
- Besides genetic factors, which are responsible for half the variation, other determining factors are nutritional status, ethnicity and the socioeconomic status. Table 3.2.1 briefly discusses the determinants of undernutrition during adolescence and their key features.

IMPLICATIONS OF UNDERNUTRITION

- Undernutrition adversely affects the physical growth, delays the pubertal development, adversely affects cognition and impairs work capacity.

Table 3.2.1: Dietary determinants of undernutrition in adolescents and their key features

Determinant	*Key features*
Energy	• The growth rate serves as the biomarker of adequacy of energy intake. • Many disease states can alter the energy requirements; interfere with nutrient availability or utilization. • Athletic activity and heavy physical work increase the energy needs. • It is crucial to determine the extent and acuity of the deficit.
Protein	• Dietary requirements are affected by age, gender, growth rate, illness, and adequacy of other nutrients. • During periods of infection and stress and subsequently during recovery phase, it would be reasonable to increase (20-30%) the protein intake. • No evidence to suggest any specific amino acid needs for adolescents.
Adolescent bone health	• Peak bone mineralization occurs during adolescence and around half of adult bone calcium is accreted. • Apart from genetic and hormonal influence, exercise, optimal calcium and vitamin D status play an important role in bone growth and accretion during these formative years.
Unhealthy eating habits	• The quest for self identity, difficulty in accepting the existing schedules, desire for peer acceptance and concern about body image tend to have a great impact on lifestyle and food behavior among adolescents. • Certain food fads also influence the eating behavior of the adolescents.
Early teen pregnancy	• The adolescents commonly have deficiency of calcium, vitamin D, folic acid, iron and zinc, which can have deleterious effect on outcome of pregnancy. • Offsprings of adolescent mothers are even at a higher nutritional risk because of inadequate nutrient stores at birth, but also due to inappropriate breastfeeding and child-care practices.

- It compromises the immune system and predisposes to increased risk of infections and chronic illnesses which in turn lead to metabolic stress, weight loss and further impairment of the immunity and nutritional status.
- Underweight adolescents may have a negative body image, particularly males who may desire a muscular physique.
- Chronic undernutrition results in stunting. Stunted women have greater risk of obstructed labor due to cephalopelvic disproportion. Undernourished adolescent girls are at high risk of preterm births and producing low birth weight babies which are at high risk of metabolic syndrome. This is discussed in detail in Chapter 3.4.

HISTORY TAKING

- It is extremely important to have a comprehensive dietary assessment with focus on current feeding practices and the development of feeding pattern since birth.
- A meticulous review of the systemic history to exclude chronic medical or surgical illness and assessment of current and potential future co-morbidities is of immense significance to plan management.
- An insight into the socioeconomic history, cultural practices and environmental factors influencing nutritional status is important to identify the risks and plan interventions accordingly.
- A detail on the salient features in history is given in Box 3.2.1.

PHYSICAL EXAMINATION

- Determine the sexual maturity rating (SMR) stage of the adolescent to assess the growth and progression of puberty.
- Anthropometry is an important measure of the nutritional status.
- Anthropometric indices in adolescence are complicated by onset and progression of puberty and the changes in body proportions with sexual development across populations.
- The pubertal stage correlates better with bone age (skeletal maturation) rather than the chronological age. Cormic index (sitting height/standing height ratio) may to some extent be used to adjust for ethnic differences in body proportions although this has not been validated.
- Physical assessment (Box 3.2.2) should begin with an accurate measurement of height and weight, and calculation of body mass index (BMI) which is an important tool to measure undernutrition or thinness.
- Periodic assessment helps to check growth velocity, which is more valuable.
- Currently WHO classifies undernutrition as "thinness" and "severe thinness" using cut offs at –2SD and –3SD of BMI for age respectively.

Box 3.2.1: Components of history in assessment of adolescent's nutritional status

Evaluation of adolescent's health concerns

- Any recent weight loss over last 6-12 months or poor gain in height.
- Is the weight loss intentional or involuntary?
- Is there a history of a known medical condition?
- Any history suggestive of acute or chronic infection or chronic underlying illness.
- What is the desired weight by the adolescent that is considered ideal?
- Preconceived ideas about nutrition and health.
- Has the dietary pattern changed over the past 6-12 months?
- Any history of starvation or induced vomiting or use of laxatives or drugs to lose weight.
- What is the level of physical activity performed by the adolescent? Has it changed recently?
- History of participation in sports and athletics.

Dietary assessment

- Elaborate the meal pattern, frequency and the proportion of food items consumed in each meal using 24 hours dietary recall.
- Vegan or dietary restrictions and history of intake of dairy products.
- Is the food intake appropriate with respect to the pubertal stage and level of activity?
- Skipping of meals, frequency per week and at what time of day or history of voluntary attempt to eat less?
- History of intake of nutritional supplement/vitamin preparations.
- Substance abuse like cigarette smoking, drugs, alcohol, or use of caffeine.

History of any definitive or suggested chronic illness

- Any acute illness or underlying chronic condition like malabsorption, chronic kidney, heart, pulmonary or liver disease, HIV infection, psychiatric illness or any other health concerns.
- Metabolic and endocrine problems like type 1 diabetes mellitus, hypo/hyperthyroidism, and celiac disease.
- History of drugs, which can alter the appetite.
- Identify the problems and complications due to undernutrition like short stature, poor work performance, delayed puberty or menstrual irregularities.

Box 3.2.2: Physical assessment in an adolescent with undernutrition

STEP 1

Assessment of growth and nutrition

a. Weight, height and body mass index (BMI).
b. Plot the parameters on a growth chart (age and gender specific) and compare it with the reference population. Calculate and plot the midparental height (MPH).
   Thinness: BMI < –2 SD for age and sex.
   Severe thinness: BMI < –3 SD for age and sex.
   Short stature: Height for age < 3rd centile or < –2 SD for age and sex.
c. Calculate the growth velocity over the past 6-12 months.
d. Determine the sexual maturity rating (SMR) stage of the adolescent and check whether it conforms to the chronological age.
e. Mid upper arm circumference (MUAC) used in emergency circumstances (famine, or refugee crises, or when reliable scales and height boards are not available) and for monitoring the response to nutritional rehabilitation.
f. Look for bipedal edema.

STEP 2

General physical examination

(a) Vital signs: Temperature, heart rate, BP and signs of dehydration.

(b) Identify signs of macro- and micronutrient deficiencies.

- Visual appearance of extreme emaciation, loss of subcutaneous fat with loose skin folds and inability to walk or perform day today activities.
- Pallor and signs of micronutrient deficiencies.

STEP 3

Thorough systemic examination to look for signs of acute or chronic illnesses that can explain the current nutritional status.

- Since linear growth continues and BMI changes with age after attaining sexual maturity, age and sex specific cut off points should be used to measure undernutrition. This is in contrast to adults in whom a single cut off value of BMI is used to classify malnutrition for both sexes; BMI > or = 18.5 kg/m^2 is considered normal.
- The distinction between acute and chronic undernutrition among adolescents is not as clear as it is among young children. Stunting is a measure of chronic undernutrition and is defined as height for age < 3rd centile or < –2 SD using population reference curves.
- Regardless of the specific index used, evaluation of nutritional status must take into account the presence or absence of bilateral pedal edema.
- Mid upper arm circumference (MUAC) can be utilized to monitor the response of nutritional rehabilitation in anorexia nervosa, as it is not influenced by fluctuations in body weight due to water content and constipation. As per Integrated Management of Adolescent and Adult Illness (IMAI), severe malnutrition in adolescents is defined by the presence of an MUAC < 160 mm or an MUAC of 161–185 mm plus one of the following criteria: pitting edema; or inability to stand; or sunken eyes. Clinical signs like visual evidence of extreme emaciation, bipedal edema, and inability to walk or work may be used to identify those in need of urgent nutritional rehabilitation.

INVESTIGATIONS

- The initial evaluation in an adolescent with undernutrition includes assessment of energy and protein deficit and accompanying micronutrient deficiencies. The investigations ordered in a particular case are guided by the history and examination (Box 3.2.3).
- The search for secondary causes of undernutrition is routinely done in all individuals directed by the clinical cues. A conscientious effort to investigate for the co-morbidities is also done.

MANAGEMENT

Nutrition interventions for adolescents should be tailored to the developmental level of each individual adolescent to respond to their needs (Table 3.2.2).

Education plays an integral role to empower the adolescents to take care of their nutritional needs.

LEARNING POINTS

- Inadequate calorie and protein intake along with subclinical micronutrient deficiencies are common because of increased requirements in adolescence.
- Iron deficiency is the most common deficiency. Other common nutrient deficiencies include that of vitamin A, folic acid, iodine, zinc and calcium.
- Assessment of nutritional status using anthropometric parameters is complicated by changes in body

Box 3.2.3: Investigations to evaluate undernutrition in adolescents
Check for macro/micronutrient deficiencies
• Complete blood counts with peripheral smear • Iron studies/Vitamin B12/Folate levels • Serum Calcium/Inorganic phosphate/Alkaline phosphatase • Serum 25(OH)D levels if needed • Thyroid Profile: Serum Free T4/TSH levels • Serum electrolytes and kidney function tests in case of bulimia • Total protein with albumin, liver function tests • DEXA scan for bone mineral density
Endocrine causes and Eating disorders
• Bone age (X-ray of left wrist joint) if short stature or delayed puberty present • Serum anti-tissue transglutaminase (tTG) levels in suspected celiac disease • Fasting blood sugar • ECG • Lipid profile
Specific Investigations
• To evaluate the etiology of chronic medical illnesses like tuberculosis, HIV, chronic kidney disease/chronic liver disease, any pulmonary or cardiac cause.

Table 3.2.2: Specific interventions in relation to health concerns in adolescent with undernutrition

Problem	*Intervention*
Thinness	Locally available nutrient-rich or fortified supplementary foods to restore normal nutritional status. Besides adequate calories (20-30% additional of recommended energy for age) and protein, vitamins and minerals including calcium, zinc, iron, and folate must be supplemented to permit catch up growth and weight gain. If malabsorption is present, supplements of fat-soluble vitamins are indicated. Determine and treat the underlying cause of malnutrition.
Severe Thinness	Manage as outpatients in a therapeutic feeding program unless there is accompanying medical/surgical illness to require hospitalization. Consider for inpatient care if infections are present or appetite is poor. During the initial phase of stabilization, therapeutic feeding options include ready-to-use food (RUTF), fortified blended flours, or formula milks (F75 or F100) as available. The recommended feeds per kg body weight for adolescents are less than that started in children for nutritional rehabilitation with the initial goal to prevent further tissue loss. Nasogastric tube feeding can be used if oral intake is poor. As the appetite returns, a diet based on the traditional foods is provided with added oil and supplemented vitamins and minerals.

proportions with age, pubertal development, environmental factors and ethnicity.

- Undernutrition in adolescent girls is detrimental to her own health, but may have poor pregnancy outcomes (increased chance of preterm birth and IUGR) and can later lead to translation into intergenerational malnutrition.
- Birth weight is an important determinant of postnatal growth and development and with regard to their predilection for major degenerative diseases in adult life.
- Principles of management of severe malnutrition are similar to young children.

SUGGESTED READING

1. American Academy of Pediatrics Committee on Nutrition. In: Klienman RE editor. Pediatric Nutrition Handbook, 6th ed. Elk Grove Village, IL: American Academy of Pediatrics; 2009.
2. Delisle E. Nutrition in adolescence: Issues and challenges for the health: Sector issues in adolescent health and development. Geneva: World Health Organization; 2005.
3. Fernandez MAL, Delchevalerie P, Van Herp M. Accuracy of MUAC in the detection of severe wasting with the new WHO Growth Standards. Pediatrics 2010;126:e195-e201.
4. IMAI District Clinician Manual: Hospital care for adolescents and adults. Guidelines for the management of common illnesses with limited resources, Volumes 1 and 2. Geneva: World Health Organization; 2011 (http://www.who.int/hiv/pub/imai/imai2011/en/).
5. International Institute for Population Sciences (IIPS) and Macro International, 2007. National Family Health Survey (NFHS-3), 2005–06: India: Volume II. Mumbai: IIPS.
6. Onis M, Onyango AW, Borghi E, Siyam A, Nishida C, Siekmann J. Development of a WHO growth reference for school-aged children and adolescents. Bull World Health Org 2007;85:660-67.
7. Martin AC, Pascoe EM, Forbes DA. Monitoring nutritional status accurately and reliably in adolescents with anorexia nervosa. Paediatr Child Health 2009;45:53-57.
8. Tang AM, Dong K, Deitchler M, Chung M, Wanke C, Tumilowicz A, *et al.* Use of cutoffs for mid-upper arm circumference (MUAC) as an indicator or predictor of nutritional and health-related outcomes in adolescents and adults: A systematic review. Washington, DC: Food and Nutrition Technical Assistance (FANTA) Project; 2013.
9. Toteja GS, Singh P, Dhillon BS, Saxena BN, *et al.* Prevalence of anemia among pregnant women and adolescent girls in 16 districts of India. Food Nutr Bull 2006;27(4):311-15.

3.3

Overnutrition and Obesity

Sandra G Hassink, Swati Y Bhave

INTRODUCTION

Obesity, defined by a body mass index (BMI) ≥ 95% for age and gender, is both a significant risk for morbidity in adolescence and for obesity and its attendant risks in adulthood. Adolescents are at high risk for unhealthy eating and physical inactivity patterns that may have become entrenched over the years resulting in the accumulation of obesity-related risk factors. Obesity has emerging co-morbidities such as type 2 diabetes, non-alcoholic steatohepatitis (NASH), obstructive sleep apnea, dyslipidemia, slipped capital femoral epiphysis and Blount disease. These add to the chronic disease burden and complexity of treatment. In addition, obesity in a young woman who becomes pregnant carries with it increased morbidity for the mother and infant as well as increased risk of obesity for the offspring, and is one of the factors perpetuating the obesity epidemic. Thus the period of adolescence is a crucial time to focus on obesity treatment for preventing adult diseases as well as intergenerational effect (Box 3.3.1).

CLINICAL FEATURES

Presenting Symptoms

An adolescent with obesity can present only with the symptom of weight gain or with symptoms of co-morbidity (Table 3.3.1).

Box 3.3.1: Risk for developing obesity

- Puberty is a sentinel event in adolescence and the physical and metabolic changes that result can enhance the risk for obesity and obesity-related co-morbidities.
  - Pubertal transition from Tanner stage 1 to stage 3 is associated with a 32% reduction in insulin sensitivity as well as increases in fasting glucose, insulin and insulin resistance.
  - Insulin resistance reaches a peak at mid-puberty coincident with peak height velocity and returns to almost prepubertal levels at the end of puberty with a strong correlation with BMI throughout.
  - These changes are similar across gender, ethnicity and obesity and are not associated with changes in body fat, visceral fat, insulin-like growth factor, androgens, or estradiol.
- The context in which lifestyle risk factors occur is also important. An increased risk for obesity and bigger barriers to treatment are seen in adolescents with:
  - Developmental delays.
  - Poverty.
  - Strong family histories of obesity.
- Such adolescents are at increased risk for obesity and may also face increased barriers to treatment.
- The shift towards positive energy balance that has occurred in the individual, within families and in the population over the past 3 decades has resulted in a series of evidence-based targets for obesity intervention both at the individual and increasingly at the population level.
- Studies have shown that the association of TV time and obesity is mediated through commercials and reduction of commercial TV may be a prime target of treatment.
- Physical activity declines as children move into adolescence and adolescents may feel inhibited about participation due to their weight, teasing and bullying, or limitations in the family's ability to support athletic involvement.
- Intergenerational effect: Malnourished mothers produce low birth weight infant who is at high risk for insulin resistance, obesity and metabolic syndrome–Barker's hypotheses.

Table 3.3.1: Signs and symptoms of co-morbidities

System	*Signs and Symptoms*	*Co-morbidity*
Ophthalmologic	Diplopia, visual field cuts	Pseudotumor cerebri
Pulmonary	Snoring, apnea, daytime somnolence, school problems, enuresis, napping	Obstructive sleep apnea
	Wheezing, nighttime cough, exercise intolerance	Asthma
Cardiovascular	Exercise intolerance	Deconditioning Cardiomyopathy of obesity
Gastrointestinal	Abdominal pain, vomiting Right upper quadrant discomfort Right upper quadrant pain	Reflux Non-alcoholic fatty liver disease Cholecystitis
Musculoskeletal	Knee pain, limp, hip pain Knee pain, bowing Foot and/or ankle pain	Slipped capital femoral epiphysis Blount disease
Neurological	Headache	Pseudotumor cerebri Hypertension
Endocrine	Thyromegaly, constipation Height deceleration, striae, centripetal obesity Amenorrhea, oligomenorrhea, weight loss, polyuria, polydipsia, vaginal infections Polyuria, polydipsia, increased appetite, weight loss	Hypothyroidism Cushing syndrome Polycystic ovarian syndrome Type 2 diabetes
Psychological	Irritability, poor school performance, anger, or other symptoms of depression, anxiety, low self-esteem, self-injury or suicidal ideation, psychotropic medication use, sleep disturbance, limited sleep, poor sleep hygiene and fatigue	Depression Anxiety

History Taking

Taking a careful history is important not only to uncover risk factors for obesity and to understand the general condition of the adolescent's health and environmental context, but also to begin establishing a positive relationship with the adolescent upon which treatment can be based.

The physician must be alert that although rare, adolescents may present with short stature, developmental delay and obesity as manifestations of a previously undiagnosed genetic syndrome that needs to be identified and treated.

Weight Gain

A detailed history of weight gain is very important. This should include risk factors which predispose to obesity in childhood:

- Beginning before birth with maternal and paternal BMI.
- Gestational weight gain, and/or history of gestational diabetes of the mother.
- Birth weight should be ascertained because both large and small for gestational age infants have a higher risk for later obesity.
- Infant feeding, whether breast, bottle or mixed, and age of transition to table food will also indicate risk factors for childhood obesity.
- Nicotine consumption, both smoking and chewable and other tobacco products in pregnancy.

Review of the pattern of weight gain can contribute to an understanding of the adolescent's obesity.

- A pattern of early adiposity rebound is a risk factor for childhood obesity.
- A normal weight gain, followed by an inflection point and rapid crossing of percentiles can indicate a shift in family dynamics and/or a change in the child's environment (e.g. divorce, move, death in the family, job loss and school change).

Detailed dietary, physical activity and sedentary activity history are critical to understanding energy balance and setting realistic lifestyle treatment goals with the adolescent and family.

- A 24-hour diet history, asking about the preceding day, is the best way to get an accurate snapshot of intake and dietary patterns.
- Often asking about both a weekday and a weekend day can elicit even more accurate information about eating patterns.
- Maintaining a weekly diet history helps is a useful monitoring tool.
- Food insecurity is also associated with obesity and should be identified as part of a nutrition assessment in economically deprived adolescents.

- Understanding patterns of activity and sedentary behavior is important. It is not unusual for adolescents to have patterns of excessive screen time and limited physical activity.

In addition to understanding dietary patterns and intake, it is important to understand the adolescent's relationship with food.

- Breakfast skipping is a common eating pattern that begins at puberty and may relate to the adolescent's shifting sleep cycle.
- Meal skipping is often an adolescent strategy for weight loss, as are limited food item diets.
- Questions about stress eating, comfort eating, food as a reward, distracted eating while watching TV or working on the computer, and night eating, if present can be the focus of patient goals for change.
- Adolescent's choice of food can also be affected by peer group, impact of media and advertisement and what is available in the school canteen.

These eating patterns often require the assistance of a dietician. Binge eating is not unusual and may be best approached through the use of a questionnaire. If present it requires intervention by a trained professional experienced with disordered eating.

A detailed *family history* can be an important motivator for change:

- It is important to understand the family's response to obesity and obesity-related co-morbidities and modeling of healthy behavior to understand the context for treatment of the adolescent.
- Family eating patterns, food available in the house, home cooking vs. processed and packaged food, parents' activity level, exercise habits etc. are factors that contribute to an obesogenic environment.
- Focus on obesity-related co-morbidities such as type 2 diabetes, hypertension, cardiovascular disease, hyperlipidemia, non-alcoholic hepatosteatosis (NASH), obstructive sleep apnea, polycystic ovarian syndrome and obesity as well as family members who have had bariatric surgery.

Physical Examination and Review of Systems

A thorough review of systems is critical to understand the adolescents overall health, identify health problems that may have been previously unrecognized and to identify obesity-related co-morbidities. Table 3.3.1 offers suggestions for an obesity focused review of systems and Table 3.3.2 illustrates findings on physical examination.

Body Mass Index (BMI)

The first step in performing a physical examination is to make sure accurate height and weight are measured and the BMI is calculated and plotted on a growth curve.

Severe obesity is not uncommon in the adolescent age group and BMI percentiles and Z scores may have limited utility because of the contraction of values that occurs at the upper range of the growth curve.

- BMI as a percentage of the 95th BMI percentile has been recommended for characterizing and tracking children with high BMI.
- A threshold of BMI ≥120% of the 95th percentile has been proposed as the definition of severe obesity. Growth charts have been published which reflect this definition which may help in further defining BMI as a risk factor.

Table 3.3.2: Physical examination in obese adolescents

Head	Thinning hair/male pattern baldness
Eyes	Visual field cuts, diplopia, papilledema
Ears, Nose and Throat	Tonsillar hypertrophy, thyromegaly
Puberty	Tanner staging
Lungs	Wheezing, chest tightness
Cardiovascular	Murmur, elevated blood pressure
Gastrointestinal	Enlarged liver
Musculoskeletal	Limitation of motion of the hips or knees, limp, bowing of knees
Skin	Hirsutism, acne, acanthosis nigricans, striae, cervical fat pad
General	Weight loss if associated with other signs of type 2 diabetes

- An absolute BMI of 35 kg/m^2, can also be used if it is lower based on age and gender.
- The inclusion of an absolute BMI threshold (35 kg/m^2) aligns the pediatric definition with class II obesity in adults, a high-risk category of obesity associated with early mortality in adults.

Due to genetic predisposition in Asian population the BMI cut-offs are different for Asia that includes the Indian population (Table 3.3.3).

Blood Pressure

It is important to measure blood pressure accurately and at every visit. The proper size cuff should be used and blood pressure measurement classified as normal, pre-hypertensive or hypertensive in order to make sure it is properly managed.

Obesity-Related Co-morbidities

Obesity-related co-morbidities increase as obesity persists into adolescence. Sleep apnea and hypertension are commonly diagnosed and are linked to BMI. Features of the metabolic syndrome, such as hyperinsulinemia, obesity, hypertension, hyperlipidemia and dyslipidemia are much more common in adolescents who have obesity.

- Elevated BMI in adolescence, even with normalization of weight as an adult had an independent association with the onset of coronary artery disease in young adulthood.
- Elevated BMI is also related to depression; adolescents with obesity with the highest depression scores had the greatest increase in BMI.

Unhealthy weight control behaviors are associated with obesity in both boys and girls and are associated with low life satisfaction for both genders and negative affect, and body size dissatisfaction in boys. It is important to screen for and identify obesity-related co-morbidities in all adolescents with elevated BMI. Table 3.3.4 illustrates obesity-related emergencies and Table 3.3.1 signs and symptoms of common co-morbidities of obesity.

Investigations

These will basically depend upon the associated co-morbidities as outlined in Table 3.3.1. Every adolescent with obesity and/or with family history of risk factors should undergo screening for metabolic syndrome as outlined in Chapter 3.4 as well as other obesity-related co-morbidities.

MANAGEMENT

The basis of obesity treatment is lifestyle change, with a focus on optimal nutrition, physical activity and a reduction in sedentary time. The lifestyle changes to reduce obesity risk are listed in Table 3.3.5.

Treatment strategies should take into consideration the developmental stage of the adolescent (early, mid or late adolescence).

- Knowledge of adolescent development, family dynamics, and communication techniques such as motivational interviewing along with specific strategies to help the family and adolescent to make healthy lifestyle changes are key components of treating obesity.
- The role of the family is very important in transitioning the adolescent into young adulthood and in restricting the severity of obesity and the related co-morbidities.

Treatment also occurs in the context of factors that can either promote successful weight loss or present barriers such as:

- Previous successful or unsuccessful attempts to lose weight.
- Family history of obesity and role modeling of healthy lifestyle.
- The extent of bullying and teasing.
- Co-existing mental or behavioral health problems and the health promoting nature of the adolescent's home, school and social environment.

Some of the important aspects of successfully managing obesity in adolescents are listed in Box 3.3.2.

Table 3.3.3: BMI cut-offs for Asian population

	Overweight		*Obesity*	
	Percentile	**BMI (kg/m^2)**	**Percentile**	**BMI (kg/m^2)**
WHO	> 85%	>25	>95%	>30
WHO, Asian	–	22-25		≥28
IOTF (revised 2012), Unofficial Asian	–	23		≥28

Table 3.3.4: Emergencies related to obesity

Emergency and Co-morbidity	*Clinical Features*	*Supportive Evidence*
Diabetic Ketoacidosis	Polydipsia Polyuria Weight loss Abdominal pain Confusion	• Hyperglycemia (blood glucose >11 mmol/L (200 mg/dl) • Venous pH <7.3 and/or bicarbonate <15 mmol/L • Ketonemia and ketonuria
Hyperglycemic Hyperosmolar State	Vomiting Abdominal pain Dizziness Weakness Polyuria/polydipsia Weight loss Diarrhea Confusion	• Plasma glucose >600 mg/dl • Serum CO_2 >15 mmol/L • Small ketonuria • Absent to low ketonemia • Effective serum osmolality >320 mOsm//kg • Stupor or coma
Pulmonary Emboli	Chest pain Dyspnea Hemoptysis	Hypoxia Risk factors • Obesity • Hypoventilation/Obstructive sleep apnea • Coagulation disorder • Complication of bariatric surgery
Cardiomyopathy of Obesity	Dyspnea Orthopnea	• Cardiomegaly • Left ventricular hypertrophy (LVH) • Left ventricular diastolic dysfunction
Complications of Bariatric Surgery	Bleeding Bowel perforation Deep vein thrombosis (DVT), pulmonary embolism (PE) Dehydration Dysphagia Nausea/vomiting Small bowel obstruction, anastomotic leak Peritonitis	

Table 3.3.5: Lifestyle changes to reduce obesity risk
(Evidence-based lifestyle changes are in **bold.** Author's comments are in *italics*)

Evidence for Improving Obesity/Energy Balance	*Evidence for Support of a Healthy Weight*
Limit consumption of sugar sweetened beverages *Encourage drinking of plain water*	**Eat a diet rich in calcium**
Limit TV *and all screen time* • *0 hours for <2 years old* • *<2 hours for >2 years old*	**Eat a diet high in fiber**
Remove TV from primary sleeping area *But now with mobiles, IPads, tablets etc. children are having increasing screen time that parents find difficult to monitor*	**Eat a diet with balanced macronutrients (food groups)**
Eat breakfast daily	**Encourage breastfeeding**
Limit eating out *Encourage home cooked meals*	**Promote moderate/vigorous activity (60 minutes/day)** *Reduce sedentary lifestyle*
Encourage family meals	**Limit consumption of energy dense foods**
Limit portion size *This has been shown to be the best way to reduce excess intake and maintain healthy nutrition*	**Encourage adequate sleep** *Sleep deprivation as well as excess sleeping have been shown to promote obesity*

Box 3.3.2: Important aspects of obesity treatment in adolescents

Obesity is a chronic disease and as such requires:

- A proactive and prepared clinical team.
- A family equipped with the knowledge and skills to achieve ongoing lifestyle change.
- A community that supports healthy choices and encourages a healthy lifestyle.
- A health system that promotes integrated and multidisciplinary care with communications and it support.

Evidence shows that multidisciplinary obesity treatment can be successful. Components of a clinical team include physicians, nurses, dieticians, exercise specialists and psychologists. Obesity treatment in primary care is less well studied but early evidence shows that a clinical team prepared to identify, classify and categorize BMI, engage in motivational interviewing and goal setting with families and patients and commit to frequent follow-up has the best chance of success. Partnership with community based dieticians and psychologists can provide added benefit.

Box 3.3.3 lists some of the important treatment interventions with adolescents.

Involvement of the Family

Involvement of the family is crucial in weight reduction of adolescents. It is important to evaluate all the environments that the adolescent is in and work with them on the specifics of achieving their goals in each venue.

- For example: If the goal is to reduce or eliminate sugared beverages, plans will need to be made for home, school, friends and extended family in order to carry out this goal.

Box 3.3.3: Treatment interventions with adolescents

- After a complete review of all risk factors and investigations, the physician should explain to the adolescent and family the health implications of having an elevated BMI.
- Motivational interviewing is helpful in opening up the conversation to help the adolescent and the family to identify goals that are important for them.
- Based on the dietary, physical and sedentary activity assessment, the physician can help the adolescents and their families determine small achievable goals that they can self-monitor and review on follow-up.
- Family support is crucial for the adolescent and this should be emphasized especially when the family has engaged in blaming the adolescents for their weight gain.
- If the family is willing to create a healthy nutrition and activity environment at home for all family members, the adolescent will have a 'safe haven' where making the healthy choice is the easy choice and will have positive role modeling and support from family members.

- Often parents will need help in understanding how best to support their adolescent and creating a healthy home environment is a powerful way to start.
- Parents may also want to decide with the adolescent how they will intervene if the adolescent is not achieving their goals.
- Families can discuss who might be able to partner the adolescent in increasing physical activity and how screen time can be reduced by the whole family.
- The family can be supportive of the adolescent and the challenges of keeping their goal behaviors at school and when with peers.
- Talking through the anticipated situation and debriefing afterward can be helpful in teaching the adolescent strategies to make healthy changes.
- Self-monitoring is an important tool that is associated with successful lifestyle change.
- Diet records, records of screen time, and physical activity are all helpful in keeping teens and families on track.
- Frequent visits and contact are important in maintaining motivation. Brief, frequent visits to check weight, review goals and trouble shoot can avert relapse.

Surgical Options

For adolescents with severe obesity and attendant co-morbidities, bariatric surgery may be an option, but should only be performed in a center with a strong adolescent weight management program, a multidisciplinary team which includes a surgeon, pediatric weight management physician, psychologist, dietician, and exercise professional at a minimum and has the ability to perform a through pre-surgical assessment of physical and mental health and carry out appropriate follow-up.

LEARNING POINTS

1. Adolescence is an important time to break the cycle of obesity.
2. Screening of obesity-related co-morbidities should be a routine part of every practice.
3. Health care providers should be prepared to identify obesity-related emergencies.
4. Obesity is a chronic disease and requires a long-term coordinated approach to manage obesity in adolescents.

5. Obesity is often a multi-generational disease and requires a family-focused approach.
6. Adolescents with obesity are often the subject of bullying and teasing and need to be approached in a positive and compassionate manner.

SUGGESTED READING

1. Barlow SE. Expert committee recommendations regarding the prevention, assessment, and treatment of child and adolescent overweight and obesity: Summary report. Pediatrics 2007;120(Suppl 4): S164-92.
2. Bhave SY (Ed). Obesity in Children and Adolescents. New Delhi; IJCP Group of Publications; 2014.
3. Hassink S. Pediatric Obesity: Prevention, Intervention and Treatment Strategies for Primary Care; 2nd edition. Elk Grove Village, Illinois, USA; American Academy of Pediatrics; 2014.
4. Kelly AS, Barlow SE, Rao G, Inge TH, Hayman LL, Steinberger J, Urbina EM, Ewing LJ, Daniels SR: Severe obesity in children and adolescents: Identification, associated health risks, and treatment approaches: A scientific statement from the American Heart Association. Circulation 2013;128:1689-712.
5. Spear BA, Barlow SE, Ervin C, *et al.* Recommendations for treatment of child and adolescent overweight and obesity. Pediatrics 2007:120 (Suppl4):S254-88.
6. Tanofsky-Kraff M, Wilfley DE, Young JR, *et al.* Preventing excessive weight gain in adolescents; Interpersonal psychotherapy for binge eating. Obesity (Silver Spring) 2007;15(6);1345-405.
7. Whitlock EP, O'Connor EA, Williams SB, Beil TL, Lutz KW. Effectiveness of weight management interventions in children: A targeted systematic review for the USPSTF. Pediatrics 2010; 125(2): e396-e418.
8. Woo JG. Using body mass index Z-score among severely obese adolescents: A cautionary note. Int J Pediatr Obes 2009;4:405-10.

Metabolic Consequences of Obesity

3.4

Vaman V Khadilkar, Prashant P Patil

INTRODUCTION

Metabolic syndrome also known as "Syndrome X" first coined by Reaven in 1920 represents a constellation of metabolic derangements consisting of hyperinsulinemia, high triglycerides and apolipoprotein B, low high-density lipoprotein-cholesterol (HDL) and hypertension. Central obesity and insulin resistance (IR) plays a pivotal pathogenic role in development of metabolic syndrome. It is postulated that programming of these disorders begin in fetal life and manifest due to complex interactions of multiple risk factors, throughout life. Out of various criteria for metabolic syndrome the most widely accepted criteria are by International Diabetes Federation (IDF-2005) which takes into account age group and ethnicity (Box 3.4.1).

Interventions such as early screening of at-risk population, health education and community participation are very vital to prevent future epidemic of diabetes and cardiovascular diseases in already at-risk population.

DEFINITION

Since the first description of the metabolic syndrome by Reaven in 1920, multiple attempts have been made to define metabolic syndrome in children (WHO 1998, NCEP: ATPIII 2001). All these definitions have a common component of obesity (waist circumference or body mass index [BMI]), component of dyslipidemia (elevated triglycerides and low HDL cholesterol), hypertension, and altered glucose homeostasis (impaired fasting glucose or impaired glucose tolerance; Table 3.4.1).

Box 3.4.1: International Diabetes Federation (IDF) definition of metabolic syndrome in adolescents

- Abdominal obesity (waist circumference >90th percentile) according to age and gender (NHANES)
- Presence of 2 or more of the following 4:
  1. Hypertriglyceridemia ≥ 150 mg/dL
  2. High density lipoprotein (HDL) cholesterol ≤ 40 mg/dL
  3. High blood pressure ≥ 90th percentile according to age, gender and height (NHANES)
  4. Fasting blood glucose ≥ 100 mg/dL

Table 3.4.1: Components of metabolic syndrome
Hypertension
Dyslipidemia
Insulin resistance
Type 2 diabetes mellitus
Glucose intolerance
Atherosclerosis/heart failure
Liver cirrhosis
Steatosis (non-alcoholic fatty liver disease)
Non-alcoholic steatohepatitis (NASH)
Obstructive sleep apnea

The International Diabetes Federation (IDF) criterion in 2005 is the most recently published and widely accepted criteria to define metabolic syndrome. The IDF definition is stratified as per different ethnical background and age-groups with central obesity. The IDF particularly emphasized on waist measurement as a simple screening tool as adopted by American Heart Association (AHA).

CLINICAL FEATURES

History Taking

History taking for an obese or overweight adolescent has already been covered in the previous Chapter 3.3 on Overnutrition and Obesity.

For screening for metabolic syndrome additional important points in history taking are:

- Asian ethnicity.
- Family history of obesity in one or both parents
- Type 2 diabetes mellitus.
- Coronary heart disease or early death due to heart ailment.
- Gestational diabetes mellitus and/or ovarian hyperandrogenism such as polycystic ovarian syndrome (PCOS).

Physical Examination

The height and weight should be carefully taken to calculate the body mass index (BMI).

BMI as a Diagnostic Tool

BMI expressed in terms of kg/m^2, is used as a surrogate marker for adiposity; however it has its limitations. Firstly it is an absolute value which can only be used as a statistical tool. Secondly it does not take sexual maturity and ethnicity into consideration. BMI is an indirect measure of adiposity distribution in the body. Therefore BMI when used alone as a marker may falsely overlook proportion of adolescents with high inherent risk for metabolic syndrome.

Other Parameters

Apart from height, weight and BMI measurements, waist circumference is most important in the clinical examination.

Look for signs of insulin resistance such as acanthosis nigricans and signs of polycystic ovarian syndrome such as acne and hirsutism.

The height and weight are taken to calculate BMI using the formula–weight in kg divided by height in meter squared (Wt/Ht^2). Hence is it very important to use the correct techniques to take these parameters.

Steps for Accurate Height Measurement

- Set the modified measuring board (e.g. Harpenden stadiometer) vertically on stable level surface.
- Remove footwear, hair bands and other hair accessories. The adolescent should stand on a flat and uncarpeted floor against a flat wall.
- Make the adolescent stand against a flat wall while looking ahead in such a way that the chin is perpendicular to the scale and the line of vision is parallel to floor with shoulders at level, arms at sides, feet straight and touching together and flat.
- Four bony prominences–external occipital protuberance (occiput), scapula (back), ischium (pelvis) and calcaneus (heels) should touch the flat surface of the wall.
- Use a flat surface (headpiece) perpendicular to wall and lower the headpiece till it firmly touches the crown of the head with examiners visual axis at the same level as that of the headpiece.
- Faintly mark the wall where lower end of headpiece firmly touches the wall, and then use a metallic tape to measure height.
- Read and announce the measurement to the nearest 0.1 cm or 1/8th of an inch.
- Record and repeat the measurement to the measurer to make sure it has been correctly heard.

Weight Taking

- Ask the teenager to remove footwear and heavy clothing, such as sweaters and accessories (e.g. mobile phone).
- Measure the weight with the help of a digital scale placed on a hard, and even surface with feet placed in the center of scale and adolescent looking straight.
- Measure the weight to the nearest decimal fraction (e.g. 34.7 kg).

Waist Circumference

- Waist circumference, a direct measure of abdominal obesity, is considered a potential marker in place of or in combination with BMI to identify adolescents with increased metabolic risk. It provides more valuable information than BMI alone and may be used as very important tool for identifying children and adolescents at risk for metabolic syndrome.
- Waist circumference is an independent marker of insulin sensitivity and increased visceral adiposity tissue (VAT) and thereby all components of metabolic syndrome in children and adolescents. IDF (2005) uses waist circumference > 90th percentile for particular ethnicity as part of the criteria for diagnosis of metabolic syndrome in adolescents.
- There are few limitations for using waist circumference as a diagnostic tool. There is no universal method for measurement of waist circumference. While WHO recommends waist circumference should be measured at the midpoint between the superior iliac crest and inferior most rib, the NIH and NHANES advocates its measurement immediately above the iliac crest.
- Second, there is lack of standardized waist circumference percentiles in adolescence as well as for different ethnicity as opposed to absolute waist circumference values used as cut-offs in adulthood. Thus interpretation of waist circumference is all the more a difficult task in adolescents.
- When performed correctly elevated waist circumference measurement can be used as an important yardstick for developing overall risk for complications of obesity and metabolic syndrome.

- Indian waist circumference percentiles are given in Table 3.4.2.
- Authors recommend that 70th percentile of Indian waist circumference as screening cut-off for metabolic syndrome.

PATHOGENESIS AND INVESTIGATIONS

Pathogenic mechanisms of various components of metabolic syndrome are explained in the Table 3.4.3 and Figure 3.4.1.

Investigations in Adolescent with Obesity and Suspected with Metabolic Syndrome

- Overnight fasting lipid profile, liver enzymes and abdominal ultrasound should be done for non-alcoholic fatty liver disease.
- For suspected type 2 diabetes, fasting glucose and insulin ratio are measured and an oral glucose tolerance test performed with 1.75 g/kg (or 75 g whichever is higher) of glucose along with insulin measurements.
- Glycosylated hemoglobin (HbA1c) is not yet accepted by WHO as a single diagnostic test of diabetes in children and adolescents although American Diabetes Association is in favor of it as a screening test.
- Mild elevation of TSH and T3 are common in obese children and adolescents and is an effect of leptin drive and peripheral thyroid resistance imposed by obese state and not hypothyroidism. Such mild elevation of TSH should not be treated with thyroxine.

Table 3.4.2: Waist circumference values for Indian boys and girls

Age (yr)	*3rd*	*10th*	*15th*	*25th*	*50th*	*70th*	*75th*	*85th*	*90th*	*95th*
Boys										
9+	54.7	56.5	57.8	59.9	64.2	**68.0**	69.2	72.3	74.6	78.2
10+	57.0	59.0	60.4	62.6	67.3	**71.4**	72.7	76.0	78.4	82.3
11+	59.3	61.5	63.0	65.4	70.4	**74.9**	76.2	79.7	82.3	86.4
12+	61.5	63.8	65.4	68.0	73.3	**78.0**	79.4	83.1	85.8	90.1
13+	63.4	65.8	67.6	70.3	75.8	**80.7**	82.2	86.0	88.8	93.2
14+	64.9	67.5	69.3	72.2	78.0	**83.0**	84.5	88.4	91.2	95.6
15+	66.2	68.9	70.8	73.8	79.8	**84.9**	86.5	90.4	93.2	97.6
16+	67.4	70.2	72.1	75.2	81.3	**86.5**	88.1	92.1	94.9	99.2
17+	68.4	71.3	73.3	76.5	82.7	**87.9**	89.6	93.5	96.3	100.6
Girls										
9+	54.5	56.3	57.6	59.7	64.0	**67.9**	69.1	72.3	74.6	78.4
10+	56.8	58.8	60.3	62.5	67.2	**71.3**	72.6	75.9	78.3	82.2
11+	59.3	61.5	63.1	65.5	70.5	**74.8**	76.2	79.6	82.1	86.0
12+	61.7	64.0	65.7	68.3	73.5	**78.1**	79.5	83.0	85.5	89.5
13+	63.6	66.1	67.9	70.6	76.1	**80.8**	82.2	85.7	88.3	92.2
14+	65.0	67.6	69.5	72.3	78.0	**82.7**	84.2	87.8	90.3	94.2
15+	66.0	68.7	70.6	73.5	79.3	**84.1**	85.6	89.1	91.6	95.4
16+	66.6	69.5	71.4	74.4	80.3	**85.1**	86.5	90.1	92.5	96.3
17+	67.1	70.1	72.1	75.2	81.1	**85.9**	87.4	90.9	93.3	96.9

Table 3.4.3: Manifestations and principal pathogenic mechanisms

Manifestations	*Principal pathogenic mechanism*
Hypertension	Oxidative stress, chronic sodium retention
Dyslipidemia	Hyperinsulinemia decreases HDL-C and increases hepatic synthesis of VLDL, and TG and LDL-C
	Reduced uptake of glucose and free fatty acids (FFA) from adipose tissue
	Rates of lipolysis are increased
	Reduced triglyceride (TG) clearance due to down-regulation of lipoprotein lipase
Steatohepatitis	Hepatic inflammation and a transient rise in serum transaminases due to accumulation of TG in liver (hepatic steatosis)
Type 2 diabetes mellitus	Oxidative stress with dysregulation of insulin secretion leads to impaired fasting glucose (IFG) and impaired glucose tolerance (IGT) and then overt diabetes in genetically susceptible adolescents

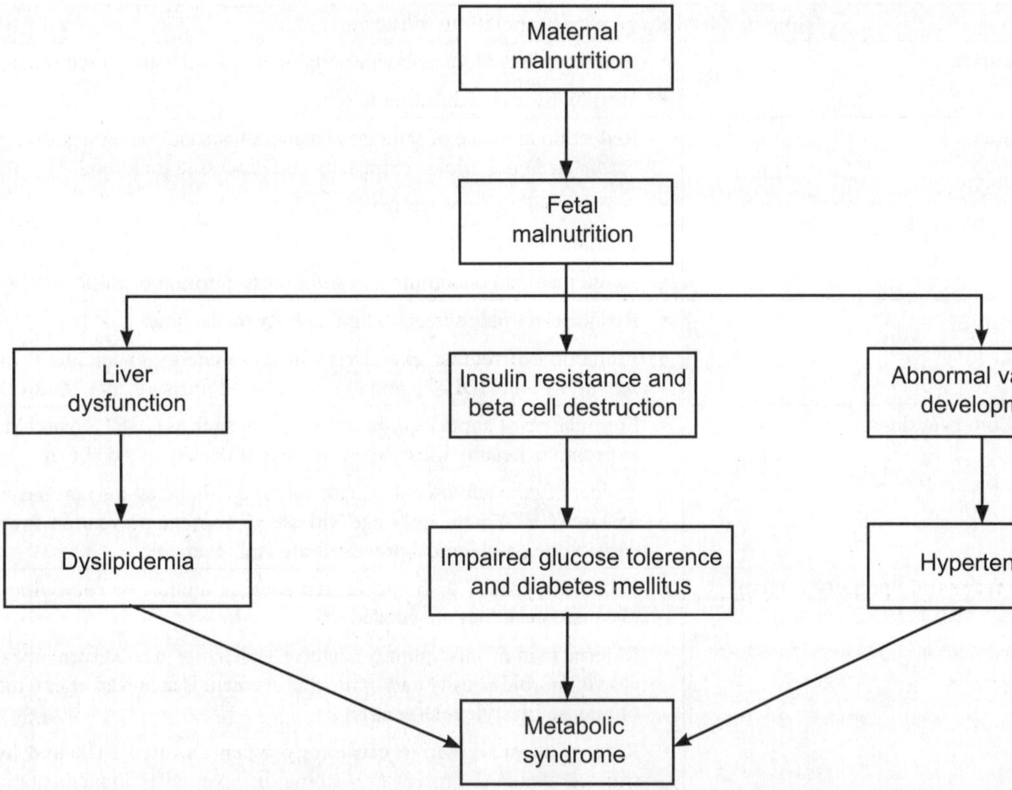

Figure 3.4.1: Fetal origins of adult onset disease (Barker hypothesis)

**Source:* Modified from Nair L, Nair MKC, Chacko DS. Markers of fetal onset adult disease; Indian Pediatr 2009;46:s48-s54.

MANAGEMENT OF METABOLIC SYNDROME

Prevention of Metabolic Syndrome

The old saying "Prevention is better than cure" holds good for metabolic syndrome. Since the origin of adult disease begins in fetal life, care of maternal nutrition is of paramount importance as malnutrition in mother may lead to development of metabolic syndrome as stated in Barker hypothesis. Similarly overfeeding of the children should be strictly avoided especially those who are born small for gestational age (SGA). Pediatricians and clinicians dealing with adolescents have an important role to play in the prevention of metabolic syndrome. The main emphasis should be regular monitoring and tracking BMI to prevent obesity and overweight in children and adolescents. In addition screening should be done for all suspected cases of metabolic syndrome.

Performing screening in schools and colleges will also be an important extension activity.

Treatment of metabolic syndrome in obese adolescents needs a multi-disciplinary approach and is best treated in a multi-disciplinary specialized clinic. Metformin is an attractive and effective option in some (Box 3.4.2).

Principles of Management

The basic principles of management are listed in the Table 3.4.4.

Box 3.4.2: Important points to remember for metformin treatment in adolescents

- **Class of Drug:** Biguanide
- **Use:** Approved for the use in children >10 years
- **Mechanism of action:**
  - Increases insulin sensitivity by direct anorectic effect or indirectly by stimulating secretion of glucagon-like peptide 1 (GLP-1)
  - Increases hepatic glucose uptake, decreases gluconeogenesis, and reduces hepatic glucose production.

Advantages:
- Helps in weight loss by its anorectic action
- Significant reduction in macro-vascular complications
- Decreases waist circumference, BP, triglycerides and total cholesterol
- Well tolerated by most of the adolescents

Side effects:
- Nausea, flatulence, bloating sensation (most common)
- Lactic acidosis (most serious especially seen in patients with renal insufficiency)

Dose:
- 10-18 years: 500 mg orally q12 hourly then titrate the dose 500 mg weekly
- Maximum dose: 2000 mg/day in divided dose

- **Peak plasma concentration**-regular-2-3 hours; extended release 4-8 hours
- **Half-life:** 4-9 hours
- **Contraindications**
  - Concurrent use of iodinated contrast media
  - Alcohol ingestion: Disulfiram like reaction

Table 3.4.4: Management of metabolic syndrome	
Behavioral modification	• Correct maladaptive behavior pertaining to food habits, food faddism • Healthy lifestyle education in school
Dietary modifications	• Reduction in intake of saturated fat and refined carbohydrates, sweetened carbonated cold drinks, extra salty and processed junk food • Avoid snacking between major meals • Encourage intake of low-fat (PUFA) food, dietary fiber, salads and fruits • Avoid maternal undernutrition and excess nutrition in child
Physical activity	• Reduce electronic screen to half an hour to one hour • Promotion of regular exercise to increase energy expenditure, insulin sensitivity and HDL-C; and to reduce blood pressure and TG levels
Community-based interventions	• Formulation of population-based programs such as CHETNA and MARG to promote healthy lifestyle, awareness of obesity and diabetes • To identify the adolescents at risk for type 2 diabetes and coronary heart disease (CHD) at an early age and use appropriate prevention strategies early while pathological processes are still reversible
Multi-disciplinary team and Specialty referral	• Holistic approach with specialized such as dieticians, counselors, and exercise specialists are needed • Referral to multi-disciplinary centers specializing in adolescent obesity in case of morbid obesity and/or no improvement is achieved after 6 months of intense lifestyle intervention • Referral to preventative cardiology–when elevated LDL and hyper-triglyceridemia is present (> 400 mg/dL) even after implementation of healthy lifestyle interventions • Formal somnography sleep apnea study–when signs of obstructive sleep apnea are present
Pharmacological interventions	• Metformin is considered when insulin resistance evidenced by impaired glucose tolerance, HbA1c in the pre-diabetes range or higher (> 5.7%), or persistently elevated fasting insulin levels after 6 months of intensive lifestyle modification • Cardiovascular morbidity and mortality (as described in Box 3.4.2) • Use of statins for dyslipidemia is not recommended in children <10 years of age
Newer drugs: Metabolic inhibitors and cytokine therapy	• Adiponectin, the cannabinoid-1 receptor antagonist rimonabant; satiety agents like extending 4; dipeptidyl peptidase IV inhibitors; peptide YY; and analogs of amylin • Efficacy is yet to be proven children and adolescents
Policy formulation	• Creation of national task force and national programs for obesity • More playgrounds, parks and walking and bicycle tracks • Restriction on TV commercial advertisement junk or processed foods during children's programs

LEARNING POINTS

- Indians are particularly at higher risk for developing metabolic syndrome even at lower waist circumference owing to their genetic make-up, high percentage of body fat, rising prevalence of abdominal obesity.
- Waist circumference, a direct surrogate marker of abdominal obesity and metabolic syndrome should be used as potential cost-effective screening tool.
- Clustering of cardiovascular risk factors, secondary to adipocyte dysfunction leading to inflammation and peripheral insulin resistance, in genetically prone individuals develops into metabolic syndrome later in life.
- Indian waist circumference percentiles are available for use in Indian children and adolescents and 70th percentile is the suggested cut-off for metabolic risk in Indian children and adolescents.
- Obese adolescents with two or more risk factors should have BP monitoring; undergo testing for type 2 diabetes from the age of 10 years; and fasting lipid profile.

- Metformin can be used in appropriate adolescents to treat insulin resistance and cardiovascular health.
- A multi-pronged approach is essential to prevent metabolic syndrome; India should formulate population-based community intervention programs like western countries to prevent the epidemic of metabolic syndrome.

SUGGESTED READING

1. Alberti KG, Eckel RH, Grundy SM, *et al.* Harmonizing the metabolic syndrome: A joint interim statement of the International Diabetes Federation Task Force on Epidemiology and Prevention; National Heart, Lung and Blood Institute; American Heart Association; World Heart Federation; International Atherosclerosis Society; and International Association for the Study of Obesity. Circulation 2009;120:1640-45.
2. Barker DJP. Mothers, babies and health in later life. Edinburgh: Churchill Livingstone; 1998.
3. Barker DJP, Osmond C, Goding J, Kuh D, Wadsworth MEJ. Growth in utero, blood pressure in childhood and adult life, and mortality from cardiovascular disease. BMJ 1989;298:564-67.
4. Barker DJP, Osmond C, Simmonds SJ, Wield GA. The relation of small head circumference and thinness at birth to death from cardiovascular diseases in adult life. BMJ 1993:306:422-26.
5. Glueck CJ, Fontaine RN, Wang P, *et al.* Metformin reduces weight, centripetal obesity, insulin, leptin and low-density lipoprotein cholesterol in nondiabetic, morbidly obese subjects with body mass index greater than 30. Metabolism 2001;50:856-61.
6. Khadilkar AV, Ekbote V, Chiplonkar S, *et al.* Waist Circumference Percentiles in 2-18 Years Old Indian Children. J Pediatr 2014;164:1358-62.
7. Misra A, Misra R, Wijesuriya M, Banerjee D. The metabolic syndrome in South Asians: Continuing escalation and possible solutions. Indian J Med Res 2007;125:345-54.
8. Mohan V, Mathur P, Deepa R, *et al.* Urban rural differences in prevalence of self-reported diabetes in India–The WHO-ICMR Indian NCD risk factor surveillance. Diabetes Res Clin Pract 2008;80:159-68.
9. Neel JV. Diabetes mellitus: A "thrifty" genotype rendered detrimental by "progress". Am J Human Genet 1962;14: 353-61.
10. Yajnik CS, Lubree HG, Rege SS, *et al.* Adiposity and hyperinsulinemia in Indians are present at birth. J Clin Endocrinol Metab 2002;87:5575-80.

4.1

Adolescent Sexuality

Deepak K Jumani, Swati Y Bhave

INTRODUCTION

Today's generation is exposed to several erotic materials—be it films, television, billboards, newspapers, magazines or internet. The adolescents with their bubbling sex hormones have to cope with negative peer pressure, ambivalence about gender identity and inadequate information or guidance on sexuality with hardly any proper sex education. These are triggers for confusion in the minds of adolescents and naturally adolescents today have several unanswered questions about sex and sexuality.

It is very important to have careful parenting to create a sense of security—where all questions dealing with sexuality are addressed openly and honestly; factual information about sex and sexuality are provided whenever asked; and parents are always open to answer every query in a non-judgemental manner. This will help the growing adolescent make appropriate choices and not become a prey to hasty and reckless sexual experimentations.

HOW DO WE ASSESS ADOLESCENT SEXUALITY ISSUES?

Adolescents have a variety of sexual health-related unsolved issues, and the current adolescent health programs are not adequate or optimum to deal with these issues. Even the primary health care physicians are incompetent and untrained to address these issues. The need of the hour is "Adolescent Friendly Clinics" run by trained personnel who can provide psychological and mental health services, offering facilities for appropriate behavior changes, communication skills and awareness for an overall healthy lifestyle.

PRESENTATION IN ADOLESCENT CLINIC

Most adolescents especially those in the early and middle stages, do not present with symptoms directly related to sexuality. For example an adolescent who has started indulging in masturbation may present with falling academic grades or is brought by parents for alteration of behavior of wanting excessive privacy, day dreaming etc. It will require the skills of an experienced clinician to get to the real underlying issues.

On the other hand an older adolescent may directly come to a sexuality clinic especially if he or she has indulged in a risky sexual behavior. However, most adolescents report to a clinician with symptoms that are not directly related to any risky sexual behavior. The most common sexuality issues affecting adolescent boys and girls are listed in Tables 4.1.1 and 4.1.2.

Table 4.1.1: Common sexuality problems associated with adolescent boys

Issues	*Comments*	*Management*
Masturbation	I have done a big sin. I feel I am not fit for marriage. My penis is bent. My semen has become less and thin.	Reassurance. Explain that masturbation is normal, healthy and beneficial. Loosing semen does not make one infertile as semen is produced from 9 to 90 years and it has to flow out, and cannot be stored. There are less incidences of cancer of prostate in all who masturbate. Disciplined masturbation does not change the shape or size of the penis. Concentration of semen has nothing to do with fertility.
Night falls or wet dreams	My undergarments get stained every third or fourth day. I lose all my semen and I am feeling weak and tired all the time.	Reassurance. Production of semen is constant from 9 to 90 years, and once it is formed it always has to flow out. Similar to urine, semen also cannot be stored.

Contd.

Contd.

Size of the genitals	My penis is very small. I can't think of marrying as I don't want to spoil her life.	Reassurance. It is not the length, but strength in the penis that is important. The normal length of penis required for optimum sexual pleasure is about 5 cm and more in an erect state.
Performance anxiety	I ejaculate just when I touch her or even if she kisses me or hold me tight.	Reassurance. You are becoming self-conscious. Be fearless, carefree and playful.
Worry about sexual attractiveness	I don't have a sex appeal. I have a 'paunch'. I have lot of hair. I am short and I am thin.	Reassurance. Every person is a sexual human being. Height and weight are just mere numbers. Never compare yourself to anyone.
Erectile issues	Whenever I get intimate with her I don't get erection, but when I masturbate I get good erection. I also get morning erections.	Reassurance. These erectile dysfunction problems are situational and psychogenic. Advice on stopping smoking, excess of alcohol. Anyone below 40 years of age and getting morning erections is normal.
Experimentation with commercial sex workers	I have no girlfriend and I feel the urge to have sex. I wish to visit some call girl or go to a commercial sex worker.	Visiting sex workers can be risky. You can get sexually transmitted infections (STI) or other contagious skin diseases. Abstinence is ideal until you are in a committed relationship. If you still want to experiment, use barriers like condoms and safeguard yourself from viral infections such as HIV.
Confusion about premarital relationships	I have friends who have had sexual relationship with girls and are much experienced before they got married. I also wish to do so. I am confused.	Counseling on making right choices in life. Many a times indulging in such relationships and not being committed leaves mental scars for a life time. The shame and guilt are very difficult to cope with. Mutual trust and safe health practices are ideal choices.
Fear of STI due to high risk behavior	I have unprotected sex with many partners–some of them I know and some of them I am not close to. I fear I may have or get STI.	This fear is natural, but this can be avoided by using protective barriers like condoms. To overcome fears of STI, one can get all the blood tests for HIV, hepatitis and other venereal diseases (VD) to rule them out. If negative, one is fortunate. If positive we have treatment for the same.
Addiction to pornography	I watch porn every day and I enjoy. I don't get erections when I am with my partner. I get turned off when I am with my committed partner.	Counseling and cognitive behavior therapy help. Pornography is a business; everything shown is fabricated and edited so that it sells. One enjoys watching the variety shown; women are shown as dehumanized. This also raises the threshold of arousals. Watching too much porn also makes one believe that a girl or a boy should be of a particular shape or color to have a good enough sex. This is a myth and one who watches porn gets victimized with these thoughts and mindsets.
Addiction to phone sex and sexting	I don't have a girlfriend but I enjoy phone sex. I get aroused by sending sexy remarks and sex images.	Counseling and cognitive behavior therapy is a must. Sexting is a risky behavior; it can cause emotional problems and also can lead to legal problems. Online sex addiction is being web entangled. It is because there is anonymity, easily accessible and affordable. One can conceal age, marital status or any health related issues. Usually the internet addicts have anxiety, depression and relationship issues in marital life, career or other forms of stress.

Contd.

Contd.

Sexual abuse	I am scared to go near her. I hate being intimate. I feel sad, helpless and hopeless.	Counseling. Anxiety, shock and fear lead to post-traumatic stress disorders and need group therapy.
Filmed and MMS sent	I like to watch live erotic activities and enjoy women surrendering and begging me for help.	Counseling and cognitive behavior therapy. These are sadomasochistic acts. These adolescents derive pleasure from feeling the power and authority by playing a dominant role. 12 step de-addiction programs do help.
Confusion about sexual orientation (LGBT)	I think I am in a wrong body as I am attracted to boys more. I get aroused with guys. I don't want to get married. I want to have my sex changed.	Intensive counselling and psychotherapy are tried to reverse their orientations. It is not hereditary or genetic.

Table 4.1.2: Common sexuality associated with adolescent girls

Issues	***Comments***	***Management***
Masturbation	I like to play with my clitoris and feel nice and wet. I don't get wet as I used to before. I don't enjoy it any more. I am scared it may affect my married life.	Reassurance. Explain that masturbation is normal, healthy and beneficial. Masturbation leads to release of feel good endorphins. It eases post-menopausal sexual problems. One may try water based lubricants.
Size of the breast	My breasts are too small and I am not attractive. My breasts are too big and I am not confident that this will attract or appeal or be a turn off.	Reassurance and counseling help in body image issues. A committed relationship doesn't look for anything which is physical. Everyone is a sex subject and not a sex object. If it's too much of a concern certain plastic surgeries such as breast implants and mammopexy may be helpful.
Shape and size of genitals	I feel I am not at all attractive down and I don't want to be intimate. I have had too much sex. I feel my passage has become big.	Reassurance and counseling. It's a myth that the size of vulva or vagina changes with lot of sex. If there is no pain during intercourse and have no penetration issues, all is well. If there is too much of a concern, plastic surgeons can perform labiaplasty and there is a fashion of designer vagina.
Performance anxiety and fear of being frigid	I don't think I will be able to enjoy or give joy to my partner. I think I am too cold.	Reassurance and counseling. Cognitive behavior therapy also helps. Coping of every fear can be done by actually being in that situation. One needs to be fearless, carefree and playful in bedroom.
Worry about sexual attractiveness	My figure is such that I feel I am not sexually attractive. I may be a turn-off to my partner.	Reassurance and counseling. Every person is a sexual human being. Being sexually fit is being sexually committed. Spontaneity and being sex positive make everyone sexually attractive.
Confusion about entering premarital relationship	I have friends who have had sexual relationship with guys and are experienced much before they get married. I also wish to do so. I am confused.	Counseling on making right choices in life. Many a times indulging in such relationship and not being committed leaves mental scars for life time. The shame and guilt are very difficult to cope with. Mutual trust and safe health practices are ideal choices.
Confusion about sexual orientation (LGBT)	I think I am in a wrong body as I am attracted to girls more and I don't get aroused with guys.	Intensive counseling and psychotherapy are tried to reverse their orientations. It is not hereditary or genetic.
Addiction to pornography	I watch porn every day and I enjoy. I don't get orgasms when I am with my boyfriend. I get turned off when I am with my committed partner.	Counseling and cognitive behavior therapy helps. Pornography is a business; everything shown is fabricated and edited so that it sells. One enjoys watching the variety shown. Internet addiction can be managed by avoiding watching porn and psychotherapy.

Contd.

Contd.

Fear of STI due to high risk behavior	I have unprotected sex with many partners—some of them I know and some of them I am not close to. I fear I may have or get STIs	This fear is natural, but this can be avoided by making the partners use protective barriers like condoms. To overcome fears of STI, one can get all the blood tests for HIV, Hepatitis, VD etc. and rule out these. If negative one is fortunate. If positive we have treatment for the same.
Addiction to phone sex, sexting	I enjoy phone sex. I feel safe with it. I can have it with any one and many. I get aroused by sending sexy remarks and sex images.	Counseling and cognitive behavior therapy is a must. Sexting is a risky behavior; it can cause emotional problems and also can lead to legal problems. Online sex addiction is being web entangled. It is because there is anonymity, easily accessible and affordable. One can conceal age, marital status or any health related issues. Usually the internet addicts have anxiety, depression and relationship issues in marital life, career or any form of stress.
Sexual abuse	I hate men. I don't like the touch of a man. I feel sad and helpless and hopeless when I hear my friends talk about they enjoying their sexual relationship.	Counseling. Anxiety, shock and fear are due to some childhood molestations. It can lead to post-traumatic stress disorders and need group therapy.
Filmed and MMS sent	I feel shy and ashamed to meet men. I am scared and my life is ruined.	Counseling and cognitive behavior therapy are needed. Rape and sexual assault leads to fear, shame and depression in victims. Being raped and then filmed result in mental trauma. Long-term counseling and motivations to move on is encouraged.

HISTORY TAKING

A complete history taken using the HEEADSSS approach gives very useful information including sexual activity (see Chapter 1.3). In addition a detailed sexual history should be taken. This needs to be done in complete privacy and in a non-judgemental and unbiased manner. Some tips are given in Box 4.1.1.

Box 4.1.1: Tips for dealing with sexuality issues with adolescents

- Always greet him/her in a friendly manner–be open, flexible and relaxed.
- Be honest and simple and respect her/his point of view.
- During examination inform him/her what is not normal in a soft tone.
- Never make him/her feel that you are judgemental or disapproving–but explain risks in a scientific manner.
- Always answer his/her calls and modestly ask him/her to visit you as often as possible.
- Keep your counseling sessions short–give medical facts and never scare him/her.

The ambience and environment of the clinic where the therapist is present, has to be safe and conducive to let the adolescent submit for proper history taking and examination, and receptive.

History should include the following details:

- Risk taking behaviors such as consumption of alcohol, tobacco, smoking, drug use, and substance abuse.
- Altered behaviors, depression, attempted suicides, dietary habits, sleep pattern, patterns of watching television and watching porn, use of mobile phones and other screen time.
- How is his/her performance in school, attendance and behavior with peers?
- What are the dating and driving habits?
- What is the pocket money he or she gets and how is it spent?

If an adolescent gives history of being sexually active, the clinician needs to ask some direct questions to understand the pattern of sexual behavior (Box 4.1.2).

Box 4.1.2: Questions for sexually active adolescents

1. Do you stay alone or with one or both parents?
2. Do you indulge in sex with men or women or both?
3. In the past 12 months how many partners you have had sex with?
4. During these relationships has your sex partner had relationship with someone else?
5. Do you have vaginal, oral and/or anal sex?
6. Do you use protections while having sex (e.g. condom, I-pill)?
7. Have you ever had an abortion?
8. Have you or your partners ever injected drugs or exchanged money for drugs?
9. Have you taken human papilloma virus (HPV) or hepatitis B vaccinations?

PHYSICAL EXAMINATION

A complete physical examination should be done with measurement of vital parameters, height, weight, body mass index (BMI), and Tanner staging for puberty. All medical illnesses need to be dealt with appropriate detailed system examination. Details of these aspects are covered in subsequent chapters. In this chapter we will focus on physical examination which is relevant to sexuality issues.

- Check if the adolescent is well groomed with good personal hygiene. Neglect can be pointer to substance abuse or depression.
- Check for tattoo marks or piercings on the various parts of the body like lips, nipples, labia, umbilicus etc. This gives some idea about the lifestyle of the adolescents. However one must avoid being prejudiced—tattooing, piercing and hep dressing styles need not be always associated with free lifestyle and could be just peer pressure and wanting to fit in the crowd.

Sexuality problems may often be associated with depression and self-harming behavior. Examine for self-inflicting injuries–check for cut marks on hands, chest etc.

Examination of External Genitalia and Perianal Region in Both Boys and Girls

- Look for skin infections (e.g. bacterial folliculitis or fungal infections such as tinea pubis and pubic lice) and pubertal progress.
- Signs of STI such as shingles of herpes or post-herpetic lesions, warts or any urethral discharge or glands in the groin (see Chapter 4.3 Sexually Transmitted Infections and Chapter 6.4 Dermatological Problems).
- Abnormalities of growth, progress of puberty, development of primary and secondary sexual characteristics are matters of concern. Thus ambiguous genitalia can give us information about congenital adrenal hyperplasia whereas tall stature, gynecomastia, delayed puberty, and/or hypogonadism provide clues for the diagnosis of Klinefelter syndrome and similar conditions.

Detailed examination in a male adolescent is outlined in Box 4.1.3.

INVESTIGATIONS

The adolescent may need routine investigations and specific tests for suspected sexually transmitted infections (STIs) depending on the history and physical examination. These include tests for human immunodeficiency virus (HIV), hepatitis B (HBsAg), hepatitis C (anti-HCV), specific tests for gonorrhea, syphilis and Chlamydia. (For more details see Chapter 4.3 Sexually Transmitted Infections and Chapter 6.4 on Dermatological Problems).

MANAGEMENT

After having taken a detailed sexual history, performing the physical examination from top to bottom, and doing the laboratory studies, we as adolescent physicians should tailor anticipatory guidance and counselling on the basis of specific risk factors and/or information obtained during an individual patient's visit and his/her developmental stage.

Box 4.1. 3: Examination of external genital/Perianal region for male adolescents

- *Assessment of pubertal development:* Tanner sexual maturity rating, measurement of penile length, testicular volume, size and volume, pattern of sexual hair
- *Identification of signs for genetic diseases:* Ambiguity of external genitalia (congenital adrenal hyperplasia), firm testes (Klinefelter syndrome)
- *Evidence of structural anomalies:* Varicocele which can affect fertility, uncorrected hypospadias, which can result in significant embarrassment, problems with sexual function, and/or abnormal urine flow
- *Issues related to an uncircumcised penis:* E.g. phimosis and hygiene
- *Problems related to testes:*
  - Previously unrecognized absent testes attributable to cryptorchidism
  - Evidence of testicular atrophy secondary to central or exogenous causes (e.g. steroids or marijuana use)
  - Testicular trauma
- *Normal findings that might require reassurance:* E.g. pearly penile papules
- Examination of testis is very crucial in males with history of:
  - HIV infection
  - Klinefelter syndrome
  - Family history of testicular cancer

Counseling forms the mainstay of the treatment of adolescent sexuality issues. Counseling needs be done on many aspects:

- Reducing sexual risk including barriers to condom use.
- Counseling on use of contraceptives: This includes demonstration or providing resources (e.g. videos or handouts) for correct condom use.
- Communication with partner about sex.
- Sensitizing them about normal and abnormal behaviors; educating them to make the right choice and assess for experience of stress.
- Perils of pornography.

Family life education should replace the word sexuality education and should be propagated in all teaching institutions and in the community for out-of-school teens.

Tips for Parents to Deal with Sexuality Issues

Make an effort to know the core sexual/reproductive health knowledge about their teen and ensure that it does not adversely affect their quality of life.

1. Advise parents to educate themselves about pubertal development. They should use every opportunity to have age-appropriate discussions about sexual health with their teens e.g. TV shows, newspaper reports on sexual molestation, rape, teen pregnancy etc. on several occasions.
2. Help them to understand difference between sexual experimentation without being in a committed relationship and being abstinent and guide them to build healthy, responsible relationships.
3. Problems of sexuality can affect the emotional and psychosocial development of teens; so learn to recognize them and help.
4. Do timely referral to health care professionals without feeling stigmatised.
5. Some of the parents may not be comfortable doing counseling. They should be advised to seek the help of a trained adolescent health care professional.

Treatment of STIs and Other Medical Issues

This has been covered in other chapters in this book.

Vaccinations

Reproductive health-related vaccines, including hepatitis A and B and HPV vaccines should be administered as recommended (For details see Chapter 7.1 Immunization).

LEARNING POINTS

1. Adolescent sexuality problems can have long-term adverse effects on their physical, mental and psychosocial growth and development.
2. Clinicians should learn to pick up these issues during routine clinic visits of teens even if they have presented with other issues.
3. Anticipatory guidance and preventive counseling should be done at the first opportunity with an adolescent.
4. Parents should be educated and encouraged to discuss openly issues of sexuality with teens.
5. Parents who are not comfortable doing this, should be advised to refer the teen to a trained adolescent health care professional.
6. Family life education should replace the word sexuality education and should be propagated in all teaching institutions and in the community for out-of-school teens.

SUGGESTED READING

1. Brener ND, Billy JO, Grady WR. Assessment of factors affecting the validity of self-reported health-risk behavior among adolescents: Evidence from the scientific literature. J Adolescent Health 2003;33:436-57.
2. Cheung AH, Zuckerbrot RA, Jensen PS, *et al.* Expert survey for the management of adolescent depression in primary care. Pediatrics 2008;121:e101-07.
3. Hagan JF, Shaw JS, Duncan P, eds. Bright futures: Guidelines for health supervision of infants, children, and adolescents, 3rd edition. Illinois; American Academy of Pediatrics, 2008.
4. Institute of Medicine (IOM). The health of lesbian, gay, bisexual, and transgender people: Building a foundation for better understanding. Washington, DC: The National Academies Press; 2011.
5. Lempp T, de Lange D, Radeloff D, Bachmann C. The clinical examination of children, adolescents and their families. In: Rey JM (ed), IACAPAP e-Textbook of Child and Adolescent Mental Health. Geneva: International Association for Child and Adolescent Psychiatry and Allied Professions; 2012.
6. le Couteur A, Gardner F. Use of structured interviews and observational methods in clinical settings. In: Rutter M, Bishop D, Pine D *et al.* (Eds). Rutter's Child and Adolescent Psychiatry, 5th Edition. Oxford: Blackwell 2008; 271-88.
7. Marcell AV, Wibbelsman C, Seigel WM, Committee on Adolescence. Male adolescent sexual and reproductive health care. Pediatrics 2011;128:e1658-76.
8. Society for Adolescent Health and Medicine. The Male Genital Examination: A Position Paper of the Society for Adolescent Health and Medicine. J Adolescent Health 2012;50:424-25.

4.2

Lesbian, Gay, Bisexual and Transgender (LGBT) Issues

Donald E Greydanus, Kevin W Cates

INTRODUCTION

Biological perspectives on homosexuality conclude that sexual orientation is a result of genetics and additional biological causes. Differences in the hypothalamus and anterior commissure have been noted in heterosexual versus homosexual persons. Complicating this picture is the research noting that if an XX female fetus is exposed to excessive male hormones (e.g. as in congenital adrenal hyperplasia), she may demonstrate behavioral traits considered to be masculine (i.e. absence of doll playing and aggressive playing). Continued research and increased understanding and awareness of the biological perspective of gender and sexual orientation could help remove the stigma experienced by people with non-heterosexual orientations as well as highlight the many variations of sexual behavior.

Though etiologic considerations of sexual orientation in humans remains controversial, a major advance in sexuality was accomplished in 1973 when the American Psychiatric Association officially concluded that homosexuality is not a psychiatric disorder. This same scientific conclusion was noted by the American Psychological Association in 1975. Since then the American Academy of Pediatrics has issued a number of statements of its Committee on Adolescence in 1983, 1993 and 2013 reflecting on the normalcy of homosexuality. Research in USA shows significant population has homosexual orientation (Box 4.2.1). Some persons have both homosexual and heterosexual features.

Box 4.2.1: Sexual orientation–USA population studies

- Landmark research in USA by Kinsey *et al.* (1948, 1953) noted that 4% of the adult males and 2% of the adult females are exclusively homosexual regarding their sexual behavior and fantasy life.
- This study involved a survey of 5,000 adult males and 6,000 adult females with regard to their sexual behavior.
- This classic study reported that 50% of the adult (ages 16-55) male population had a prepubertal homosexual experience; 37% revealed such behavior with orgasm, and 10% had this same sex orientation for at least 3 years after puberty.

Despite these scientific statements, societal attitudes over many millennia as stimulated by numinous influences have been disdainful of non-heterosexual orientation. Even in societies historically amenable to non-heterosexual identity and behavior, anti-homosexual attitudes have been introduced and enforced through the impact of European colonialism from the 16th century to the mid-20th century. Though there has been some gains in tolerance of non-heterosexual identity and behavior in the American culture of the recent decade, youth still faces intense anti-gay attitudes on a day-to-day basis resulting in considerable psychological distress to these persons. In India though socially homosexuality has been accepted by many, there has been changing laws about homosexuality (see Chapter 1.5 for more details).

CLINICAL PRESENTATION

Youth who are gay, lesbian, or bisexual may present to the primary care clinician for various reasons, as listed in Table 4.2.1.

Table 4.2.1: Reasons why gay and lesbian adolescents seek medical attention*

- Information about homosexuality
- Sexually transmitted diseases (STDs): Fears, information
- Psychosocial difficulties
  - – Family
  - – School
  - – Personal problems
  - – Vocational concerns
  - – Religious conflicts
- Human immunodeficiency virus (HIV) or acquired immunodeficiency syndrome (AIDS): Infection, concerns about HIV/AIDS
- Other medical disorders
- Substance abuse
- Legal problems (including prostitution)

* Reproduced with permission from Greydanus DE, Sison AC, Guilonard KW. Homosexual attraction and sexual behavior in adolescents. In: DE Greydanus, DR Patel, HD Pratt, JL Calles Jr., Eds. Behavioral Pediatrics, 3rd edition. New York: Nova Biomedical Books, 2009; Chapter 19: 297-315.

In India parents often bring their children to a clinician requesting help to change the sexual orientation to 'normal'. Often the young person is forced to marry and produce children in order to prove his/her "sexual normalcy" to society. This results in either the person accepting the situation and living a bisexual life or it can lead to tremendous mental anguish and the frustration can make the person chronically depressed to the extent of suicide. One should not seek to change the sexual orientation of a patient since this is unethical and can result in long-term psychological harm.

HISTORY TAKING

Clinicians should provide a safe environment for adolescent patients where they can present confidential information about their sexual and medical issues. These youth can learn from non-prejudicial health care professionals regarding risks for sexually transmitted diseases (STDs), substance abuse, disclosure of sexual orientation, and avoiding negative effects of societal animadversion (criticism or censure) regarding homosexuality i.e. bullying, depression and suicide. The Kinsey scale of sexual orientation helps to assess the type and degree of sexual orientation (Box 4.2.2).

Gay and lesbian youth may have few places for accurate and safe health care if their clinician does not provide a safe place for them to be seen and treated as necessary.

- When counseling youth, clinicians need to have open conversations about sexuality.

Box 4.2.2: The Kinsey scale of sexual orientation

Rating	*Description*
0	Exclusively heterosexual (in sexual behavior and fantasy)
1	Essentially heterosexual with incidental or limited homosexual history
2	Largely heterosexual with distinct homosexual history
3	Equal heterosexual and homosexual orientation–'ambisexuality'
4	Largely homosexual with distinct heterosexual history
5	Essential homosexual with limited heterosexual history
6	Exclusive homosexual (in sexual behavior and fantasy)

Interpretation: *Exclusively heterosexual* (rating 0) to *exclusively homosexual* (rating 6) to various mixtures (ratings 1-5).

In studying homosexuality, it is beneficial to distinguish between *sexual behavior and sexual fantasy.*

The Kinsey scale has helped to illustrate that human sexual behavior does not lie on a dichotomy consisting of heterosexual or homosexual behavior; but rather, on a continuum with many variations in between.

- Clinicians should emphasize that late adolescence or early adulthood is a normal time when many become aware of as well as accepting of their gay or lesbian sexual orientation.
- It is critical to stress with youth that experimentation with one's sexuality is normal and does not determine one's orientation.
- In fact, there can be homosexual experimentation in early adolescence in some who later identify as heterosexual.
- Sexual orientation may be established in some by middle childhood but can be confirmed in puberty or later depending on various factors. Humans are complex living beings and each can take his or her own path in life.

Stages in Different Sexual Orientation

In history taking it is important to identify at what stage the adolescent is in as the management will vary greatly. The psychosocial support and referral will also vary. Youth who have not yet started sexual activity need to be given anticipatory guidance about the medical issues involved and those who are already sexually active have to be examined and treated for the well-known medical problems that come with those that eventually identify as gay or lesbian. The Green's classification describes the various stages acceptance of sexual orientation (Box 4.2.3).

Troiden has outlined 4 stages of gay identity development, as outlined in Table 4.2.2.

Early Stages

In the initial phase the adolescents may have some homosexual experiences and have the knowledge about the negative views of the society about homosexuality. In subsequent stages they are in constant struggle with the society's application of negative views on homosexuality as applied to them. These reactions include despair, denial, avoidance of sexual activity, and eventually, development to stages 3 and 4.

Some of these youth develop limited social skills and have limited access to healthy adult role models. The need for secrecy and paucity of comprehensive sexuality

Box 4.2.3: Green's classification of sexual orientation

1. First, there is a sense of being "different"
2. Then, one develops an infatuation with one of the same sex
3. Finally an eventual phase called "coming out" in which the person reveals this same sex orientation to family, peers, or others.

Table 4.2.2: Troiden's stages of gay identity development*

Stage	*Gay identity development*	*Characteristics*
1	Sensitization	Gains homosexual experiences in childhood and adolescence while learning of general society's negative view on homosexuality.
2	Dissociation and Signification: Sexual Identity Confusion	Struggles to reject the concept that society's negative views on homosexuality applies to one's self.
3	Coming Out: Sexual Identity Assumption	Identifies one's self as "gay" and reaches out to become involved in some aspect of the gay society culture; begins to consider homosexuality as a viable lifestyle option.
4	Acceptance: Integration and Commitment	Fuses one's concepts of sexuality and emotionality as an adult; some are "arrested" at stage 3 while others will eventually arrive at stage 4.

* Reproduced with permission from Greydanus DE, Sison AC, Guilonard KW. Homosexual attraction and sexual behavior in adolescents. In: DE Greydanus, DR Patel, HD Pratt, JL Calles Jr., eds. Behavioral Pediatrics, 3rd Edition. New York: Nova Biomedical Books; 2009; Chapter 19;297-315.

education may lead to considerable physiological and psychological complications including self-hate, bullying, STDs, depression and suicide.

Often adolescents will rely on the internet for information regarding sexuality; however, sometimes this information can be false and/or dangerous, highlighting the importance of knowledgeable and accessible clinicians. Unfortunately, LGBT youth can find the school environment very hostile leading to increased drop-out rates and fear of bullying and violence.

Research notes that gay youth represent 30% of completed suicides in this age group and that 30% of surveyed gay as well as bisexual males have had at least one suicide attempt. Though some have denied the accuracy of such studies, other research confirms a high level of suicidality among gay males.

Youth who are thrown out of their homes or who run away because of domestic violence often live on the streets as homeless victims. These youth are subject to hate crimes that can include verbal assaults as well as physical attacks. Street life is very dangerous with physical and emotional sequelae from violence, drug abuse and prostitution.

The Disclosure of Sexual Orientation– 'Coming Out' Phase

The adolescent can experience intense fear which can be very problematic depending on his/her perception of the reaction of family, peers and society.

- This adolescent may feel s/he has no one to talk with about this and, become very depressed, and may even experience suicidal thinking.
- Parents or others may dismiss this as a passing phase or parents may blame themselves for having a child with a gay or lesbian sexual orientation.
- Some parents are convinced that this orientation may change while some may become so angry that the adolescent is physically abused and thrown out of the home.
- Parents may forbid the youth from talking to others about this issue.
- Many parents are concerned with how their child will fare in an anti-gay world, become concerned that their child will not become a well-adjusted adult, and/or may mourn the loss of becoming grandparents in a way honored by their own tradition.
- In some cultures 'coming out' as gay or lesbian is seen as a rejection of one's religious upbringing and culture leading to intense psychological distress for all involved.

These factors (and many others) may result in a sense of isolation for a youth considering 'coming out'. Adolescents who are in various stages of homosexual identity development should have strong, non-biased support from their primary care pediatrician to help deal with rejection as well as bullying from peers and potential parental rejection.

CLINICAL EXAMINATION

A complete physical examination should be done. Sexually active youth can acquire a wide variety of STDs and gay males can be infected with a number of additional organisms that can cause enteric diseases (perianal and rectal infections).

Young gay adolescents may preferentially engage in sexual activities in public or semi-public places where limited access to condoms increases risks for STDs (including HIV infection).

Lesbian youth may have sex with males and increase their risks for various STDs as well.

Homeless youth of any sexual orientation may rely on sex work to acquire money for food, housing and clothing.

A summary of medical evaluation principles when seeing these youth is presented in Table 4.2.3.

Table 4.2.3: Medical evaluation of gay and lesbian adolescents*

History taking (ensure confidentiality, privacy) • Social • School • Family • Employment • Substance use • Assessment of psychosocial problems, including suicidal ideations • Sexual history (non-prejudicial; do not assume heterosexual orientation)
Clinical examination • General • Systemic review all systems • Close inspection for sexually transmitted diseases (STDs) • Other procedures as indicated (pelvic examination, anoscopy)
Laboratory evaluation (see text) • Rapid plasma reagin • Gonorrhea • *Chlamydia trachomatis* • Human immunodeficiency virus (HIV) • Pap smear
Treatment • Hepatitis B immunization (if not already taken) • Appropriate treatment of STDs (including partners) and any medical problems
Counseling • Discussion of risk reduction, abstinence, contraception
Further management • Referral to support groups as necessary • Follow-up visit(s) with primary care physician (including family)

* Adapted and modified with permission from Greydanus DE, Sison AC, Guilonard KW. Homosexual attraction and sexual behavior in adolescents. In: DE Greydanus, DR Patel, HD Pratt, JL Calles Jr., eds. Behavioral Pediatrics, 3rd edition. New York: Nova Biomedical Books, 2009; Chapter 19: P. 297-315.

INVESTIGATIONS

In addition to routine investigations, all LGBT youth must be screened for sexually transmitted infections (STIs) (See Box 4.2.4 and Table 4.2.4).

Box 4.2.4: US Centers for Disease Control and Prevention (CDC) recommendations-2015

- Males having sex with males receive annual screening that includes HIV serology (if HIV-negative or not previously tested), syphilis serology, and screening for *Neisseria gonorrhoeae* as well as *Chlamydia trachomatis*.
- This includes pharyngeal culture for gonorrhea in males with oral-genital exposure and rectal culture for gonorrhea and chlamydia for males with receptive anal coitus.
- Men having sex with men should be vaccinated with hepatitis A, hepatitis B, and human papillomavirus vaccines if recommended age guidelines are met.
- Screening for drug abuse and as noted, for various STDs as well is recommended. The frequency of this screening is dependent on the patient's history and STD screening for some should be every 3 to 6 months.

Table 4.2.4: Sexually transmitted diseases in gay adolescents*

Urethritis • *Neisseria gonorrhoeae* • *Chlamydia trachomatis* • *Mycoplasma hominis* • *Ureaplasma urealyticum*
Acquired immunodeficiency syndrome (persons with HIV infection may acquire various other opportunistic infections not listed)
Genital warts (infection with human papilloma virus)
Ectoparasites
Hepatitis
• Hepatitis A, B, C, D, and/or E virus • Cytomegalovirus • Epstein-Barr virus
Ulcerative lesions • Syphilis *(Treponema pallidum)* • Herpes simplex • Chancroid *(Haemophilus ducreyi)* • Lymphogranuloma venereum *(Chlamydia trachomatis)* • Granuloma inguinale *(Calymmatobacterium granulomatis)*
Enteritis/proctocolitis • Giardia lamblia • Salmonella enteritidis • Entamoeba histolytica • Cryptosporidium species • Campylobacter species • Shigella species

* Reproduced with permission from Greydanus DE, Sison AC, Guilonard KW. Homosexual attraction and sexual behavior in adolescents. In: DE Greydanus, DR Patel, HD Pratt, JL Calles Jr., Eds. Behavioral Pediatrics, 3rd Edition. New York: Nova Biomedical Books, 2009; Chapter19: pages 297-315.

MANAGEMENT OF LGBT YOUTH

Management includes medical treatment, education and counseling. Regular screening of sexually active youth for STDs should be done and treatment is given as needed (Box 4.2.4). For more on STI management please see section 4: Chapter 4.3.

The American Academy of Pediatrics reaffirms the physician's responsibility to provide comprehensive health care and guidance for all adolescents, including gay and lesbian adolescents and those young people struggling with issues of sexual orientation (American Academy of Pediatrics, Pediatrics, 1993).

Anticipatory Guidance and Preventive Counseling

- All youth, including heterosexual, gay, lesbian, and bisexual, should be given accurate information about

STDs, condoms, contraception, and other aspects of comprehensive sexuality.

- Information may also be found via professional or reliable internet sources as well as coalitions of parents of gay and lesbian adolescents.
- Education should be provided to all regarding biomedical pharmacologic interventions, including pre-exposure prophylaxis (PrEP) and post-exposure prophylaxis (PEP) for HIV prevention (refer to www.cdc.gov/hiv).
- If appropriate and available, youth at increased risk for HIV acquisition (including those who refuse condom use, engage in sex work, or have a partner or partners known to be HIV-positive) should be provided PrEP or PEP, and referred to appropriate services.
- Clinicians caring for adolescents should be part of this education as well as providers of comprehensive medical care.
- Health care professionals can screen gay and lesbian youth for potential bullying from others, depression, anxiety and suicidality.
- Primary physicians like the pediatricians can provide as well as refer to others for non-prejudicial counseling, educate about social skills, and consider the need for family counseling.
- Clinicians can provide these youth and their families with neutral information about same sex orientation. LGBT youth want professional clinicians who are accessible to them and provide them with needed care.
- Unfortunately, clinicians charged with providing professional care to their patients often fail to inquire about sexual orientation of their patients as well as fail to manage these issues.
- Youth should always be educated that the only way to fully avoid risks for STDs and, with heterosexual activity, unwanted pregnancy is to be abstinent from sexual activity. Youth usually have limited understanding of risks of such sexual behavior such as the acquisition of STDs. Youth should also be taught that condoms can be beneficial in prevention of many STDs.

Acknowledgement

Roger W. Apple PhD, Assistant Professor and Director, Division of Developmental-Behavioral Pediatrics, Department of Pediatric and Adolescent Medicine, Western Michigan University, Homer Stryker MD School of Medicine, Kalamazoo, Michigan USA for his valuable inputs for this chapter.

SUGGESTED READING

1. American Academy of Pediatrics. Homosexuality and Adolescence. Committee on Adolescence. Pediatrics 1993;92:631-34.
2. American Psychiatric Association. Diagnostic and Statistical Manual of Mental Disorders 5th edition (DSM-5), 2013.
3. Committee on Adolescence. Office-based care for lesbians, gay, bisexual, transgender and questioning youth. Pediatrics 2013;132(1):196-203.
4. Green R. 1987. The "Sissy Boy Syndrome" and the Development of Homosexuality. New Haven: Yale University, 1987.
5. Greydanus DE, Sison AC, Guilonard KW. Homosexual attraction and sexual behavior in adolescents. In: DE Greydanus, DR Patel, HD Pratt, JL Calles Jr, eds. Behavioral Pediatrics, 3rd edition. New York: Nova Biomedical Books, 2009;297-315.
6. Kinsey A, Pomeroy W, Martin C. Sexual Behavior in the Human Male. Philadelphia: W.B. Saunders, 1948.
7. Kinsey A, Pomeroy W, Martin C, Gebbard P. Sexual Behavior in the Human Female. Philadelphia: WB Saunders, 1953.
8. Kitts RL. Barriers to optimal care between physicians and lesbian, gay, bisexual, transgender, and questioning adolescent patients. J Homosexual 2010;57(6):730-47.
9. Stahl MA, Greydanus DE, Truba N, Cates K, Pratt HD. Sexuality and the LGBT youth. In: DE Greydanus, DR Patel, HD Pratt, J Calles Jr., A Nazeer, J Merrick (Eds.), Behavioral Pediatrics, 4th edition. New York: Nova Biomedical Books, 2015, Chapter 30, 439-55.
10. Steever JB, Cooper-Serber E. A review of gay, lesbian, bisexual, and transgender youth issues for the pediatrician. Pediatr Ann 2013;42(2):34-39.

Sexually Transmitted Infections Including HIV/AIDS

4.3

Newton Luiz, Swati Y Bhave

INTRODUCTION

Sexually transmitted infections (STIs) are among the most serious infections of adolescence, and their incidence is increasing. They are a major preventable cause of infertility in both genders.

The term 'sexually transmitted infection' (STI) is preferred to the former term 'sexually transmitted disease' (STD), as it is frequently asymptomatic and often subsides without causing any disease (e.g. human papilloma virus [HPV] infection). 'Reproductive tract infection' (RTI) includes both STIs and non-sexually transmitted infections such as bacterial vaginosis. Some STIs may also be transmitted non-sexually e.g. by blood transfusion and from mother to child.

One in four new human immunodeficiency virus (HIV) infections occurs in persons under 22 years of age. About 10 years elapse from the time of infection to the first acquired immune deficiency syndrome (AIDS)–defining illness. According to National AIDS Control Organization (NACO) statistics, India has 2.1 million people living with HIV infection, and 34% of the reported cases are in the age group of 15-29 years. While the other STIs have low intrinsic mortality, they predispose a person to HIV infection.

There are two groups of HIV-infected adolescents:

- A perinatally transmitted group who have often been exposed to anti-retroviral therapy (ART) and have an increased chance for treatment failure.
- Those who later acquire HIV through the sexual route or transfusions.

Adolescents are ill-equipped in terms of both information and life-skills and hence they are at high risk for STI and HIV due to their likelihood of sexual experimentation. Adolescents who start having sex early are more likely to have sex with high risk partners or multiple partners, and less likely to use condoms, and hence they are more vulnerable than adults (Box 4.3.1). STIs are also more common in girls due to various other factors (Table 4.3.1).

Box 4.3.1: Why are STIs more common in adolescents?

- Sexual abuse is an important cause of STI in adolescents.
- The incidence of premarital sex is increasing in both urban and rural areas of India.
- Since the subject is taboo, adolescents have poor knowledge of STIs, especially about the transmission and prevention of STIs.
- They are more prone to high risk behavior and believe themselves to be invincible.
- Early sexual debut, substance use, lack of condom use, and frequent change of sexual partners increase the risk of STI.
- They often do not correlate symptoms like dysuria, vaginal discharge, urethral discharge, lower abdominal pain and vulval itch with STI.
- Even when adolescents do recognize an STI, they face many financial and social obstacles to access health facilities.
- Delay in seeking treatment for STIs is common among adolescents, and increases the opportunities for transmitting the infection to others.
- STIs increase transmission of HIV, which occurs most commonly during adolescence and early adulthood; early detection and treatment of STIs reduces the prevalence of HIV infection.

In India the four most common STIs are trichomoniasis, chlamydiasis, gonorrhea and syphilis. *Herpes simplex virus* (HSV) and HPV are probably under-reported due to lack of awareness about them among physicians. Unlike the bacterial STIs, the viral STIs are not curable. Table 4.3.2 lists the most common STIs seen in adolescents.

SEXUALLY TRANSMITTED INFECTIONS

History Taking

Adolescent STI is best managed in an adolescent clinic that is manned by non-judgmental personnel who guarantee confidentiality. History taking should include a detailed sexual history, and an enquiry into their behavioral

Table 4.3.1: Why are adolescent girls more vulnerable to STIs?

Issue	*Factors*	*Comments*
The immature adolescent girl	• Very often asymptomatic • Ignorant of STI and its consequences • Mistakes STI for normal vaginal discharge • Fears pregnancy but not STI	• Requires education and awareness
The immature vagina	• Simple columnar epithelium is more susceptible to trauma and infection	• Gradually converted under the influence of estrogen into stratified squamous epithelium
	• Throughout adolescence 70% of girls will have some columnar epithelium at the junction of the vagina with the uterine cervix	• This 'cervical ectopy' predisposes to cervical infection
	• Low mucus production • Higher pH	• There is increased mucous production and lower pH as the girl becomes older making her more resistant to infection
	• The smaller introitus is more prone to physical trauma	• This happens with an adult abusing immature girls
Difficulty accessing health care	• No financial resources • Embarrassed to discuss sexual behavior or ask contraceptive advice • Fear of adult disapproval • Fear that parents will find out • No access to adolescent health clinics	• Need more accessible adolescent health services and education and community awareness
Other factors	• Victim of sexual abuse • Multiple and high-risk older partners • Commercial sex episodes • Human papilloma virus (HPV) infection in adolescence predisposes to future cervical cancer	• Greater social awareness and protection of adolescents

Table 4.3.2: STIs in adolescents

STIs	*Common*	*Less Common*
Bacterial	Gonorrhea Chlamydiasis Syphilis	Chancroid Lymphogranuloma venereum (LGV) Donovanosis
Viral	Human immunodeficiency virus (HIV) Human papilloma virus (HPV) *Herpes simplex virus* 2 (HSV2) Hepatitis B virus (HBV)	*Herpes simplex virus* 1 (HSV1) Hepatitis A virus
Others	Trichomoniasis Candidiasis	

risk status. This is followed by a systemic and genital examination.

The adolescent clinic should have both male and female staff. The consulting room should offer privacy for genital examination, and one should ensure that conversations cannot be overheard. Adolescents should not be expected to visit an 'STI clinic'.

- Clinicians should emphasize confidentiality right at the start.
- They should be non-judgmental and reassuring, even when they notice obvious untruths in the history.
- Most adolescents are not frank or open initially, due to shyness or fear of stigma, and one should expect them to be unwilling or embarrassed to share information initially.
- They often mention minor problems, and hope that the clinician will find the major diagnosis.
- History taking should initially focus on the presenting complaints.
- Next ask about immunization with hepatitis B, HPV and hepatitis A.

- Enquire whether the adolescent frequently stays away from home due to study or work (e.g. in a hostel), uses alcohol or drugs, or has a tattoo.

Leading Questions About Symptoms that Could Possibly be Due to An STI

- Does the girl have normal and regular menstrual cycles, dysmenorrhea, dysuria and/or frequency of micturition?
- Does she have vaginal discharge; and if so what is the amount, odor and color?
- Does she have genital itch or rash or ulcers?
- Does the boy have dysuria, frequency of micturition, discharge of pus from the penis, genital itch/rash/ ulcers, scrotal pain/swelling, or groin swelling?
- Have these symptoms occurred in the past, and if so was any treatment taken?
- Anal STI can cause anal discharge, tenesmus, diarrhea, blood in stool, abdominal cramps and local ulcers or vesicles.

Finally One Should Take a Sexual History

- When did the adolescent last have sex, and has he/she had sex earlier, and if so with how many partners?
- How often; is it with a person of the opposite or same gender; is it genital, oral or anal sex?
- Has the adolescent ever been tested for, diagnosed with, or treated for STI?
- What about the partner?
- Is any protection against pregnancy or STI used, and if so what, and how regularly?

Clinical Examination

The clinician should explain what is to be done and why. If the patient is below 18 years, parental permission is needed. Ask the adolescents if they wish someone trusted to be present. If examining a member of the opposite sex, an assistant of the same sex as the patient should be present.

Start with a general examination, including the vital signs, inspection of the skin and mucous membranes. Do a systematic search for enlarged lymph nodes, and record their number, size, consistency, and whether tender. Use gloves during genital examination.

Examination of the Male Adolescent

- Look for penile ulcers.
- Retract the foreskin and systematically examine the glans penis, coronal sulcus, frenulum and urethral meatus.
- If there is no obvious discharge, milk the urethra 3-4 times from the base towards the urethral meatus.
- Palpate the testis, epididymis, and spermatic cord.

Examination of the Female Adolescent

- Separate the labia majora with both hands, and inspect the labia majora and minora, the Bartholin glands, and the introitus.
- Pressing under the urethra with one finger might cause a drop of urethral discharge to come out.
- Holding the labia majora apart and pulling them towards the examiner permits internal examination.
- If there is vaginal discharge, do a speculum examination to differentiate between vaginitis and cervicitis.
- If there is cervicitis do a bimanual palpation.

Oral and Anal STIs

Adolescents may indulge in oral or anal sex to avoid pregnancy. A high degree of suspicion is required to diagnose these STIs.

- There may be ulcers or pharyngeal inflammation.
- Separate the buttocks with two hands to visualize the perineal area properly.
- Do a rectal examination and proctoscopy if there is rectal discharge or history of anal intercourse.

Investigations

Most laboratory tests for STIs have limited sensitivity and specificity, but one should do available and affordable tests as they reduce over-diagnosis and over-treatment.

Examination of vaginal discharge is very important in girls.

- Vaginal fluid is collected with a swab inserted deep into the lateral or posterior fornices of the vagina, or from the tip of the speculum after a speculum examination of the vagina.
- The use of jelly or disinfectant will interfere with the results.

Flowchart 4.3.1 describes the investigations necessary in cases of vaginal discharge syndrome in girls. The tests described in Table 4.3.3 will give a diagnosis in up to 80% of cases of vaginal discharge.

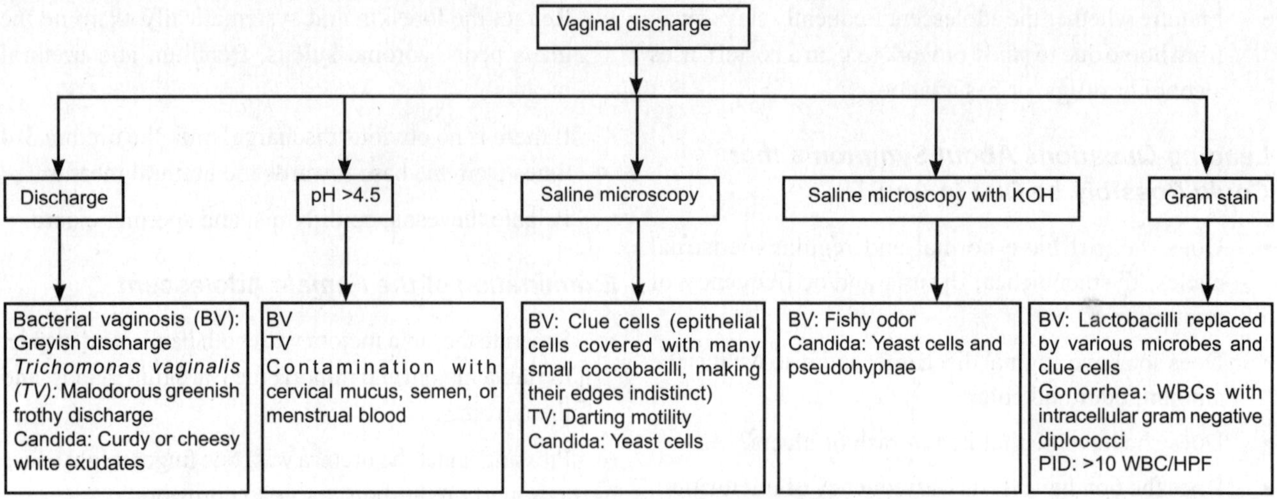

Flowchart 4.3.1: Investigations for vaginal discharge syndrome

Table 4.3.3: Useful investigations in STI

STIs	*Tests*	*Interpretation*
Chlamydiasis and gonorrhea	• Gram stain of urethral discharge	• Shows WBCs with intracellular gram negative diplococci in *N. gonorrhoeae*
	• NAATs (Nucleic acid amplification tests): These are sensitive tests	• These sensitive tests are costly and not easily available
Non-gonococcal urethritis	• Gram stain of urethral discharge	• >5 neutrophils per oil immersion field
	• First-void (NOT mid-stream) urine sample	• >10 neutrophils/HPF
Syphilis	• Rapid Plasma Reagin (RPR) and VDRL tests	• Sensitive tests with occasional false positives
	• *Treponema pallidum* Hemagglutinin test (TPHA)	• Confirmatory
Chancroid	• Gram stain of urethral discharge	• Gram negative coccobacilli
	• Culture	• *H. ducreyi* isolated
HSV	• Tzanck test	• Neither sensitive nor specific
	• Serology, PCR and culture	• Costly, limited accuracy
Pelvic inflammatory disease (PID)	• MRI, laparoscopy and Ultrasonography (USG)	• May reveal thickened, fluid-filled tubes, free fluid in the pelvis and/or a tubo-ovarian mass

Treatment

Principles of Treatment

- The drug used should be at least 95% effective, low-cost, with low toxicity, and not contraindicated in pregnancy.
- A single-dose, oral, directly observed regimen is preferred.
- The patient and partner should practice sexual abstinence until 7 days after completing treatment.

Syndromic Approach

The majority of STIs are asymptomatic; when symptomatic the manifestations are variable and usually non-specific. A syndromic approach is useful because:

- Etiologic diagnosis is often not possible clinically.
- Mixed infections are common.
- Laboratory diagnosis is often costly, difficult, time-consuming, with limited sensitivity and specificity, and facilities are limited.

Management of Specific Syndromes

Vaginal Discharge due to Bacterial Vaginosis: (See Flowchart 4.3.2).

- The most common cause of vaginal discharge in adolescent girls is bacterial vaginosis (BV), which is not an STI but is often mistaken for one.

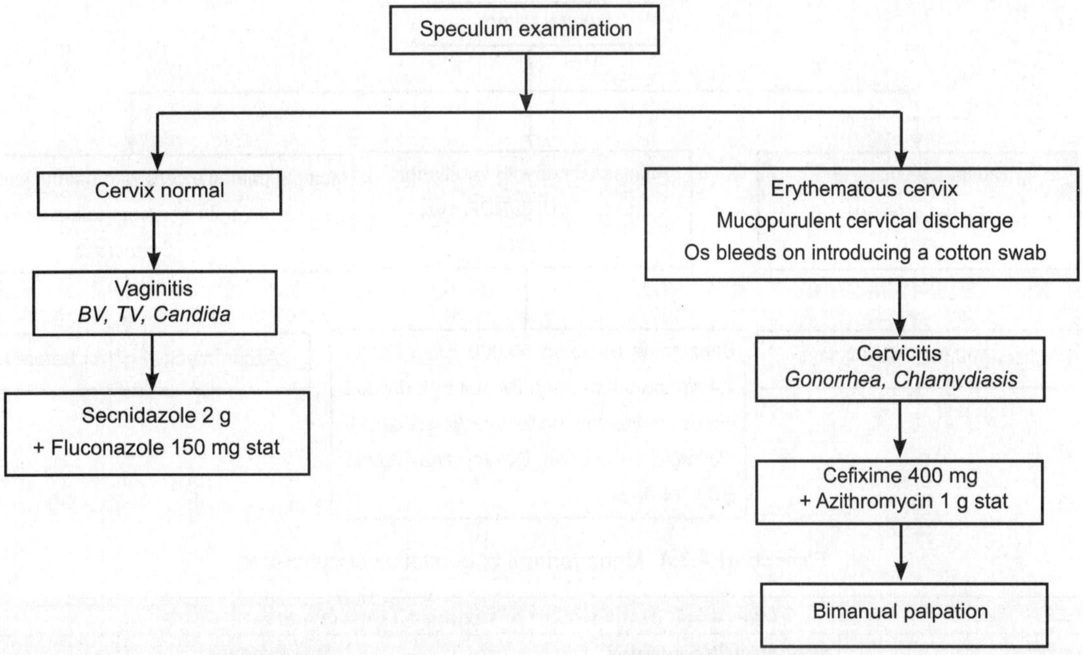

Flowchart 4.3.2: Management of vaginal discharge syndrome

- It presents as a sticky greyish vaginal discharge with a foul odor. It does not cause local itching or soreness.
- It occurs when lactobacillus, which is the normal vaginal flora of the vagina, is replaced by an overgrowth of mobiluncus (an anaerobe), often in association with *Gardnerella vaginalis, Ureaplasma urealyticum or Mycoplasma genitalium*.
- Secnidazole 2 g as a single dose is effective.

Urethral Discharge in Males: (See Flowchart 4.3.3)

- Urethral discharge, dysuria or frequency of micturition in an adolescent male is due to an STI until proved otherwise.
- The usual cause is *N. gonorrhoeae* or chlamydia; dual infection is common.
- *Trichomonas vaginalis, Mycoplasma genitalium,* HSV, enteric bacteria and adenovirus are less common.

Management of genital ulcers is shown in Flowchart 4.3.4. Table 4.3.4 describes briefly the management of various STI syndromes in adolescents. Table 4.3.5 summarizes the clinical profile of various STIs seen in adolescents including the causative agents, manifestations in boys and girls and their management.

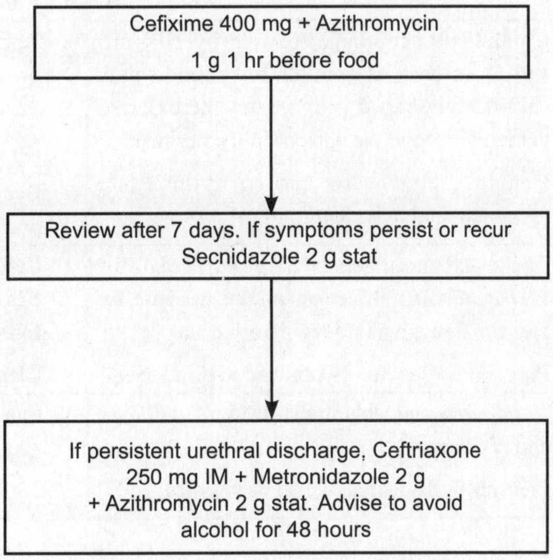

Flowchart 4.3.3: Management of urethral discharge syndrome in males

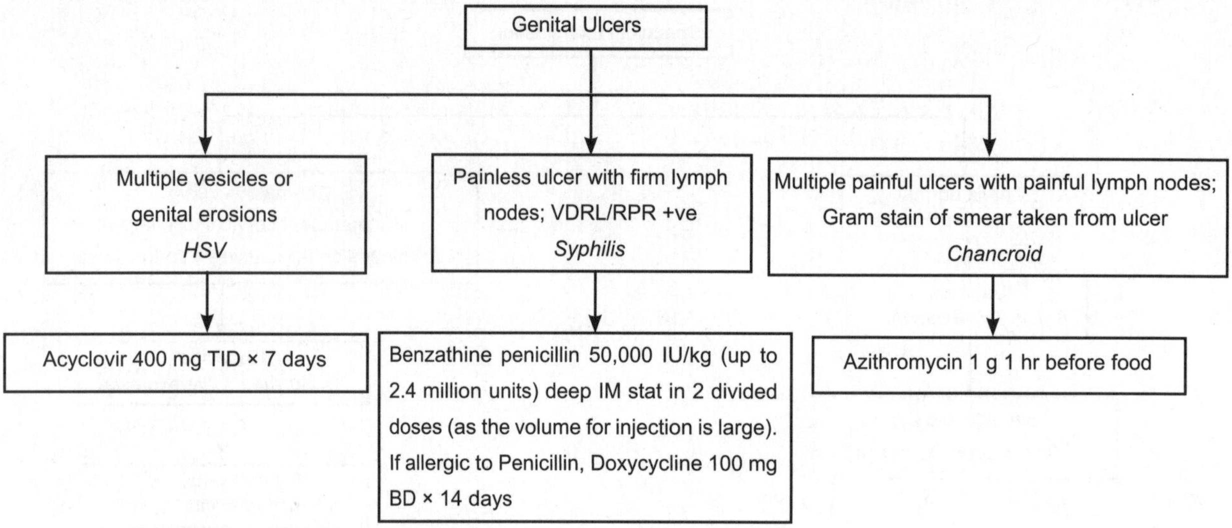

Flowchart 4.3.4: Management of genital ulcer syndrome

Table 4.3.4: Management of various STI syndromes

Syndromes	*Organism/Presentation*	*Management*
Scrotal pain or swelling	• Both chlamydia and gonorrhea can cause epididymo-orchitis. • D/D: Other causes are mumps, filaria, tuberculosis, and infection by coliform bacteria. • Rule out torsion of the testis and trauma.	• As the infection can reduce fertility, treatment should cover both. • Cefixime 400 mg + Azithromycin 1 g (supervised) 1 hour before food. • Advise bed rest, scrotal elevation with T-bandage and analgesics.
Genital ulcers	• Vesicles are seen.	• Treat for HSV.
	• If unsure of causative agent.	• Treat all three together: HSV, syphilis and chancroid.
Chronic inguinal lymphadenitis (buboes)	• Can be caused by lymphogranuloma venereum (LGV), granuloma inguinale (GI) and chancroid. • D/D: Acute inguinal adenitis due to local bacterial infections, and chronic adenitis due to tuberculosis or filariasis.	• Doxycycline 100 mg every 12 hours for 21 days at least + Azithromycin 1 g as a single dose. • Avoid procedures such as incision and drainage, which leads to chronic sinus formation. • If fluctuant, aspirate.
Genital skin lesions	• Condyloma acuminata, caused by HPV 16 and 18, presents as multiple soft painless pink cauliflower-shaped growths on the external genitalia, around the anus or in the perineum. • Benign genital warts and condyloma lata (syphilis) tend to be flatter.	• Apply 20% podophyllin on the wart after protecting the surrounding areas with Vaseline; wash it off after 3 hours. • Do this weekly till the lesions resolve. • Cervical lesions cannot be treated with podophyllin, and cryotherapy is needed.
Ophthalmia neonatorum	• The usual pathogen is *N. gonorrhoeae* or *C. trachomatis* infection of the neonate by passage through an infected birth canal. • Purulent conjunctivitis can lead to blindness.	• Ceftriaxone 50 mg/kg IM stat (maximum 125 mg) + erythromycin 50 mg/kg/day in four divided doses for 14 days. • Clean the eyes with distilled water or saline.
Oral or anal STIs	• *N. gonorrhoeae,* chlamydia, HSV, *T. pallidum* and *H. ducreyi.* • Presents as discharge, ulcers or vesicles.	• Syndromic management. • May also require antidiarrheal agents.

Table 4.3.5: Overview of STIs in adolescence

Infection	*Gonorrhea*	*Chlamydiasis*	*Trichomoniasis*	*Candidiasis*	*Primary Syphilis*	*Genital Herpes*	*Chancroid*	*Lymphogranuloma Venereum (LGV)*	*Donovanosis or Granuloma Inguinale (GI)*
Organism causing it	***Neisseria gonorrhoea***	***Chlamydia trachomatis***	***Trichomonas vaginalis***	***Candida albicans***	***Treponema pallidum***	**Herpes simplex virus (HSV) 2, rarely HSV 1**	***Hemophilus ducreyi***	***Chlamydia trachomatis* (L1, L2 and L3 serovars)**	***Klebsiella granulomatis***
Males	Urethritis, may lead to strictures or abscess; epididymo-orchitis; proctitis; 10% asymptomatic	Non-gonococcal urethritis (NGU); epididymo-orchitis; often asymptomatic	Chronic prostatitis; occasionally NGU; often asymptomatic		Single painless ulcer with an indurated border and a clean base; firm painless lymph nodes	Multiple vesicles or painful shallow ulcers; >50% have lifelong recurrent episodes	Multiple painful ulcers with non-indurated undermined borders and a purulent base, painful bubo	Painful buboes with draining sinuses; may cause rectal strictures, urethral damage, elephantiasis of the lower limbs or genitals	Painless, slowly progressive ulcers; no lymph nodes; subcutaneous granulomas (pseudo-buboes) that are vascular (beefy red) and bleed easily on contact.
Females	85% are asymptomatic; vaginal discharge, urethritis, vulval itch; cervicitis may lead to pelvic inflammatory disease (PID)	Majority are asymptomatic; irregular bleeding; cervicitis; silent PID; 20% have chronic pelvic pain; 20% become infertile	Vulvovaginitis with malodorous greenish frothy discharge; cervicitis; occasionally PID; 30% asymptomatic	Vulvar pain, itching, and erythema, especially during periods; curdy or cheesy white exudate	As in males	As in males	As in males	Painful buboes with draining sinuses; may cause rectal strictures, urethral damage, rectovaginal fistulas	As in males
Treatment	Cefixime 400 mg OR Ceftriaxone 250 mg IM	Azithromycin 1 g 1 hr before food OR Doxycycline 100 mg BD × 7 days	Secnidazole 2 g stat orally	Fluconazole 150 mg stat OR Clotrimazole 500 mg intravaginally	Benzathine penicillin 50,000 IU/kg (up to 2.4 million units) deep IM stat in 2 divided doses (as the volume for injection is large). If allergic to penicillin, Doxycycline 100 mg BD × 14 days	Acyclovir 400 mg TID × 7 days	Azithromycin 1 g orally OR Ceftriaxone 250 mg IM OR Erythromycin 500 mg QID × 7 days OR Ciprofloxacin 500 mg BD × 3 days	Doxycycline 100 mg BD × 21 days preferred OR Azithromycin 1 g weekly for 3 weeks. Avoid incision and drainage	Doxycycline 100 mg BD × 21 days or until all lesions heal OR Azithromycin 1 g weekly × 3 weeks at least OR Ciprofloxacin 750 mg BD × 3 weeks at least

Special Issues in Adolescent Girls

Since adolescent sex is often unplanned, impulsive, unprotected or under sexual coercion or exploitation, unwanted pregnancy can occur and hence it is important to ask a female adolescent with STI if she is pregnant or is there a risk of being pregnant. Table 4.3.6 lists the impact of STI at various stages of pregnancy and childbirth. Pelvic inflammatory disease (PID) is a complication of STI in females (Box 4.3.2).

Table 4.3.6: Interactions between STI and pregnancy

Issue	*Comments*
Intra-uterine infection	Maternal syphilis causes intrauterine growth restriction (IUGR) or severe fetal damage, resulting in stillbirth and neonatal death in at least one-third of cases.
Premature labor	Incidence is increased if mother has an STI.
Perinatal infection	• *Gonorrhea:* Neonatal conjunctivitis or sepsis. • *Chlamydia:* Neonatal conjunctivitis or pneumonia at 1-3 months. • *HSV:* Cutaneous infection, encephalitis, disseminated infection.
Drugs	• Quinolones (e.g. ofloxacin, ciprofloxacin), doxycycline and fluconazole are contraindicated in pregnancy. • Erythromycin stearate is acceptable, but not the estolate. • Podophyllin should be avoided.
Maternal candidiasis, anogenital warts and chancroid	Worsen during pregnancy.
Bacterial vaginosis	May cause low birth weight, chorioamnionitis, premature rupture of membranes, premature delivery and puerperal sepsis.

Box 4.3.2: Pelvic inflammatory disease (PID)

- This term is preferred for infection of the female upper genital tract.
- An ascending infection of the internal genitalia can result in any combination of endometritis, salpingitis, tubo-ovarian abscess and pelvic peritonitis.
- The infecting agent is usually *N. gonorrhoeae* or chlamydia; other causes include anaerobic bacteria like mobiluncus, gardnerella and *Mycoplasma genitalium.*
- *PID may be asymptomatic, especially in chlamydial infection, or it may present with pelvic or low abdominal pain, along with high fever, tenderness and guarding of the lower abdomen, or a pelvic mass.*
- Bimanual palpation may reveal tenderness of the adnexa or uterus or on cervical motion.
- There may also be vaginal discharge, menorrhagia, dysmenorrhea, dyspareunia, dysuria or tenesmus.
- ESR is raised.
- The differential diagnosis includes ectopic pregnancy, threatened or septic abortion, urinary tract infections and gastrointestinal disorders such as appendicitis and inflammatory bowel disease.
- A pregnancy test should always be done to rule out an ectopic pregnancy.
- Treatment consists of cefixime 400 mg every 12 hours for 7 days along with doxycycline 100 mg every 12 hours for 14 days and metronidazole 400 mg 12 hourly for 10 days.
- Careful follow-up is essential to confirm cure.

HIV/AIDS

Further History Taking

Soon after acquiring infection, the patient develops a temporary 'flu-like illness' of acute seroconversion that is often missed clinically and by routine antibody testing. P24 antigen/DNA-PCR may help in diagnosis in this early phase. After this phase the adolescent undergoes a slow progressive destruction of the immune system before manifesting with illness. Young adolescents with HIV infection may have delayed growth and development, often resulting in late puberty and, in girls, delayed or irregular menstrual cycles. These may be further worsened by progressing HIV illness and malnutrition.

After confirming HIV infection a further medical history and physical examination should be performed.

- The purpose is to determine the clinical stage of the infection, identify HIV-related illnesses that require treatment, identify coexisting medical conditions that may influence therapy, note past illnesses related to HIV, and decide about the need for anti-retroviral therapy (ART) and prophylaxis of opportunistic infection (OI).

- Enquire into the health of the parents to rule out perinatally acquired infection and to identify a caregiver.

  Details should be asked about the following:

1. *HIV tests:* Whether tested earlier for HIV, when, why, and the results and exposure to ART.
2. *HIV risk factors:* Unprotected sexual contact, injection drug use, men having sex with men, sex with a commercial sex worker (CSW), or partner HIV positive.
3. Detailed system-wise symptom review for HIV and OIs.
4. Past history of OIs, tuberculosis or STI.
5. History of menstrual irregularity, vaginal discharge and contraceptive use.
6. History of alcohol or drug use.
7. Social, economic and educational status.

Physical Examination

This is done to determine the clinical stage of the disease, and to rule out opportunistic infections using the WHO clinical staging (Table 4.3.7). A detailed discussion of these conditions is beyond the purview of this chapter.

Table 4.3.7: WHO clinical staging of HIV/AIDS for adults & adolescents, 2010

Clinical stages	***Signs and symptoms***
Clinical Stage 1	Asymptomatic
	Persistent generalized lymphadenopathy (multiple, bilateral, soft, non-tender, mobile cervical nodes, and less often in the axillae and groin)
Clinical Stage 2	Unexplained moderate weight loss (<10% of presumed or measured body weight)
	Recurrent respiratory tract infections (sinusitis, tonsillitis, otitis media, pharyngitis)
	Herpes zoster infection
	Angular cheilitis
	Recurrent oral ulceration
	Papular pruritic eruptions
	Seborrheic dermatitis
	Fungal nail infections
Clinical Stage 3	Unexplained severe weight loss (>10% of presumed or measured body weight)
	Unexplained chronic diarrhea for longer than one month
	Unexplained persistent fever (above 37.5°C intermittent or constant for >1 month)
	Persistent oral candidiasis
	Oral hairy leukoplakia
	Pulmonary tuberculosis
	Severe bacterial infections (e.g. pneumonia, empyema, pyomyositis, bone or joint infection, meningitis, bacteremia)
	Acute necrotizing ulcerative stomatitis, gingivitis or periodontitis
	Unexplained anemia (<8 g/dl), neutropenia ($<0.5 \times 10^9$/L) and/or chronic thrombocytopenia ($<50 \times 10^9$/L)
Clinical Stage 4	HIV wasting syndrome
	Pneumocystis pneumonia
	Recurrent severe bacterial pneumonia
	Chronic *Herpes simplex* infection (orolabial, genital or anorectal of more than one month's duration or visceral at any site)
	Esophageal candidiasis (or candidiasis of trachea, bronchi or lungs)
	Extra-pulmonary tuberculosis
	Kaposi sarcoma
	Cytomegalovirus infection (retinitis or infection of other organs)
	Central nervous system toxoplasmosis
	HIV encephalopathy
	Extra-pulmonary cryptococcosis including meningitis
	Disseminated mycosis (extra-pulmonary histoplasmosis, coccidioidomycosis)
	Recurrent septicemia (including non-typhoidal salmonella)
	Lymphoma (cerebral or B cell non-Hodgkin)
	Invasive cervical carcinoma
	Atypical disseminated leishmaniasis
	Symptomatic HIV-associated nephropathy or symptomatic HIV-associated cardiomyopathy

Investigations

HIV is diagnosed by doing a blood ELISA or rapid HIV test. A person who tests HIV positive should be tested twice more using different kits. Reports are given as follows:

- Reactive if a person tests positive thrice.
- Equivocal if a person tests positive twice.
- Non-reactive if the last two tests are negative.
- If the report is equivocal, the person should be subjected to a DNA-PCR test.

An HIV positive patient has to undergo the following laboratory evaluation:

- Complete blood counts: Hemoglobin, total and differential leukocyte counts.
- Serum alanine aminotransferase (ALT or SGPT), creatinine, fasting blood sugar and lipid profile.

  (These are repeated at least every 6 months while on ART).
- VDRL, HBsAg, urine routine and microscopic examination.
- Chest X-ray.
- CD4 counts.
- Investigations to rule out OIs, as directed by clinical features.

Management

Disclosure

Disclosure of HIV status to one's sexual partner should be encouraged though it is often the most challenging issue. The fear of rejection after disclosure is great, especially if the partner is the most supportive and loving person in the adolescent's life. Parents of perinatally infected children fear that their child will reject them, but have less depression after disclosure.

There are well established guidelines for starting ART therapy (Table 4.3.8). Adolescents over 13 years and above 30 kg are prescribed the adult dose. Maximum pediatric dose permissible is the adult dose (Table 4.3.9).

Table 4.3.8: Anti-retroviral therapy (ART)

Issues	*Indications*	*Details*
Pre-ART care	Offered to the HIV positive person who does not require ART	• Regular follow-up. • Intermittent CD4 screening. • Advice to return if new symptoms develop. • Counseling of the family and partner.
When to start ART	ART is given to all patients in stage 3 or 4 and patients with CD4 <350 cells/mm³ Patient must be registered in an ART center	• A comprehensive package of care including prevention and treatment of OIs, nutritional programs, psychosocial support, and HIV prevention efforts. • OIs should be treated before starting ART. • If the patient has tuberculosis, ART is started 2 weeks to 2 months after starting ATT. • However, ART is not postponed for unexplained anemia (Hb <8 g/dl), CMV infection, *Mycobacterium avium* complex, or skin conditions like pruritic papular eruptions, seborrheic dermatitis, psoriasis or HIV-related exfoliative dermatitis.
Choice of ART	The first-line regimen is a 3-drug combination i.e. • Lamivudine + • Zidovudine/Tenofovir, a Nucleoside reverse transcriptase inhibitor [NRTI] + • Nevirapine/Efavirenz, a Non-nucleoside reverse transcriptase inhibitor [NNRTI]	• Zidovudine is preferred unless Hb is <9 g/dl. • Nevirapine is preferred unless patient has hepatic dysfunction or hepatitis B or C infection or is on Rifampicin for ATT. • Injecting drug users are switched to methadone, but they may need higher doses as NNRTIs reduce plasma levels of methadone.
Preventive therapy	Cotrimoxazole 960 mg OD is given to all patients in stage 3 or 4 and all patients with CD4 <250 cells/mm³	This is effective against PCP, toxoplasma, bacterial pneumonia and many organisms that cause diarrhea.
For a detailed discussion on ART please see reference 4		

Table 4.3.9: Drugs used in ART

Drug	*Adult dose*	*Pediatric dose*	*Comments, Side-effects*
Nucleoside RTI (NRTI)			
Zidovudine (AZT/ZDV)	300 mg BD	240 mg/m²/dose	Severe anemia or neutropenia
Lamivudine (3TC)	150 mg BD	4 mg/kg/dose	Effective against hepatitis B
Didanosine (DDL)	400 mg OD	–	Pancreatitis, peripheral neuropathy
Abacavir (ABC)	300 mg BD	8 mg/m²/dose	Occasionally severe hypersensitivity
Tenofovir (TDF)	300 mg OD	8 mg/kg OD	Occasionally metabolic acidosis, lipoatrophy, renal dysfunction
Non-nucleoside RTI (NNRTI)			
Nevirapine (NVP)	200 mg OD for 14 days; then 200 mg BD	120–200 mg/m²/dose	Hepatotoxic; blood levels decreased by rifampicin; Stevens-Johnson syndrome
Efavirenz (EFV)	600 mg OD	300-400 mg OD	Potentially teratogenic
Protease inhibitors (PI)			
Saquinavir (SQV) + Ritonavir (RTV)	SQV 1000 mg RTV 100 mg BD	Not available	Gastrointestinal side-effects

Adherence to Antiretroviral Therapy

HIV-infected adolescents commonly cope poorly with their illness due to low self-esteem, chaotic lifestyles, and a lack of family support. The concrete thought processes of adolescence make it difficult for them to take medications, especially because they do not want to feel different from their peers. Further difficulties are faced by adolescents who live with parents to whom they have not yet disclosed their HIV status and those who are homeless and have no place to store medicine.

Without good counseling compliance with ART is very poor among adolescents, as it is required even when asymptomatic, and multiple drugs are prescribed, and side-effects are common. One study from a multidisciplinary adolescent HIV clinic indicated that only 61% of patients reported >90% adherence to their medications in the past 90 days. The most common reason for non-adherence in this cohort was "too many pills". Strategies have to be employed to improve adherence (Box 4.3.3).

Box 4.3.3: Strategies to improve adherence

- Establish trust and identify mutually acceptable goals for care.
- Obtain explicit agreement on need for treatment.
- Identify depression and low self-esteem. Treat prior to starting ART, if possible.
- Identify family, friends, health team members, or others who can help with adherence support.
- Educate them about HIV and its manifestations, and the benefits and side effects of medications.
- Identify the adherence target: 95% of prescribed doses.
- Educate them that poor adherence leads to drug resistance, which may permanently result in a need for more toxic and/or less effective regimens.
- Choose the simplest regimen possible, reducing dosing frequency and number of pills.
- Choose drugs with the fewest side effects.
- Use discrete pill boxes to store and organize medicines.
- Use reminders and alarms.
- Monitor adherence at each visit, and in between visits by telephone or letter as needed.
- Provide access to a nurse or social worker for counseling and support.

Counseling

Counseling an Adolescent with HIV/AIDS

Counseling provides psychosocial support to patients, improves compliance to ART, and helps them to modify lifestyle so as not to spread the disease to others; it is required lifelong. The counselor should guarantee confidentiality and should be totally accepting and non-judgmental. Counseling is also important for their intimate contacts, their families and friends, and for health workers in regular contact with them.

Counseling begins right from the time one suspects HIV/AIDS or when an adolescent requests an HIV test. Consent for testing can be given by the adolescent himself/herself if above 18 years. HIV testing should not be treated like any other diagnostic laboratory testing as the results have a lot of psychosocial implications and can create havoc in a patient's life. Pre-test and post-test counseling are essential, and will also take care of medicolegal issues. One should prepare for proper referral and follow-up if needed. Table 4.3.10 describes the major steps in counseling an adolescent with HIV/AIDS.

Table 4.3.10: Counseling in HIV/AIDS infection in adolescents

Period	*Comments*
PRE-TEST COUNSELING	• Obtain the personal history of the client. • Explore why the client wants the test, and assess the risk of HIV exposure. • Find out what the client already knows about HIV, and give appropriate information. • Anticipate the client's response to the result. • Anticipate the effect on relationship with others.
POST-TEST COUNSELING **A negative result:** *Relief or euphoria*	• Make him/her aware that it may be falsely negative due to the window period of three months. • Explain the need for a repeat test. • Discuss how to prevent further exposure by avoiding high risk behavior. • Discuss safer sex practices. • Discuss avoidance of needle sharing.
A positive result: *Fear, guilt, grief, denial, anxiety, anger, suicidal thoughts*	• First discussion should be private and confidential. • Explain the result. • Discuss the medical and social implications. • Do not speculate about prognosis. • Provide information on how to prevent further transmission. • Offer psychosocial support.
An equivocal test result: *Anxiety, confusion*	• Explain that it may occur in up to 10% of samples. • Explain the need for further tests. • Clarify that a clear result may take 3 months. • Offer psychological support until then. • Provide information on how to prevent further transmission.

Counseling Adolescents with Other STIs

Counseling is vital for treatment and to prevent recurrence.

- The physician should explain how and why they got the infection, the manifestations and complications of the infection, the mode of spread and how it can be prevented in future, and how it can be cured, so that they understand why drugs are needed, and how to minimize the risk of acquiring or transmitting STIs.
- The correct use of condoms should be taught, and condoms should be provided free or at subsidized rates.
- All patients should be encouraged to get screening for HIV and syphilis.
- There should be a return visit after 7 days to ensure treatment compliance, to see the reports of tests done, and to confirm cure.
- Counseling should be tailored to the adolescent's needs. The counselor should help the patients to develop critical thinking skills, promote their self-esteem, and encourage positive values. The importance of partner therapy should be emphasized (Box 4.3.4).

Box 4.3.4: Partner therapy in STI

- Partner therapy is important to cure the partner (who may be asymptomatic and so does not seek treatment) to prevent the primary patient from being re-infected, and to prevent other persons from being infected by the partner.
- The patient should be convinced of the importance of partner management, and should be asked to bring the partner along.
- Both of them should be treated for any STIs found in either of them.
- If it is not possible to examine the partner, a prescription is given without evaluation: this is known as *'expedited partner therapy'*.
- Partner therapy is not needed for vaginal candidiasis or bacterial vaginosis unless the patient does not improve with treatment or the partner is symptomatic.

Prevention

Factors such as lack of maturity, peer pressure, alcohol and drug abuse put adolescents at an increased rate for HIV and other STIs. Many adolescent girls equate sex with love and/or peer acceptance. There is need to make adolescents aware of HIV/AIDS and other STIs, dangers of alcohol and drugs, how to handle peer pressure, sex and value education, risks of pre-marital sex, prevention of sexual abuse, and contraception. Trained peer educators are effective teachers of adolescents.The strategies that can be used are:

- Educate adolescents about STIs and HIV/AIDS, preferably in school family life education (FLE) programs. Teach life-skills.
- Make available adolescent friendly health services. They should be situated close to schools, open soon after school hours, and offer multiple activities such as evening classes and sports facilities.
- Sexually active adolescents should be screened confidentially for chlamydiasis and gonorrhea every year.
- HIV testing should be done in adolescents at high risk. This is a tricky issue if they are below 18 years of age as permission from parents is essential.
- Promote condom use among sexually active adolescents, and teach correct use.
- Encourage immunization against HPV and hepatitis B.

LEARNING POINTS

- STIs are often asymptomatic or mild, yet cause considerable long-term morbidity and promote transmission of HIV infection.
- Adolescents are very vulnerable due to various psychosocial factors. Special attention has to be given to the girls.
- A syndromic approach to STI management is preferred as dual infections are common and sensitive low-cost diagnostic tools are not available.
- The recommended drug should be given as a single-dose directly-observed regimen; it should be at least 95% effective, low cost, oral, and with low toxicity.
- Partner therapy is very important, as also counseling to prevent recurrence and follow-up to ensure cure.
- There is a high incidence of HIV/AIDS in adolescents and the best method of prevention is by creating awareness and empowerment through life-skills training in school programs, and community programs for out of school adolescents.
- Challenges in diagnosing and treating HIV in adolescents include the requirement for parental permission for testing in minors, the difficulty in disclosing one status to one's sexual partner, and the need for lifelong polytherapy using drugs with significant side-effects even when asymptomatic.

SUGGESTED READING

1. Burstein GR. Sexually Transmitted Infections. In: Kliegman RM, Stanton BF, St. Geme III JW, Schor NF, Behrman RE. Nelson Textbook of Pediatrics, 19th ed. Philadelphia: Elsevier; 2011; 705-14.
2. Greydanus DE, Bhave SY, Patel D. Reproductive Tract Infections and Sexually Transmitted Diseases. In: Bhave's Textbook of Adolescent Medicine, 1st edition. New Delhi; Jaypee Brothers Medical Publishers 2006; 46-61.
3. McManus A, Dhar L. Study of knowledge, perception and attitude of adolescent girls towards STIs/HIV, safer sex and sex education: A cross sectional survey of urban adolescent school girls in South Delhi, India. BMC Women's Health 2008; 8:12.
4. Ministry of Health and Family Welfare, Government of India. Antiretroviral therapy guidelines for HIV-infected adults and adolescents. New Delhi, India; May 2013.
5. Ministry of Health and Family Welfare, Government of India. National Guidelines on Prevention, Management and Control of Reproductive Tract Infections and Sexually Transmitted Infections. New Delhi, India; July 2014.
6. Shekhar M, Ghosh S, Panda P. Exploring Safe Sex Awareness and Sexual Experiences of Adolescents in Patna. Economic and Political Weekly, December 1, 2007, 48-55.
7. WHO Fact sheet on STI. Available from: http://www.who.int/mediacentre/factsheets/fs110/en/Accessed June 25, 2015.
8. World Health Organization. Sexually transmitted infections in adolescence. Geneva, World Health Organization; 2004.
9. Yogev R, Chadwick EG. Acquired Immunodeficiency Syndrome (Human Immunodeficiency Virus). In: Kliegman RM, Stanton BF, St. Geme III JW, Schor NF, Behrman RE. Nelson Textbook of Pediatrics, 19th ed. Philadelphia: Elsevier 2011;1157-77.

Contraception in Adolescents and Youth

4.4

Ashwini Bhalerao Gandhi, Rajani Vaidya

INTRODUCTION

Many adolescents of this generation are becoming sexually active without adequate knowledge of sexuality, reproduction, contraception and sexually transmitted diseases (STIs) and human immunodeficiency virus (HIV) infection. Thus adolescents and young people are prone to unintended pregnancies and STIs. Complications during pregnancy and childbirth are the second cause of death for 15 to 19-year-old girls globally. Though sexual activity starts early in life, adolescents and young people do not use contraceptives regularly due to a variety of reasons (see Table 4.4.1):

- *Psychosocial factors:* Unexpected and unplanned nature of sexual activity, peer pressure, impulsive behavior, fear of medical procedures and fear of violence from partner or parents.
- *Lack of information and knowledge* regarding the availability and access to the contraceptive methods.
- *Judgmental attitude from health care providers* in public health services.
- Accessing contraceptive services from private sectors is expensive.
- Political, religious and cultural barriers.

HISTORY TAKING

- While prescribing contraception it is important to know the prevailing laws of the country related to provisions of different contraceptive methods.
- The history taking should be done in a safe, non-threatening environment with non-judgmental attitude and with confidentiality ensured.
- In order to advise proper contraceptive method, personal factors like partner's attitude, lifestyle, compliance etc. have to be taken into account.
- A detailed history of sexual behavior whether unplanned, sporadic or regular is also important.

Table 4.4.1: National family health survey (NFHS) 3

Characteristic	*Percentage*
Age at marriage	15–17 years (19%)
Age at childbearing	15–24 years (39%)
Sexual intercourse before the age of 15	Urban–4.5%
	Rural–12.7%

CLINICAL EXAMINATION

World Health Organization (WHO) recommends a careful personal, family and medical history (with important attention to cardiovascular risk factors) and an accurate blood pressure measurement before the initiation of oral contraceptive pills. If the patient is in WHO category 1 or 2, then combined oral contraceptive (COC) pills can be safely used without detailed pelvic or breast examination (Table 4.4.2).

WHO Medical Eligibility Criteria

- **Category 1:** A condition for which there is no restriction for the use of the contraceptive method.
- **Category 2:** A condition where the advantages of using the method generally outweigh the theoretical or proven risks.
- **Category 3:** A condition where the theoretical or proven risks usually outweigh the advantages of using the method.
- **Category 4:** A condition which represents an unacceptable health risk if the contraceptive method is used.

MANAGEMENT

Once puberty has been achieved, contraceptive methods that are physiologically safe for adults are also physiologically safe for adolescents (Table 4.4.3).

In order to make well informed and voluntary choices, full information regarding various methods including their effectiveness, advantages and disadvantages etc. should be provided (Table 4.4.4).

Over the years, the concentration of ethinyl estradiol in the pill is being reduced and newer progestogens have been added to minimize the side effects.

Table 4.4.5 provides the various choices of contraception for young people. Table 4.4.6 lists the available progestins for contraceptive use. Table 4.4.7 provides the details of proprietary names and compositions of combined OCPs.

Table 4.4.2: Medical eligibility criteria for some conditions and contraceptives

Condition	*Combined oral contraceptive (COC) pills*	*Progestogen only pills (POP)*	*Depot medroxyprogesterone acetate (DMPA)/ Norethindrone enanthate (NETen)*	*Copper-intrauterine device (Cu-IUD)*
Sexually transmitted infections (STIs)				
Current purulent cervicitis/chlamydial/gonorrheal infection	1	1	1	4
Vaginitis (including bacterial vaginosis)	1	1	1	2
WHO stage 1 or 2 HIV (asymptomatic or mild)	1	1	1	2
WHO stage 3 or 4 HIV (severe or advanced stage)	1	1	1	3
Breastfeeding				
<6 weeks postpartum	4	2	3	
≥6 weeks to ≤6 months	3	1	1	
≥6 months postpartum	2	1	1	
Postpartum (non-breastfeeding women)				
<21 days		1	1	
–Without other risk factors for venous thromboembolism (VTE)	3			
–With other risk factors for VTE	4			
≥21 days to 42 days		1	1	
>42 days	1	1	1	
Postpartum (breastfeeding/non-breastfeeding women)				
<48 hours of delivery				1
≥48 hours to <4 weeks				3
≥4 weeks				1
Puerperal sepsis				4

* The number against each contraceptive in the columns indicate the WHO medical eligibility criteria category.

Table 4.4.3: Various contraceptive methods
1. Abstinence and non-penetrative sex
2. Natural/Fertility awareness based and behavioral methods
3. Barrier contraceptives
- Diaphragm
- Vaginal spermicides
- Diaphragm with spermicides
- Cervical cap
- Female condom
- Male condom
4. Hormonal pills
- Combined oral contraceptive (COC) pills
- Mini pills
5. Transdermal hormonal contraception
6. Injectable contraception
- Combined injectable
- Progesterone only injectable
7. Intrauterine devices
8. Emergency contraception (EC)

Table 4.4.4: Information about contraceptives to be provided to adolescents
A. Provide information on all available methods to enable well-informed choices
• Effectiveness in pregnancy
• Effectiveness in STI/HIV prevention
• Possible risks and benefits to health
• Ease of obtaining supplies for use
• Return of fertility after discontinuing method
B. Once a choice has been made, provide additional information on the method
• Regarding correct use
• Signs and symptoms, which will require a visit to the clinic
• Ease of obtaining supplies for future use

Table 4.4.5: Choice of contraception in young people

Method	*Important aspects*	*Relevance in young people*
Abstinence	Premarital sexual activity is banned by most religions and abstinence is advocated by the society; hence this is practiced by some unmarried young people.	Not acceptable to many young people today. Many have earlier sexual debut due to peer pressure and urge to experiment and experience the sexual activities. The age of marriage is also delayed due to higher education and other socioeconomic factors; hence abstinence for such a prolonged period is not considered as practical or feasible.
Behavioral and Fertility Awareness Based Methods	Depends on user recognition of the fertile days of menstrual cycle as intercourse must be avoided or barrier contraception should be used during this unsafe time. Non-penetrative sex, oral sex, mutual masturbation or self sex are used as alternative methods to protect from pregnancy.	Irregularity of the menstrual cycle and the timing of ovulation in adolescents–barrier for successful implementation. Degree of personal motivation, involvement of both partners required to practice the methods correctly–a challenge for many adolescents. Most are not aware that these have risk of STIs and HIV. Need to be cautioned that barrier contraceptives should be used even while indulging in anal/oral sex.
Barrier Methods	These are simple to use and are available across the counter. In fact, in many countries condom vending machines are placed in public areas. Male and female condoms prevent pregnancy as well as STIs, but in the event of condom slippage, breakage or failure to use–emergency contraceptives should be used. *Dual protection:* E.g. condom use can be combined with use of chemical contraceptives like spermicidal jelly, pessary by the female partner. Still better option would be that the female partner takes oral contraceptive (OC) pills while the male partner continues to use condom.	These methods are coital related; require user comfort, familiarity with his/her genitalia. Self-assurance is needed to purchase condoms over the counter and the cost may be prohibitive. Use of dual method of contraception has the added advantage of minimizing the failure rates.
Combined Oral Contraceptives (COC)	The COCs act by: • Inhibiting the ovulation by suppressing FSH and LH. • Alteration of endometrium making it unsuitable for implantation and making cervical mucus scanty and viscous. The regime followed for COC is usually 21 active pills + 7 placebo pills. Nowadays 24+4 regime is followed for some very low dose and ultra-low dose pills. This regime is more forgiving for forgotten pills. Thus it improves success rate. As pill free interval is reduced to only 4 days, hormonal withdrawal symptoms are minimal. Drospirenone containing pills are also used to treat acne and premenstrual disorders.	Multiple non-contraceptive benefits e.g.: • Less chances of endometrial/ovarian/colorectal cancer. • Less prone to ectopic pregnancies. • Menstrual cycles become more regular with less pain and less flow. • Reduced incidence of pelvic inflammatory disease (PID), endometriosis, benign breast disease and ovarian cyst. They are also used as a therapeutic measure for treating DUB, dysmenorrhea, premenstrual syndrome (PMS), polycystic ovarian syndrome (PCOS), acne, hirsutism, bleeding disorders etc.

Contd.

Contd.

Instructions for Use of COC	**Initiation of use** (Choose any one option given below) • Begin taking pill on the first day of menstrual bleeding. • On first Sunday after the menstrual bleeding starts. • Take the pills immediately if definitely not pregnant and has not had unprotected sex since last menstrual period. **Stop pills** In case of abdominal pain, chest pain, headaches, eye problems and severe leg pain.	**Missed pill** If<24 hours after last pill–take one that pill immediately and then return to normal schedule. If>24 hours after last pill– take both the missed pill and the next scheduled pill at the same time. If <48 hours after last pill (i.e. 2 or more missed pills), take only the last missed pill, discard the other missed pill and continue the schedule with additional contraception for the remainder of the cycle.
Intrauterine Devices (IUD)	Current evidence demonstrates the safety of modern IUDs. It suggests that the relative risk of pelvic inflammatory disease (PID) is increased only in the first 20 days after IUD insertion and then returns to baseline, while the absolute risk remains small. Bacterial contamination associated with the insertion process is the likely cause of infection, not the IUD itself. The development of no touch technique for insertion has reduced the infection rate.	Frameless IUD adapts to any uterus, including the smaller uterus of nulliparous adolescent and young women. Equally effective as in adults. As it does not offer protection against STIs, not recommended for women who are likely to have multiple partners unless used in conjunction with barrier contraceptives. Properly inserted it reduces the incidence of bleeding and pain in abdomen. Low expulsion rate with high efficacy.
Injectable Hormonal Contraception	**Available in India:** • Depot medroxyprogesterone acetate (DMPA) and norethindrone enanthate (NETen). • Depot medroxyprogesterone acetate (DMPA)– Long acting progesterone given once in every 3 months: single 150 mg intramuscular dose. • Norethindrone enanthate (NETen)–Dose 200 mg intramuscularly every 2 monthly. To ensure effective contraception, the first injection is given within first 7 days of the menstrual cycle. However if the injections are started after day 7 of regular cycle, a backup method is necessary for next 7 days.	Especially good for married parous young women after postpartum period. The Society for Adolescent Health and Medicine (SAHM) guidelines for DMPA: • Duration need not be restricted to 2 years. • Bone density monitoring individualized. • Use should not be routinely restricted based on skeletal health concerns, as the BMD returns to pre-use level after stopping the injectable contraception. • Supplementation with 1,300 mg calcium and 400 IU Vitamin D. • Exercise regularly.

EMERGENCY CONTRACEPTION (EC)

Since September 2005, EC pills are available in India as over the counter drugs (OTC). They are also available free of cost at municipal and government hospitals. Widespread advertising through electronic and print media has led to their indiscriminate use.

The I Pill–Emergency contraceptive pill (ECP) outsells both condoms and other regular contraceptive pills. Male partners are refusing use of condoms and forcing females to use EC pills instead. Some couples use them even before indulging in sexual activity, reflecting irresponsible, unethical usage. A complete ban on advertising EC pills was imposed in January 2010. It was subsequently lifted by the Government of India–Drug Technical Advisory Board with the caveat that advertisements promoting EC pills should specifically emphasize on their usage during emergency only.

All adolescents and youth should be informed regarding EC as unplanned and impulsive sexual activity is the most common feature in this age group. The other indications are slippage of condom, missing pills or sexual activity against will. Using EC is any day better than undergoing MTP or unwanted pregnancy.

Table 4.4.6: Available progestins for oral contraceptives
First Generation–No longer used
Second Generation • Norgestrel • Ethnodiol diacetate • Norethindrone • Levonorgestrel
Third Generation • Norgestimate • Desogestrel
Fourth Generation • Spironolactone Derived–Drospirenone

Table 4.4.7: Proprietary names and compositions of combined OCP
1. Standard Dose Ovral G/Duoluton–EE 0.05 mg, Levonorgestrel 0.25 mg
2. Low Dose Ovral L/Mala N–EE 0.03 mg, Norgestrel 0.15 mg Novelon–EE 0.03 mg, Desogestrel 0.15 mg Mala D–EE 0.03 mg, Norethisterone acetate 1 mg Yasmin–0.3 mg, Drospirenone 3 mg
3. Very Low Dose Femilon–EE 0.02 mg, Desogestrel 0.15 mg Loette–EE 0.02 mg, Levonorgestrel 0.10 mg Yaz–EE 0.02 mg, Drospirenone 3 mg (24+4 regime)
4. Ultra Low Dose Minesse–EE 0.15 mg, Gestodene 0.6 mg (24+4 regime)

Important Points to Remember in Emergency Contraception (EC)

1. Use of hormonal ECs as a regular contraceptive has not been found to provide adequate contraceptive efficacy. Frequent use invariably leads to irregular excessive required.
2. Levonorgestrel (LNG) can be used more than once in the same cycle. If another exposure happens within 12 hours of a dose of LNG, then further ECP is not required.
3. Sexual activity during the safe period is extremely unlikely to result in pregnancy; the patient's anxiety level should determine the use of EC.
4. Available scientific data suggests that there should not be any increased risk of teratogenic effects as ECP are taken long before organogenesis.
5. Liver enzyme inducing drugs lower the efficacy of LNG. Consideration should be given to increase the amount of hormone either by giving a double dose in one or both pills or an extra pill.
6. To seek medical advice if they vomit within two hours of taking LNG. A repeat dose of same pill or Copper IUD may be offered if appropriate. Vomiting after two hours does not necessitate repeat dose.
7. ECP taken immediately before is as effective as taken afterwards. A method other than ECP such as barrier method is a better choice.
8. ECP acts either prior to implantation or prevent implantation therefore, ECP is not an abortifacient.
9. Patient should be counseled properly at the time of prescription regarding the lower efficacy and higher cost of ECPs as compared to the currently available contraceptive methods for regular use. Also ECPs can cause unpleasant side-effects, which discourage their use as a regular method.
10. There is no evidence in western countries to suggest that knowledge of EC promotes sexual activity among young people. Instead the need for EC often brings sexually active young people into family planning clinics where they can receive other services and counseling.

Table 4.4.8 details the various emergency contraception methods available for young people. Table 4.4.9 provides the steps to be followed during evaluation before starting EC and during follow-up.

SITUATION IN INDIA

The legal age of consent for sexual activity varies by jurisdiction across Asia, from age 12 to age 21. The specific activity engaged in or the gender of its participants can also be affected by the law.

At present by Indian laws, sexual activity with or without mutual consent below 18 years of age is illegal amounting to rape (see Table 4.4.10). Thus medical practitioners cannot advocate or advise contraceptive methods to adolescents whose age is less than 18 years. Many professionals are of the opinion that this age limit should be lowered to 16 years as before. This reversal will respect sexual rights of the adolescent population and will also empower the health professionals to protect them against unwanted pregnancy as well as STIs including HIV.

According to the Protection of Children from Sexual Offences Act (POCSO Act) 2012 Section: A man is said to commit "rape" if he (...) sixthly—with or without her consent, when she is under eighteen years of age. There is an exception clause under Section 375, which stipulates: "Sexual intercourse or sexual acts by a man with his own wife, the wife not being under fifteen years of age, is not

Table 4.4.8: Various emergency contraception methods

Method	*Timeframe*	*Dose*	*Pregnancy rate*	*Comments*
High dose estrogen	72 hours	Diethylstilbestrol (DES) 50 mg × 5 days Ethinyl Estradiol (EE) 5 mg × 5 days	0.3–1.6%	Nausea, vomiting. Failure to complete regimen because of side effects.
Yuzpe method	72 hours	2 tablets 50 μg EE + 0.25 mg LNG. Repeat after 12 hours	0.2–3.2%	Low efficacy. Nausea and vomiting.
Levonorgestrel (LNG)	72–120 hours	1 tablet of 0.75 mg Repeat dose 0.75 mg after 12 hours Single dose–1.5 mg	1.1%	Less cost. Fewer incidences of nausea and vomiting. Safe and effective.
Copper T	5–7 days	—	<1%	Continued contraception. Need infrastructure and training for the procedure.
Mifepristone	72–120 hours	Single dose–600 mg	1.3%	High cost.
Danazol	72 hours	800 mg–3 doses 1200 mg–2 doses	1.7% 0.8%	Androgenic side effects. High cost.
Centchroman (Ormeloxifene)	120 hours	50 mg–2 tablets	To be evaluated	Controlled trials needed.

Table 4.4.9: Evaluation before starting EC and during follow-up

History–Last menstrual period (LMP), duration of cycle, timings of all unprotected acts in relation to the current cycle, medical history, contraception used
Examination–Blood pressure (BP), per speculum (PS), per vaginal (PV) not mandatory
Contraindications for E+P–Current focal migraine, current hepatocellular jaundice, past history of thrombotic disease
Contraindications for IUD–Nulliparity, PID
Instructions: Antiemetic 1 hour before the dose
Barrier method/abstinence till next period
Follow-up visit: Advised within 3-4 weeks of treatment
Advised to come earlier if there is delay in menses of more than 1 week, lower abdominal pain, and heavy bleeding/scanty next periods.

Table 4.4.10: Historical aspects of age of consent for sexual activity in India

1892	The marital rape and subsequent death of an 11-year-old girl caused the age of consent to be raised from 10 to 12 years of age.
1949	Raised to 15 years of age after agitation from women groups about the adverse effect of early pregnancy.
1982	Raised to 16 years of age.
2012	The Protection of Children from Sexual Offences (POCSO) Bill raised the age to 18. Although, the Criminal Law (Amendment) Act, 2013 initially sought to lower the age to 16, it was set at 18 due to political and social pressure.

LEARNING POINTS

1. Once puberty has been achieved, contraceptive methods that are physiologically safe for adults are also physiologically safe for adolescents.
2. Education and awareness is needed to prevent misuse of emergency contraception.
3. Contraception to major adolescents should be selected with care as all methods may not be suitable.

SUGGESTED READING

1. Adolescents and long-acting reversible contraception: implants and intrauterine devices. Committee Opinion No. 539. American College of Obstetricians and Gynecologists. Obstet Gynecol 2012;120:983-88.
2. Parasuraman S, Kishor S, Singh SK, Vaidehi Y. A Profile of Youth in India. National Family Health Survey (NFHS-3), India, 2005-06. Mumbai: International Institute for Population Sciences; Calverton, Maryland, USA: ICF Macro.
3. Society for Adolescent Health and Medicine. Sexual and reproductive health. Updated Feb 2015. Available at: https://www.adolescenthealth.org/Topics-in-Adolescent-Health/Sexual-Reproductive-Health.aspx.

4. World Health Organization. Adolescent pregnancy [Internet] Updated Sept 2014; cited July15]. Available from: http://www.who.int/mediacentre/factsheets/fs364/en/.
5. World Health Organization. Contraception–Issues in Adolescent Health and Development. Geneva: WHO; 2004. Available at http://whqlibdoc.who.int/publications/2004/9241591447_eng.pdf.
6. World Health Organization. Medical eligibility criteria wheel for contraceptive use. Fifth edition 2015. Available at: www.who.int/reproductivehealth/publications/family.../mec-wheel.../en.

Pregnancy in Adolescents 4.5

Harish K Pemde, Kamlesh Harish

INTRODUCTION

Pregnancy in adolescence is a major global issue with the prevalence rate varying from 2 to 25% in different communities. In recent years, the prevalence is increasing probably due to low puberty age, early onset of sexual activity in girls and lack of education on contraceptive methods. Pregnancy in adolescents contributes to high maternal and perinatal mortality and morbidity in our country. Infants born out of these pregnancies are at a high risk of developing various prenatal, natal, and postnatal complications.

National Family Health Survey–NFHS-3 found that 43.9% of 15–19 years old women were already mothers, 14.4% were currently pregnant with first child, and 58.2% began child bearing in this age group. These figures translate to a large number of adolescents having pregnancy and present a challenge to health services.

HISTORY TAKING

When an adolescent is married and pregnancy is suspected they will directly go to an obstetrician. A young adolescent girl may not even know that she has become pregnant as during early adolescence due to anovulatory cycles, many girls may have irregular periods. Due to some intermittent spotting they may also report normal periods during pregnancy. Hence unmarried adolescent may not be even aware that she is pregnant and may come to clinicians of other speciality with various symptoms.

Early detection of pregnancy will help in adequate care of adolescent girl in both situations, if she desires to terminate the pregnancy or decides to continue it. Some victims of sexual abuse may not have adequate knowledge about how pregnancy occurs. Sexual abuse in the form of rape or incest should be ruled out in all adolescents with pregnancy.

Even when a girl suspects to be pregnant, if she is unmarried she may try to hide it. When an adolescent presents with secondary amenorrhea, pregnancy should always be ruled out. Very often adolescents do not seek medical help until several periods are missed.

Adolescents may also present with vomiting, vague pains, or change in behavior.

History taking for suspected pregnancy is a very sensitive issue in unmarried adolescents. Environment in health facilities should be such that adolescents can share their concerns and problems without any fear of harm to their body, reputation and image in society (Table 4.5.1). If not handled with empathy the adolescent is likely to get scared and not come for follow-up. But at the same time it is important to remember the law of the land. Pregnancy in an adolescent below the age of 18 years is legally a rape or sexual abuse and it is mandatory for health care providers (HCP) to report this (for more details please see Chapter 4.7 for POCSO Act).

Table 4.5.1: Points to remember while interacting with an unmarried pregnant adolescent
• Be comfortable with her sexuality aspect and avoid being judgmental.
• Provide adequate privacy and ensure confidentiality.
• Use simple and clear language.
• Encourage her to ask questions.
• Make her comfortable in talking difficult subjects like fear of parents, disapproval of other significant adults, social stigma, etc.
• Support her in taking an appropriate decision on continuation or termination of pregnancy.
• Explain her questions and concerns related to, peer pressure, forming relationships, and social stigma.
• Help her to make decisions best suited for her including birth planning, institutional delivery, prevention of STI or HIV/AIDS (by using condom), and spacing the next pregnancy by at least 2 or 3 years.

If the health care provider (HCP) suspects the likelihood of pregnancy based on the history in a married adolescent then a detailed history should be taken (see Table 4.5.2). Though legal age of marriage is 18 years for a girl in India, in a rural set up often girls are married

Table 4.5 2: Model questions to ask about suspected pregnancy
• When did you have your last period? Is it late this time?
• Do you have (1) vomiting or feelings like vomiting in morning, and (2) swelling or heaviness or soreness in your breasts?
• Do you have (1) pain in lower abdomen, and (2) bleeding from vagina?
• Did you have sex in past few weeks? If yes, whether in last 5 days? Did you (or your partner) use any contraceptive? If yes, what? and how?

before they are major. Take a detailed history to find out if she is sexually active and did not use any contraceptive correctly and consistently during sexual intercourse.

HCPs should also look for early signs of pregnancy like nausea and history of unprotected sex (Table 4.5.2).

PHYSICAL EXAMINATION

- A general physical examination should be done to detect if there is anemia or features of any other deficiency disease.
- Blood pressure recording for detection of hypertension.
- Height and weight are also taken to find if any high risk factors for poor outcome of pregnancy like short stature or under-nutrition are present.
- An abdominal palpation is done to look for enlarged uterus.
- The pelvic examination remains the same as for older women. One should also check for signs of sexually transmitted infections. If she has vaginal bleeding or moderate or severe lower abdominal pain and pregnancy or possible pregnancy, she may have complications of pregnancy. Such adolescents require immediate care by a trained obstetrician; so refer appropriately.

INVESTIGATIONS

- *Confirm Pregnancy:* The suspected pregnancy has to be confirmed by a pregnancy test.
- *Urine pregnancy test (UPT)* is easy to perform and can detect pregnancy as early as 6 weeks after the first day of last menstrual period or 2 weeks after her missed period. If she comes before 2 weeks of missed period and urine pregnancy test is negative, repeat the test more than 2 weeks after the missed period. UPT may become positive 7-10 days after conception.
- *Ultrasound examination of uterus* is confirmatory in advanced pregnancy.
- When adolescent decides to continue the pregnancy, then all the routine investigations as in the case of any other pregnancy have to be done. These include complete blood counts, urine routine and culture, HBSAg, HIV, and VDRL, etc.

MANAGEMENT OF PREGNANT ADOLESCENT

Counselling of Pregnant Adolescent

If the adolescent is married, it is important to discuss the pregnancy and its various consequences with the couple together.

In case the adolescent girl is not married, discuss about various options of termination of pregnancy and about the MTP Act too. If she desires to terminate pregnancy, do help her and refer her to legal and safe abortion services.

Medical Management

General principles of management of pregnancy in adolescent are similar to that in case of an adult with pregnancy. IMPAC Guidelines by WHO provides standard care during pregnancy, childbirth and of neonate. Care of adolescent during pregnancy is described in brief below.

Antenatal Care

- Ensure privacy and confidentiality and use the antenatal visits for counselling about nutrition, exclusive breastfeeding and care of the neonate.
- Atleast four antenatal visits should be ensured.
- First visit should be as early as possible after detection of pregnancy and preferably within 4 months of gestation. Second, third and fourth visits should be ensured at 6, 8, and 9 months of pregnancy.
- Antenatal visits should be used to evaluate adolescent for likelihood of early delivery, and of difficult labor.
- Several complications like pregnancy induced hypertension, anemia, STIs etc. can be detected and managed by primary care physician (see Table 4.5.3). Counsel adolescent to go to hospital when certain signs are present (Table 4.5.4).

Postpartum Care

This includes early detection and management of postnatal complications in mother and baby. It also includes counselling for postponing next pregnancy and use of contraceptives, care of the neonate, exclusive breastfeeding, and care of the infant.

Adolescent mothers require lots of support from immediate family members. Pregnancy is very difficult for an unmarried mother.

Table 4.5.3: Complications and consequences of pregnancy in adolescents
During Antenatal Period • Pregnancy induced hypertension • Anemia • Higher severity of malaria
During Labor and Delivery • Pre-term birth • Obstructed labor
During Postpartum Period • Anemia • Pre-eclampsia • Postpartum depression • Too early repeat pregnancy
Care of the Neonate and Young Child
• Low birth weight • High perinatal and neonatal mortality • Inappropriate care of neonate and young child • Inadequate breastfeeding practices

Table 4.5.4: Advise on danger signs during pregnancy
Advise to go to hospital immediately without waiting, when one or more of the following are present: • Vaginal bleeding • Convulsions • Severe headache and blurred vision • Fever • Too weak to get out of bed • Severe abdominal pain • Fast or difficult breathing
Advise to go to hospital as early as possible when one or more of the following are present: • Feels ill • Fever • Abdominal pain • Swelling fingers, face or legs
Discuss plan for transport to go to chosen hospital, time to reach hospital and difficulties in availing medical help.

These visits can be utilized to counsel for adequate diet during pregnancy and breastfeeding, care of neonate including prevention of hypothermia and sepsis, exclusive breastfeeding and infant feeding, and prevention of next pregnancy for 2-3 years.

Labor and Delivery

If adolescent does not have any complications of pregnancy, she is likely to have a normal vaginal delivery at term without any risk.

In presence of severe anemia, postpartum hemorrhage may occur.

Continuous empathic support during labor by a technically qualified HCP benefits mother and baby both.

FETAL AND NEONATAL OUTCOME OF TEENAGE PREGNANCIES

- The teenage period is very vulnerable and constitutes a high-risk group for pregnancy.
- Special attention and high priority services are required for them.
- It is well known fact that teenagers face greater risks related to childbearing than women in their twenties.
- A pregnant teenager is literally "a child in a child", and has to meet the growing demands of her fetus in addition to her own growing needs, thus putting her in a stressful situation.
- They have an increased incidence of low birth weight, preterm and of babies dying during the first year of life.
- Post-neonatal mortality rates are approximately twice as high for infants of adolescents under 17 years of age compared to older women.

LEARNING POINTS

- Pregnancy in adolescents is quite common in India.
- These adolescents require friendly services for detection of pregnancy, for taking an informed and supported decision about continuation or termination of pregnancy, and for availing prenatal, perinatal and postnatal services.
- When dealing with pregnancy in minor unmarried adolescent, the HCP should follow the law of the land which has mandatory reporting.
- Management of adolescent pregnancy is more or less similar to that of pregnancy in adults except that some complications occur more in adolescents.

SUGGESTED READING

1. Ministry of Health and Family Welfare, Government of India. Rashtriya Kishor Swasthya Karyakram (RKSK), Resource Book, 2014.
2. World Health Organization. Adolescent Job Aid. Geneva; WHO. available at (http://www.who.int/maternal_child_adolescent/documents/9789241599962/en/)
3. World Health Organization. Integrated Management of Pregnancy and Childbirth (IMPAC) Available at (http://www.who.int/maternal_child_adolescent/topics/maternal/impac/en/)

The Protection of Children from Sexual Offences (POCSO) Act

4.6

Rajeev Seth, Swati Y Bhave

INTRODUCTION

Medical professionals are often the first point of contact with abused children, adolescents and their families. They have a key role in detecting abuse and providing immediate and long-term care and support to the children, adolescents and their families. The purpose of this chapter is to sensitize our health professionals on how to use Protection of Children from Sexual Offences (POCSO) Act of 2012 (Box 4.6.1) and respond to this large societal and public health problem, with a multi-disciplinary approach. The basic understanding of POCSO Act aims to serve as a guide to ensure a prompt and adequate response to victims of child sexual abuse by all medical professionals.

The POCSO Act envisages a multi-disciplinary approach (Box 4.6.2 and Figure 4.6.1).

An algorithm depicting components of comprehensive health care response to sexual violence as per guidelines and protocols of Ministry of Health and Family Welfare is illustrated to simplify medico-legal care of survivors/victims by medical professionals (Figure 4.6.2).

It is very important to connect the child and family to the socio-legal services which they may not be able to afford or may feel embarrassed to approach. Government of India has a telephone helpline for this. Medical professionals should be aware and use this telephone helpline to refer cases of child abuse (Box 4.6.3).

Box 4.6.2: Multi-disciplinary approach of POCSO Act

- The POCSO Act envisages a multi-disciplinary approach that will be conducive to medical care and justice delivery.
- This can be achieved through coordination and convergence between all key stakeholders such as juvenile police units, child welfare committees, district child protection units, health professionals, mental health professionals (including psychiatrists, psychologists and counselors), child developmental experts, medical social workers, advocates, magistrates and members of legal profession.
- The model guidelines under the POCSO Act, published by the Ministry of Women and Child Development, contain descriptions of the function of each of these above mentioned professionals under the Act.
- They also lay down guidelines for how these duties are to be discharged.

Box 4.6.3: Childline 1098

- **Childline 1098:** This is an emergency telephonic helpline, which helps link children in situations of abuse/neglect with rehabilitation services.
- This has become an exceptional model of public private partnership, operational in more than 400 cities/districts across the country.

Box 4.6.1: Protection of children from sexual offences Act (POCSO), 2012 in India

- The UN Convention on the Rights of the Child (UNCRC), ratified by India in 1992, urges states to ensure the right of children to protection from abuse, violence, neglect and exploitation.
- India has adopted POCSO Act in 2012.
- This is the first comprehensive law on sexual abuse which expands the scope and range of forms of sexual offences, makes reporting of abuse mandatory and defines guidelines for child-friendly police and procedures.
- Together with the Juvenile Justice Act (2000), POCSO Act has created an opportunity to ensure greater protection to children who have suffered abuse.
- It makes doctors an even more important piece of the puzzle in ensuring a prompt and adequate response to child victims. POCSO Act provides safeguards to the best interest and wellbeing of the child at every stage of the judicial process, in collection of evidence, investigation and trial of the offender.
- It provides protection of children from sexual offences (both penetrative and non-penetrative), sexual harassment and pornography.
- The POCSO Act defines sexual assault to be aggravated when the abuse is committed by police, army personnel, doctor, management or staff of a hospital/educational institution or if the abused child is mentally ill or disabled. More needs to be done to raise awareness and capacity of the medical sector to be in the position to offer high quality services to children and to work together with the rest of the child protection machinery.
- Since the act defines child as anyone below 18 years of age, adolescents are also included.
- For full details of the Act see www.wcd.nic.in/childact/childprotection31072012.pdf

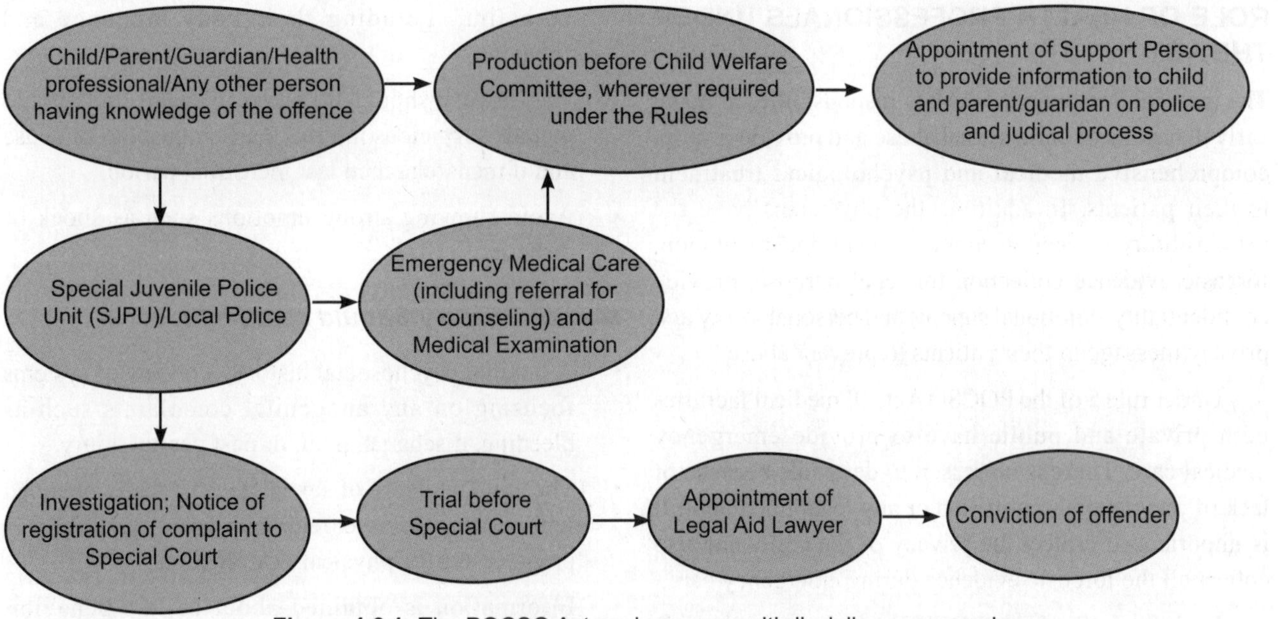

Figure 4.6.1: The POCSO Act envisages a multi-disciplinary approach

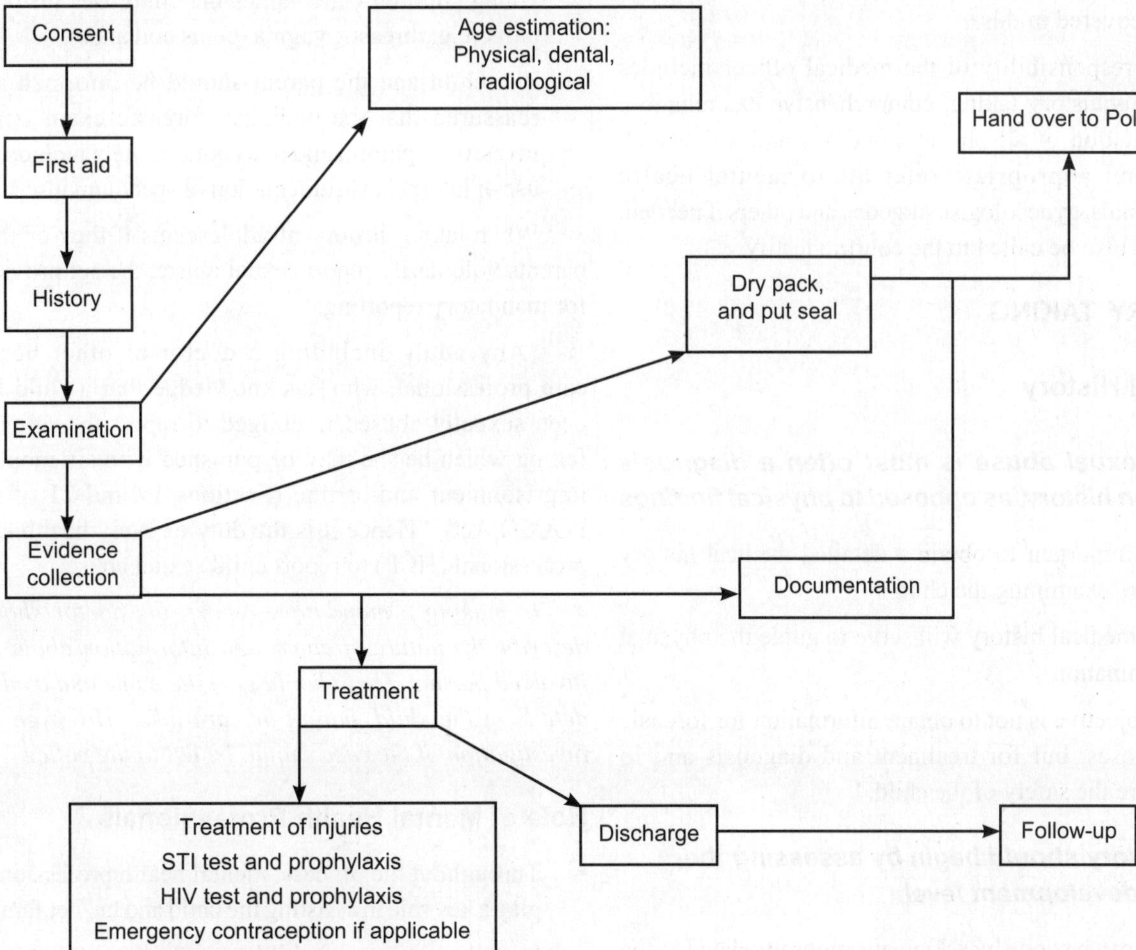

Figure 4.6.2: Algorithm depicting components of comprehensive health care response to sexual violence

Source: Guidelines and Protocols. Medico-legal care of survivors/victims of sexual violence 2014.www.http://mohfw.nic.in

(STI: Sexually transmitted infections)

ROLE OF HEALTH PROFESSIONALS UNDER THE ACT

The medical doctors have the key responsibility to make early diagnosis of child sexual abuse and provide prompt comprehensive medical and psychological treatment to their patients. In addition, the physicians have the responsibility to keep accurate medical documentation, forensic evidence collection for legal purpose, provide confidentiality, emotional support and personal safety and privacy message to their patients to prevent abuse.

Under rule 5 of the POCSO Act, all medical facilities both private and public have to provide emergency medical care. There is no reason to deny this because of lack of magisterial requisition or any legal document. It is important to protect the privacy of the child and also collect all the forensic evidence during emergency care.

Under rule 7 of the POCSO Act compensation is awarded to the child and the expenses of medical care, are also covered in this.

The responsibility of the medical officer includes meticulous history taking, comprehensive examination, documentation of all physical findings and a thorough report and appropriate referrals to mental health professionals, gynecologist/surgeons and others if needed. They can also be called to the court to testify.

HISTORY TAKING

Medical History

Child sexual abuse is most often a diagnosis based on history, as opposed to physical findings

- It is important to obtain a detailed medical history before examining the child.
- The medical history will serve to guide the physical examination.
- Its objective is not to obtain information for forensic purposes, but for treatment and diagnosis and to ensure the safety of the child.

The history should begin by assessing the child's development level

- This can be done by asking questions unrelated to the abuse, such as favorite colors, school activities, and likes and dislikes.
- The history should be taken in a non-judgmental and empathetic manner. It is best to avoid leading questions. The child's response should be documented verbatim, including their body language and behavior.
- Past history should be taken in detail and should include suspicious injuries, earlier episodes of abuse and if menarche then last menstrual period.
- Avoid showing strong emotions such as shock or disbelief.

Medical History Should also Include

- A familial psychosocial history; a review of systems focusing on any anogenital complaints such as bleeding, discharge, pain, or past genital injury.
- The child's history of sexual abuse, ideally obtained without the parent/caregiver present; and child is prepared for the physical examination.
- Information is obtained about child's behavior, specifically sexualized behaviors, and especially in young children—the names the child uses for body parts (e.g., breasts, vagina, penis and anus).
- The child and the parent should be informed and reassured that the pediatric forensic exam is not invasive or painful and does not routinely include the use of internal instrumentation or speculum insertion.

When taking history of adolescents if they or their parents voluntarily report sexual abuse, the act provides for mandatory reporting:

"Any adult, including a doctor or other health care professional, who has knowledge that a child has been sexually abused is obliged to report the offence, failing which he/she may be punished with six months' imprisonment and/or fine (Sections 19 and 21 of the POCSO Act)." Hence it is the duty of every health care professional (HCP) to report child sexual abuse.

In making a mandatory report, the doctor should describe the nature of abuse and information about the involved parties. They should give the name and contact details of the child, parent or care taker. However, the investigation of the case should be left to the police.

Role of Mental Health Professionals

- Throughout the process, mental health professionals play a key role in assisting the child and his/her family.
- Usually victims of child sexual abuse (CSA) are vulnerable to considerate psychological distress and hence tend towards self-harming behavior.
- Professionals can help the child narrate the incident and undergo complete catharsis to reduce the burden of trauma.

- In many cases of CSA, the child may not receive proper medical care, counseling and adequate legal assistance.
- Therefore, there is a need for action to prevent further abuse, trauma and re-victimization. It is important to have detailed assessment of psychosocial issues, including family background with specific emphasis on parental practice and types of family interaction.

CLINICAL EXAMINATION

Medical Examination

Under section 27 of the POCSO Act, doctors are legally bound to examine the survivors of sexual violence. The doctor should conduct the medical examination in accordance with the section 164A of the Code of Criminal Procedure, 1973 (2 of 1974), whether or not the First Information Report or complaint has been registered for the offence.

The medical examination has to be conducted by a woman officer if the victim is a girl.

The parent guardian or an adult whom the child trusts should be present during the medical examination. In the absence of these it has to be conducted in the presence of a woman nominated by the head of the medical institution.

Consent

Consent should be taken for the following purposes:

- Examination.
- Sample collection for clinical and forensic examination.
- Treatment.

As per the Indian Penal Code (IPC)

- Where the child is over 12 years old, consent should be sought from the child himself/ herself.
- Where he/she is below the age of 12, a parent or the guardian is required to give consent for the medical examination.
- Such consent should be informed, i.e. the person giving the consent should be told about the purpose, expected risks, side effects, and benefits of the examination, and the amount of time it will take.
- This information should be given before the examination is conducted, in a form, language and manner that the child and his parent/guardian can understand.

Informed Consent

Consent should be informed, i.e. the person giving the consent should be told about the purpose, expected risks, side effects and benefits of the examination and amount of time it will take.

The information is given before the examination is conducted, in a form, language and manner that the child and his/her parents/guardian can understand.

A survivor has the right to approach a medical facility under the following situations:

1. Survivors can come on their own or with parent of guardian if minor, for medical treatment for the effects of the assault.
   (a) A hospital has to provide emergency care even if there is no police requisition.
   (b) A person has come for medical treatment but has not filed an FIR– first information report–and does not want to report to the police. It is mandatory for the doctor to inform the police but has to give the emergency care. A medicolegal case (MLC) has to be registered by the doctor. If the victim or guardians refuse to put in an FIR, this refusal must be documented. Medical examination for forensic evidence can be refused by the victim. The court and/or police cannot force it.
2. They can come with a police requisition. The MLC number and the police station should be recorded. They can lodge a complaint later.
3. They can come with a court directive.

Physical Examination

There are guidelines given for medical examination of suspected sexual abuse. Please see wcd.nic.in/childact/childprotection31072012.pdf and for more details please see Table 4.6.1.

The general approach to the physical examination follows the standard head-to-toe approach. Elements of the examination include the following:

- Determination of structures of interest– mons pubis, labia majora and minora, clitoris, urethral meatus, hymen, posterior fourchette, and fossa navicularis.
- Choice of positioning for optimal exposure of prepubertal genital structures–Frog-leg supine position, knee-chest position, or left lateral decubitus position.
- Calming the child during examination.
- General observation and inspection of the anogenital area, looking for signs of injury or infection and noting the child's emotional status.

Table 4.6.1: Type of evidence to be collected			
History of Sexual Violence	*Type of Swab*	*Purpose*	*Points to Consider*
Peno-vaginal	Vaginal	1. Semen/sperm-detection 2. Lubricant 3. DNA	1. Whether ejaculation occurred inside vagina or outside 2. Use of condom
	Body	1. Semen/sperm detection 2. Saliva (in case of sucking/ licking)	1. If ejaculation occurred outside
Peno-anal	Anal	1. Semen/sperm detection 2. DNA 3. Lubricant 4. Fecal matter	1. Whether ejaculation occurred inside anus or outside 2. Use of condom
	Body	1. Semen/sperm detection 2. Saliva (in case of sucking/licking)	1. If ejaculation occurred outside
Peno-oral	Oral	1. Semen/sperm detection 2. DNA 3. Saliva	1. Whether ejaculation occurred inside mouth or outside 2. Use of condom
	Body	1. Semen/sperm detection 2. Saliva (in case of sucking/licking)	1. If ejaculation occurred outside
Use of objects	Swab of the orifice (anal, vaginal and/or oral)	1. Lubricant	1. Detection of lubricant used if any
Use of body parts (fingering)	Swab of the orifice (anal, vaginal and/or oral)	1. Lubricant	
Masturbation	Swab of the orifice or body part	1. Semen/sperm detection 2. DNA 3. Lubricant	1. Whether ejaculation occurred or not 2. If ejaculated in orifice or body parts

Source: Ministry of Health and Family Welfare (MHFW) Guidelines available at www.http://mohfw.nic.in

- Visualization of the more recessed genital structures, using handheld magnification or colposcopy as necessary.
- Collection of specimens for STD screening and forensic evidence collection.

There may be some findings of acute injury or residual effects of repeated episodes of genital contact.

The physical examination can be normal in majority of survivors of child sexual abuse as many forms of violence do not cause physical injury if there is no penetration and involves fondling or genital contact only. Physical force also may not have been used if the perpetrator is known to the child and/or family and the child is gradually groomed by the perpetrator into acceptance before the abuse starts. Also in children the mucosal tissue is elastic and heals quickly or there is delay in seeking medical care.

Investigations

The following investigations are routinely done:

- Gram stain of vaginal or anal discharge
- Genital, anal, and pharyngeal culture for gonorrhea
- Genital and anal culture for chlamydia
- Serology for syphilis
- Wet preparation of vaginal discharge for *Trichomonas vaginalis*
- Culture of lesions for herpes virus
- Serology for human immunodeficiency virus (HIV), based on suspected risk.

Other tests that may be considered include the following:

- Collection of forensic evidence via rape kit and
- Urine toxicology screen (if the abuse or assault was substance-facilitated).

MANAGEMENT

The basic treatment of child sexual abuse (CSA) involves the following:

- Treat sexually transmitted infections (STIs) with appropriate medications.
- In post-menarcheal children, consider the possibility of pregnancy and the need for emergency contraception.
- Recognize the overriding need for emotional support and attention.
- When sexual abuse is seriously suspected or has been diagnosed, ensure that it is reported to the appropriate authorities.

- Keep well-documented medical records; these are essential in legal proceedings, which may occur over long periods.
- A referral to a mental health specialist should be made in all cases. Mental health consultation is warranted to evaluate and treat acute stress reaction and, later, post-traumatic stress disorder (PTSD).

FORENSIC EXAMINATION

Forensic medical examination is an important part of comprehensive evaluation of survivors of child sexual abuse to provide appropriate care, medical evidence to prosecute offenders and support legal decision making. It is usually conducted within 72–96 hours of sexual assault, because with passage of time the healing process may obscure medical evidence. It also enables to assess the age of the child and whether child was given alcohol or drugs. The forensic evidence is collected from blood, serum, semen, hair or skin fragments and other debris like fibers from clothes etc. that could link the sexual assault to an offender. The doctors can provide expert testimony in court based on the finding of forensic evidence.

Forensic Evidence Helps to Ascertain

- Age of the survivor specially in case of minors.
- If the survivor has been drugged or given alcohol.
- Whether a sexual act has been completed or an attempt has been made.
- Sexual act includes penetration of genital, oral and or anal penetration by penis or any other object. It also includes any type of sexual touch which is forced.
- If the sexual act is recent.
- If any injuries are present or not. Absence of injuries does not mean the survivor has given consent for the act.

For the types of evidence to be collected, as per the guidelines and protocols of Ministry of Health and Family Welfare for medico-legal care of survivors/victims of sexual violence, please refer to Table 4.6.1.

LEARNING POINTS

- The POCSO Act makes multi-disciplinary agencies of the state, such as the police, medical professionals, judiciary and child welfare committee under Juvenile Justice Act, social workers and collaborators work together, in securing justice for a sexually abused child.
- This child friendly act is a welcome legislation. It aims to ensure that the child is given an opportunity to obtain justice for the harm suffered, and begins the process of rebuilding the child's life and future.
- Since it is now mandatory for all clinicians to report and to deal with child sexual abuse victims in their clinical setup whether they are working in a private or public sector, it is important for us to read this act and its guidelines very carefully and follow them so that we can do full justice to these patients and also be legally safe ourselves.

SUGGESTED READING

1. Integrated Child Protection Scheme (ICPS) (2009), available from www.wcdhry.gov.in/icps01.htm. Accessed July30, 2015.
2. Ministry of Health and Family Welfare, Government of India. Guidelines and Protocols. Medico-legal care of survivors/victims of sexual violence 2014. www. http://mohfw.nic.in. Accessed August 15, 2015.
3. Ministry of Women and Child Development, Government of India. Study on Child Abuse: India (2007). Available from www.wcd.nic.in/childabuse.pdf. Accessed August 16, 2015.
4. National Policy for Children (2012). Available from http://pib.nic.in/newsite/erelease.aspx?relid=94782. Accessed August 15, 2015.
5. Seth R. Child Abuse and Neglect in India. Indian J Pediatr. 2015;82:707-14.
6. Srivastava RN. Child Abuse and Neglect: Asia Pacific Conference and the Delhi Declaration. Indian Pediatr 2011; 49:11-12.
7. The Criminal Law (Amendment) Act, 2013 -www. indiacode.nic.in/acts-in-pdf/132013.
8. The Protection of Children from Sexual Offences Act, 2012, available from wcd.nic.in/child act/childprotection31072012.pdf.Accessed August 4, 2015.
9. UN Convention on the Rights of the Child (with Optional Protocols), available from www.unicef.org/crc. Accessed August 15, 2015.
10. UNICEF and Indian Medical Association (IMA). Child Sexual Abuse: Prevention and Response. Information for doctors and health care professionals (2014) booklet.

5.1.1

Headache

Sujata Kanhere, Swati Y Bhave

INTRODUCTION

Neurological problems in adolescence range from seizures, neuromuscular disorders, neurodegenerative disorders to inflammatory conditions of the central nervous system (Box 5.1.1.1). It is not possible to cover all the diseases due to space constraint, hence we are focusing on the common adolescent problems of headaches and seizure disorders (see Chapter 5.1.2) which occur specifically in adolescence, or become worse during these years. Both these disorders can adversely affect the academic performance, emotions, psychosexual development and social life of adolescents and are very challenging to manage in this age group.

Box 5.1.1.1: Common neurological problems in adolescence
Headaches
Seizure disorder–Epilepsy
Neurodegenerative disorders
Neuromuscular disorders
Inflammatory disorders

HEADACHE

Almost every adolescent suffers from a headache at some time or other; and this is a common reason for missing school days and in many it is severe enough to seek help from a physician. High levels of anxiety related to academic stress and achievement are noted in the majority of cases. An adolescent's performance, memory, personality, interpersonal relations and school/college/work place attendance are adversely affected by recurrent or chronic headaches and the degree depends on the cause of headache, frequency and severity. These also lead to restriction in daily activities affecting the psychosocial and emotional status.

Headache can be benign; chronic low-grade headache without any associated symptoms, intermittent headache from which the adolescent recovers completely (migraine) or due to local inflammation like sinusitis or otitis media.

Headache can be due to serious intracranial pathology which comes on as persistent chronic headache or severe unusual headache of recent onset which is associated with other signs and symptoms suggestive of brain tumor, meningitis, brain abscess or hydrocephalus. Parents are often most worried about this serious possibility. Therefore, every adolescent with persistent, recurrent, severe headaches or unusual headaches (Box 5.1.1.2 and Table 5.1.1.1) must be assessed carefully by history and physical examination and investigated thoroughly.

Box 5.1.1.2: Types of Headaches - Etiopathogenesis
1. Vascular–Migraine, cluster headache, toxic headache due to fever
2. Muscle contraction (tension)–Tension-type headache
3. Traction–Secondary to raised intracranial pressure
4. Inflammatory–Meningitis, sinusitis

Table 5.1.1.1: Causes of headaches in adolescents

Type	*Causes*
Acute generalized headache	• CNS infection • CNS hemorrhage • Electrolyte imbalance • Hypoglycaemia • Hypertension • Systemic infection • Trauma
Acute localized headache	• Refractive errors • Otitis media • Sinusitis • Temporomandibular joint dysfunction
Acute recurrent headache	• Migraine – Classic – Common – Complicated–Basilar, hemiplegic, etc. – Migraine variants–Cyclic vomiting syndrome, Abdominal migraine, Benign paroxysmal vertigo • Tension type headache • Cluster headaches
Chronic progressive headache	• CNS tumor • Brain abscess • Hydrocephalus • Pseudotumor cerebri
Chronic non-progressive headache	• Anxiety • Stress • Depression • Conversion reaction • Malingering

HISTORY TAKING

History is of paramount importance in the diagnosis of the type of headache and its etiology. Detailed history must be obtained about the following:

- Frequency, duration, location and time of onset of the headache.
- Description–Whether throbbing, pounding, dull aching, excruciating or unbearable, and location whether unilateral or diffuse or confined to one area.
- The number of school days missed will indicate severity and disability,
- Duration of headache-free intervals will help in identifying the pattern of headache and if more than one type of headache occurs it may suggest medicine related rebound headache.
- Treatment history should be specifically asked for as this may assist in establishing diagnosis.
- History of eyestrain, sinusitis, head trauma, earache and other causes of headache must be asked for.
- Ascertaining etiology is imperative as the treatment of different types of headaches is specific and depends on the cause (see Box 5.1.1.2 and Table 5.1.1.1).

The following History is Very Suggestive of Migraine (see Box 5.1.1.3)

- Recurrent headaches with symptom free intervals.
- History of nausea, vomiting, abdominal pain, photophobia and phonophobia.
- Presence of aura which may be visual, sensory or motor.
- Triggering food factors–cheese, nuts, chocolates, coffee and Chinese food.

Box 5.1.1.3: Migraine

- It is the most important and the most common type of headache in adolescence.
- Migraine headaches may begin in childhood or adolescence.
- Childhood-onset migraines may resolve before adulthood but those that start in adolescence tend to continue lifelong.

Migraine and the Adolescent Girl–Puberty, Contraceptives and Pregnancy

- The higher incidence of migraine in post-pubertal girls supports the observation that hormonal changes in the menstrual cycle can trigger attacks of migraine.
- Similarly, the effect of oral contraceptives on headaches varies.
- Some adolescents will experience more frequent and severe attacks of migraine on oral contraceptives whereas others will show an improvement.
- Pregnancy may remit or aggravate migraine.

- Associated symptoms such as neck and shoulder pain, abdominal pain, back pain and otalgia are more common in migraine than other headaches.
- The pain in migraine is often excruciating and unbearable.
- Other triggers include bright flashing lights, glare, hunger, unusual smells, stress and alcohol.
- Relieving factors such as sleep, and effect of exercise should be asked for to diagnose migraine.
- Family history of migraine in one or both parents supports the diagnosis. Migraine is three times more common in girls: in girls hormonal changes, oral contraceptives or lack of sleep may play a role.

CLINICAL EXAMINATION

General physical examination reveals whether the child is looking well or sick. A sick looking child with photophobia or phonophobia suggests migraine.

Neurological Examination

- A normal neurological examination usually indicates a benign cause of headache.
- Higher functions including change in behavior could point towards a space occupying lesion in the brain.
- Cranial nerve palsy such as sixth cranial nerve palsy suggests raised intracranial pressure.
- Diplopia, head tilt, other cranial nerve palsies, focal neurological deficit or ataxia should alert one to the possibility of a brain tumor.
- Fever and neck stiffness with photophobia with acute illness are suggestive of meningitis.
- Fundus examination is essential to rule out raised intracranial pressure.
- Other examinations such as vision testing or ENT check-up should be done only if suspected on history or examination.

INVESTIGATIONS

Often a good history followed by a detailed general physical as well as neurological examination is sufficient to make a diagnosis.

- CSF examination is restricted to situations where meningitis is suspected.
- EEG in headaches may be done to exclude the possibility of benign occipital epilepsy.

- A routine CT scan is not necessary in every adolescent with a chronic headache and most definitely not indicated if the neurological examination is normal in a migraine type of headache.

Neuroimaging is required only in certain situations such as:

- Abnormal neurological signs.
- Early morning intense headache waking the adolescent from sleep.
- Recent school failures associated with behavioral change.
- Focal neurological symptoms or signs which persist after the headache.
- Headache and seizure occurring in the same episode.

MANAGEMENT PROTOCOL

It is important to follow well established protocols to get good results. For approach to headache see Figure 5.1.1.1 and Table 5.1.1.2 and for migraine see Box 5.1.1.4.

LEARNING POINTS

- Headache is a common problem and one of the most distressing of symptoms resulting in loss of school days, work days and adding to the already stressed life of an adolescent.
- Migraine, tension-type headache and cluster headaches are the important primary headaches at this age.
- Avoidance of triggers, changes in lifestyle and appropriate medical therapy are the principles of management.

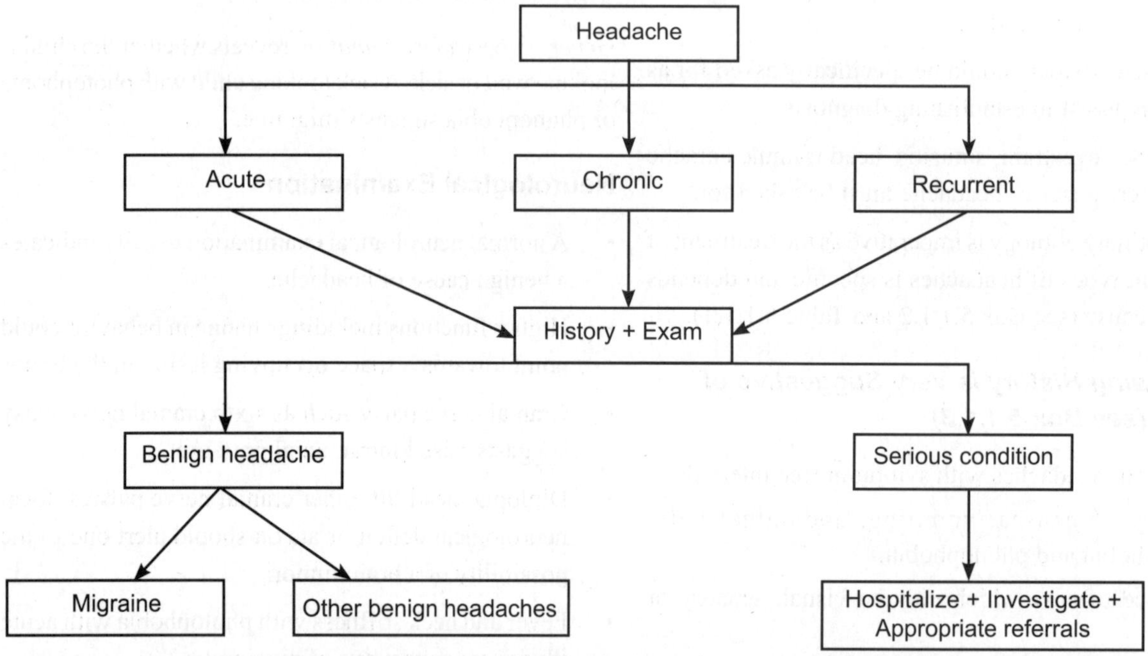

Figure 5.1.1.1: Approach to management of headache

Table 5.1.1.2: Different types of headaches and their management

Type	*Description*	*Management*
Tension-type headache (TTH)	Most prevalent type of primary headache 3 forms: • Infrequent episodic (<1 attack/month) • Frequent episodic (1-14 attacks/month) • Chronic TTH (>15 attacks/month) Headaches last 30 min to 7 days Bilateral, non-throbbing Mild to moderate intensity Lack of aggravation by physical activity Photophobia, phonophobia alone Not associated with nausea Not linked to hormones or food No genetic basis Brought on by depression, anxiety and stress Contraction of neck, face and scalp muscles	Analgesics like acetaminophen for acute headaches Non-drug therapy for chronic TTH: • Biofeedback • Relaxation training • Counseling • Cognitive restructuring Antidepressants may help

Contd.

Contd.

Cluster headache	Primary headache Onset exclusively after 10 years of age Affects boys Clusters of headaches recur over weeks or months with intervals of 1-2 years Headache starts during sleep Pain occurs in bursts lasting 30-90 min Every two to six times each day Headache starts around one eye Spreads to the hemicranium Pain is intense enough to make the adolescent keep pacing the floor Nausea and vomiting do not occur Symptoms of hemicranial autonomic dysfunction are seen	Prednisolone suppresses bouts of cluster headaches Dose: 1 mg/kg/day For 5 days Tapered over 2 weeks Acute attacks can be treated with Sumatriptan Oxygen inhalation (100% O_2 at 8-10 liters/min) In chronic cluster headache lithium is used Ergotamine can be added
Medication overuse headache	Secondary headache Very important entity Most common cause of a chronic migraine-like syndrome Frequent and regular use of anti-migraine medication or analgesics by adolescents with migraine or TTH, aggravate the primary headache	Stop overuse of medications

Box 5.1.1.4: Management of migraine

Step 1: Explain diagnosis of migraine to adolescent and parents
Allay fears + Reassure
Step 2: Counseling regarding
Lifelong condition – no cure, only treatment
Lifestyle changes, Avoid precipitants
Step 3: Medical treatment
a. Treatment of acute attack
b. Prevention of future attacks-Prophylaxis

(a) Treatment of the acute attack

Symptomatic relief

1. Sleep–Ideal treatment
2. Headache–Analgesic and NSAID
3. Nausea–Promethazine if required

Specific Therapy to abort the acute migraine attack

1. Triptans*, substituted indoles, selective serotoninin agonists e.g. Sumatriptan–SC Injection, Oral, Nasal spray effective.
2. Dihydroergotamine: Available as a nasal spray and is effective.
3. Narcotics should not be used for recurrent headaches.

* No sedation; side effects–dizziness, flushing, vasospasm, angina, cardiac arrhythmias

(b) Prevention of future attacks

Prevention of migraine by simple measures:

1. Keeping a headache diary: Note down:
   Triggers including food
   Time of onset of headache
   How long they last
   What provides relief
   Which medications help
2. Lifestyle changes:
   Avoid triggers
   Get enough sleep
   Plan regular exercise, rest and relaxation
   Avoid oral contraceptives.
3. Strategies to improve quality of life:
   Join support groups
   Counseling for managing stress.

If frequency >3 times a month: ***Preventive therapy is recommended***

Beta blockers—#Propranolol–1 mg/kg/day in 3 divided doses
Calcium channel blockers—Verapamil, Flunarizine
Antiepileptic drugs—Valproic acid
Others—Cyproheptadine and Amitriptyline
#Contraindicated in adolescents with asthma
#Rebound headaches if stopped abruptly.

SUGGESTED READING

1. Bendtsen L, Evers S, Linde M, *et al.* EFNS guideline on the treatment of tension type headache: Report of an EFNS Taskforce. Eur J Neurol 2010;17:1318-25.
2. Bhave SY, Kanhere S. Handbook of Management of Headaches in Children and Adolescents. IJCP Group of Publications; 2009.
3. Headache Classification Committee of the International Headache Society: Classification and diagnostic criteria for headache disorders, cranial neuralgias and facial pain, 2nd edition. Cephalalgia 2004; (Suppl 1):1-160.
4. Headaches: Diagnosis and management of headaches in young people and adults. NICE Guidelines 2012.
5. Kanhere S, Bhave SY. Headache in Adolescents. In: Bhave SY, Nair MKC, Parthasarathy A, Menon PSN (Eds.) Bhave's Textbook of Adolescent Medicine, 1st edition. New Delhi: Jaypee Brothers; 2006; 394-402.
6. Lewis D, Ashwal S, Hershey A, *et al.* Practice parameter: Pharmacological treatment of migraine headache in children in children and adolescents: Report of the American Academy of Neurology Quality Standards Subcommittee and the Practice Committee of the Child Neurology Society. Neurology 2004;63(12):2215-24.

5.1.2

Seizure Disorders

Sujata Kanhere, Swati Y Bhave

INTRODUCTION

Seizure disorder is the most common neurological problem encountered in adolescence which hampers the quality of life of an individual and has major social implications. Seizures affect education, career decisions, peer interactions, social life and reproductive life of adolescents. The fear of loss of control due to uncertainty of when a seizure may occur is particularly unsettling at an age where a child is making a transition from the dependence of childhood to the autonomy of adult life. Adolescents already have to deal with issues of developing self-identity and self-esteem. Social stigma associated with seizures and epilepsy, which is a major deterrent, compounds these. Moreover, diagnosis and management of seizures in this age group is a big challenge. The need for regularity in taking medications, their side effects, associated educational difficulties and parental over-protection, add to stress in adolescents with epilepsy.

In this chapter it is not possible to cover the whole spectrum of seizure disorders; so we will be focussing on epilepsy. Epilepsy is defined as a condition characterized by at least two or more unprovoked (reflex) seizures more than 24 hours apart or one unprovoked (reflex) seizure plus evidence of likelihood of further seizures or diagnosis of an epilepsy syndrome.

Adolescents may present for the first time with seizures or come with a childhood diagnosis of epilepsy (Box 5.1.2.1). Various issues and challenges in management are covered in this chapter.

Box 5.1.2.1: Epilepsies of adolescence

Adolescent onset epilepsy
- Seizures that start during adolescence

Epilepsy syndromes
- Idiopathic generalized epilepsies (IGE)
  - IGE with generalized tonic-clinic seizures only (Epilepsy with GTC seizures on awakening)
  - Juvenile myoclonic epilepsy (JME)
  - Juvenile absence epilepsy
- Benign partial seizures of adolescence

- Reflex seizures and reflex epilepsies
- Late onset benign occipital epilepsy
- Idiopathic photosensitive occipital lobe epilepsy
- Progressive myoclonic epilepsies

Other causes of seizures occurring for the first time in adolescence
- Head injury
- Infection: Intracranial granulomas
- Cortical brain tumors
- Subacute sclerosing pan-encephalitis (SSPE)
- Drug-related

Generalized Epilepsy with Febrile Seizures plus and Mesial Temporal sclerosis may begin before adolescence, but are seen mainly in adolescence

HISTORY TAKING

Taking a detailed and meticulous history from the adolescent and his/her parents is of utmost importance to ensure that a correct diagnosis is made as seizures have to be differentiated from a number of other conditions. Description of the event/episode is crucial to confirm that it is a seizure. If possible, the patient's parents or friends should be instructed to record seizure-like events with a mobile phone camera. Teachers, classmates and friends can also be asked about the event, because the diagnosis depends a lot on the account of a witness. They should be able to describe the type of seizure whether generalized tonic-clonic or myoclonic or absence seizures or focal seizure and the duration.

Family history of seizures, must be asked for. Past history of prolonged febrile seizure or febrile status epilepticus is relevant in mesial temporal sclerosis or hippocampal sclerosis.

For proper control of seizures, compliance from the adolescent is very necessary; so good rapport needs to be established with the adolescent. History of precipitants of seizures such as lack of sleep, alcohol, flickering lights in discos and menstrual period should be asked for.

See Figure 5.1.2.1 for approach to an adolescent with epilepsy.

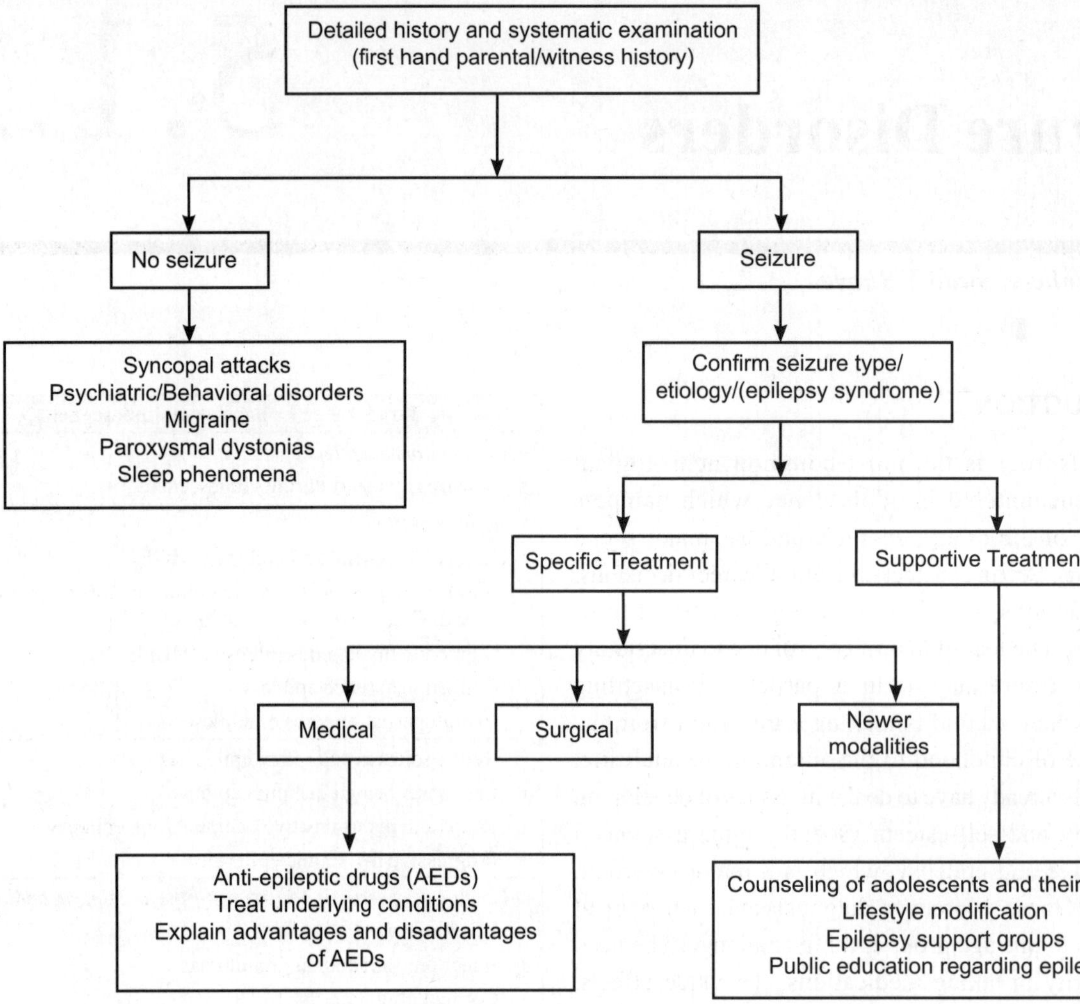

Figure 5.1.2.1: Approach to an adolescent with epilepsy

A detailed history and careful physical examination is necessary to decide whether it is a seizure or not, to confirm the seizure type and the etiology (Table 5.1.2.1).

The characteristic features of idiopathic generalized epilepsies including seizure type, EEG, medication, response to treatment and prognosis are given in Table 5.1.2.1.

CLINICAL EXAMINATION

General physical examination may give clues to the etiology of the seizure. In progressive myoclonic epilepsies such as neuronal ceroid lipofuscinosis, early onset visual loss is the first indicator of the disease; in MERFF syndrome, short stature and hearing loss are seen. Presence of neurocutaneous markers may point towards neurocutaneous syndrome. However, in the majority of epilepsies, general physical examination may be normal.

Neurological examination is normal in most of the epilepsy syndromes.

In progressive conditions such as SSPE, brain tumors, progressive myoclonic epilepsies, neurological examination correlates with the symptoms.

INVESTIGATIONS

The investigations to be carried out in an adolescent with epilepsy consist of EEG, neuroimaging and certain special tests as indicated by the etiology. See Figure 5.1.2.2 for details.

MANAGEMENT PROTOCOL

The epilepsies of adolescence should not be grouped together as a single entity. Knowing which epilepsy syndromes of childhood will remit before adolescence, which will persist into adolescence, which will begin and remit in adolescence and which will continue into adulthood is most important for the treatment of this age group. No treatment may be required for single benign partial seizures of adolescence, however, treatment of juvenile myoclonic epilepsy (JME) with sodium valproate is essential and usually needs to be continued long-term.

Table 5.1.2.1: Diagnostic clues on history taking for seizures	
Description of seizure	*Interpretation–suggestive of*
Timing 1. On awakening from sleep or within 2 hours of waking up from night or daytime sleep 2. Twitching movements of the shoulders and arms which occur soon after awakening and history of flinging movements and dropping of toothbrush or spilling tea shortly after waking up 3. After a late night or after playing a video game or watching television	1. GTCs on awakening 2. Juvenile myoclonic epilepsy 3. Photosensitive epilepsy
Early generalized or focal seizures followed by myoclonic and clonic seizures and later by cognitive decline, ataxia, pyramidal and extrapyramidal features including chorea	Progressive myoclonic epilepsies
Staring spells lasting for 30-40 secs or more accompanied by automatisms as well as history of visual seizures or visual symptoms	Juvenile absence epilepsy
Abnormal movements which start at adolescence with decline in school performance, poor concentration, poor short term memory, behavioral disturbances, absences, clumsiness, myoclonic, tonic-clonic seizures, dysphagia, dysarthria, increased involuntary movements and cortical visual impairment, coma and death with a past history of measles by 2 years of age	Subacute sclerosing pan-encephalitis (SSPE)
1. Visual hallucinations with deviation of eyes and head or blindness which terminate in either a hemi-convulsion or a generalized tonic-clonic convulsion 2. Sometimes, there may be no tonic-clonic movements, but only consciousness may be lost	1. Late onset occipital epilepsy 2. Loss of consciousness only has to be differentiated from vasovagal syncope. Involuntary urinary incontinence a feature of epileptic seizures, can be seen with syncope
1. Young healthy adolescents first seizure 2. Partial seizure with no other symptoms	1. Head trauma, drugs or alcohol should not be missed 2. Intracranial granuloma

Management of Psychological Aspects is as Important as Medications

Adolescence is a very sensitive period in an individual's life when one wants freedom and independence, a desire to establish one's own identity and sexuality. Adolescence is itself a difficult time and the onset of epilepsy at this stage further complicates the situation. Denial may lead to lack of compliance, aggravating the problem. The fear

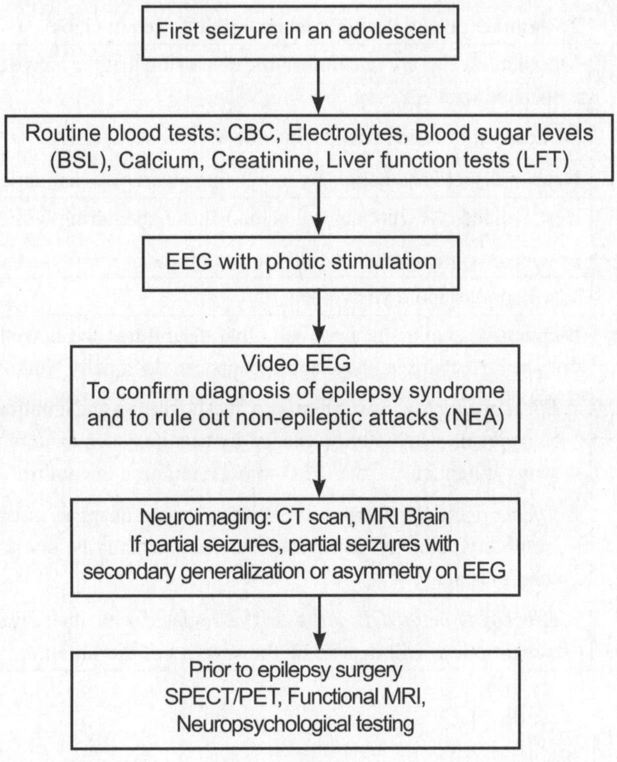

Figure 5.1.2.2: Step-wise investigations in an adolescent with seizures

of having a seizure in a public place or fear of injury may lead to social withdrawal and isolation resulting in anxiety, depression and loss of self-esteem and confidence. This restricts them from developing friendships and relationships which are normal at this age (Box 5.1.2.2 and Table 5.1.2.2).

Awareness and education of peers and school and college authorities and community programs are very important to remove the stigma associated with epilepsy.

Community Education to Improve Quality of Life in Adolescents

1. Public awareness
2. Family counseling
3. Roles of support groups
4. Need for specialized care for severe cases

There should be education to general public also to deal with a seizure (Box 5.1.2.3).

Box 5.1.2.2: What makes epilepsy in adolescence more difficult to control?

- Social difficulties prove a greater problem than the seizures themselves.
- Adolescents with epilepsy usually go through the same common phases like any chronic disease before coming to terms with a diagnosis. Denial, non-compliance and refusal to take precautions are common reactions.
- A strong desire to meet approval of their peers, reluctance to be seen taking medication and rebellion against authority are some factors that make control of epilepsy in adolescence more challenging.
- Damage to the fragile self-esteem is a vital issue at this age and they have to be counseled on gaining control of their life in spite of epilepsy with compliance of drug therapy, monitoring lifestyle and avoiding triggers.
- The specific issue of supervised swimming and care in bath tub to prevent drowning in the bath tub must be discussed.
- Independence versus safety must be considered in other areas such as sport, driving and employment.
- These situations carry risk, as do the very basic daily functions such as taking a bath.

Table 5.1.2.2: Issues: Challenges of an adolescent with epilepsy–areas of counseling

Issues	*Comments*
Social life	Communication is vital Smoking, drugs and alcohol are best avoided Lifestyle effects: 1. Lack of sleep or disturbed sleep pattern 2. Another potential trigger is the lighting used in clubs
Peer interactions	Most adolescents are uncomfortable disclosing that they have epilepsy due to the social stigma associated with epilepsy Difficulty in forming friendships due to poor self-esteem Need to dispel false beliefs by increasing awareness that epilepsy is a medical condition
Bicycling and driving vehicles	Best avoided if seizure control is inadequate and during withdrawal of medication Driving possible if seizure-free for 12 months
Sports	Water sports should be avoided
Education, cognition and behavior	If epilepsy is not associated with other disabilities and is well controlled with an appropriate drug in correct doses, these adolescents can do equally well as those without epilepsy 1. *Effect of epilepsy:* Seizures may affect cognition and emotional behavior. Sometimes certain behavior may actually be caused by seizures such as unresponsiveness in non-convulsive status epilepticus. Video-EEG may be required to confirm 2. *Effects of AEDs:* Certain AEDs may cause changes in cognition and physical abilities. Irritability, lethargy, confusion, etc. may actually be due to the AED but often blamed on substance abuse 3. *Effect of associated disabilities:* If associated with other disabilities, education and therefore career options will depend on the severity of the situation

Box 5.1.2.3: Emergency management–What to do?
Parents, teachers and peers need to be educated in general basic management of a seizure before taking to a doctor
• Do not panic. • Loosen clothes, neck tie and buttons. • If in safe place do not move the adolescent–move furniture away. • Do not crowd around the patient. • Note down when the seizure started. • Be there with the patient. Gently guide him/her away from any danger. • Cushion the head with something soft. • Don't hold him/her down. • Don't make him/her smell anything. • Nothing should be put in their mouth. • Call an ambulance, if a convulsion doesn't stop on its own in 5 minutes. • Stay with the patient until complete recovery.

Comprehensive management of epilepsy in an adolescent girl, has a lot of issues (Box 5.1.2.4).

Box 5.1.2.4: Epilepsy and the adolescent girl–Puberty, contraceptives and pregnancy
Menarche: The association between seizures and the menstrual cycle is known. • Menstrual cycle-related (catamenial) seizures occur in 35-50% women with epilepsy. • Seizures usually occur during a period due to progesterone withdrawal and at ovulation due to estrogen surge. • Many women experience seizures in anovulatory cycles as the estrogen to progesterone ratio remains high.
Contraception: *This must be discussed because of the impact of epilepsy and AED on pregnancy and the fetus.* • Certain anti-epileptic drugs such as carbamazepine can compromise the efficacy of some methods of contraception, such as the pill, so it is important for teenagers to be aware of this. • Adolescent girls taking enzyme-inducing antiepileptic drugs should use contraceptives containing a higher estrogenic component of 50 microgram or more. • Switching over to antiepileptic drugs that are non-inducers of liver enzymes may be considered in some patients.
Pregnancy • In a third of women with epilepsy, there is an increase in the seizure frequency during pregnancy which may be due to changes in the pharmacokinetics of the antiepileptic drugs as well as poor compliance.
Other Family Planning Issues Risk posed to a developing fetus by certain doses of particular AEDs and how to reduce the risk need to be considered. The American Academy of Neurology (AAN) practice parameter advocates the following: 1. Monotherapy that controls seizures effectively, at the lowest dose. 2. Periconceptional folic acid supplementation is recommended to all women of childbearing age. The recommended dose in women taking antiepileptic drugs is 4 mg per day. 3. Mothers should receive10 mg of oral vitamin K per day during the last month of pregnancy to bring down the risk of neonatal hemorrhage. In addition, intramuscular vitamin K should routinely be given to the neonate at birth.
Marriage Until recently, epilepsy was considered as a mental illness by law and was therefore used as a ground for divorce. But now with these changes, adolescents with epilepsy can look forward to a happy married life.

Medical management of epilepsy is detailed in Box 5.1.2.5 and Table 5.1.2.3.

Box 5.1.2.5: Medical management of a seizure in a clinic set-up
• Maintain airway, breathing and circulation (ABCs) • Nasal or buccal midazolam (single dose) dosage depending on age/weight of adolescent • IV benzodiazepine (1st line): Only one dose Diazepam/Lorazepam/Midazolam, if already received one dose by any route • IV phenytoin/phosphenytoin (2nd line): 20 mg/kg given slowly • If seizure continues, shift to a hospital ICU for further management

Table 5.1.2.3: AEDs for adolescent seizure disorders

Name of drug	*Indications*	*Important points to remember*
Sodium valproate	Drug of choice for a number of epilepsies of adolescence	• Weight gain–Female adolescents, may refuse to take the drug. • The association of polycystic ovary syndrome has been debated. • In mothers being treated with valproate, there is an increased risk of neural tube defects and of cognitive deficits in their children. But the use of prophylactic folic acid has reduced this effect.
Lamotrigine	Newer drug Increasingly being used as a first-line drug It has a wide spectrum of action Well tolerated, no weight gain and safer in pregnancy	It has life-threatening rashes or skin reactions–SJ syndrome and toxic epidermal necrolysis (TEN).
Vigabatrin	Second line drug	Potential side effect of possible visual field constriction. Visual fields should be regularly checked every 6 months and decision on continuing the drug made based on the results.
Levetiracetam	Effective as add-on therapy for idiopathic generalized epilepsy syndromes and has a broad spectrum of efficacy	Headache, somnolence, impulsiveness and severe behavioral side effects such as psychosis and confusion are reported.

In 2015, a new guideline on the prognosis and treatment of first unprovoked seizures in adults was released by the American Academy of Neurology (AAN) and the American Epilepsy Society (AES), which states that the recurrence risk within the first two years is reduced if, antiepileptic drug (AED) therapy is started immediately as against, if started after a second seizure. However, quality of life may not improve.

Antiepileptic Drugs (AEDs)–The Mainstay of Treatment

The AED chosen should be the most appropriate for the type of seizure/epilepsy and have the least impact on quality of life of the adolescent. For success of any regime, the adolescents must understand the full extent of their condition and the need for regular medication. They should also be aware of the effect of irregular sleep, high risk of unsupervised bath, driving, sport, employment, marriage, contraception and genetic implications.

Points to Keep in Mind While Prescribing AEDs in Adolescents (see Table 5.1.2.3)

Choice of Drugs

1. The first-line drugs sodium valproate and phenobarbitone are effective and should be used.
2. Carbamazepine may work in certain symptomatic partial seizures and can be continued. However absence and myoclonic seizures worsen with carbamazepine.
3. Phenytoin is not effective in idiopathic generalized epilepsy (IGE). A change of AED is warranted when a child enters adolescence.
4. Sodium valproate is the drug of choice for JME and absence seizures and also effective for generalized tonic-clonic seizures. *But it has side effects pertinent to the adolescent age group.*

Role of Surgery

Role of surgery is mainly for cases of operable intracranial space occupying lesions and seizures that are resistant or refractory to medical treatment. The earlier the surgery is done, the better the results for adolescent normal development. Presurgical evaluation includes neuroimaging, nuclear imaging, neuropsychological testing and specialized EEG studies.

LEARNING POINTS

- Seizure disorder is the most common neurological problem in adolescence which affects education, career decisions, peer interactions, social life, sexual and reproductive life of adolescents.
- Antiepileptic drugs are the mainstay of treatment. Choice of antiepileptic drugs depends on the cause of seizure, diagnosis of epilepsy syndrome as well as the efficacy and safety profile of the drug in adolescents.
- The need for regularity in taking medications, their side effects, associated educational difficulties, social stigma and parental over-protection add to stress in adolescents with epilepsy.
- Issues such as alcohol, driving, sport, contraception, genetic implications and 'safety versus independence',

imply that the management of epilepsy in adolescence requires skill and sensitivity.

- The role of the family, pediatrician and support groups is very important in the management of epilepsy in adolescents in terms of quality of life.
- If epilepsy in adolescents is managed in a systematic manner, it can lead to providing a better and satisfying life in most and a normal life in many.

SUGGESTED READING

1. Andermann F, Berkovic SF. Idiopathic generalized epilepsy with generalized and other seizures in adolescence. Epilepsia 2001;42:317-20.
2. Fischer RS, Acevedo C, Arzimanoglou A, *et al.* A practical clinical definition of epilepsy: ILAE Official Report. Epilepsia 2014;55(4):475-82.
3. Kanhere S, Bhave SY. Epilepsy in Adolescence. In: Bhave SY, Parthasarathy AS, Nair MKC, Menon PSN, Eds. Bhave's Textbook of Adolescent Medicine, 1st edition. New Delhi: Jaypee Brothers Pvt Ltd 2006;394-420.
4. Krumholz A, Wiebe S, Gronseth G, *et al.* Evidence-based guideline: Management of an unprovoked first seizure in adults. Neurology 2015;84(16):1705-13.
5. Rosalind WF, Benbadis S, Edrich P, Tassinari CA, Hirsch E. Levetiracetam as add-on therapy for idiopathic generalised epilepsy syndromes with onset during adolescence: Analysis of two randomized, double-blind, placebo-controlled studies. Epilepsy Res 2009;85(1):72-80.

5.2 Respiratory Problems

TU Sukumaran, Mathew Varghese

INTRODUCTION

The respiratory problems in children, adolescents and adults are similar in many respects. This chapter will focus on some of the common respiratory problems that are seen in adolescents: allergic diseases such as bronchial asthma and allergic rhinitis; and acute respiratory infections such as mycoplasma pneumonia, pertussis and tuberculosis. More than 99% of adolescent asthmatics have associated allergic rhinitis as a part of united airway disease. Compliance to inhalers is poor in adolescents. There is a high prevalence of reactivation tuberculosis in adolescents which manifests as cavitatory tuberculosis. Among the acute respiratory tract infections (ARI), *Mycoplasma pneumoniae* is very common in adolescent age and accounts for 25% of all pneumonias. Pertussis is underdiagnosed in adolescents because of its atypical clinical presentations and its prevalence is increasing throughout the world.

HISTORY TAKING

Bronchial Asthma

Adolescents with asthma may present with classical features of asthma such as persistent cough, wheezing and dyspnea or with any of the following atypical features (Box 5.2.1):

- Cough variant asthma
- Nocturnal asthma
- Activity induced asthma
- Persistent cough after an acute upper respiratory tract infection (AURI)
- Recurrent pneumonia at different sites.

A detailed history will also be needed to classify the grade of asthma (Table 5.2.1).

Box 5.2.1: Bronchial asthma in adolescents

- Asthma is a chronic inflammatory disorder of airway.
- It is characterized by 3 features:
  - Airway obstruction–This is reversible spontaneously or with medications.
  - Airway inflammation.
  - Airway hyperresponsiveness.
- Diagnosis:
  - Episodic symptoms of airflow obstruction, more than 3 episodes are present.
  - Airway obstruction that is at least partially reversible spontaneously or with drugs.
  - All possible alternative diagnoses are excluded clinically.

Table 5.2.1: Classification of severity of asthma

Grade	*Day symptoms*	*Night symptoms*	*Peak expiratory flow rate (PEFR)*
Intermittent Grade 1	< Once a week	< Twice a month	> 80% and < 20%
Mild persistent Grade 2	> Once a week but < Once a day	> Twice a month	> 80% and 20-30% variation
Mod persistent Grade 3	> Once a day; Attack affects activity	> Once a week	60-80% and 20-30% variation
Severe persistent Grade 4	Continuous; Limited physical activity	Frequent	< 60% and 20-30% variation

History should be obtained to rule out the comorbid conditions of asthma which can often exist in adolescents. These include:

- Gastroesophageal reflux disease
- Allergic rhino-sinusitis
- Obesity
- Adenoid hypertrophy
- Depression.

The questions to be asked are:

- Is there any diurnal variation for cough and wheezing?
- Is there any seasonal variation of symptoms?
- Are the symptoms aggravated after exercise or any activity?
- Is there a family history or personal history of other atopic diseases?

Allergic Rhinitis

Allergic rhinitis is manifested by:

1. Nasal block
2. Running nose (rhinorrhea)
3. Sneezing
4. Itching.

To diagnose allergic rhinitis, any 2 of the above 4 symptoms must be present for >1 hour every day for >2 weeks. It is also important to take a detailed history to elicit *possible triggers of asthma and allergic rhinitis*:

- Allergens like pollen, dust mite, pet, dander, cockroach, and/or mold
- Respiratory tract infections due to rhinovirus and influenza virus
- Inhaled irritants (cigarette smoke, pollution and chemicals)
- Physical activity (running and sports)
- Environmental factors (temperature and humidity)
- Menstrual cycle
- Drugs like aspirin and, beta blockers
- Stress and anxiety.

Tuberculosis

Tuberculosis in adolescents differs in the clinical presentation when compared to younger children (Box 5.2.2). Adolescents are more likely to present symptomatically, as opposed to being identified during contact investigations. Contact tracing is difficult in adolescents as they are more socially active than younger children.

Box 5.2.2: Tuberculosis in adolescents

- Increasing prevalence of tuberculosis in adolescents is due to increased incidence of reactivation tuberculosis.
- Tuberculosis commonly seen in adolescents is cavitatory tuberculosis.
- Adolescents are more likely to be infectious to others.
- Diagnosis and management of adolescents with tuberculosis should follow Revised National Tuberculosis Control Program (RNTCP) guidelines.

Pertussis

Pertussis will present in the *catarrhal stage* with mild fever, cough, running nose and sneezing. In the *paroxysmal stage*, the characteristic cough with whoop and lacrimation and post-tussive vomiting are often present. In the *convalescent stage*, spasms become much less and cough decreases (Box 5.2.3).

Box 5.2.3: Pertussis in adolescents

- The prevalence of pertussis is increasing in adolescents.
- The reason for increasing incidence is the waning immunity.
- Pertussis remains an underestimated and under-reported disease in adolescents and adults due to atypical clinical presentation in these age groups.
- **Causative organism:** *B. pertussis and B. parapertussis.*
- **Transmission:** Person to person by close contact with aerosolized droplets.
- **Complications:** Subconjunctival bleeds, umbilical hernia and inguinal hernia, pneumonia, otitis media, seizures, encephalopathy and polyneuropathy.

Mycoplasma Pneumonia

We should suspect mycoplasma pneumonia, if an adolescent comes with sore throat, fatigue, fever, headache and slowly worsening cough lasting for weeks or months. It can present as interstitial pneumonia and lobar pneumonia and even bilateral pneumothorax (Box 5.2.4).

Box 5.2.4: Mycoplasma pneumonia in adolescents

- Mycoplasma pneumonia is most commonly seen in the school-going children and adolescents.
- It mainly affects the lung, central nervous system (CNS), liver, skin and hemopoeitic system.
- The various clinical presentations range from acute upper respiratory infection to lobar pneumonia.
- **Transmission:** Airborne droplets.
- **Spread:** Coughing or sneezing while in close contact.
- **Incubation period:** 1 to 4 weeks.
- **Complications:** Severe pneumonia, encephalitis, acute disseminated encephalomyelitis, hemolytic anemia and renal dysfunction.

CLINICAL EXAMINATION

- In adolescents with asthma, examination of respiratory system may be normal during remission.
- During acute exacerbation, adolescents usually have fast breathing, chest retractions, bilateral wheezes and crackles.
- Presence of clinical features suggestive of chronic lung disease as growth retardation, cyanosis, clubbing and chest deformity are unusual in asthma.
- In tuberculosis, look for evidence of wasting and clubbing in general physical examination.
- Look for clinical evidence of consolidation, cavity and fibrosis on examination of chest and respiratory system.
- For allergic rhinitis, a detailed examination should be done (Box 5.2.5).

Box 5.2.5: Nasal examination in allergic rhinitis

- A deviated nasal septum can sometimes be apparent externally.
- Gross nasal polyps can produce expansion of nasal bones.
- A horizontal crease above the tip of the nose called 'Darrier's line' is characteristic feature of marked allergic rhinitis.
- 'Allergic salute' is done to relieve itching and free edematous turbinates from the septum.
- The patient may exhibit facial grimaces like nose wrinkling and mouth wrinkling which relieves the nasal itching of the rhinitis (allergic mannerism).
- With the worsening of symptoms, many children may develop bluish-black discolorations under the lower eye lids which are termed 'allergic shiners'.

INVESTIGATIONS

Diagnosis of Asthma

1. Routine blood counts are not usually done. Peripheral smear may suggest eosinophilia.
2. X-ray chest may be normal or may show emphysematous changes or enhanced vascular marking. It helps mainly to rule out tuberculosis.
3. Sputum examination for eosinophils and Curschmann's spirals.
4. Pulmonary Function Test
    - Peak expiratory flow rate (PEFR)
    - Spirometry

Diagnosis of Allergic Rhinitis

This is mainly clinical and investigations are not routinely done.

Diagnosis of Tuberculosis

- Positive *Mantoux (tuberculin)* test.
- *The radiographic findings:* X-ray findings in the apices of the lungs suggestive of reactivation disease; or intrathoracic adenopathy as seen in younger children; and higher rates of extrapulmonary disease than those seen in adults (Figures 5.2.1 and 5.2.2).
- *Examination of sputum:* Adolescents are more likely to have acid-fast bacilli (AFB) smear-positive sputum than younger children, which facilitates earlier diagnosis.

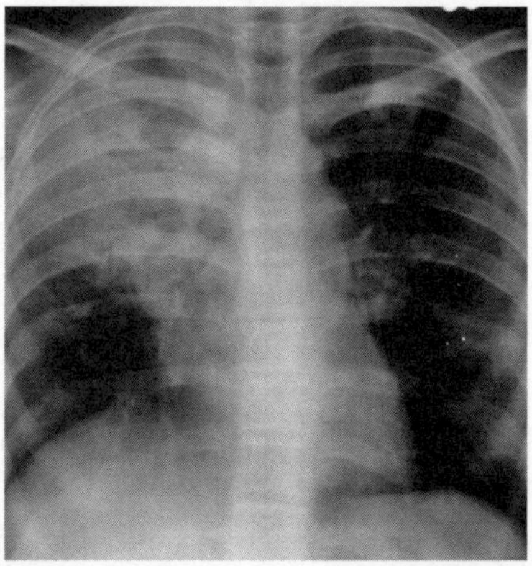

Figure 5.2.1: X-ray chest showing right upper lobe pneumonia with cavitation–Cavitatory tuberculosis

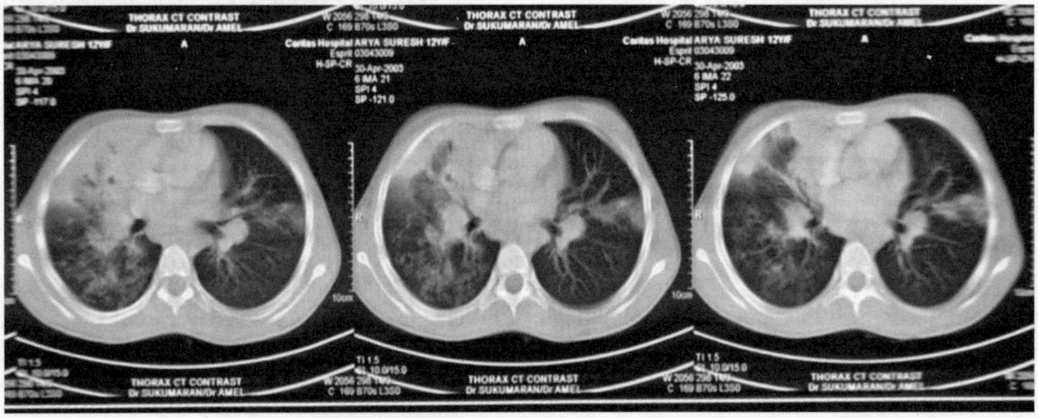

Figure 5.2.2: CT scan of the same patient showing pneumonia with cavitation

- *Positive interferon-gamma release assay:* This is not advised in developing countries.
- *Course of the disease:* There is a relatively paucity of data on the clinical course of tuberculosis in immunocompetent adolescents.
- The clinical diagnosis of tuberculosis in adolescents should not be made solely by microbiologic findings alone. Instead, the diagnosis should be made based on clinical correlation, radiographic or histopathologic findings and positive tuberculin skin test.
- For diagnosis of tuberculosis, see Revised National Tuberculosis Control Program (RNTCP) Guidelines provided in Figure 5.2.3.

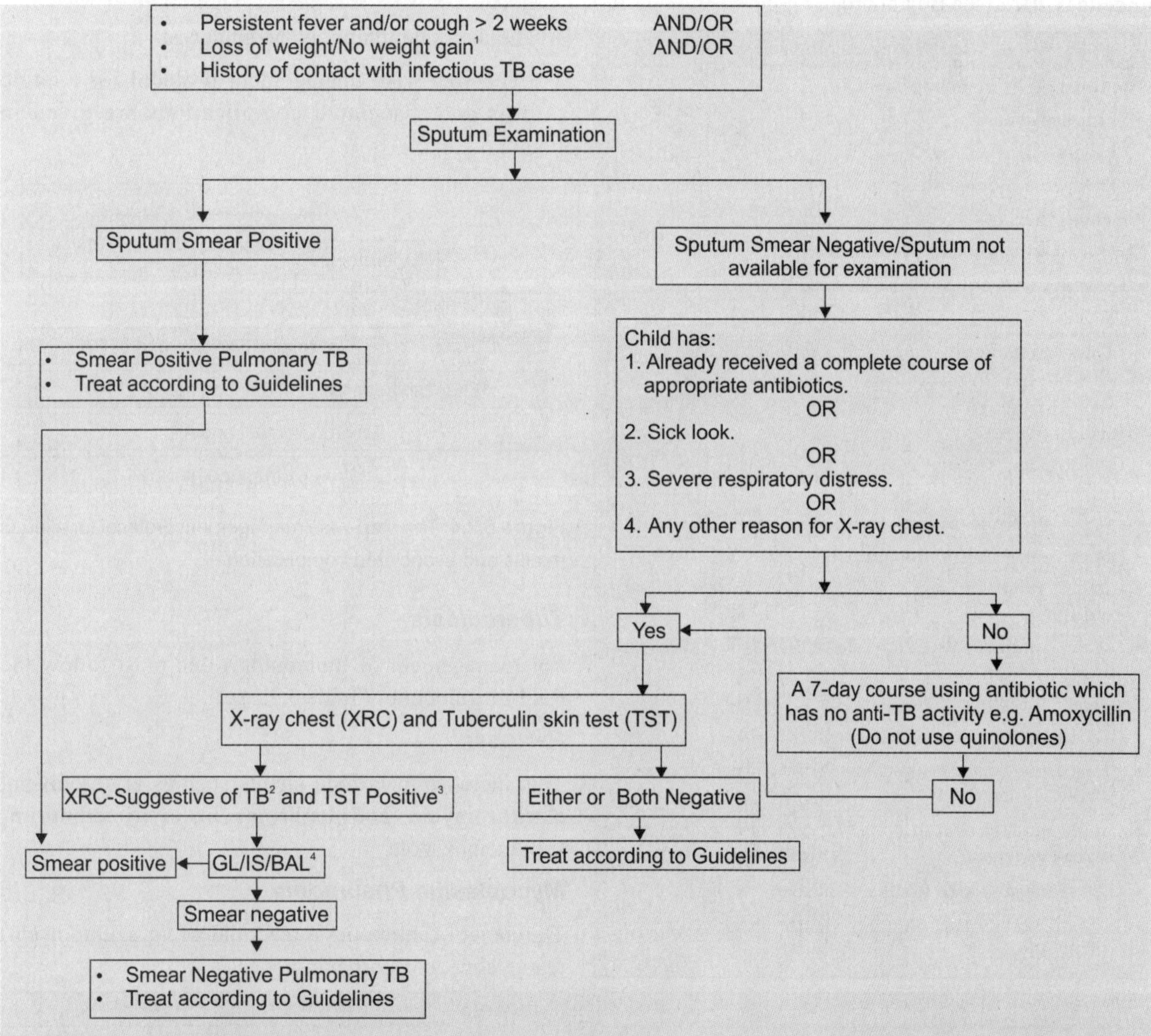

1. History of unexplained weight loss or no weight gain in past 3 months; Loss of weight defined as loss of more than 5% body weight as compared to highest weight recorded in last 3 months.
2. Radiological changes highly suggestive of TB are Hilar/paratracheal lymphadenitis with or without parenchymal lesion, miliary TB, fibro-cavitatory pneumonia.
3. If the radiological picture is highly suggestive of TB, then proceed to do further investigations irrespective of the TST result as the sensitivity of the test is not 100%.
4. All efforts including Gastric Lavage (GL)/Induced sputum (IS) or Bronchoalveolar lavage (BAL) should be made to look for Acid fast bacilli (AFB) depending upon the facilities.
   All efforts including Gastric lavage (GL)/Induced sputum (IS) or Bronchoalveolar lavage (BAL) should be made to look for Acid fast bacilli (AFB) or for M TB rapid culture or Gene Xpert® wherever facilities are available.

Figure 5.2.3: Flowchart for diagnosis of tuberculosis (RNTCP Guidelines)

Source: Kumar A, Gupta D, Nagaraja SB, *et al.*, Updated National Guidelines for Pediatric Tuberculosis in India, 2012. Indian Pediatr 2013;50:301-06.

MANAGEMENT

Asthma

Compliance to treatment is poor in adolescent asthma. A lot of patient education and motivation is needed as now they have to take care of their own disease and not depend on parents. Management should be done as per GINA guidelines 2015 (see Box 5.2.6).

Box 5.2.6: Management of asthma

The three (3) Ps in management:
- Pharmacotherapy
- Patient education and
- Prevention of trigger factors

Pharmacotherapy

Long-term management: Preventers
- *Step 1:* Consider low dose inhaled corticosteroids (ICS)
- *Step 2:* Preferred choice: Consider low dose ICS
- *Other option:* Leukotriene receptor antagonists (LTRA), Low dose theophylline
- *Step 3:* Preferred choice: Low dose ICS/long-acting $beta_2$-agonist (LABA)
- *Other option:* Medium/high dose ICS, Low dose ICS + LTRA (or + theophylline)
- *Step 4:* Preferred choice: Medium/high ICS/LABA
- *Other option:* Add tiotropium, High dose ICS + LTRA
- *Step 5:* Preferred choice: Refer for add-on treatment, e.g. anti-IgE
- *Other option:* Oral corticosteroids (OCS) low dose, Add tiotropium

Relievers
- As needed short-acting $beta_2$-agonist (SABA)
- Long acting $beta_2$ agonists, Montelucast and theophylline are steroid sparing agents

For acute management of bronchial asthma at home and in the emergency room
- Use salbutamol MDI (multidose inhaler)
- Nebulizers are used only in pediatric intensive care unit (PICU) set-up.

Allergic Rhinitis (ARIA Guidelines)

The pharmacotherapy for allergic rhinitis includes the following:

1. Second generation antihistamines (SGA)–Cetirizine, Levocetirizine, Fexofenadine and Loratidine.
2. Intra-nasal steroids (INS)–Budesonide, Beclomethasone, Fluticasone Propionate and Mometasone.
3. Leukotriene Inhibitors–Montelucast.

The step-wise management protocol for allergic rhinitis and associated complications are given in Figure 5.2.4.

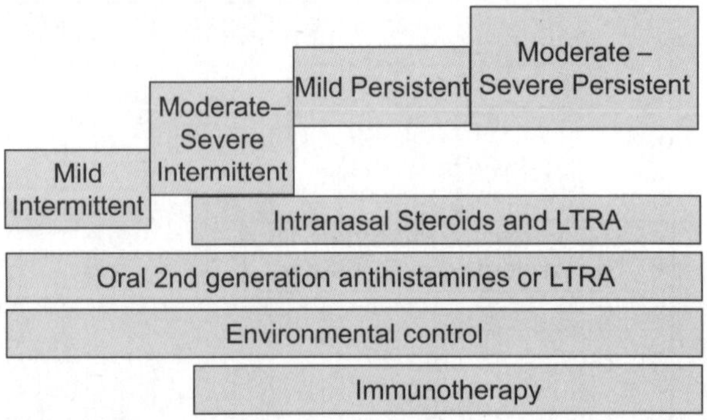

Figure 5.2.4: The step-wise management protocol for allergic rhinitis and associated complications

Tuberculosis

For management of tuberculosis one must follow the RNTCP guidelines (Table 5.2.2).

Pertussis

This includes macrolide agents such as erythromycin, clarithromycin, and azithromycin, or trimethoprim-sulfamethoxazole.

Mycoplasma Pneumonia

The choice of antibiotics is macrolides (e.g. azithromycin) tetracycline, or fluoroquinolones.

Table 5.2.2: Treatment of tuberculosis–RNTCP guidelines

Category of treatment	*Type of patients*	*Tuberculosis treatment regimens*	
		Intensive phase	*Continuation phase*
New cases	• New smear-positive pulmonary tuberculosis (PTB) • New smear-negative PTB • New extra-pulmonary tuberculosis	$2H_3R_3Z_3E_3$*	$4H_3R_3$
Previously treated cases	• Relapse, failure to respond or treatment after default • Re-treatment • Others	$2S_3H_3R_3Z_3E_3 + 1H_3R_3Z_3E_3$	$5H_3R_3E_3$

H=Isoniazid, R= Rifampicin, Z= Pyrazinamide, E= Ethambutol, S= Streptomycin.
*The number before the letters refers to the number of months of treatment.

LEARNING POINTS

- Asthma is a chronic inflammatory disorder of airway manifesting in adolescents as well.
- The controller of choice is inhaled corticosteroids.
- Compliance to treatment is poor in asthma in adolescents.
- Around 99% of adolescent asthmatics have associated allergic rhinitis as a part of united airway disease.
- Prevalence of tuberculosis in adolescents is increasing due to increased incidence of reactivation of tuberculosis.
- For diagnosis and management of adolescent tuberculosis, RNTCP guidelines should be preferred.
- The prevalence of pertussis is increasing in adolescents; this may be due to waning immunity.
- Mycoplasma pneumonia is a multi-systemic disease affecting lung, CNS, liver, skin and hemopoeitic system.

SUGGESTED READING

1. Atkinson W, Wolfe S, Hamborsky J. Centers for Disease Control and Prevention. Epidemiology and Prevention of Vaccine-Preventable Diseases, 12th edition. Washington DC: Public Health Foundation; 2012.
2. Chauhan LS, Arora VK, Central TB Division Directorate General of Health Services, Ministry of Health and Family Welfare; Indian Academy of Pediatrics. Management of pediatric tuberculosis under the Revised National Tuberculosis Control Program (RNTCP). Indian Pediatr 2004;41(9):901-05.
3. Global Initiative for Asthma. Global Strategy for Asthma Management and Prevention (2015). Available at www.ginasthma.org/documents/
4. Kumar A, Gupta D, Nagaraja SB, *et al,* Updated National Guidelines for Pediatric Tuberculosis in India, 2012. Indian Pediatr 2013;50:301-06.
5. Marconi GP, Ross LA, Nager AL. An upsurge in pertussis: Epidemiology and trends. Pediatr Emerg Care 2012;28(3): 215-19.
6. Sharma S. Tuberculosis. In: Parthasarathy A, Kundu R, Agarwal R, Eds. Textbook of Pediatric Infectious Diseases, 1st edition. New Delhi: Jaypee Brothers Medical Publishers, 2013; 242-46.
7. Sukumaran TU. Management of Childhood Asthma, 2nd edition. New Delhi: Jaypee Brothers Medical Publishers; 2014.
8. World Health Organisation. Treatment of Tuberculosis in Children. Rapid Advice. Geneva; WHO; 2010. Available at WHO/HTM/TB/2010.13.
9. Worldwide variation in prevalence of symptoms of Asthma, Allergic rhinoconjuctivitis and atopic eczema: ISAAC. The International Study of Asthma and Allergies in Childhood. Lancet 1998;35:1225-32.

Cardiology Problems

5.3

Vikas Kohli

INTRODUCTION

Cardiac disease manifesting with a new cardiac symptom is rare in teenagers. Most heart diseases presenting in this age group are either:

- Late presentations of pre-existing disease (e.g. atrial septal disease).
- Manifestation of a slowly progressive condition (e.g. hypertrophic cardiomyopathy).
- Acute and sudden onset (e.g. fulminant myocarditis).

The aim of this chapter is not to cover all the cardiac problems in adolescents but the common problems which are likely to present first to a practicing clinician or detected during routine physical examination of an adolescent like cardiac murmur or hypertension (Table 5.3.1). An adolescent can also be brought with history of syncope/pre-syncope which is common in this age group. There is a high incidence of syncope in school-going children with 15% of all children having least one episode of fainting or presyncope. Positional vasovagal syncope is the most common cause. In contrast, the frequency of seizures, a close differential at this age is only 1% and loss of consciousness from cardiac arrhythmia less common. Lastly an obese adolescent needs to be assessed for cardiovascular risk including hypercholesterolemia.

Table 5.3.1: Cardiac conditions diagnosed for the first time in adolescence

Congenital Heart Disease	Atrial Septal Defect (ASD) Bicuspid Aortic Valve Coarctation of Aorta
Acquired Heart Disease	Rheumatic Heart Disease Myocarditis Dilated Cardiomyopathy Athlete's Heart Kawasaki Disease
Heart Muscle Disease	Hypertrophic Cardiomyopathy Dilated Cardiomyopathy Restrictive Cardiomyopathy Left ventricle (LV) Non-compaction

HISTORY TAKING

Any new cardiac symptom should be evaluated completely in an adolescent. The symptoms may vary from being a minor chest discomfort (which could be the presenting symptom of a new onset myocarditis or an older dilated cardiomyopathy) or could be shortness of breath and exertional dyspnea (which might be presenting symptom of something as innocuous as exercise deconditioning or may be presenting symptom of a congenital heart condition like atrial septal defect, ASD).

Chest Pain

Symptoms of chest pain in a child may be considered benign in majority of the patients originating from chest wall, muscle or ribs or even gastritis, but, in adolescents, it may be the clue to a major problem like pericarditis, congenital coronary anomaly or cardiomyopathy.

Hypertension

On the other hand, hypertension may be completely asymptomatic. Incidental pickup of hypertension in adolescents is not uncommon. It would less likely be a surprise if screening blood pressure checks are performed annually on all teenagers. Occasionally one may get the history of headaches on and off retrospectively in adolescents with hypertension. In such patients where hypertension has been documented, a family history may be valuable (see Box 5.3.1).

Syncope

Symptoms of pre-syncope or syncope have to be taken seriously and life-threatening conditions ruled out. The significant difference in history whether the problem is benign or not depends on when the symptom happened. If the syncope/pre-syncope happened while the teenager was exercising, then likelihood of a life-threatening problem is more; while if it happened while at rest or positional change, then the likelihood of vasovagal is much more.

Box 5.3.1: Hypertension in adolescents: Etiology and risks

- Incidence: 1-5%.
  - Obese teenagers are 3 times more likely to have hypertension
- Etiology linked to:
  - Sympathetic hyperactivity
  - Insulin resistance
  - Vascular structure change
- Increased sodium content of cerebrospinal fluid (CSF)
  - Triggers increased sympathetic drive
  - Decreases urinary sodium excretion
- Parental risk of hypertension is linked to 2 times higher risk in children
- Genetic determinants:
  - Family studies have shown that 20–40% of cases seen are genetically determined.
  - Monogenic mutations in the corticosteroidogenic genes and polymorphisms in the renin-angiotensin-aldosterone system have been demonstrated. These mutations are thought to have an autosomal recessive pattern of inheritance and patients who are homozygous for the mutations have a higher likelihood for developing hypertension associated nephropathy, and focal segmental glomerulosclerosis.
- Birth weight: There is a growing body of evidence on the inverse relationship between birth weight and hypertension in children and adolescents.
- Sodium intake correlated directly with hypertension with high sodium correlating to two times higher incidence of hypertension.
- Overweight or obese children with high sodium intake had a three times higher risk of hypertension than obese low sodium intake patients.

- Teenagers are able to give a clear history and the sequence of events leading upto the syncope. This facilitates rather quick diagnosis based on history itself.
- Syncope during exercise should be differentiated from syncope after exercise. If syncope happened during physical activity it may be the clue towards a more serious arrhythmia which if confirmed could be potentially fatal also. On the other hand post-exercise vasodilatation could be associated vasovagal syncope which is benign. Teenagers with exercise-induced syncope should undergo echocardiography to rule out cardiomyopathy and arrhythmia as the cause of the syncope.
- *Pseudosyncope* should be suspected in teenage girls especially during stresses secondary to social issues or academic activities. The frequency is usually higher than vasovagal. They never tend to injure themselves. If they have a prior history of true vasovagal, the differentiation may be rather challenging.

A detailed history of hypertension in the family and dietary history especially sodium intake should be taken .

CLINICAL EXAMINATION

Critical to evaluation of a cardiac symptom is clinical examination. This should focus on the following points:

- General physical examination giving clues to a multi-systemic disease e.g. Marfan syndrome.
- Brachial blood pressure measurement.
- Femoral and radial pulses being compared for evidence of coarctation or Takayasu disease (in which subclavian arteries may be affected more than femoral).
- Cardiac auscultation may provide a clue to cardiac murmur. The presence of new murmurs may indicate a late manifestation of a previous illness (rheumatic fever in past with severe mitral regurgitation presenting now) or new onset disease (hypertrophic cardiomyopathy manifesting its obstructive element now).
- Cardiac murmurs are more difficult to auscultate in teenagers than in pediatric patients. A suspicion of a cardiac murmur is enough to warrant a workup to rule a cardiac problem.

Cardiac murmurs would be the most obvious physical sign to start suspecting a cardiac condition. Murmurs, though, may be difficult to detect in teenagers as compared to children.

The first-time appearance of a murmur in an adolescent can create a substantial amount of anxiety in the parents and the teenager. In an athlete, the onset of a cardiac murmur may be ominous. The appearance may be suggestive either hypertrophic cardiomyopathy or may suggest the onset of a close differential: the athlete's heart. The differentiation of athlete's heart from hypertrophic cardiomyopathy can be made on the basis of the factors mentioned in Table 5.3.2.

Table 5.3.2: Differentiation between athlete's heart and hypertrophic cardiomyopathy (HCM)

	Athlete's heart	*Hypertrophic cardiomyopathy*
Left ventricular (LV) Hypertrophy	<45 mm	>55 mm
Left atrial (LA) Enlargement	Absent	Present
LV Filling–Abnormal	Absent	Present
Decreasing thickness with conditioning	Yes	No
Family history of HCM	No	Yes

INVESTIGATIONS

- **Echocardiography:** The basic cardiac modality for investigation remains to be echocardiography. Echo is reliable for cardiac anatomy, function and for hemodynamics including valvular regurgitation or stenosis. The echocardiographic window remains limited in teenagers as compared to pediatric patients.
- **ECG:** This remains to be the primary modality for electrical problems. The rhythm, rate and chamber enlargement can be evaluated by this modality.
- **Holter:** For further evaluation of rhythm problems e.g. supraventricular tachycardia, one may need to perform a 24-hour recording of the ECG. Loop recorders offer the option of instantaneous recording when a rare event happens infrequently.
- **Cardiac MRI and CT Angiography:** CT angiography is good for evaluating peripheral structures like pulmonary arteries and aorta and its branches and coarctation of aorta. Renal artery stenosis, a known cause of hypertension can also be best evaluated by this modality. CMRI (cardiac MRI) is useful for evaluation of right ventricular (RV) function in late Tetralogy of Fallot where RV volume calculations are critical for deciding interventions like pulmonary valve replacement or implantation.

Diagnosis of Vasovagal Syncope and Paroxysmal Orthostatic Tachycardia Syndrome (POTS)

Historically one can suspect the diagnosis of POTS though a Tilt-Table-Test can be confirmatory in this scenario.

- During a Head-Up-Tilt Table (HUT) test one needs to document hypotension and associated increase in heart rate by at least 40 bpm. The HUT test involves standing for 10 minutes at an 80 degree angle on a special table with measurement of blood pressure and heart rate during the test.
- A 24-hour Holter monitor would help in differentiating inappropriate sinus tachycardia from POTS.

Considering the reliability of history towards the diagnosis, and the associated variability in results of HUT test, there is a clinical trend to forgo the Tilt test and manage the patients without testing.

- Electrocardiogram provides a simple cardiac assessment and could provide clues to sinister diagnoses or rule out such causes of syncope e.g. myocarditis, cardiomyopathies, long QT, and other arrhythmias.
- If a subtle arrhythmia is suspected e.g. a bradycardia or if the patient is not responding to medical treatment, one can consider an implantable loop recorder which can be used to monitor the patient's rhythm over a prolonged period of time (6 months).

MANAGEMENT

Management of Hypertension

1. Therapeutic Lifestyle Modification

- This is the first line of management of pediatric hypertension and can be the sole modality of therapy in patients diagnosed with pre-hypertension and stage I hypertension.
- It focuses on dietary management, increased physical activity, stress reduction and avoidance of illicit drug and tobacco use.
- Dietary management should include an age appropriate, salt restricted diet with emphasis on weight loss in the overweight or children with obesity.
- To have a better chance of success, the entire family should adopt these lifestyle modifications.

2. Pharmacological Therapy

Table 5.3.3 describes the common antihypertensive agents used for therapy in children and adolescents.

3. Other Forms of Therapy

- Bariatric surgery has a role in the treatment of hypertension in the morbidly obese adult and might become an option in the obese pediatric adolescent in the future. A recent study demonstrated an improvement in metabolic syndrome including hypertension with up to 30% reduction in weight.

Table 5.3.3: Antihypertensive therapy in children and adolescents			
Medication	*Initial dose*	*Max dose*	*Frequency*
Angiotensin-converting enzyme inhibitors			
Benazepril ≥ six years of age	0.2 mg per kg, up to 10 mg	0.6 mg per kg or 40 mg	Once daily
Enalapril	0.08 mg per kg, up to 5 mg	0.6 mg per kg or 40 mg	Once or twice daily
Fosinopril ≥ six years of age and weighing > 50 kg	5 to 10 mg	40 mg	Once daily
Lisinopril ≥ six years of age	0.07 mg per kg, up to 5 mg	0.6 mg per kg or 40 mg	Once daily
Angiotensin II receptor blockers			
Losartan ≥ six years of age	0.7 mg per kg, up to 50 mg	1.4 mg per kg or 100 mg	Once daily
Valsartan ≥ six years of age	1.3 mg per kg, up to 40 mg	2.7 mg per kg or 160 mg	Once daily
Beta blockers			
Metoprolol, extended release, ≥ six years of age	1 mg per kg, up to 50 mg	2 mg per kg or 200 mg	Once daily
Propranolol	1 to 2 mg per kg	4 mg per kg or 640 mg	Two or three times daily
Vasodilators			
Hydralazine	0.75 mg per kg	7.5 mg per kg or 200 mg	Four times daily
Minoxidil	0.2 mg per kg, up to 5 mg (< 12 years of age), 5 mg (≥ 12 years of age)	50 mg (< 12 years of age), 100 mg (≥ 12 years of age)	Once or twice daily
Others			
Calcium channel blocker: Amlodipine ≥ six years of age	2.5 mg	5 mg	Once daily
Central alpha agonist: Clonidine 12 years of age	0.2 mg	2.4 mg	Twice daily
Diuretic: Hydrochlorothiazide	1 mg per kg	3 mg per kg, up to 50 mg	Once daily

Source: Riley M, Bluhm B. High blood pressure in children and adolescents. Am Fam Physician. 2012 Apr 1;85(7):693-700.

- Renal nerve denervation is a therapeutic option in adults with resistant hypertension, which refers to uncontrolled hypertension despite therapy with 3 or more antihypertensives.

Treatment of Children with Vasovagal Syncope or POTS

There is no specific evidence proving the benefit of one form of treatment over the other. Increasing salt and fluid intake and medical management with midodrine or pacemakers are the medical options. But, placebos have shown as much benefit from intervention as other forms of treatment. The natural course of the problem is of spontaneous resolution over time as the teenager gets over the adolescent years.

This fact decreases the enthusiasm of both parents and physicians for use of measures as medical management and pacemakers.

SUGGESTED READING

1. Crawford MH. Screening athletes for heart disease. Heart 2007;93:875-79.
2. Maron BJ. Distinguishing hypertrophic cardiomyopathy from athlete's heart: A clinical problem of increasing magnitude and significance. Heart. 2005;91(11):1380-82.
3. Misra M, Mittal M, Verma AM, Rai R, Chandra G, Singh DP *et al.* Prevalence and pattern of congenital heart disease in school children of eastern Uttar Pradesh. Indian Heart J 2009;61(1):58-60.
4. Naik RJ, Shah NC. Teenage heart murmurs. Pediatr Clin North Am 214;61(1):1-16.
5. Riley M, Bluhm B. High blood pressure in children and adolescents. Am Fam Physician 2012;85(7):693-700.
6. Roberts KV, Brown AD, Maguire GP, Atkinson DN, Carapetis JR. Utility of auscultatory screening for detecting rheumatic heart disease in high-risk children in Australia's Northern Territory. Med J Aust. 2013;199(3):196-99.
7. Sheldon RS, Grubb BP 2nd, Olshansky B, Shen WK, Calkins H, Brignole M *et al.* 2015 heart rhythm society expert consensus statement on the diagnosis and treatment of postural tachycardia syndrome, inappropriate sinus tachycardia, and vasovagal syncope. Heart Rhythm 2015;12(6):e41-63.

8. Singer W, Sletten DM, Opfer-Gehrking TL, Brands CK, Fischer PR, Low PA. Postural tachycardia in children and adolescents: What is abnormal? J Pediatr 2012;160(2):222-26.
9. Task Force for the Diagnosis and Management of Syncope of the European Society of Cardiology (ESC); European Heart Rhythm Association (EHRA), Heart Failure Association (HFA); Heart Rhythm Society (HRS); Moya A Sutton R, Ammirati F, *et al.* Guidelines for the diagnosis and management of syncope (version 2009) European Heart J.2009;30(21):2631-71.

Genitourinary Problems

5.4

RN Srivastava

INTRODUCTION

Very few studies in India, or in fact elsewhere, have focused on renal diseases exclusively in the adolescents. The pattern of these may not be very different in India from that in developed countries, but their management is influenced by a paucity of the necessary expertise and socioeconomic conditions. In that context, poor compliance with therapeutic regimens (except for financial reasons), rebellion and obsession with body image may not be major constraints.

Renal and urinary tract disorders in adolescents can be grouped into (a) those starting earlier and continuing beyond the age of 14 years and (b) developing or first detected during adolescence. Several common conditions are mostly observed in younger children or resolve before the age of 14 years. Thus post-streptococcal acute glomerulonephritis (GN) is very uncommon during adolescence and a large majority of children with corticosteroid responsive nephrotic syndrome achieves permanent cure well before adolescence. The problems of urinary tract infection, vesicouretric reflux and obstruction in the urinary tract are also usually resolved with appropriate management. Comparatively few renal problems originate during adolescence. Various diseases observed during adolescence are shown in Table 5.4.1.

Table 5.4.1: Common diseases of kidney and urinary tract observed during adolescence

A. Conditions starting earlier (infancy or later childhood) and recurring or continuing during adolescence • Congenital abnormalities of kidney and urinary tract • Chronic kidney disease of various etiologies • Nephrotic syndrome • Renal vasculitis conditions
B. Conditions that also may first appear during adolescence • Nephrotic syndrome • Post-infectious glomerulonephritis • Collagen vascular diseases • Renal vasculitis conditions • Atypical hemolytic uremic syndrome • IgA nephropathy • Acute kidney injury • Chronic kidney disease • Urinary tract infections and voiding dysfunction • Renal calculus disease • Hypertension

HISTORY AND CLINICAL ASSESSMENT

A detailed history is of utmost importance. The age at onset of the disease should be inquired into. Whereas features such as gross hematuria, abdominal pain, dysuria, and oliguria, are readily observed by the parents and suggest the likelihood of an underlying renal disease, often the features are mild and subtle and diagnosis of the underlying condition is delayed (see Table 5.4.2).

Congenital renal anomalies (e.g. autosomal dominant polycystic kidney disease and renal ectopia) are usually asymptomatic and detected on incidental ultrasonographic examination.

Family history of renal disease should be obtained especially when renal involvement occurs as a part of a syndrome with dysmorphic features and multisystem anomalies. However, unless the adolescent has not had access to medical facilities in childhood, most syndromes with dysmorphic features would have been investigated much before adolescence.

PHYSICAL EXAMINATION

- Edema, hematuria and hypertension are the chief features of acute GN. The extent of edema (ascites and pleural effusion) should be noted.
- A rapid increase in weight (as determined from the difference in weight between present weight and a recent value, taken before the illness) gives an indication of accumulation of fluid.
- Accurate measurements of weight, height and blood pressure are recorded.

Table 5.4.2: Common symptoms of diseases of kidney and urinary tract	
Symptoms	***Comments***
Hematuria	The color of the urine should be noted. Urine is smoky, cola- or tea-colored when the hematuria is of glomerular origin. The color in bleeding from pelvis, ureter or lower urinary tract is usually bright red.
Pain abdomen	In acute glomerular diseases significant pain is absent. Flank pain with fever suggests pyelonephritis. Pain over lower abdomen and dysuria suggest cystitis or urethritis. Colicky pain is indicative of renal calculus disease.
Facial edema It is often mistaken for allergy or some eye problem, until it increases and becomes persistent. Urine should be examined for protein in a child with suspicion of even slight facial edema.	Facial edema is an early feature in acute glomerulonephritis. It is turgid and remains persistent throughout the day. In nephritic syndrome edema is of insidious onset, initially appearing on the face. It is prominent in the morning but tends to disappear after the child has been up and about. Edema is soft and easily pits on pressure. Its intensity may initially fluctuate, but gradually it increases and may become generalized with ascites and fluid collection in serous cavities.
Hypertension	Headache and vomiting and rarely encephalopathy and ocular symptoms are characteristically seen in severe hypertension of acute onset.
Delayed growth, obscure anemia, rickets, unexplained fever and fatigue	Chronic kidney disease very often presents with vague, nonspecific features. Gradual decline of renal function is usually asymptomatic. Urinalysis and renal function tests should be examined in when a diagnosis is unclear.
Voiding dysfunction	Serious forms of urinary tract infections usually present during infancy and early childhood, but voiding disorders are occasionally seen in adolescence, especially in girls. A history of frequency, urgency, delaying of voiding and holding maneuvers, straining while voiding, dribbling of urine, adequacy of local hygiene and constipation should be obtained.

- Examination of optic fundus may show the severity of hypertension as well as abnormalities seen in several syndromes (e.g. anterior lenticonus in Alport syndrome, retinitis pigmentosa in nephronophthisis).
- The back is examined for any spinal deformity and tuft of hair (suggesting spinal dysraphism). "Saddle" region is examined for sensations if neuropathic bladder is suspected.
- The presence of fever, rash, joint involvement, hepatosplenomegaly, and abdominal mass (enlarged kidney, ectopic kidney and enlarged bladder) is looked for.
- Characteristic abnormalities are seen in Henoch-Schönlein purpura and systemic lupus erythematosus. Physical growths are evaluated. Delayed growth, anemia and skeletal abnormalities would suggest chronic kidney disease.

Table 5.4.3: Laboratory investigations	
Tests	***Comments***
Urinalysis A meticulous urine analysis is the most important examination	A properly collected, mid-stream specimen is examined for specific gravity, protein, and formed elements. Characteristic abnormalities are observed in AGN, nephrotic syndrome and UTI.
Biochemical tests in urine	In suspected tubulopathies, urine concentration defects and urolithiasis.
Urine culture and sensitivity	A freshly voided sample with precautions to prevent contamination.
Blood tests Complete hemogram, platelet counts and RBC morphology Renal function tests–electrolytes, urea and creatinine ASLO titre, C'3 ANA, anti-dsDNA Anti-cytoplasmic antibodies	 Anemia and neutrophilic leucocytosis. Degree /Extent of renal disease Post streptococcal AGN For SLE For vasculitis
Ultrasonography	Should be carried out in most cases.
Standard micturating cystourethrogram	Suspected vesicouretric reflux.
Radionuclear studies: Uroflowmetry	Evaluate obstructive uropathy and renal scarring and congenital renal anomalies.
Bladder function studies Cystometry	If voiding dysfunction is suspected. Neurogenic bladder.
Renal biopsy	Unresolving acute GN. Suspected collagen vascular disease.

Diagnostic Approach and Referral

Evaluation of a careful, detailed history of the illness and physical very often suggest the underlying diagnosis (see Tables 5.4.3 and 5.4.4). The initial laboratory tests and imaging should be accurate and reliable. Whereas, urgent treatment measures should be undertaken, prompt referral to a pediatric nephrologist facility is essential. Some forms of glomerular diseases, vasculitis and renal microangiopathy require prompt renal biopsy and aggressive management since a delay would adversely affect the outcome. Table 5.4.5 details some specific issues related to adolescent girls briefly.

Table 5.4.4: Various renal conditions in adolescent age group laboratory investigations

Disease	*Comments*
Acute Post-streptococcal Glomerulonephritis	This is most commonly seen in older children, but occasionally it may occur after the age of 14 years.
Nephrotic Syndrome (NS)	NS occasionally develops in an adolescent and it is likely to be steroid resistant, usually with a "non-minimal" glomerular morphology. Cases of focal segmental glomerulosclerosis and membranoproliferative GN may also be seen.
Systemic Lupus Erythematosus (SLE), Polyarteritis Nodosa and Takayasu Disease	These are only occasionally observed in the adolescent age group.
Asymptomatic Microscopic Hematuria	Is occasionally detected during screening of school children or incidentally. Proteinuria is absent. Hypercalciuria should be excluded and an ultrasonographic examination may be performed. In the absence of a family history of renal diseases, and normal blood pressure further evaluation may not be necessary.
Enuresis and Disorders of Micturition	Primary, monosymptomatic nocturnal enuresis (NE) mostly resolves by the age of 14 years. However, in about 1% of cases it may persist beyond that age.
Chronic Renal Failure (CRF)	Due to a wide variety of underlying conditions, CRF often leads to death during early childhood. However, with earlier detection and better management the decline in renal function may be very gradual and CRF may extend beyond the age of 14 years. The required drug therapy and dietary modifications must be continued along with other supportive measures. Serious complications of CRF such as bony deformities and severe anemia can be avoided with strict adherence to the therapeutic regimen. Normal schooling and physical activity are encouraged.
Renal Replacement Measures	Renal replacement measures include: • Maintenance hemodialysis • Chronic peritoneal dialysis • Renal transplantation Various forms of dialysis are feasible but involve considerable expenditure and stress on the family. These modalities can only be considered as short term measures while awaiting renal transplantation, which is the definitive treatment of end stage renal disease. The issues of donor availability in the family, cost of long-term immunosuppressive therapy and the need for medical supervision should be discussed and explained to the family. The outcome from transplantation should also be clearly informed.

Table 5.4.5: Special issues in adolescent girls

Condition	*Comments*
Lower urinary tract infections (UTIs)	Lower UTIs are common in adolescent girls; more so if they are sexually active. Girls should be explained the importance of a liberal intake of water, local toilet and wiping action (in anteroposterior direction) after defecation. Micturition should not be postponed and the bladder promptly emptied. The need for provision of clean toilets in schools is obvious. Constipation should be avoided.
Asymptomatic bacteriuria	Routine examination of girls (occasionally boys). who have no urinary complaints occasionally shows significant bacteriuria (> 100,000/ml). Microscopic examination may show 2 to 3 'pus cells'. No treatment is necessary.
Teenage pregnancy	Besides standard obstetric care, special attention is necessary if there is a pre-existing problem such as reflux nephropathy, hypertension or impairment or renal function. The incidence of prematurity is high in such situations.

LEARNING POINTS

- A few diseases of the kidney and urinary tract have their onset during adolescence, but a majority start in early childhood and continue thereafter. The former require detailed evaluation (e.g. for suspected collagen vascular diseases) whereas others present specific problems of management.
- These conditions should be jointly managed by pediatrician and the concerned pediatric specialist, both being equally responsible.
- A majority of renal diseases are recurrent or chronic and specific curative treatment is often not possible. However, the progression of renal damage can be slowed by strict adherence to the prescribed therapeutic regimen.
- The treatment of chronic kidney disease (the term "chronic renal failure" is no longer used) involves several other disciplines (e.g. nutritionist, endocrinologist and family counsellor) and teamwork.
- Psycho-emotional and social factors are very important in the management and should be adequately addressed.
- Some of the side effects of drugs (e.g. acne, hirsutism, cushingoid facies, and short stature) may be very troublesome.
- Constant reassurance and emotional support must be provided and compliance with treatment ensured.

SUGGESTED READING

1. Cooper CC, Condron M. Voiding dysfunction. emedicine. medscape.com/article/101698.
2. Gulati A, Bagga A. Renal vasculitis and systemic lupus eryrhematosus. In: Srivastava RN, Bagga A, Eds. Pediatric Nephrology, 6th edition. New Delhi, Jaypee Brothers Medical Publishers 2015;149-65.
3. Harambat J, van Stralen KJ, Kim JJ, Tizard EJ. Epidemiology of chronic kidney disease in children. Pediatr Nephrol 2012; 27:363-74.
4. Hari P, Srivastava RN. Urinary tract infections. In: Srivastava RN, Bagga A, Eds. Pediatric Nephrology, 6th edition New Delhi, Jaypee Brothers Medical Publishers 2015;267-89.
5. Kanitkar M. Disorders of micturition. In: Srivastava RN, Bagga A, Eds. Pediatric Nephrology, 6th edition. New Delhi, Jaypee Brothers Medical Publishers 2015;503-27.
6. Moudgil A, Jordan SC. Renal transplantation. In: Srivastava RN, Bagga A, Eds. Pediatric Nephrology, 6th edition. New Delhi, Jaypee Brothers Medical Publishers 2015;449-75.
7. Pruthi PK. Nephrotic syndrome. In: Gupte S, Ed. Recent Advances in Pediatrics, Vol 23. New Delhi, Jaypee Brothers Medical Publishers 2015;273-307.
8. Srivastava RN, Menon S. Acute glomerulonephritis revisited. In : Gupte S, Ed. Recent Advances in Pediatrics, Vol 23. New Delhi, Jaypee Brothers Medical Publishers 2015;262-72.

Gastrointestinal and Hepatobiliary Problems

5.5

Malathi Sathiyasekaran, Sumathi Bavanandam

INTRODUCTION

Gastrointestinal (GI) and hepatic diseases presenting in adolescence comprises a spectrum of disorders. The luminal GI problems could be a manifestation of the lifestyle changes which are common in the teens and are influenced both by the media and the pressure of the peer group. These include binge eating, snacking, sedentary lifestyle, exposure to tobacco, alcohol and substance abuse. These youngsters are also prone to stress, anxiety, depression and psychosocial dysfunction which may trigger suicidal tendencies. These two preventable problems affect not only the quality of a blossoming young life but shatter the family's happiness and also the health status of the nation. Hormonal changes also play a role especially in girls who experience GI symptoms during their menstrual cycles. This age group is also susceptible to the communicable diseases prevalent in the community such as tuberculosis and parasitic infestations. The incidence of two pediatric GI disorders—inflammatory bowel disease and irritable bowel syndrome—peaks during adolescence and these conditions should be considered and evaluated in affected adolescents.

Hepatic disorders may be those with onset in infancy and childhood either congenital or acquired, which may have progressed with age. These include the various causes of portal hypertension, hepatitis B and C infections, and metabolic liver diseases such as glycogen storage disease, Wilson disease, tyrosinemia and hereditary fructose intolerance. On the other hand autoimmune liver disease and non-alcoholic liver disease are more prevalent in adolescence and should be considered in the differential diagnosis.

The aim of this chapter is to focus only on the common GI symptoms and liver diseases seen in the adolescent age group (Table 5.5.1).

Table 5.5.1: Common gastrointestinal (GI) and hepatic problems in adolescence

Common GI symptoms/ Liver disease	*Various diseases*
Recurrent vomiting	• Gastroesophageal reflux disease • Cyclical vomiting syndrome • Corrosive injury of GI tract with esophageal stricture
Bleeding per rectum	• Fissure in ano • Solitary rectal ulcer syndrome • Colonic polyps • Inflammatory bowel disease
Abdominal pain	• Peptic ulcer disease • Pancreatitis • Intestinal tuberculosis (TB) • Irritable bowel syndrome
Liver disorders	• Non-alcoholic fatty liver disease • Chronic hepatitis B virus (HBV) infection • Atypical manifestations of hepatitis A • Autoimmune liver disease • Wilson disease

HISTORY TAKING

A detailed history should be taken separately from the adolescent and the parent/caretaker with due caution and respect to protect the personal feelings of the adolescent. When the youngster presents with vomiting details regarding whether it is bilious or nonbilious; and associated with retching, bleeding, loss of weight, headache and menstrual cycle should be noted. The presence of red flag signs and certain characteristics of abdominal pain will point towards organic cause. Constipation and bleeding per rectum are common symptoms and the presence of pain, streaks of blood, mucorrhea, straining, systemic symptoms and weight loss will help in the evaluation. History of jaundice, itching, pale stools, GI bleed, altered sensorium and abdominal distension will assist in the evaluation of liver disease whether compensated or decompensated. In this era details regarding liver transplant should be noted in the small subset of post-liver transplant adolescents. More details are covered in the tables and boxes for individual diseases.

CLINICAL EXAMINATION

A thorough clinical examination of the adolescent in the supine position should be done while the parent is by the side. Pallor, jaundice, petechiae and bruises should be noted. All the quadrants of the abdomen should be examined carefully including the scrotum in boys. The presence of organomegaly, fluid, tenderness, distension and features of liver cell failure should be recorded. More details are covered in the tables and boxes for individual diseases.

INVESTIGATIONS

The diagnostic armamentarium for luminal GI diseases includes upper GI and lower GI endoscopy which help in evaluating the mucosa and aids in tissue diagnosis. The various imaging modalities such as ultrasonography (USG), contrast enhanced computerized tomography (CECT), magnetic resonance imaging (MRI) and endoscopic ultrasound (EUS) have improved the sensitivity of diagnosis of GI and hepatic diseases. Liver function tests and specific serological tests for viral and autoimmune diseases may be necessary for diagnosis. Liver biopsy though an invasive test is essential before definitive therapy of some liver disorders. More details are covered in the tables and boxes for individual diseases.

MANAGEMENT

The definitive management of GI and hepatic diseases depends on the diagnosis. Dietary advice should be part of the treatment protocol. Explaining the need for therapy to the adolescent should be done since poor compliance is a big drawback in this age group. These youngsters need proper counseling so that the quality of life is not affected. A multidisciplinary approach may be helpful in some diseases such as inflammatory bowel disease. Care should be taken to understand these patients during their transition to adult clinics. More details are covered in the tables and boxes for individual diseases.

RECURRENT VOMITING

Recurrent vomiting is a common and disturbing symptom in adolescence. The three most common causes of recurrent vomiting are:

1. Gastroesophageal reflux disease (GERD).
2. Cyclical vomiting syndrome (CVS).
3. Corrosive GI injury.

Gastroesophageal Reflux Disease (GERD)

This is the clinicopathological consequence of gastroesophageal reflux (GER) and may present with esophageal or extraesophageal symptoms (Table 5.5.2).

Table 5.5.2: Gastroesophageal reflux disease (GERD)

Clinical features	*Esophageal*–Vomiting, regurgitation, heart burn, retrosternal pain, dysphagia, odynophagia. *Extraesophageal*–Recurrent wheeze, nocturnal cough, pulmonary aspiration, laryngitis, hoarse voice, halitosis, dental erosions. *Alarm signs*–Anemia, weight loss, GI bleed, progressive dysphagia.
Complications	Peptic strictures, Barrett's esophagus, adenocarcinoma.
Investigations	Upper GI endoscopy for mucosal changes, hiatus hernia, strictures. 24-hour pH monitoring test and impedance manometry are the gold standard tests.
Treatment–Lifestyle modifications	Weight reduction in obese/overweight individuals. Head end elevation during sleep. Small frequent meals. Avoidance of caffeinated drinks, alcohol, smoking, chocolates, deep fried, oily and smoked food.
Drugs	*H2-receptor antagonists (H2RA) drugs:* Ranitidine 3-5 mg/kg/day. *Proton pump inhibitors (PPI):* Omeprazole 0.5-1 mg/kg Lanzoprazole 1-4 mg/kg/day given 30 minutes before breakfast for 6-8 weeks.

Cyclical Vomiting Syndrome (CVS)

This is characterized by recurrent, discrete, self-limited episodes of vomiting and is diagnosed by symptom-based criteria with negative laboratory, radiographic and endoscopic findings. North American Society for Pediatric Gastroenterology, Hepatology and Nutrition (NASPGHAN) criteria for CVS are given in Box 5.5.1.

Since dehydration, electrolyte imbalance, hematemesis, and growth failure can occur, proper evaluation and management are essential as shown in Table 5.5.3.

Box 5.5.1: NASPGHAN criteria essential for diagnosis of cyclical vomiting syndrome

1. At least 5 attacks in any interval, or a minimum of 3 attacks during a 6-month period
2. Episodic attacks of intense nausea and vomiting lasting 1 hour to 10 days and occurring at least 1 week apart
3. Stereotypical pattern and symptoms in the individual patient
4. Vomiting during attacks occurs at least 4 times/hour for at least 1 hour
5. Return to baseline health between episodes
6. Not attributed to another disorder.

Table 5.5.3: Cyclical vomiting syndrome	
Evaluation	*Step I:* Complete blood counts (CBC), Liver and Renal Function Tests, Amylase, sugar, electrolytes, ammonia (NH_3), arterial blood gas (ABG) studies, Urine gravindex, ultrasonogram (USG) abdomen and X-ray abdomen (AXR) *Step II:* Esophago-gastro-duodenoscopy (OGD), CT abdomen *Step III:* Urine porphobilinogen, EEG, MRI brain
Treatment	**Acute attack:** Dark, quiet room. Avoid triggering factors. IV fluids–D10 0.45 NS + KCl 1.5 times maintenance rates. Ondansetron 0.3-0.5 mg/kg/dose/6th hrly×24 hr IV. Lorazepam 0.05-0.1 mg/kg/dose 6th hrly×24 hr IV. Ketorolac 1mg/kg/dose 6th hrly. **Transient HT**–ACE inhibitors **Prophylactic:** > 5 years of age Amitriptyline 0.5 mg/kg/day or Propranolol or Topiramate

Corrosive Injury GIT

This is a serious and common problem in the adolescent age group especially amongst young girls who may ingest corrosives as a suicidal attempt. It may also occur during acid attacks or homicidal attempt as a part of sexual abuse or murder.

Ingestion of corrosives whether acid or alkali results in varying grades of injury to the esophageal and gastric mucosa resulting in severe morbidity (Table 5.5.4).

Table 5.5.4: Corrosive injury of the esophagus	
Clinical features	*Acute (Mucosal injury and spasm)*–Vomiting, dysphagia, odynophagia, drooling of saliva, retrosternal pain *Chronic (Stricture)*–Recurrent vomiting, dysphagia, weight loss, food bolus impaction
Investigations	Endoscopy and contrast studies to assess mucosal injury, stricture (Figure 5.5.1) and complications
Management	*Acute*–Correction of dehydration/electrolyte imbalance; no role for nasogastric tube, steroids or antibiotics
Management of complications	Sequential endoscopic dilatation Surgery–In failed endotherapy or complicated strictures

CHRONIC ABDOMINAL PAIN

Chronic abdominal pain (CAP) lasting for more than two months is still an enigma which may pose a diagnostic challenge to the pediatrician. CAP is seen in 15–17% of adolescents and comprises three main groups–organic (10-15%), functional (70-85%) and psychogenic (< 5%). Irritable bowel syndrome is an important cause of CAP in adolescents. Peptic ulcer disease, chronic pancreatitis and intestinal tuberculosis are some important organic causes of CAP. Abdominal pain that occurs in the

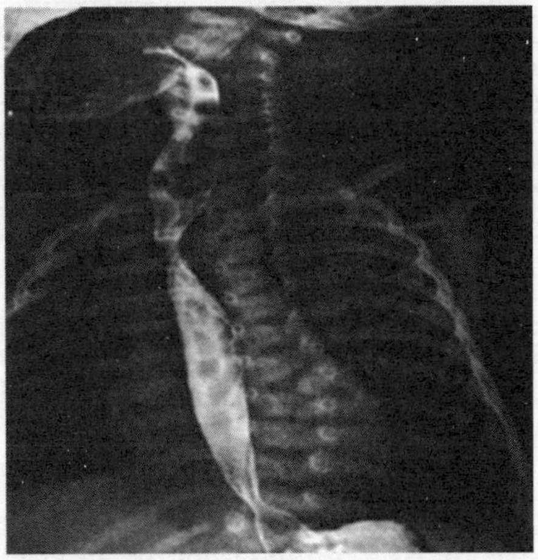

Figure 5.5.1: Barium swallow showing stricture upper third of esophagus

absence of identifiable anatomic, biochemical, metabolic, inflammatory, immunologic or neoplastic disorder is functional abdominal pain (FAP). The main problem in CAP is to differentiate organic from functional pain (Table 5.5.5).

Table 5.5.5: Differentiation of organic and functional abdominal pain

Organic pain	*Functional pain*
Localized pain; usually away from umbilicus	Periumbilical, epigastric or lower abdominal pain
Consistent pain	Paroxysmal pain
Pain lasting longer, for several minutes	Short duration of pain
Radiation of pain	Occurs in clusters
Nocturnal pain that disturbs sleep	Pain does not wake up the child during sleep
Well defined pain (burning, stabbing pain etc.)	Dull ache
Associated with sweating	May present with nausea, vomiting and anxiety

The presence of red flag signs and symptoms may indicate organic pain (Table 5.5.6). The investigations required in an adolescent with chronic abdominal pain are listed in Box 5.5.2.

Table 5.5.6: Red flag symptoms and signs for organic abdominal pain

Red flag symptoms	*Red flag signs*
Involuntary weight loss	Significant pallor
Unexplained fever	Icterus
GI bleed	Abdominal tenderness
Joint pain, skin rash	Mass abdomen
Deceleration of linear growth	Organomegaly
Significant vomiting	Low hemoglobin, elevated ESR or CRP
Chronic diarrhea	
Persistent right upper or right lower quadrant pain	

Box 5.5.2: Investigations in chronic abdominal pain (CAP)
• When functional abdominal pain (FAP) is suspected investigations are restricted to complete blood counts (CBC), urine examination and occult blood in stools.
• Ultrasound of abdomen may be done in adolescents to exclude pelvic or renal pathology.
• However if organic pain is suspected depending on the site of pain and dominant symptom e.g. in epigastric pain with dyspepsia upper GI endoscopy; and if lower abdominal pain with altered bowel habits an ileocolonoscopy may be helpful.

Peptic Ulcer Disease

Duodenal ulcer and gastric ulcer may occur secondary to *Helicobacter pylori*, non-steroidal anti-inflammatory drugs or stress (Table 5.5.7).

Table 5.5.7: Peptic ulcer disease in adolescents	
Clinical features	Abdominal pain, GI bleed, Vomiting
Endoscopy	Endoscopy shows the characteristic finding of duodenal ulcer (DU) or gastric ulcer (GU). Antral biopsy is taken for rapid urease test (for *H. pylori*)
Treatment	Proton Pump Inhibitors (PPI) × 2 months. Treat *H. pylori* infection with PPI, amoxicillin and clarithromycin or PPI with imidazole and amoxicillin for 14 days

Chronic Pancreatitis (CP)

Abdominal pain, diabetes mellitus, steatorrhea and malnutrition are the usual features of chronic pancreatitis. In adolescents abdominal pain interferes with the quality of life. The etiology of CP is diverse and may be toxic, genetic, metabolic, anatomical, tropical and idiopathic. The evaluation and management of CP are given in Table 5.5.8.

Intestinal Tuberculosis (ITB)

In India ITB should be considered when an adolescent presents with abdominal pain, fever, loss of weight and diarrhea. Crohn's disease is an important differential diagnosis though both these conditions share several similarities. There are some differentiating features which may help in diagnosis (Table 5.5.9).

Table 5.5.8: Chronic pancreatitis	
Investigations	Blood sugar, serum calcium, triglycerides and LFT Plain X-ray abdomen may show calcification (Figure 5.5.2) Ultrasound (US), CT scan, magnetic resonance cholangiopancreatography (MRCP) and endoscopic ultrasound (EUS) may show features of CP, stricture and pseudocyst Genetic studies: SPINK1 mutations
Complications	Diabetes mellitus, GI bleed and biliary strictures Rarely malignancy
Endotherapy	Stricture dilatation, stone removal, stent placement
Medical	Pancreatic enzyme replacement, analgesics
Surgery	Pancreaticojejunostomy, total pancreatectomy with islet autotransplant

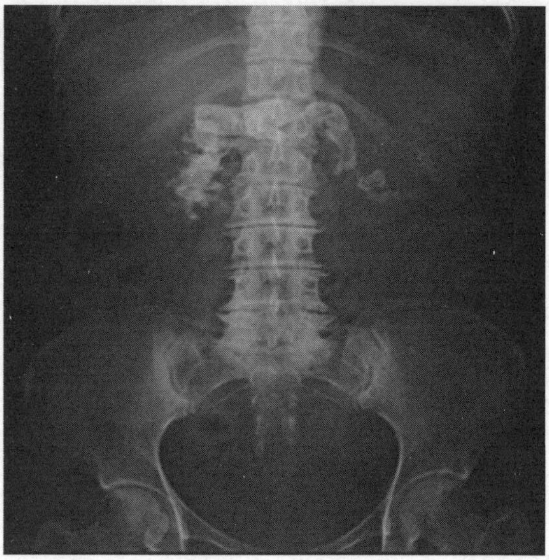

Figure 5.5.2: X-ray abdomen showing extensive pancreatic calcification

Irritable Bowel Syndrome (IBS)

This is a common functional GI disorder seen in adolescents who present with chronic abdominal pain usually related to and relieved by defecation. IBS may be associated with diarrhea, constipation or a combination of both. The symptoms may improve with psyllium seed (ispaghula or isabgol) husks. Mebeverine may help to reduce the abdominal pain. The accepted diagnostic criteria are Rome III (Box 5.5.3).

Table 5.5.9: Differentiating features between intestinal tuberculosis and Crohn's disease

Clinical features	*Intestinal tuberculosis (ITB)*	*Crohn's disease (CD)*
Fever	+++	+
Chronic diarrhea	+	++
Bleeding per rectum	+	++
Perianal sinus/ fistula	-	+++
Extra-intestinal manifestations	-	++
Duration of symptoms	Short duration	Prolonged
Ultrasound abdomen	Free fluid/lymph nodes/thickened loops	Thickened loops
Endoscopy	Ileocecal Ulcers are transverse	Any site of involvement Ulcers are longitudinal

Box 5.5.3: Rome III diagnostic criteria for IBS
This includes abdominal pain for 2 months plus 2 or more of the following at least 25% of the time.
1. Improvement with defecation.
2. Onset associated with change in the frequency of stools.
3. Onset associated with change in the form of stool.
4. No evidence of inflammatory bowel disease (IBD) or neoplasia.

BLEEDING PER RECTUM

When an adolescent presents with chronic and intermittent bleeding per rectum, the four common causes which are confirmed and diagnosed on ileocolonoscopy are given in Table 5.5.10.

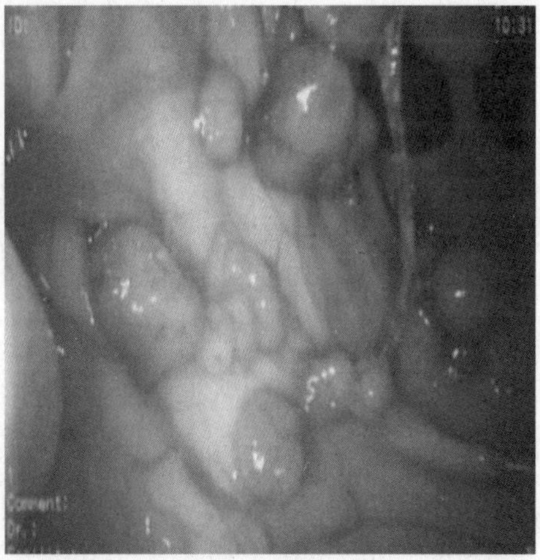

Figure 5.5.3: Familial adenomatous polyposis coli

NON-ALCOHOLIC FATTY LIVER DISEASE (NAFLD)

NAFLD is an important cause of chronic liver disease in adolescents with a prevalence as high as 40% in the obese. NAFLD comprises a wide spectrum of conditions ranging from reversible simple steatosis (non-alcoholic fatty liver/NAFL) and steatohepatitis (NASH) to irreversible fibrosis, cirrhosis (Figure 5.5.4) and even to hepatocellular carcinoma. Adolescents with NASH may present with insulin resistance and features of the metabolic syndrome such as hypertension, hyperlipidemia and type 2 diabetes. Other common

Table 5.5.10: Bleeding per rectum

Disease	*Clinical features*	*Findings*	*Treatment*
Fissure in ano	Painful defecation with blood streaked stool	Sphincter spasm and fissure at anal verge	Sitz bath, laxatives, avoidance of constipation, high fiber diet
Solitary rectal ulcer syndrome	Defecation disorder History of straining at defecation, digital evacuation, mucorrhea, blood in the stool	*Endoscopy:* Single or multiple ulcers within 10 cm of anal verge on the anterior wall of rectum *Histopathology*: Fibromuscular obliteration of the lamina propria	Bowel training and avoidance of constipation, 5-aminosalicylic acid suppositories. Rarely argon plasma coagulation or surgery if bleed is severe
Polyps	Polyps either single or multiple may occur in isolation or as part of polyposis syndromes Bleeding PR, mucorrhea or as mass descending PR	More common in the rectum They are usually juvenile polyps-hamartomatous or adenomatous	Endoscopic polypectomy Multiple polyposes should undergo surveillance because of malignant potential Familial polyposis coli: Colectomy (Figure 5.5.3)
Inflammatory bowel disease	*Ulcerative colitis (UC):* Bleeding PR *Crohn's disease (CD):* Bleeding PR, fever, abdominal pain, growth failure	*UC:* Continuous involvement and ulcerations. HPE: Glandular distortion, cryptitis and crypt abscess *CD*: Skip lesions, irregular ulcers on any part of GIT with non-caseating granuloma on histopathology	5-aminosalicyclic acid, steroids, azathioprine and biologicals: Fistulae Surgery: Stricture, perforation and obstruction

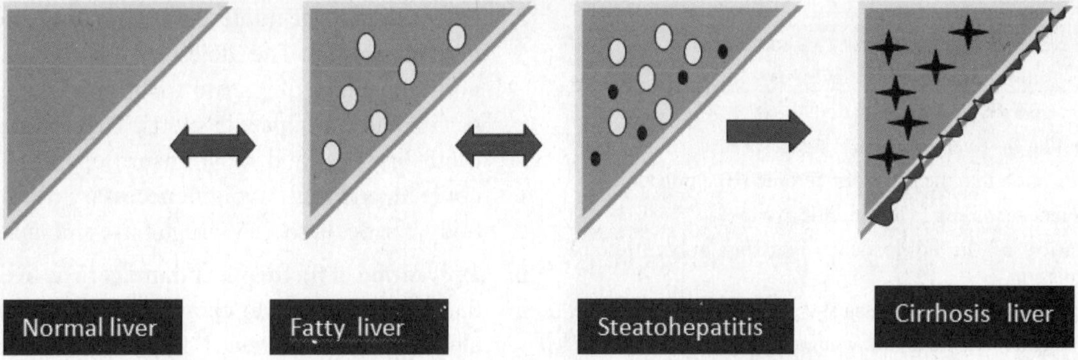

Figure 5.5.4: Diagramatic representation of stages of NAFLD

Table 5.5.11: Non-alcoholic fatty liver disease (NAFLD)

Clinical features	1. Asymptomatic. 2. Identified incidentally by elevated transaminases or fatty liver on ultrasound. 3. Right upper quadrant pain, fatigue and symptoms of metabolic syndrome. 4. Hepatomegaly is a common finding. 5. Acanthosis nigricans–hyperpigmentation and thickening of skin over the nape of neck and axilla indicates insulin resistance.
Investigations	Serum aspartate aminotransferase (AST), alanine aminotransferase (ALT) and gamma-glutamyl transpeptidase (γ-GTP) are elevated in non-alcoholic steatohepatitis (NASH). Elevated triglycerides, impaired glucose tolerance, elevated lipoproteins and markers of insulin resistance may be present. Liver biopsy shows periportal steatosis, cellular ballooning, inflammation and fibrosis.
Imaging studies	Ultrasonography (USG), computerized tomography (CT) or magnetic resonance (MR) can detect steatosis and grade the fatty liver. US cannot detect steatosis if <30%, inflammation or fibrosis. Transient elastography and fibroscan are preferred to evaluate the fibrosis.
Treatment	Lifestyle and dietary changes with regular exercise to reduce weight is the essence of effective therapy. Vitamin E may help.

associations are polycystic ovary syndrome, sleep apnea and small bowel bacterial overgrowth (Table 5.5.11).

The pathogenesis of NAFLD involves a complex interplay of several factors (inflammatory cytokines and adipokines, free fatty acids, genetic factors, oxidative stress and mitochondrial dysfunction) resulting in a cascade of events ending in cirrhosis. Table 5.5.11 highlights the steps in the evaluation and management of NAFLD in adolescents.

CHRONIC HEPATITIS B INFECTION

Hepatitis B virus (HBV) infection is an important cause of chronic hepatitis, cirrhosis and hepatocellular carcinoma though the incidence has decreased significantly in countries which have opted for universal hepatitis B immunization. In India the prevalence of hepatitis B varies from 2 to 15% and therefore it is not uncommon to encounter an adolescent who is incidentally detected to be HBSAg positive. When HBSAg is positive for more than 6 months the individual is stated to have chronic HBV infection. The 7 steps in the management of an adolescent with chronic HBV infection are given in Box 5.5.4 and described below.

Box 5.5.4: Management of an adolescent with chronic HBV infection

1. History and physical examination
2. Evaluation for liver injury/viral status
3. Classification into the phases of chronic HBV infection
4. Treatment according to the specific group
5. Education of the adolescent regarding prevention of transmission
6. Prevention of further liver damage
7. Regular and meticulous follow-up of all adolescents who are HBSAg positive

1. **History and physical examination:** Note the details of history of jaundice, antenatally detected HBSAg positivity in the mother (perinatal transmission), blood transfusions, needle pricks, tattoo and ear boring; family history of chronic liver disease or hepatocellular carcinoma (HCC); and presence of jaundice, hepatosplenomegaly, ascites and palmar erythema.
2. **Evaluation for liver injury/viral status:** This is done by estimation of serum SGOT (AST), SGPT (ALT), HBeAg, anti-HBe and HBV DNA.
3. **Classification into the phases of chronic HBV infection** should be done based on the transaminases, HBeAg and HBV DNA status (Table 5.5.12).
4. **Treatment according to the specific group:** At present treatment is only for chronic HBV infection with persistently elevated SGPT and significant viral load. Definitive therapy with peginterferon once a week for 6 months is recommended. If interferon is not administered or there is no sustained viral response nucleoside analogs tenofovir or entecavir is given indefinitely to ensure sustained viral suppression.
5. **Education of the adolescent regarding prevention of transmission:** The adolescent is encouraged to lead normal healthy life, share food with friends, attend school and participate in sports. They must not share tooth brushes, and must ensure open wounds are covered, and must avoid unnecessary needle pricks, body boring, tattoo, IV drug abuse and unsafe sex.
6. **Prevention of further liver damage:** The liver damage that may occur due to obesity, hepatotoxic drugs and alcohol should be stressed. Hepatitis A vaccine should be given to those who are HBSAg positive.

Table 5.5.12: Chronic HBV infection–Phases based on various tests

Phases	*HBSAg*	*SGPT (AST)*	*HBeAg*	*HBV DNA*	*Treatment*
1. Immune tolerant	+ve	Normal	+ve	>20,000 IU/L	No
2. Immune active (HBeAg +ve CHB)	+ve	>2 ULN	+ve	>20,000 IU/L	Yes
2a. Immune active (HBeAg –ve CHB)	+ve	>2 ULN	–ve	>2,000 IU/L	Yes
3. Inactive carrier	+ve	Normal	–ve	<2,000 IU/L	No

Abbreviations: CHB: Chronic hepatitis B; HBSAg: Hepatitis B surface antigen; HBeAG: Hepatitis B envelope antigen; >2ULN: More than twice the upper limit of the normal.

7. **Regular and meticulous follow-up of all adolescents who are HBSAg positive** since HBV disease is dynamic.

HEPATITIS A VIRUS INFECTION IN AN ADOLESCENT

Hepatitis A virus (HAV) an RNA virus which is spread by oro-fecal route is an important cause of acute sporadic hepatitis in the developing countries. The serodiagnosis is made by the detection of IgM antibodies to HAV. Acute infection does not progress to chronicity, however in less than 1% the event can progress to acute liver failure. In the majority of young children the illness is subclinical or anicteric or even if icteric is mild with complete resolution of symptoms within 7-10 days. The natural history of HAV infection in adolescents however is not as benign as in younger children (Figure 5.5.5). A spectrum of presentation resulting in increase in morbidity and mortality or requiring liver transplant, may be encountered.

1. **Atypical presentation:** Prolonged cholestasis presenting as a disturbing pruritus is often seen in adolescents and may last for 12 weeks. Relapsing hepatitis, hyperbilirubinemia, fever and ascites are other atypical features.
2. **Extrahepatic manifestations:** Due to circulating immune complexes manifestations such as evanescent skin rash, transient arthralgia, pancreatitis, vasculitis, triggering of autoimmune hepatitis, myocarditis, red cell aplasia and Guillain-Barré syndrome may occur.
3. **Acute on chronic hepatitis:** When an adolescent presents with atypical features such as firm hepatomegaly, splenomegaly and ascites, a possibility of acute on chronic liver disease should be considered.

Since HAV infection is preventable and is associated with high morbidity in older children it is necessary that active immunization is administered for all adolescents who have not received the vaccine.

AUTOIMMUNE HEPATITIS

Autoimmune hepatitis (AIH) is a chronic, progressive immunological disease of the liver characterized by the

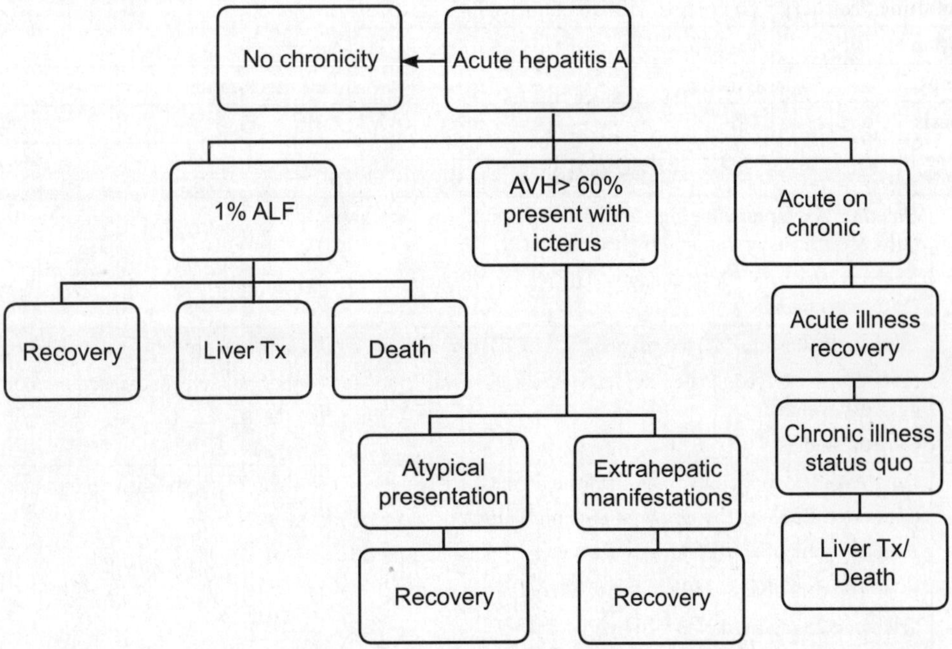

Figure 5.5.5: HAV infection in adolescent

Abbreviations: AVH: Acute viral hepatitis; ALF: Acute liver failure; Liver Tx: Liver transplant

presence of autoantibodies, hypergammaglobulinemia, elevated transaminases and interface hepatitis in the absence of viral markers, history of drug or alcohol intake or Wilson disease. AIH is common in adolescent girls and present as acute hepatitis, chronic hepatitis or cirrhosis with portal hypertension. AIH is classified into two main subtypes type I and type II based on the presence of antibody profile (Table 5.5.13).

Diagnosis: The simplified scoring system which comprises level of autoantibodies and IgG, histology and absence of viral markers may be used for diagnosis.

Treatment: Prednisolone as monotherapy or in combination with azathioprine is recommended for all adolescents with histological evidence of hepatitis with or without fibrosis or cirrhosis. The time to withdraw treatment is not definite though in type I it can be attempted once remission is attained for three years. Since relapses are common in AIH type II and puberty great caution should be taken during steroid withdrawal.

WILSON DISEASE

Wilson disease (WD) is an inherited disorder of copper metabolism presenting with a range of hepatic and neuropsychiatric manifestations either alone or in combination and is an important cause of chronic liver disease in Indian children (Table 5.5.14). WD is due to a defect in ATP7B gene on chromosome 13 which encodes for ATPase on hepatocytes and results in the toxic accumulation of copper in various tissues such as liver, brain, kidney, RBCs, cornea etc. Since WD is a treatable metabolic disorder early and prompt diagnosis will benefit the adolescent.

It is essential to screen all members of the family and treat asymptomatic siblings. The best outcome is seen in this group of asymptomatic siblings who have good quality of life and normal lifespan if they are compliant with medication.

LEARNING POINTS

- GERD and cyclical vomiting syndrome are common causes of recurrent vomiting in adolescents.
- In India corrosive injury to the GIT is an important preventable cause of morbidity in adolescents.
- The incidence of inflammatory bowel disease peaks during adolescence and should be considered when an adolescent presents with abdominal pain, bleeding per rectum and fever.
- Irritable bowel syndrome, a functional GI disorder is common in this age group.

Table 5.5.13: Types of autoimmune hepatitis

	Type I	*Type II*
Autoantibodies	Anti-nuclear, anti-smooth muscle and anti-actin antibodies	Liver/kidney microsomal antibody type 1 (LKM1) and liver cytosol antibody type 1 (LC1)
Age of onset	Any age	Children and young adults
Associated autoimmune disorders	Thyroiditis, vitiligo, diabetes ++	+
Clinical presentation	Variable	Severe
Response to therapy	Excellent	Failure common
Progress to cirrhosis	45%	80%

Table 5.5.14: Wilson disease (WD)

Clinical features	*Hepatic:* Asymptomatic hepatomegaly, elevated transaminases, acute hepatitis, chronic hepatitis, acute liver failure, cirrhosis with portal hypertension (PHT) *Neuropyschiatric:* Early changes: Grimacing (Figure 5.5.6), slurred speech and difficulty in writing. Later: Dystonia, chorea
Investigations	Low ceruloplasmin <20 mg/dl, presence of KF ring (Figure 5.5.7), and elevated 24 hours urine copper >40 µg *Liver biopsy:* Glycogenated nuclei, steatosis, special stains for copper positive. Increased copper content >250 µg/g/dry weight. Genetic studies
Management	*Diet:* Avoid copper containing diet such as nuts, cocoa, shell fish, organ meat, mushroom, spinach. *Chelators*: Lifelong therapy with D-penicillamine: • < 10 years of age: 250 mg twice a day 1 hour before food • > 10 years of age: 250 mg thrice a day before food Trientene 25 mg/kg/day in 3 divided doses Oral Zinc: 25-50 mg of elemental zinc before meals *Liver transplant :* This is the definitive therapy for those presenting with acute liver failure, end stage liver disease, non-responsive to chelation

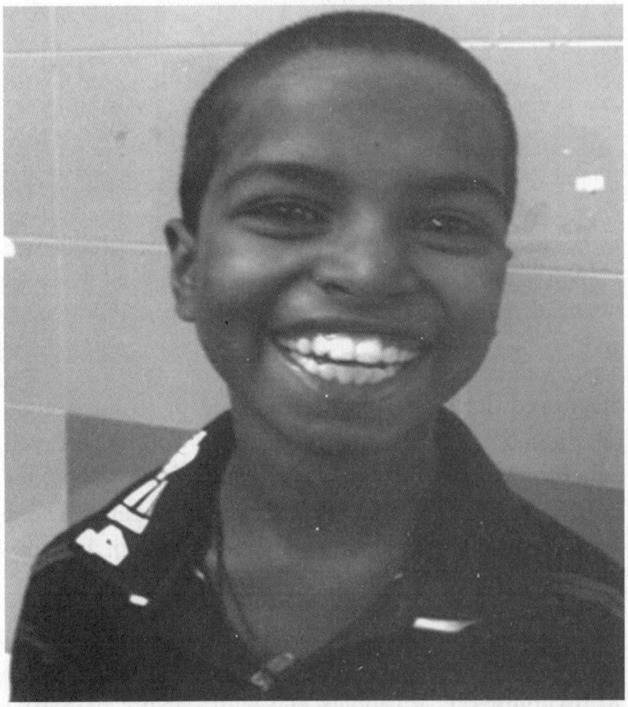

Figure 5.5.6: Grimace in neuropsychiatric Wilson's disease

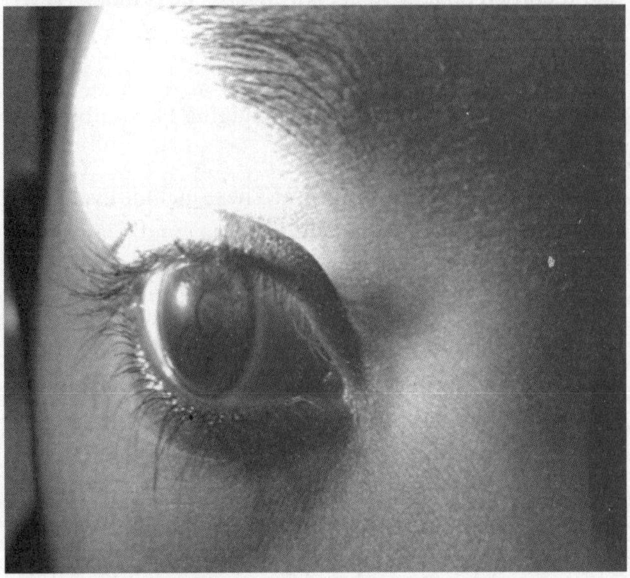

Figure 5.5.7: KF ring in Wilson's disease

- Non-alcoholic liver disease should be considered when an adolescent presents with obesity and steps should be taken to reduce weight.

SUGGESTED READING

1. American Academy of Pediatrics Subcommittee on Chronic Abdominal Pain. Chronic Abdominal Pain in Children. Pediatrics 2005;115(3):812-15.
2. Chalasani N, Younossi Z, Lavine JE, Diehl AM, Brunt EM, Cusi K, *et al.* The Diagnosis and Management of Non-Alcoholic Fatty Liver Disease: Practice Guideline by the American Association for the Study of Liver Diseases, American College of Gastroenterology, and the American Gastroenterological Association. Hepatology 2012;55:2005-23.
3. Hennes EM, Zeniya M, Czaia AJ, Dalekos GN, Krawitt EL, Bittencourt PL, *et al.* Simplified criteria for the diagnosis of autoimmune hepatitis. Hepatology 2008;48(1):169-76.
4. Kamath SR, Sathiyasekaran M, Raja TE, Sudha L. Profile of Viral Hepatitis A in Indian Pediatr 2009;46:642-43.
5. Li BU, Lefevre F, Chelimsky GG, Boles RG, Susanne P. Nelson SP, Donald W. Lewis, *et al.* North American Society for Pediatric Gastroenterology, Hepatology, and Nutrition Consensus Statement on the Diagnosis and Management of Cyclic Vomiting Syndrome. J Pediatr Gastroenterol Nutr 2008;47:379-93.
6. Makharia GK, Srivastava S, Das P, Goswami P, Singh U, Tripathi M, *et al.* Clinical, endoscopic, and histological differentiations between Crohn's disease and intestinal tuberculosis. Am J Gastroenterol 2010;105(3):642-51.
7. Roberts EA, Schilsky ML, American Association for Study of Liver Diseases (AASLD). Diagnosis and Treatment of Wilson Disease: An Update. Hepatology 2008;47(6):2089-111.
8. Suresh N, Ganesh R, Sathiyasekaran M. Solitary rectal ulcer syndrome: A case series. Indian Pediatr 2010;47(12):1059-61.
9. Vanderplas Y, Rudolph CD, Di Lorenzo C, Hassall E, Liptak G, Mazur L, *et al.* Pediatric Gastroesophageal Reflux Clinical Practice Guidelines: Joint Recommendations of the North American Society for Pediatric Gastroenterology, Hepatology, and Nutrition (NASPGHAN) and the European Society for Pediatric Gastroenterology, Hepatology, and Nutrition (ESPGHAN). J Pediatr Gastroenterol Nutr 2009;49:498-547.
10. Walker LS, Caplan-Dover A, Rasquin-Weber A. Questionnaire on pediatric gastrointestinal symptoms, Rome III version (QPGS-RIII). In: Drossman DA, Corazziari E, Delvaux M, Spiller RC, Talley NJ, Thompson WG, Whitehead WE, eds. Rome III: The Functional Gastrointestinal Disorders, 3rd ed. McLean, Virginia: Degnon Associates, Inc 2006; 963-90.

5.6.1

Thyroid Disorders

M Vijayakumar, PSN Menon

INTRODUCTION

Thyroid disorders constitute probably the most common endocrine problem in adolescence affecting mostly the girls. Hypothyroidism by far leads the list and chronic autoimmune thyroiditis is the most common disorder causing thyroid dysfunction in adolescents. Even though rare, hyperthyroidism is also prevalent in this age group with Graves disease predominating in the list. In comparison thyroid tumors are rare. Diagnosis is often delayed due to nonspecific clinical presentations; fortunately diagnosis can be made and confirmed quickly. Often management requires life-long monitoring.

HYPOTHYROIDISM

The common causes of hypothyroidism in adolescents are listed in Table 5.6.1.1.

History Taking

Usual presentation is insidious and the symptoms are nonspecific. Hence diagnosis is often delayed, unless there is a high index of suspicion. Most adolescents are diagnosed during a routine check-up or in the course of evaluation for short stature, neck swelling, delayed puberty, menstrual irregularities, and gain in weight for height, and less often with precocious puberty. These adolescents often seek consultation for dry skin, lethargy or constipation.

Table 5.6.1.1: Causes of hypothyroidism in adolescence
A. Disorders of Thyroid Gland (Primary Hypothyroidism)
• Chronic lymphocytic thyroiditis (CLT)
• *Late onset congenital hypothyroidism:* Thyroid dysgenesis, ectopic thyroid
• Inborn errors of thyroid hormonogenesis
• Iodine deficiency (endemic goiter)
• *Drugs:* Anti-thyroid drugs (PTU, methimazole, carbimazole), anticonvulsants, lithium, amiodarone
• *Goitrogens:* Cabbage, cassava, cauliflower, broccoli
• Surgery, irradiation, radioactive iodine therapy
B. Disorders of Pituitary or Hypothalamus
• *Tumors:* Craniopharyngioma
• Head trauma
• *Neuro-infections:* Meningitis, encephalitis
• Infiltrative diseases
• Cranial irradiation

Clinical Examination

Anthropometry: All adolescents with a suspected thyroid disorder should have their weight and height measured and recorded on a growth chart. Body mass index (BMI) should be calculated and body proportions should be recorded.

Pubertal assessment: Pubertal staging should be done according to Tanner staging.

General physical examination: These include evaluation for pallor, skin changes, myxedema, and features of underlying genetic dysmorphisms and autoimmune disorders.

System review: All systems should be evaluated for an underlying abnormality and possible etiology including features of hypothyroidism. The adolescent may appear euthyroid or hypothyroid. Neck should be examined for fullness, goiter, nodules and lymphadenopathy. Simple goiter is a common cause of euthyroid goiter in adolescent girls. An enlarged ectopic thyroid or thyroglossal cyst may be palpated. The goiter should be evaluated for consistency, nodularity and bruits. The signs of neurologic and cardiac involvement should be looked for.

Autoimmune Thyroiditis

The most common cause of thyroid dysfunction during adolescence is chronic lymphocytic thyroiditis (CLT, autoimmune thyroiditis). Both goitrous (Hashimoto thyroiditis) and non-goitrous (primary myxedema) varieties are described. Girls outnumber boys in this disorder. Family history of CLT is present in about 30% of cases. It causes 80% of euthyroid goiters in adolescents (Figure 5.6.1.1).

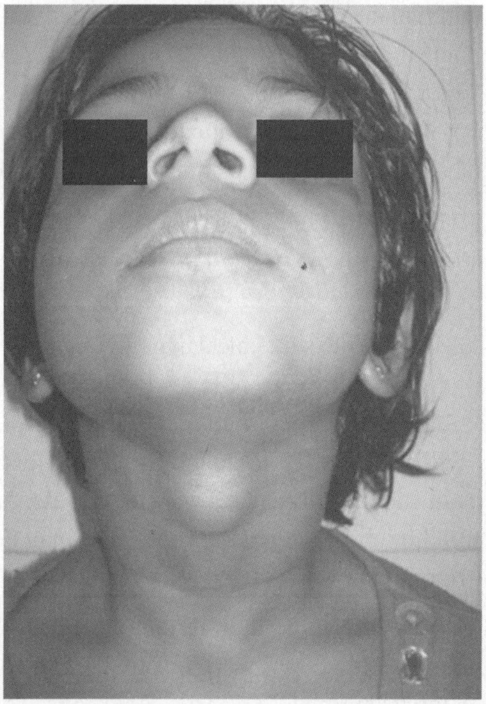

Figure 5.6.1.1: Adolescent girl with enlarged ectopic thyroid

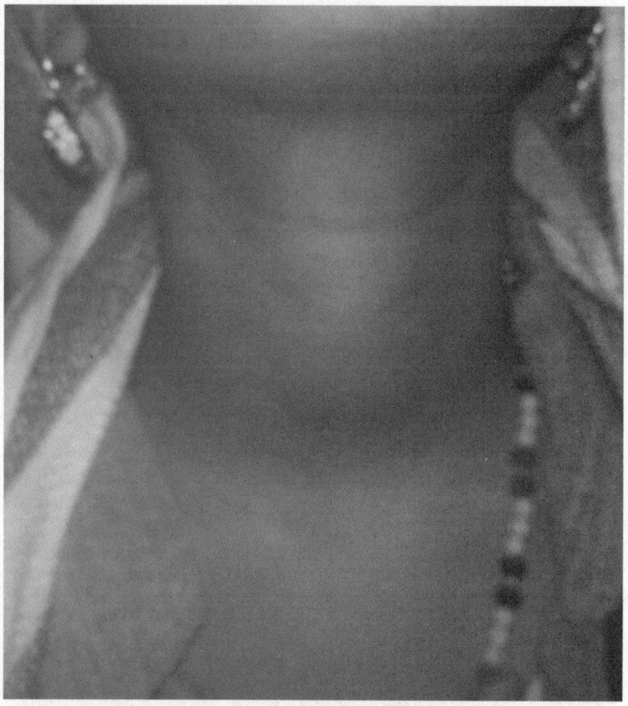

Figure 5.6.1.2: Adolescent girl with autoimmune thyroiditis

Some characteristic features of CLT are given in Box 5.6.1.1.

Box 5.6.1.1: Characteristic features of chronic lymphocytic thyroiditis (CLT)

- Autoimmune thyroiditis is seen in isolation or as a part of other diseases; majority is autoimmune disorders.
- Often there is a positive family history.
- About 25% of children and adolescents with type 1 diabetes mellitus will develop associated thyroiditis.
- Autoimmune polyglandular syndrome (APS) type 1 (APECED- Autoimmune Poly Endocrinopathy, Candidiasis, Ectodermal Dystrophy) is characterized by thyroiditis in 10% of cases.
- APS 2 (Schmidt syndrome) is more common in older children and adults; and is characterized by CLT, diabetes mellitus, with/without adrenal insufficiency.
- There is increased incidence of thyroiditis in Down syndrome, Turner syndrome, Klinefelter syndrome and Noonan syndrome.
- Thyroid enlargement (goiter) is present in around 75% of all patients at the time of diagnosis, usually resulting from lymphocytic infiltration.
- Most complain about pressure or fullness in the neck for weeks or months. Goiter is usually nontender, firm and clinically euthyroid.
- Adolescents with autoimmune thyroiditis may be euthyroid, or have compensated or overt hypothyroidism.
- Some present initially with features of thyrotoxicosis. This is due to the discharge of thyroxine from the damaged gland.
- In some cases stimulation by TSH receptor stimulatory antibodies will result in thyrotoxicosis (Hashitoxicosis).
- Thyroid scintiscan: Irregular distribution of radiotracer agent.

Late-Onset Congenital Hypothyroidism

Some congenital forms of hypothyroidism secondary to thyroid dysgenesis, dyshormonogenesis and ectopic thyroid may not be detected in early childhood. They are often detected while evaluating an adolescent with short stature, developmental delay, delayed puberty or scholastic backwardness. Children having thyroid dyshormonogenesis or ectopic thyroid may present with goiter (Figure 5.6.1.2).

Micronutrient Deficiencies

Iodine deficiency is widely prevalent in India. Endemic cretinism is the most severe form of this spectrum. In regions of moderate iodine deficiency, hypothyroidism as a result of iodine deficiency is common in adolescents. Ingestion of goitrogenic foods (sweet potato, cabbage, cauliflower, broccoli, and cassava) aggravates this condition. Selenium is important for de-iodination of thyroid hormone; hence its deficiency aggravates hypothyroidism.

Clinical Manifestations

The clinical features are insidious and non-specific to begin with. Hence majority of cases are diagnosed late. A high index of suspicion is needed for early diagnosis and management. The major clinical symptoms are described in the Table 5.6.1.2.

Table 5.6.1.2: Clinical features of hypothyroidism
• Poor linear growth–Height is more affected, hence children appear relatively overweight
• Thyroid swelling (goiter)–Diffuse, firm, usually non-nodular
• Thyroid facies in long-standing cases–myxedema of face
• Delayed dental and skeletal maturation
• Lethargy
• Cold intolerance
• Constipation
• Dry skin
• Pallor
• Periorbital edema
• Poor scholastic performance (rare)
• Delayed puberty
• Precocious puberty (rare)
• Bradycardia
• Cold extremities
• Delayed relaxation of deep tendon reflexes
• Muscular hypertrophy (Kocher–Debre–Semelaigne syndrome, rare)

Diagnostic Evaluation

- **Thyroid stimulating hormone (TSH):** Usually measured by chemiluminescent assay. TSH is elevated in primary hypothyroidism. TSH levels are low in pituitary and hypothalamic lesions.
- **Total or free thyroxine:** Free thyroxine (FT4) levels are normal in subclinical hypothyroidism and low in overt hypothyroidism. In secondary or tertiary (pituitary or hypothalamic) forms FT4 and TSH are low.
- **TRH stimulation test:** In secondary (pituitary) hypothyroidism, TRH administration will not elicit TSH response. In tertiary (hypothalamic) hypothyroidism, increased TSH response is seen after TRH administration.
- **Autoantibodies:** CLT is diagnosed by elevated titers of thyroperoxidase (TPO) and thyroglobulin (TG) antibodies.
- **Thyroid ultrasonography/radioisotope studies:** They help to identify the presence and location of thyroid gland and also the presence of a thyroid nodule.
- **Histology:** Fine needle aspiration cytology (FNAC) is not indicated in a straightforward thyroiditis. If done, it demonstrates lymphocytic infiltration, lymphoid follicles and follicular cell hyperplasia.

Management

- Sodium levo-thyroxine (l-thyroxine) is the treatment of choice.
- Rapid replacement should not be initiated (unlike in neonates). Since these adolescents are accustomed to chronic hypothyroid state for a long time, rapid normalization leads to headache (pseudotumor cerebri), hyperactivity, insomnia, tremors, tachycardia, short attention span and behavioral problems.
- Start with a small dose and increase the dose slowly over months.
- Adolescents with subclinical hypothyroidism (normal T4, slightly elevated TSH (5-10 mU/L) need not be treated. But they should be closely followed up with serial thyroid function tests. Most cases remain subclinical, but a few (with elevated thyroid antibodies and enlarged thyroid gland) may develop overt hypothyroidism later.
- In adolescents with other chronic illnesses, thyroid function tests show low T3, free T4 and total T4 with low or normal TSH. This condition is called as sick euthyroid syndrome and these patients do not require treatment. Elevated reverse T3 (rT3) confirms the diagnosis. This condition is due to deficiency of 5'-deiodinase and resolves once the primary condition is cured.
- The aim of the treatment is to keep TSH in a low normal (0.3–1 mU/L) range and total T4/free T4 at a high normal range.
- Average optimal doses in different age groups:
  - 6–10 years: 3–4 μg/kg
  - > 11 years: 2–3 μg/kg
- The patients should be monitored once in a month till optimal dose has been reached. Once s/he has reached euthyroid state, s/he should be followed up every 4–6 months.
- Growth, pubertal development, bone age, and scholastic performance should be assessed in every visit, apart from monitoring thyroid function tests (T4, freeT4 and TSH).
- Monitoring is life-long.

HYPERTHYROIDISM

Hyperthyroidism is a rare disorder in children compared to adults. However older children and adolescents are commonly affected. The common causes of hyperthyroidism are given in Table 5.6.1.3.

Table 5.6.1.3: Causes of hyperthyroidism in adolescents

- Graves disease (diffuse toxic goiter)
- Functioning thyroid adenoma
- Toxic multinodular goiter
- McCune-Albright syndrome
- Toxic phase of autoimmune thyroiditis
- Thyroid hormone ingestion (thyrotoxicosis factitia)
- Central hyperthyroidism (TSH producing adenoma)
- Thyroid hormone resistance

History Taking

Even though many hyperthyroid adolescents have classical features of thyrotoxicosis including involvement of the eye, most are picked up during evaluation of hyperactivity, short attention span and other neurobehavioral problems.

- Majority of cases of hyperthyroidism are caused by Graves' disease (90%).
- This is an autoimmune disorder with a strong female predilection (6:1).
- Major histocompatibility antigen complexes associated with Graves' disease are HLA B8, HLA-DR3 and HLA DQA1.
- Graves' disease occurs as an isolated disease entity or may be associated with other autoimmune diseases like diabetes, Addison disease, vitiligo, systemic lupus erythematosus, idiopathic thrombocytopenic purpura and rheumatoid arthritis.
- Down syndrome and DiGeorge syndrome have increased risk of Graves' disease.
- The mechanism is due to production of TSH receptor stimulating antibodies that will mimic the action of TSH on its receptor thus stimulating the production of thyroid hormones.

Clinical Manifestations

Symptoms are often non-specific and because of the rarity of this disease, the diagnosis is often delayed. Usual clinical features are given in the Table 5.6.1.4. Deterioration of behavior and school performance in an adolescent who previously was doing well may be the earliest warning signal. The combination of thyrotoxicosis and ophthalmopathy makes the diagnosis of Graves' disease relatively easy (Figure 5.6.1.3).

Investigations

- **Thyroid function tests:** Elevated levels of thyroid hormones and suppressed TSH are suggestive of hyperthyroidism.

Table 5.6.1.4: Clinical features of hyperthyroidism

- *Thyroid enlargement:* Diffuse soft, smooth. Bruit often present. A thyroid nodule is suggestive of toxic adenoma
- *Eye signs:* Prominent eyes, mild proptosis lid lag, lid retraction
- *Neurologic:* Headache, tremor, insomnia, fatigability, fidgetiness
- Weight loss in spite of excessive appetite
- Diarrhea
- Heat intolerance
- Proximal muscle weakness
- *Cardiac:* Tachycardia, precordial over-activity, hypertension
- Shortened attention span
- *Behavioral:* Emotional lability, behavior problems
- Delayed puberty
- Advancement in bone age
- Warm moist hands
- Café-au-lait spots in McCune-Albright syndrome

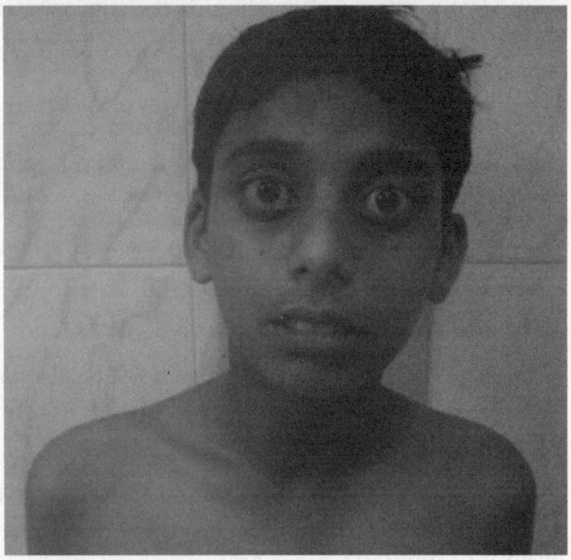

Figure 5.6.1.3: Graves disease in an adolescent boy with ophthalmoplegia

- Measurement of *TSH receptor antibodies* helps in the diagnosis of Graves' disease. TSH receptor antibodies are negative in toxic phase of chronic lymphocytic thyroiditis.
- Baseline complete and differential WBC counts along with ALT (SGPT) are essential before starting the treatment.
- **Imaging:** Ultrasound scan of neck with radio-uptake study helps to confirm the diagnosis.

Management

Choice of therapy varies between medical, surgical and radioiodine therapy. Medical therapy is preferred in adolescents.

Medical Therapy

- Commonly used drugs are thiouracil derivatives like methimazole, carbimazole, and propylthiouracil

(PTU). These drugs inhibit organification of iodine and the coupling of iodotyrosine on the thyroglobulin molecule thus decreasing the production of T3 and T4. Carbimazole is converted into methimazole for its action. PTU has an added advantage of inhibiting the peripheral conversion of T4 to T3.

- PTU can cause serious liver injury leading to fatal liver cell failure. Hence it is used as a second line of drug. In first trimester, methimazole and carbimazole are associated with increased risk of embryopathy including aplasia cutis.
- The starting dose of carbimazole/methimazole is 0.5 mg/kg/day given twice a day. The starting dose of PTU is 5 mg/kg/day and should be given thrice a day.
- The dose is titrated depending on the concentration of T4/free T4. The smallest effective dose to produce a euthyroid state should be used.
- A beta-blocker (propranolol) in a dose of 1-2 mg/kg/day in 2-3 divided doses is added to control tremor or tachycardia.
- Serum T4 and T3 normalize within 4-6 weeks, much ahead of TSH.
- The median time of remission is 3-4 years.
- Drugs can be tapered and stopped if the is adequate response, but relapse is frequent. Hence life-long follow up is mandatory.
- Some experts prefer 'block-therapy'–suppression of T4 and T3 and supplementation of thyroxine along with anti-thyroid drugs.
- Drugs reactions are more commonly seen in children and adolescents compared to adults. These include erythematous rash, urticaria or granulocytopenia (<1500/mm^3). These are usually seen with carbimazole/methimazole and are dose-related.
- Most serious complication is agranulocytosis. This complication is more commonly seen within 3 months of starting the treatment. Lupus like syndrome and thrombocytopenia are rare. Medication should be discontinued if the granulocyte count is <1000 /mm^3. Hepatitis is commonly seen with PTU.

Surgery

- Near total thyroidectomy is preferred.
- **Indications:** Patients who have failed medical or radio-iodine treatment; who have markedly enlarged thyroid; and those with significant eye disease.
- Pretreatment with anti-thyroid medication for 4-6 weeks (for controlling the hyperthyroid state) and beta-antagonist followed by Lugol's iodine for 1-2 weeks are advised by some centers.
- Complications of surgery include transient hypocalcemia, hypoparathyroidism and recurrent laryngeal nerve palsy.
- Most of the patients become hypothyroid and require life-long thyroid replacement therapy.

Radioactive Iodine (RAI)

- **Indication:** Failure of drug therapy, or if the patient had a life-threatening adverse effect following drug therapy.
- Less commonly used in children below 8 years fearing proliferative effects of ionizing radiations.
- A dose of 50-250 μCi of ^{131} I/gram of thyroid tissue is used.
- Daily thyroxine administration is needed after radioiodine therapy.
- Worsening of ophthalmopathy is reported after RAI. Hence a course of corticosteroid is advised after the radiation for 6-8 weeks.

THYROID NEOPLASIA

- Thyroid malignancy is the third most common pediatric solid tumor (1% of all pediatric cancers) and most common pediatric endocrine malignancy.
- Girls are commonly affected (female to male ratio is 3:1).
- Unlike children, adolescents often seek consultation advice for a neck swelling in the form of goiter or lymph node enlargement.
- Tumors may arise from follicular or non-follicular epithelium.
- Major histologic types are papillary and follicular. 75% of thyroid neoplasia is constituted by papillary carcinoma.
- Another type of neoplasia is the medullary thyroid carcinoma arising from parafollicular C cells of the thyroid gland. They often occur as a part of multiple endocrine neoplasia (MEN) type 2.
- Nodular hyperplasia and follicular adenomas are other group of thyroid tumors.

Clinical Features

- Painless mass identified by routine examination or by the parent or patient.
- Characteristics of the swelling: Firm, rapid growth, fixation to skin, lack of movement while swallowing, cervical lymphadenopathy.

Investigations

- Thyroid function tests.
- Thyroglobulin levels: Elevated.
- Imaging (thyroid ultrasound): Multiple solid hypo-echogenic lesions with a peripheral halo are seen in benign tumors. Lesions with a thick or irregular halo are seen in malignant tumors.
- Thyroid scintigraphy: Most lesions show reduced uptake. Hyperfunctioning or "hot" nodules are usually malignant.
- Whole body scanning is helpful to assess metastatic disease.
- Fine needle aspiration cytology, cyst and biopsy help to confirm the pathology.

Management

- Total or near total thyroidectomy with cervical node resection is the treatment of choice.
- All adolescents should undergo radioiodine remnant ablation (^{131}I) for 4-6 weeks after thyroidectomy to destroy any remnant thyroid tumor tissue.
- Thyroid hormone replacement therapy should be started after radioiodine administration.
- Prognosis: Better with papillary of follicular and worse with anaplastic.

LEARNING POINTS

- Thyroid diseases are more common in girls.
- Onset of thyroid diseases is usually insidious and symptoms are non-specific. Hence high index of suspicion is required for early diagnosis.
- Majority of acquired thyroid disorders are of autoimmune etiology.
- Once diagnosed, dose increment should be gradual.
- Thyroxine replacement is the treatment option for hypothyroid conditions like autoimmune thyroiditis and they need life-long monitoring.
- Good compliance is essential for better outcome.
- Hyperthyroidism is a rare disorder and hence often missed.
- Graves' disease constitutes 90% of childhood and adolescent hyperthyroidism.
- For hyperthyroidism antithyroid drugs are the mainstay of treatment. Other treatment modalities are surgery and radioiodine.
- Always monitor for drug toxicities while the adolescent is on antithyroid drugs.
- For evaluating a thyroid nodule, FNAC and ultrasound are the best tools.
- Thyroid cancers require total thyroidectomy and radioablation.

SUGGESTED READING

1. Desai M. Hypothyroidism, Goiter and thyroid neoplasia. In; Desai MP, Menon PSN, Bhatia V, eds. Pediatric Endocrine Disorders, 3rd edition. Hyderabad; Universities Press 2014; 194-211.
2. Kumar S. Hyperthyroidism. In: Gupta P, Menon PSN, Ramji S, Lodha R, eds. PG Textbook of Pediatrics, 1st edition. New Delhi; Jaypee Publishers 2015; 2319-20.
3. Ravikumar K. Hypothyroidism in childhood and adolescence. In: Shah NS, Rao S, eds. IAP Subspeciality Series on Pediatric Endocrinology. New Delhi; Jaypee Medical Publishers 2013; 43-51.
4. Thomas I. Thyroid diseases. In: Jain V, Menon RK, eds. Case Based Reviews in Pediatric Endocrinology, 1st edition. New Delhi; Jaypee Publishers 2015; 49-56.
5. Zacharin M, Simon A. Thyroid disorders. In: Zacharin M, ed. Practical Pediatric Endocrinology in a Limited Resource Setting; 1st edition. Merck Serono; 2011; 56-78.

Diabetes Mellitus

5.6.2

PSN Menon, M Vijayakumar

INTRODUCTION

Diabetes mellitus is a heterogeneous group of disorders with different etiological and pathophysiological mechanisms, genetic patterns, age distribution, clinical features, management options and prognosis. All these group of disorders result in impairment of glucose tolerance and manifest as hyperglycemia.

The criteria for diagnosis of diabetes mellitus are given in Box 5.6.2.1. It is important to identify adolescents as early as possible in pre-diabetic stage as lifestyle modifications can slow down the progression of the disease and improve outcome. There is a tremendous economic burden of the disease on the society and the nation as reflected in global efforts to decrease disease burden.

Adolescent with diabetes have distinct characteristics that require different standards of care. The management of diabetes should take into consideration the major differences between children, adolescents and adults.

These include:

- Insulin doses based only on body size are likely to be incorrect.
- The consequences of hypoglycemia are distinctly different between children, adolescents and adults.
- The risks for diabetic complications are likely to be influenced by puberty.
- The targets of diabetes education need to be adjusted for an adolescent and must include the parent or caregiver.

Box 5.6.2.1: Diagnostic criteria for diabetes mellitus (American Diabetic Association 2013)

Diabetes mellitus

- Classic symptoms of diabetes with plasma glucose concentration > 200 mg/dl (>11.1 mmol/L)
- Fasting (no caloric intake for at least 8 hours) plasma glucose > 126 mg/dl (> 7.0 mmol/L)
- 2 hours post-load glucose > 200 mg/dl (11.1 mmol/L) during an oral glucose tolerance test (OGTT). (The test should be performed using a glucose load containing the equivalent of 1.75 g/kg to a maximum of 75 g of anhydrous glucose dissolved in water.)
- HbA1C >6.5%

Impaired glucose tolerance and impaired fasting glucose

- Impaired fasting glucose (IFG): Plasma fasting glucose level between 100-125 mg/dl
- Impaired glucose tolerance (IGT): 2 hours post-load glucose level between 140-200 mg/dl

TYPES OF DIABETES MELLITUS

These are listed in Table 5.6.2.1. Type 1 diabetes was in the past labelled as insulin-dependent diabetes or juvenile-onset diabetes. Classifying diabetes various types of diabetes according to their etiology helps to optimize management and follow-up to delay the onset of chronic complications. Type 1 and 2 diabetes account for most of the diabetes seen in adolescents.

The differentiating features between type 1 and 2 diabetes are given in Table 5.6.2.2. In general type 1 diabetics are ketosis-prone, lean, and present with weight loss. On the other hand type 2 diabetes is characterized by overt obesity with increased visceral fat, hypertension, acanthosis nigricans, dyslipidemia and in females, polycystic ovarian disease, which responds to oral hypoglycemic drugs. Other forms of diabetes are rare in adolescents.

TYPE 1 DIABETES MELLITUS

History Taking

The clinical presentation of type 1 diabetes is quite typical and is listed in Table 5.6.2.3.

Clinical Examination

- In most adolescents there may not be any specific features of diabetes at initial visit except loss of weight, abdominal pain and/or distension.
- Hepatomegaly may be present due to fatty infiltration of liver.

Table 5.6.2.1: Types of diabetes mellitus		
Type	*Etiology*	*Comments*
Type 1 diabetes mellitus	Beta cell destruction leading to absolute insulin deficiency • Type 1A: Autoimmune (90%)	• Characterized by severe insulin deficiency. • Affected adolescents have to depend on exogenous administration of insulin to preserve life. • Islet cell antibodies (ICA) and antibodies to glutamic acid decarboxylase 65 (GAD65) can be demonstrated at diagnosis. • Coexistence of other autoimmune diseases: Autoimmune thyroid disease, celiac disease, pernicious anemia, Addison disease and vitiligo.
	• Type 1 B: Idiopathic (10%)	• Markers of autoimmunity are not found.
Type 2 diabetes mellitus	• Insulin resistance with relative insulin deficiency	• Increasing incidence over the years because of the obesity epidemic. • Not completely insulin dependent initially. • Oral drugs like metformin are effective. • Onset and progression of symptoms slow. • Strong family history of type 2 diabetes.
Other specific types of diabetes mellitus	• Monogenic diabetes of the young (MODY)	• Mutations in one of several genes encoding enzymes or transcription factors important for islet cell development and insulin secretion results in diabetes. • They have a dominant mode of inheritance. • Six varieties of MODY each due to a single gene defect have been identified.
	• Mitochondrial diabetes	• Maternally inherited diabetes and deafness.
	• Genetic defects of insulin action	• Single gene mutations cause resistance to the action of insulin either by affecting the insulin receptor or by affecting adipose tissue development or function.
	• Endocrine disorders	• Cushing syndrome, acromegaly pheochromocytoma and hyperthyroidism. • Disease can be reversed by treatment of the primary endocrine disorder.
	• Diseases of exocrine pancreas	• Loss of pancreatic tissue due to disease, surgical removal, toxic damage or radiation. • Examples: Cystic fibrosis, fibrocalculous pancreatopathy and pancreatitis.
	• Drug or chemical induced	• Glucocorticoids, thiazide, diazoxide and L-asparaginase.
	• Infections	• Congenital rubella, cytomegalovirus, adenovirus, mumps, Epstein-Barr virus and rotavirus.
	• Other genetic syndromes sometimes associated with diabetes	• Down syndrome, Klinefelter syndrome, Turner syndrome, Prader-Willi syndrome. • Diagnosis can be established by clinical and genetic studies.
Gestational diabetes mellitus (GDM)	• Diagnosed by a 75 g OGTT done at 24–28 weeks of gestation	• Higher birth weight increases risk of overweight in adolescence. • Being born to a mother with GDM is associated with increased adolescent overweight.

- Signs of dehydration may be present.
- There may be evidences of associated infections.
- There may be evidence of ketosis with air hunger (Kussmaul breathing) due to metabolic acidosis with acetone odor of breath.
- Breathlessness in the absence of any respiratory and cardiovascular findings should alert the physician to the possibility of diabetes.
- It is not uncommon to see an adolescent with progressive drowsiness, shock and coma due to diabetic ketoacidosis.

Management

Management of newly diagnosed type 1 diabetes requires a team approach with the primary care physician or pediatrician/pediatric endocrinologist, dietician, clinical psychologist and diabetes educator to provide up-to-date adolescent-specific diabetes education and support. The diabetes nurse educator is the core member of the team who with the physician and dietician manages the patient with frequent contacts with the patient and monitoring therapy. Adolescents with diabetes ideally should wear identification tags indicating that they have diabetes.

Table 5.6.2.2: Differentiating clinical features of type 1 and type 2 diabetes mellitus

Features	*Type 1 diabetes mellitus*	*Type 2 diabetes mellitus*
Age group	Any age group; common in children	Second decade (> 10 years)
Family history of diabetes	< 10% have family history	Common
HLA DR3/DR4 association	Common	Not present
Clinical presentation	Usually acute; may present as DKA	Usually insidious, rarely present as DKA
Insulin autoantibodies	Positive	Negative
Obesity	Uncommon; usually lean	Common
Features of metabolic syndrome	Rare	Common; usually present during initial diagnosis
Acanthosis nigricans	Rare	Common
C-peptide levels	Low	Normal or high
Islet cell antibodies (ICA)	> 85%	< 5%
Treatment	Insulin–universal requirement	Metformin with or without insulin

Table 5.6.2.3: Clinical features of type 1 diabetes mellitus in adolescents

Diabetes mellitus should be suspected if an adolescent presents with the following symptoms:

- Classical triad of polyuria, polydipsia and polyphagia
- General weakness, lethargy and weight loss despite good food intake
- Recent onset of nocturia or enuresis
- Polyuria despite dehydration
- Recurrent or persistent genital fungal infections (vaginal candidiasis)
- Recurrent urinary tract infections
- Persisting pruritus
- Blurring of vision
- Recurrent abdominal pain with no focus of etiology
- Progressive worsening of sensorium and development of coma

Box 5.6.2.2: Principles of insulin therapy

- Insulin must be started as soon as possible after the diagnosis (preferably within 6 hours if ketonuria is present) to prevent metabolic decompensation and ketoacidosis (DKA).
- Since in our body, insulin is secreted in the basal state and also after each meal, insulin replacement should mimic this basal-bolus secretion.
- Intensive insulin regimen is always preferred.
- Commonly used basal insulins are NPH and insulin analogs (glargine and detemir).
- Rapid acting or bolus insulins are regular insulin, and rapid acting analogs (aspart, lispro and glulisine).
- Premixed insulin is not preferred for type 1 diabetes.

Insulin Therapy

Parenteral insulin is the only treatment option for type 1 diabetes. The principles of insulin therapy are outlined in Box 5.6.2.2.

Table 5.6.2.4 highlights the various types of insulin preparations available in India and their action profile. Table 5.6.2.5 provides the general guidelines for insulin therapy in adolescents with type 1 diabetes using various regimens such as basal-bolus, split-mix or insulin pumps.

The precautions to be taken while using insulin are given in Table 5.6.2.6.

Assessment and Monitoring

Monitoring of glycemic control is the cornerstone in the management of diabetes.

- In adolescents need close monitoring because they may manipulate the results.
- Monitoring includes daily home monitoring of glucose as well as periodic monitoring of overall glycemic status.

Table 5.6.2.4: Types of insulin preparation and their action profile

Insulin type	*Onset of action (hours)*	*Peak action (hours)*	*Duration of action (hours)*
Rapid acting analogs – Ultra-short acting (Aspart, Glulisine, Lispro)	0.15–0.30	1–3	3–5
Regular–Short acting	0.30–1	2–4	5–8
NPH	2–4	4–12	12–24
Long acting analogs –			
Glargine	2–4	None	24
Detemir	1–2	6–12	20–24
Degludec	1–2	None	>24

Table 5.6.2.5: Guidelines for insulin therapy

Type of regime	*Principles*	*Comments*
Basal-bolus regimen	• Total insulin is calculated initially. • To begin with the total daily dose is calculated as 0.5–1 units/kg body weight. • During adolescent period, requirement increases to 1–2 units/kg. Insulin requirements are usually based on body weight, age and pubertal status. • Further adjustment of the dose is based on blood glucose values.	• About 40–50% of the total dose is given as basal insulin (NPH or basal analogs). • Basal insulins are given at bedtime and in the morning (twice daily). • Glargine can be given once daily also. • The rest is given as pre-prandial regular or rapid acting (bolus) insulin in divided doses. • Regular insulin should be given 20–30 minutes before each main meal (breakfast, lunch and dinner). • Rapid acting insulin analogs can be given immediately before meals. • In rare circumstances, it can be given immediately after meals also. • Insulin dose should be adjusted to glucose levels, meal content and physical activity
Split-mix regimen	Fixed doses of intermediate and short acting insulin given at regular intervals.	• This include twice daily regimen (morning and evening) with a mixture of NPH and regular insulin. • 2/3rd of the total dose is taken as NPH and remaining as regular insulin. • 2/3rd of the total dose is given before breakfast and 1/3rd in evening.
Continuous subcutaneous insulin infusion (CSII) or insulin pump	Insulin pump is a physiological form of insulin replacement therapy.	• Newer generation pumps even calculate the dose based on insulin–carbohydrate ratios. • Treatment may be hazardous when education and adherence to therapy are not adequate.

- Accurate monitoring will help in reducing the risks of short-term complications (e.g. hypoglycemia and DKA), as well as chronic complications (e.g. microvascular and macrovascular diseases).
- Measurement of glycemic status is done by self-monitoring of blood glucose (SMBG), which will provide immediate documentation of blood glucose status.
- Continuous glucose monitoring (CGM) enables a more real-time monitoring of blood glucose values and is being increasingly used often along with CSII.
- HbA1C predicts long-term microvascular and macrovascular complications.

Details of self-monitoring of blood glucose, urinary or blood ketones and HbA1C are given in Table 5.6.2.7.

Table 5.6.2.6: Precautions while using insulin
• Insulin is available as vials and pen (cartridges).
• Insulin vials are available in different strengths, 100 Units/ml (U 100) and 40 Units/ml (U 40).
• Different types of syringes are also present.
• If you are using 100 U insulin vials, you should use only 100 U syringes (and vice versa).
• Regular insulin should be drawn first in the syringe. It should not be mixed too much.
• Insulin vials should not be kept in room temperature while not in use.
• Direct sunlight and hot climate may damage insulin.
• Unused insulin should be stored in refrigerator at 4–8°C. It should never be frozen.
• Insulin that has changed its physical appearance should be discarded.
• Abdomen, front and lateral aspects of the thigh and lateral aspects of upper arm are the preferred sites for insulin administration.
• Rotation of injection sites should be practiced to prevent lipoatrophy or hypertrophy.
• All aseptic precautions should be followed during injections to avoid infections and lipohypertrophy (Figure 5.6.2.1).

Table 5.6.2.7: Self-monitoring of blood glucose, urinary or blood ketones and HbA1C
Self-Monitoring of Blood Glucose (SMBG):
• It should be done at bed time and prior to meals and 2 hours after each major meal. • It should also be done frequently if hypoglycemia is suspected, and during exercise and during intercurrent illness. • The target should be to maintain blood glucose value between 70–150 mg/dl. • A dairy should be maintained and the readings should be verified both by the parents and the treating physician.
Urinary or Blood Ketones:
• Measurement of urinary or blood ketones should be done during impending ketoacidosis, sick days, or during episodes of uncontrolled hyperglycemia. • High urinary/blood ketone levels in the presence of hyperglycemia are suggestive of insulin deficiency and the patient is at risk for metabolic decompensations like ketoacidosis. • Urine ketone testing (which assesses acetone) is less specific than blood tests (which assess β-hydroxybutyrate). Blood ketone level < 0.6 mmol/L is normal and > 3.0 mmol/L is associated with acidosis.
HbA1C:
• It measures the glycemic status over the preceding 4–12 weeks. • A target of < 7.5% is recommended for young diabetics (< 18 years). • Lower the HbA1C values, fewer and more delayed will be the long-term complications.

Medical Nutritional Therapy

Nutritional advice should be individualized. The help of a trained dietician should be sought. Monitor weight and height regularly and maintain appropriate measurements. The basic principles are summarized in Box 5.6.2.3.

Physical Activity

Physical activity is an important aspect of management of diabetes. Adjustments to be made to the diet and insulin dose are given on Box 5.6.2.4.

Management During Sick Days

It is a common practice to omit insulin when the young diabetic is sick and not eating properly. But most illnesses associated with fever actually raise the blood sugar level because of higher levels of stress hormones promoting gluconeogenesis and insulin resistance. Chance of ketone body production is more in such young diabetics, making them more prone for DKA. Hence golden rule is "do not stop insulin when the young diabetic is sick". See Table 5.6.2.8 for details.

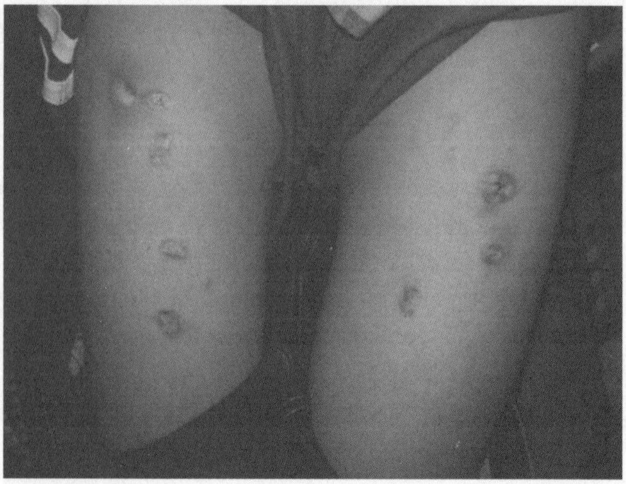

Figure 5.6.2.1: A boy with type 1 diabetes with scars of infected injection sites

Box 5.6.2.3: Nutritional advice for diabetic adolescents – basic principles

- Food, especially carbohydrate, is one of the major influences on blood sugar levels.
- There is no "ideal diabetic diet".
- Ideal diet should help the young diabetic to attain normal growth and development and at the same time, should prevent the young diabetic from major complications like hypoglycemia and hyperglycemia.
- It should also help them to avoid long-term complications.
- While selecting a "meal plan" the following should be kept in mind:
  - Food should contain optimum amount of both macro- and micronutrients (balanced diet).
  - Avoid food rich in salts.
  - Avoid simple sugars.
  - Reduce cholesterol and saturated fat intake.
  - Increase fiber intake.
- Conventionally meals are divided into 3 major (breakfast, lunch and dinner) and 3 minor (snacks) meals (mid-morning, afternoon, and at bed time).
- Meals should be taken at the same time each day.
- Consistency and regularity is the key for euglycemia.
- Balance carbohydrate intake and insulin dose carefully:
  - In the constant carbohydrate meal plan, the amount of carbohydrate is kept about the same for each meal and snack.
  - Carbohydrate exchange list should be taught based on the locally available food pattern.
  - Carbohydrate counting meal plan involves counting the gram of carbohydrate to be eaten for a matching dose of insulin. It allows greater freedom and flexibility in food choices.
  - Insulin carbohydrate ratio is calculated by dividing 500 with total units of insulin used per day (500/total daily insulin = the rule of 500). If it is say 15, it means that one unit of insulin for every 15 grams of carbohydrate. This should be adjusted based on blood glucose levels.
  - Generally food with low glycemic index is preferred over those with high glycemic index.
- Parents should be taught about exchange meal plan.

Complications

Type 1 diabetes is associated with both short and long-term complications as a result of the disease and often due to treatment. Patient and family characteristics predicting difficulty with diabetes management should be sought and addressed. The adolescent should be encouraged to gradually assume greater responsibility for diabetes management tasks.

Box 5.6.2.5 highlights the features of hypoglycemia, the most common acute complication seen in type 1 diabetes.

Box 5.6.2.4: Adjustments during exercise

- Adolescents should be encouraged to participate in regular sports activities and exercise programs which will increase their insulin sensitivity.
- Certain precautions and preparations should be carried out before planning exercise.
- Any form of exercise should be avoided if blood glucose levels are > 250 mg/dl especially if there is associated ketonemia.

- It is recommended to reduce the rapid acting insulin before exercise.
- A carbohydrate diet is given one hour prior to the event.
- If the activity is of longer duration (more than 60 minutes), a snack in the interval time or immediately after the exercise will prevent an attack of hypoglycemia.
- Since the chance of nocturnal hypoglycemia is high after exercise, bed time blood glucose measurement is a must and if found to be low, a bed time snack and reduction of evening insulin is advised.

Table 5.6.2.8: Sick day guidelines for adolescent diabetics

- More frequent (every 2 hours) blood glucose monitoring and ketone body estimation are warranted in adolescents who are sick.
- Normal fluid and water balance should be maintained.
- If the young diabetic has hyperglycemia, short or rapid acting insulin should be given in a dose of 0.05–0.1 U/kg every 2–4 hourly according to blood glucose response.
- If s/he has elevated ketones and is in impending DKA, the insulin dose should be doubled (0.1–0.2 U/kg).
- Aim of the treatment is to keep the blood glucose level within 80–150 mg/dl.
- Some infections like gastroenteritis are associated with hypoglycemia. Careful management to keep the fluid and electrolyte balance should be undertaken.
- If blood glucose levels are low, insulin can be reduced.
- Patients with severe hypoglycemia may require mini glucagon injection (0.15 mg).

Box 5.6.2.5: Acute complications: Hypoglycemia

- Hypoglycemia is the most common acute complication. In clinical practice, a glucose value below 70 mg/dl (3.9 mmol/L) is used as the threshold value for initiating treatment.
- Hypoglycemic events are classified as symptomatic and asymptomatic.
- Main clinical features are tremor; sweating or increased heart beat (adrenergic activation), headache, drowsiness or loss of consciousness (neuroglycopenia).
- A hypoglycemic episode can be precipitated by excess dose of insulin, missed meals or increased physical activity.
- In adolescent group, alcohol ingestion should be enquired.
- Adolescents with severe hypoglycemia (hypoglycemia associated with seizure and loss of consciousness) should be admitted and treated with intravenous glucose (10% glucose 2–3 ml/kg).
- Inj glucagon in a dose of 1 mg given IM/SC is also effective.
- Milder events should be treated with oral glucose (10–15 g). This should be followed by additional carbohydrates to prevent recurrence.
- Blood glucose should be re-checked 10–15 minutes after an episode.
- Food with high fat content is not preferred for treatment since fat will decrease the absorption of glucose.

Diabetic Ketoacidosis (DKA)

DKA is a life threatening acute complication of type 1 diabetes. It is a common initial presentation because of late diagnosis. It can also happen to a young diabetic already on treatment when insulin dose is omitted or during an episode of intercurrent illness. Incidence of DKA is very high in adolescents. Some management aspects of DKA are given in Table 5.6.2.9.

Long-Term Complications

- Lipodystrophy is a common complication following insulin therapy. Both lipoatrophy and lipohypertrophy occur following human insulins.
- Limited joint mobility (LJM) is a bilateral painless contracture of finger joints and large joints with tight skin. The patient has difficulty in approximating the palmar surfaces of interphalangeal joints resulting in the characteristic 'prayer sign' (Figure 5.6.2.2).
- The long-term vascular complications include retinopathy, nephropathy, neuropathy, and macro-vascular diseases, the latter leading to cardiac diseases, stroke and peripheral vascular diseases.

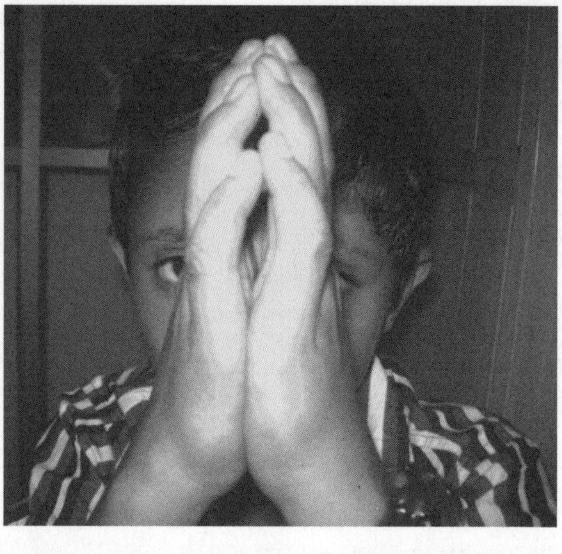

Fig 5.6.2.2: "Prayer sign", bilateral painless contracture of finger joints, a complication of type 1 diabetes due to limited joint mobility

- Improvement in glycemic control is the most important factor which will reduce the risk of onset and progression of vascular complications.

The schema for screening for long-term complications is given in Table 5.6.2.10.

Table 5.6.2.9: Management of DKA in adolescents

Biochemical Criteria for DKA
- Hyperglycemia (blood glucose > 200 mg/dl or 11 mmol/L
- Acidosis (venous pH < 7.3) or bicarbonate < 15 mmol/L
- Ketonemia and ketonuria

Clinical Features of DKA

The patient presents with dehydration, vomiting, respiratory distress, deep sighing respiration (Kussmaul respiration), tachycardia, abdominal pain, drowsiness or unconsciousness.

Principles of Management
- Correction of dehydration is of paramount importance and should be initiated even before insulin administration.
- Estimated fluid deficit should be replaced evenly for 48 hours.
- Volume expansion should be initiated with 0.9% saline, in the dose of 10–20 ml/kg over 1-2 hours.
- Subsequent deficit replacement is given for 4–6 hours.
- Deficit replacement after 6 hours is done with a solution with 0.45% saline.
- Insulin therapy is started 1–2 hours after initiation of fluid replacement in the dose of 0.05–0.1 U/kg/hr.
- Potassium replacement should be started if the patient is not hyperkalemic and good urine output is documented. It should be given with 20–40 mmol/L of infusate.
- Once the ketosis is controlled, IV insulin should be changed to subcutaneous basal-bolus regimen.

Table 5.6.2.10: Schema for screening for long-term complications

Complications	*Time of screening*	*Screening methods*	*Possible intervention*
Retinopathy	Annually after 10 years	Ophthalmoscopy or fundal photography	Laser therapy
Nephropathy	Annually after 10 years	Urine microalbuminuria, albumin creatinine ratio	Angiotensin converting enzyme inhibitors (ACEI) or angiotensin receptor blockers (ARB)
Neuropathy	Annually	History and physical examination	–
Macrovascular diseases	Annually after 10 years	Blood pressure, lipid profile	Control hypertension, statins
Screening for other autoimmune diseases	Annual	Thyroid, celiac disease	

Psychological Issues

- Adolescents with diabetes have a greater incidence of depression, anxiety, and other psychological problems compared to other age groups.
- Young diabetics with poor metabolic control are more likely to have these complications.
- Those with frequent hypoglycemic attacks have higher incidence of learning problems and scholastic backwardness.
- These young diabetics require more social and psychological support.
- Patient and family characteristics which predict difficulty with diabetes management should be sought and addressed.

For other psychological issues associated with chronic illnesses please see Chapter 1.3.

TYPE 2 DIABETES MELLITUS

Type 2 diabetes has become a major concern in younger age including adolescents, mainly because of increasing incidence of obesity in this age group. Obesity leads to metabolic syndrome, details of which are given in Chapters 3.3 and 3.4 (see Figure 5.6.2.3).

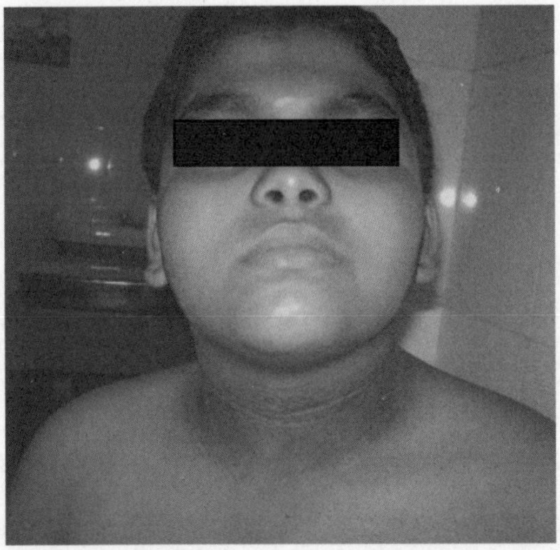

Figure 5.6.2.3: An adolescent with type 2 diabetes. His father is a known diabetic. Note acanthosis nigricans around neck

The usual age of presentation is during second decade, usually between 12–15 years, which is the age of peak physiological insulin resistance. A strong family history of type 2 diabetes is common in these young diabetics. Routine testing for autoantibodies should be done since a small percentage of type 1 diabetes may be obese at presentation. Lab tests should include fasting lipid profile, liver enzymes and an ultrasonography of abdomen.

An integrated approach, including lifestyle modification should be initiated along with drug therapy at the very beginning of treatment. Metabolically stable infants (HbA1C <9%) with no symptoms should be started on metformin monotherapy. Young diabetics, who are not stable, require insulin therapy along with metformin.

These young diabetics should be regularly assessed for other co-morbid conditions. Urine albumin-creatinine ratio (ACR) should be done at the time of diagnosis and then every year. If this is abnormal, angiotensin-converting enzyme inhibitors (ACEI) should be initiated.

MONOGENIC DIABETES

Among adolescents with diabetes, monogenic diabetes represents a small group (1–2%). A variety of monogenic diabetes is called as maturity onset diabetes in young (MODY). This group of diseases results from single gene defects and is often inherited as dominant or recessive fashion or as a non-Mendelian manner. Many cases occur as de-novo mutation. In young diabetics, majority of cases result from mutations in genes causing beta cell dysfunction or mutations resulting in severe insulin resistance.

Most cases of monogenic diabetes are initially diagnosed as having type 1 or type 2 diabetes. Usual pattern is a familial form of diabetes with milder clinical features compared to type 1 diabetes. Islet cell antibodies are absent in these young diabetics. In some young diabetics it may mimic type 2 diabetes. If adolescents present with clinical features suggestive of type 2 diabetes without obesity, acanthosis nigricans and features of metabolic syndrome, and with a strong family history of diabetes monogenic diabetes should be suspected.

Common subtypes of MODY in adolescents are described in Table 5.6.2.11.

Table 5.6.2.11: Common subtypes of MODY in adolescents

Gene defect	*Locus*	*Clinical features*	*Glycemic pattern*	*Management*
HNF1A	12q24.2	Renal glycosuria	Postprandial hyperglycemia initially, progressing to general hyperglycemia	Sulphonylurea
HNF1B	17q12	Renal developmental abnormalities, genital tract malformations	Postprandial hyperglycemia initially, progressing to general hyperglycemia	Insulin
HNF4A	20q13.12	Macrosomia, Fanconi syndrome	Postprandial hyperglycemia initially, progressing to general hyperglycemia	Sulphonylurea
GCK	7p15.3-p15.1	Mild asymptomatic hyperglycemia	Stable, mild fasting hyperglycemia	Diet control

LEARNING POINTS

- Type 1 diabetes accounts for > 90% of cases of diabetes in adolescents. Type 2 diabetes is being increasingly diagnosed now.
- Lifelong insulin injections and strict monitoring of blood sugar are essential for survival.
- Basal-bolus regime is the most accepted regime for good glycemic control.
- Hypoglycemia (blood glucose < 70 mg/dl) is the most common acute complication of type 1 diabetes.
- Diabetic ketoacidosis is the most common cause of death in young diabetics.
- Continuous insulin infusion with adequate hydration is the standard of care for young diabetics with DKA.
- Metformin is the only approved oral antidiabetic drug for management of Type 2 diabetes in young diabetics and adolescents.

SUGGESTED READING

1. Brink SJ, Rhen W, Lee W. Diabetes in young children and adolescents; CDIC Training Manual, 2011.
2. Craig ME, Jefferies C, Dabelea D, Balde N, Seth A, Donaghue KC. Definition, epidemiology, and classification of diabetes in young children and adolescents. Pediatric Diabetes 2014:15 (Suppl. 20): 4-17.
3. Irani A. Type 1 Diabetes. In: Gupta P, Menon PSN, Ramji S, Lodha R, Eds. PG Textbook of Pediatrics, 1st edition. New Delhi; Jaypee Publishers 2015: 2378-83.
4. Irani AJ, Menon PSN, Bhatia V. Type 1 diabetes mellitus in young children and adolescents in India. Clinical Practice Guidelines 2011. Indian Society for Pediatric and Adolescent Endocrinology. Lucknow; Army Printing Press, 2011.
5. Kordonouri O, Klingensmith G, Knip M, Holl RW, Aanstoot HJ, Menon PS, Craig ME; International Society for Pediatric and Adolescent Diabetes. ISPAD Clinical Practice Consensus Guidelines 2014. Other complications and diabetes-associated conditions in children and adolescents. Pediatric Diabetes 2014;15(Suppl. 20):270-78.
6. Menon PSN, Bajpai A. Diabetes mellitus in adolescents. In: Bhave SY, Parthasarathy A, Nair MKC, Menon PSN, Eds. Bhave's Textbook of Adolescent Medicine, First edition. New Delhi: Jaypee Brothers Medical Publishers Pvt. Ltd. 2006; 363-75.
7. Rubio-Cabezas O, Hattersley AT, Njølstad PR, Mlynarski W, Ellard S, White N, Chi DV, Craig ME. The diagnosis and management of monogenic diabetes in young children and adolescents. Pediatric Diabetes 2014:15(Suppl. 20):47-64.
8. Silverstein J, Klingensmith G, Copeland K, *et al.* care of children and adolescents with type 1 diabetes. A statement of the American Diabetes Association. Diabetes Care 2005;28(1):186-212.
9. Svovren BM, Jospe N. Type 2 Diabetes Mellitus. In: Kliegman RM, Stanton BMD, St Geme J, Schor NF, Eds. Nelson Textbook of Pediatrics, 20th edition. New Delhi; Elsevier India Ltd 2015; 2783-86.

Hematological Problems 5.7

Bharat R Agarwal, Vinod Gunasekaran

INTRODUCTION

This chapter does not cover all the hematological manifestations that can present in the adolescent age group, but will be covering those that are commonly seen in the adolescent age group e.g. nutritional deficiency anemias, thalassemia, aplastic anemia, thrombocytopenia and systemic illnesses with hematological manifestations. Adolescents may present with inherited hematological disorders for the first time or may come to a pediatrician with adolescent specific complications of conditions present since childhood e.g. thalassemia major, hemophilia, Fanconi anemia etc. Some inherited hematological conditions may manifest only in adolescence e.g. MYH9 related thrombocytopenia syndromes, gray platelet syndrome, Wiskott-Aldrich syndrome and X-linked thrombocytopenia. A meticulous clinical approach is essential to reach a correct diagnosis and manage these adolescents appropriately (see Table 5.7.1).

Hematological manifestations may come along with specific disorders or with many disorders. Both infectious and non-infectious disorders can have derangements in hematological parameters and at times, these may be the initial presenting features. Some of them are shown in Table 5.7.2.

Deficiency of iron, folic acid and vitamin B12 are the major causes of nutritional anemia, of which iron deficiency is the most common cause in adolescents. WHO cut-offs are provided in Table 5.7.3. Important aspects in adolescents are covered in Boxes 5.7.1 and 5.7.2.

HISTORY TAKING

Approach to anemia in adolescents is outlined in Figure 5.7.1.

Iron Deficiency Anemia

- Weakness, excess lethargy, dizziness, exercise intolerance, pagophagia and exertional dyspnea are some of the initial presenting features.
- Ringing in ears, taste disturbances and restless leg syndrome are other known symptoms.

Table 5.7.1: Special features of various hematological diseases in adolescents

Disease	*Unusual presentation in adolescents*	*Specific points to remember in investigations and management*	*Prognosis as compared to pediatric or adults*
Immune thrombocytopenia (ITP)	Collagen disorders must be ruled out in all adolescents.	If there are atypical features like fever, bone pains or tenderness, pallor, lymphadenopathy, arthritis, enlarged testes or organomegaly, one should always doubt the diagnosis of ITP. Chronic ITP should be evaluated for autoimmune diseases (DCT, ANA and dsDNA tests), immunodeficiency (immunoglobulin levels) and chronic viral infections (HIV).	Chances of long-term remission in adolescents are much less as compared to ITP in children.
Bleeding disorders	Moderate (factor level 1–5%) and severe (factor level <1%) varieties usually manifest in early childhood. However, certain milder variants may be detected during adolescence incidentally on preoperative evaluation or with menorrhagia or milder bleeds.	Mild variety (factor level 5–40%) develop severe bleeding only with major trauma or surgery.	Prognosis remains the same.

Table 5.7.2: Hematological manifestations of systemic diseases

Systemic diseases	*Hematological manifestations*
Malaria	1. Anemia (may be severe and fatal in complicated cases) - Hemolysis (intravascular and immune-complex mediated) - Hypersplenism - Decreased erythrocyte deformability - Defective marrow response 2. Coagulation abnormalities 3. Thrombocytopenia
Kala azar	1. Anemia (hemolysis) 2. Pancytopenia (due to hypersplenism) 3. Bone marrow hyperplastic with dyserythropoietic changes 4. LD bodies in bone marrow 5. Erythrophagocytosis
Tuberculosis	1. Normocytic normochromic anemia 2. ESR elevated 3. Bone marrow–granuloma formation 4. White blood cells (WBC) and platelets–decreased or increased 5. Hemophagocytosis
Hookworm infestation	1. Iron deficiency anemia 2. Eosinophilia
Human immunodeficiency virus (HIV) infection	1. Thrombocytopenia 2. Microangiopathic hemolytic anemia 3. Lymphopenia 4. Pancytopenia 5. Lymphoma
Celiac disease	1. Iron deficiency anemia 2. Megaloblastic anemia 3. Pancytopenia 4. Coagulopathy (vitamin K malabsorption) 5. Gastrointestinal (GI) blood losses
Dengue	1. Hemoconcentration 2. Thrombocytopenia 3. Disseminated intravascular coagulation
Snake bite	1. Consumptive coagulopathy 2. Thrombocytopenia 3. Intravascular hemolysis

Table 5.7.3: Cut-off values given by WHO for classification of anemia

Reference group	*Cut-off (mg/dL)*	*Cut-off for categories of anemia (mg/dL)*		
		Mild	*Moderate*	*Severe*
Pregnant women	11	10-11	7-9.9	<7
Non-pregnant women	12	10-11.9	8-9.9	<8
Men	13	11-12.9	8-10.9	<8
Children 6–59 months of age	11	10-10.9	7-9.9	<7
Children 5–11 years of age	11.5	11-11.4	8-10.9	<8
Children 12–14 years of age	12	11-11.9	8-10.9	<8

CLINICAL EXAMINATION

Iron Deficiency Anemia

- Paleness of palms and mucosa on examination are used for screening, though they have low sensitivity and specificity.
- Other signs include brittle and flattened or spoon shaped nails (koilonychia), angular stomatitis and glossitis. Cardiac flow murmurs and tachycardia are seen in severe anemia (Hb <5 g/dL).

Box 5.7.1: Important aspects of iron deficiency in adolescents

- Adolescent girls become a high risk group for nutritional anemia due to increased requirements (corresponding to rapid growth in body mass) and due to increased losses (menstruation, worm infestations).
- These factors are compounded by poor dietary intake (vegetarian diet), poverty, incidence of adolescent pregnancies, chronic infections, etc.
- Absorption of heme iron in meat and fish is better (15%) as compared to that in vegetarian diet (5%). Presence of phytates and polyphenol further inhibits the absorption.
- Excessive consumption of bovine milk (low iron content, blood loss from milk protein colitis) is an important predisposing factor among younger children.
- Other rare causes to be considered especially in cases refractory to therapy include conditions with occult blood losses from gastrointestinal tract (GIT) like peptic ulcer, Meckel diverticulum, polyp, hemangioma, chronic diseases like inflammatory bowel disease; alternative diagnosis (thalassemia trait, and other nutritional deficiencies), or rarely pulmonary hemosiderosis.
- Though seemingly benign, long-term consequences include decreased exercise capacity, depressed immune function, impaired cognitive function, decreased scholastic performance and compromised physical growth.
- Iron deficiency also increases lead and cadmium absorption.
- In pregnancy, it leads to prematurity and fetal growth retardation.

Prevention

- Efforts to reduce the prevalence of iron deficiency anemia have been highly unsuccessful. The reasons have been multifactorial.
- The Centers for Disease Control and Prevention (CDC) recommends annual screening for anemia among all females with high risk factors and 5 yearly in the absence of risk factors.
- National Nutritional Anemia Prophylaxis Program is operational in India, targeting population from 6 months to 18 years of age, pregnant and nursing women. It aims at providing oral iron supplementation for 100 days per year in this vulnerable population in age appropriate doses.

Box 5.7.2: Important aspects of megaloblastic anemia

- Decreased nutritional intake–Strict vegetarian diet high risk for B12 deficiency.
- Folate deficiency in pregnant mothers leads to neural tube defects in their babies.
- Infants born to mothers with B12 deficiency develop symptoms early in life.
- Decreased endogenous B12 production due to lifestyle changes.
- Other causes: Pernicious anemia due to intrinsic factor deficiency, malabsorption resulting in folate deficiency (celiac disease, giardiasis) and certain inborn errors of metabolism e.g., methylmalonicaciduria (B12 deficiency) and methylenetetrahydrofolate reductase deficiency (folate).

Prevention

- The RDA for folate in 14–18 years old adolescents is 400 μg daily.
- Folate has been added to iron in supplementation programs especially because of the neurodevelopmental side effects.
- Strict vegetarians can be given daily supplements (>2 μg B12 daily) or food fortification to prevent B12 deficiency.

Megaloblastic Anemia

- Hyperpigmentation of knuckles and terminal phalanges (seen commonly in Asian population) and hepatosplenomegaly.
- Adolescents and adults may develop megaloblastic madness (depression, mania, delusions, etc), altered mental status and cognitive decline.
- Paresthesia and loss of proprioception are also seen.
- Cognitive decline and neurological sequelae may persist despite treatment.
- High level of homocysteine seen in this condition is a risk factor for coronary artery disease.

INVESTIGATIONS

Iron Deficiency Anemia

Measurement of hemoglobin concentration in blood by finger prick is a useful method to screen high risk population for anemia. However, a diagnosis of iron deficiency anemia is made based on a list of parameters as mentioned below:

- Hemoglobin (less than the recommended cut-offs for different age groups as mentioned in Table 5.7.1)
- Mean corpuscular volume <82 fL
- Red cell distribution width (RDW) >14%
- Transferrin saturation <16%

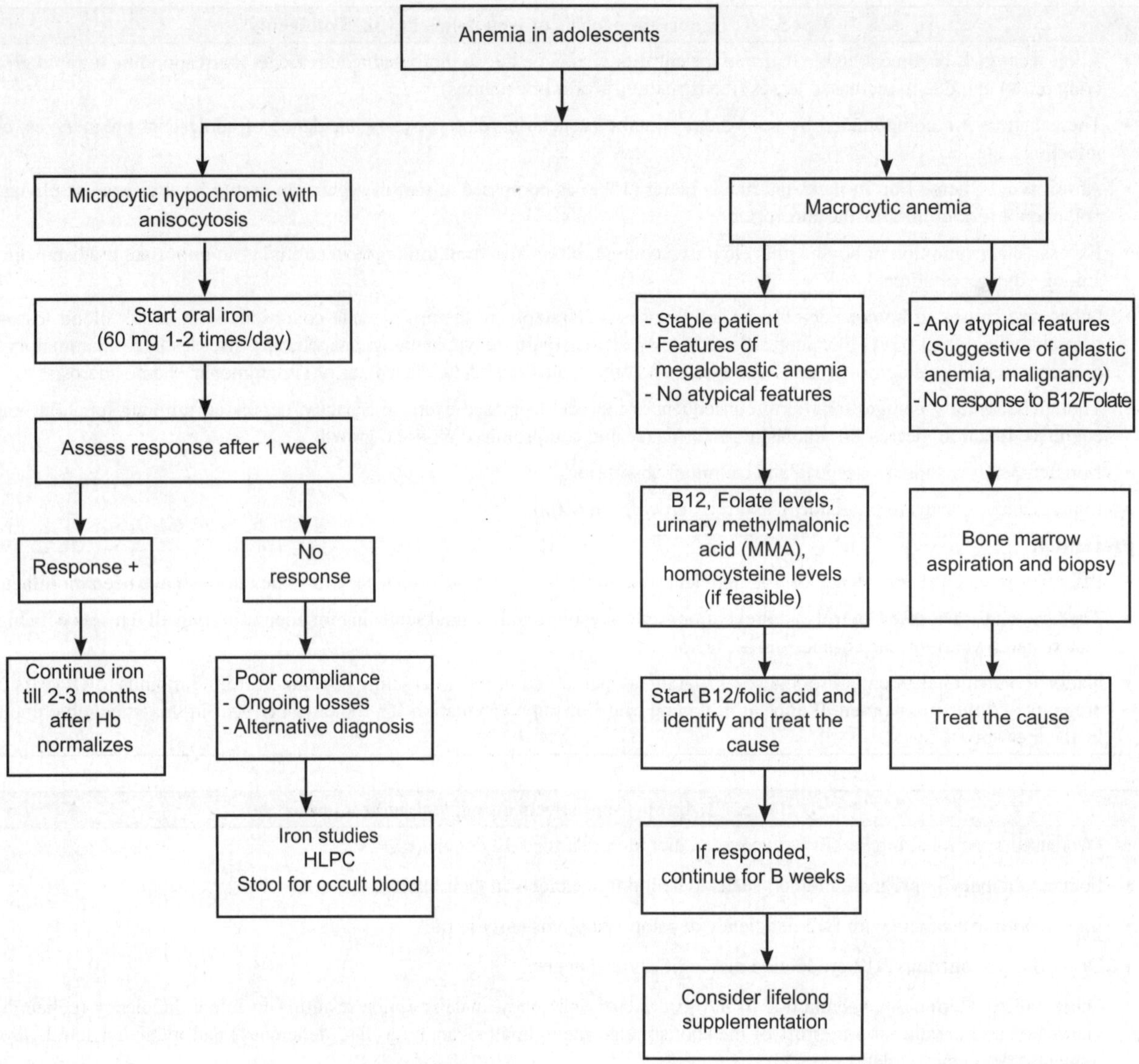

Figure 5.7.1: Approach to anemia

- Serum ferritin <15 μg/L (<12 in children <5 years of age) in the absence of infection
- Serum transferrin receptor concentration (TfR) >8.5 mg/L
- Free erythrocyte protoporphyrin (FEP) >70 μg/dL

The hematological manifestations of folate and B12 deficiency are similar.

- Macrocytic anemia, bicytopenia and pancytopenia.
- Presentation may mimic aplastic anemia and acute leukemia.
- Hypersegmented neutrophil in peripheral smear is a known feature.
- LDH and liver enzymes may be elevated.
- Serum or red cell levels of vitamin B12 and folate identify the deficiencies. However, the availability, cost, fluctuating levels and influence of hepatic dysfunction make the measurement of levels cumbersome. Reliable and feasible surrogate markers are identified.
- Increased serum homocysteine levels are seen in B12 and folate deficiency.
- Increased urinary level of methylmalonic acid (MMA) is considered diagnostic of B12 deficiency. FIGLU test is found to be specific for folate deficiency.
- Bone marrow aspiration in not required, but if done, shows hypercellular marrow with megaloblastic changes.

TREATMENT

Microcytic Hypochromic Anemia

Even in the absence of detailed iron studies, any adolescent with microcytic hypochromic anemia with elevated RDW should be given a trial of oral iron therapy. Response to therapy supports the presumptive diagnosis of iron deficiency anemia.

Elemental iron 60 mg 1–time daily is the usual treatment. Intermittent instead of daily iron has also been found to be an effective means with improved tolerance. It is absorbed in duodenum which is better in acidic environment and in the presence of vitamin C, copper and zinc. Calcium, magnesium and phosphorus impair the absorption. If intolerance is an issue, iron can be given after food or at bed time. Avoid taking multivitamins containing calcium and phosphorus together with iron.

The response after starting oral iron therapy is shown in Table 5.7.4.

Table 5.7.4: Response after initiating iron supplementation

Time since initiating iron	*Response*
12-24 hours	Subjective improvement and increased appetite
36-48 hours	Bone marrow showing erythroid hyperplasia
48-72 hours	Reticulocytosis (peaking at 5-7 days)
4-30 days	Increase in hemoglobin level
1-3 months	Repletion of stores

Though hemoglobin level normalizes in 4-6 weeks, iron should to given for another 3 months to replenish the stores and to prevent recurrences.

Oral formulations include ferrous sulphate, ferrous gluconate, ferrous fumarate, carbonyl iron and polysaccharide-iron complex. Parenteral preparations include iron dextran, iron sucrose, ferric carboxymaltose and iron isomaltoside. Dietary iron sources include meat, fish and poultry, lentils, dried beans, grain products, vegetables, dried fruit, and molasses. However, they cannot replace iron therapy in deficient states. Animal sources of iron (heme) have better bioavailability as compared to plant sources.

Megaloblastic Anemia

Treatment is mainly the replacement of the deficient nutrients along with dietary counseling. Folate is available as 5 mg tablets, which is prescribed as one tablet daily. B12 is available in oral tablets (500 μg strength) and as intramuscular and intravenous preparations. Intramuscular 1 mg injection is frequently used, which bypasses intestinal absorption. Six to eight weeks treatment is usually considered sufficient in case of nutritional deficiency. An oral or intramuscular dose of 500–1000 μg daily for 1 week, followed by weekly for 4–8 weeks and lifelong supplementation if required is commonly followed. Lifelong parenteral or high dose oral B12 is recommended in case of pernicious anemia and malabsorption. Patients should be followed up with complete blood counts to look for recovery in counts and occasionally thrombocytosis may be seen.

Immune Thrombocytopenic Purpura

Management of immune thrombocytopenic purpura (ITP) is briefly shown in Figure 5.7.2.

Thalassemia in Adolescents

Adolescents with thalassemia are now entering the adolescent age group due to better management in the pediatric age group. Apart from transfusions, the management of thalassemia is complicated by various comorbidities, which pose difficulty mainly during the adolescent age group (see Table 5.7.5 for details).

Aplastic Anemia

Approach to an adolescent with aplastic anemia is shown in Figure 5.7.3.

LEARNING POINTS

1. Commonly seen hematological problems in adolescent age are nutritional deficiency anemia, thalassemia, aplastic anemia, thrombocytopenia and systemic illnesses with hematological manifestations.
2. Adolescents may present with inherited hematological disorders for the first time or may come to a pediatrician with adolescent specific complications of conditions present since childhood e.g. thalassemia major, hemophilia, Fanconi anemia etc.
3. Some inherited hematological conditions may manifest only in adolescence e.g. MYH9 related thrombocytopenia syndromes, gray platelet syndrome, Wiskott-Aldrich syndrome and X-linked thrombocytopenia.
4. Thalassemics are now entering the adolescent age group due to better management in the pediatric age group. Apart from transfusions, the management of thalassemia is complicated by various comorbidities, which pose difficulty mainly during the adolescent age group.

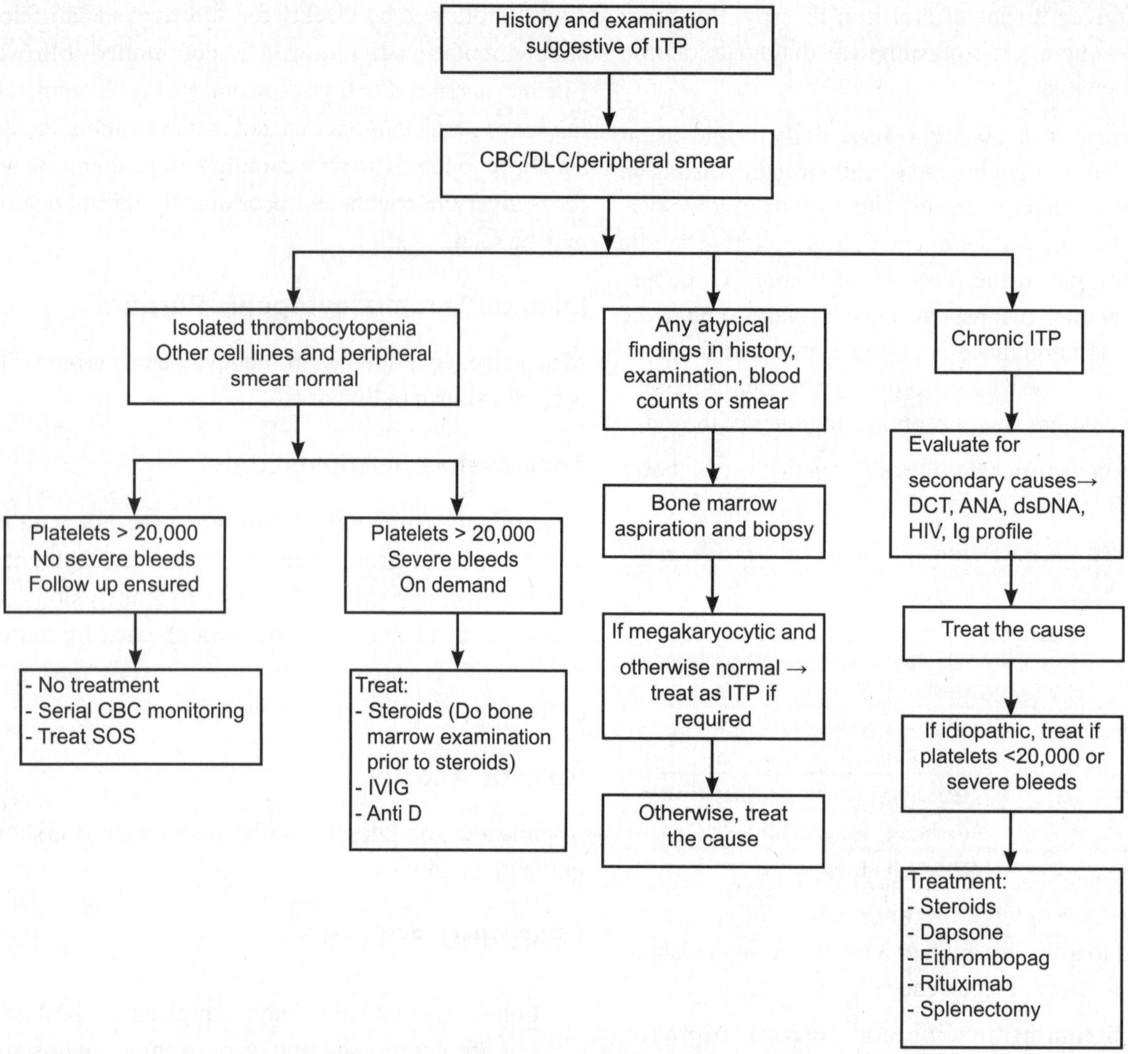

Figure 5.7.2: Approach to a case of immune thrombocytopenic purpura (ITP)

Table 5.7.5: Long-term complications of thalassemia

System	*Manifestations*	*Investigations and management*
Iron overload	Skin hyperpigmentation Hepatic failure Cardiac failure Endocrine symptoms	Recommended transfusion of 100-200 ml/kg/year is equivalent to 116-232 mg iron/kg/year. Iron chelation is initiated after first 10-20 transfusions or ferritin level above 1,000 µg/l • Deferiprone–oral-75 mg/kg/day in 3 divided doses • Deferasirox–oral-20 mg/kg/day; once a day before a meal, dissolved in water (or apple juice), using a non-metallic stirrer • Desferrioxamine–IV/SC-20-40 mg/kg; infuse over 8-12 hours 6 nights minimum per week
Endocrine complications	• Short stature • Primary hypothyroidism • Insulin-dependent diabetes mellitus • Impaired glucose tolerance • Hypoparathyroidism • Hypogonadism • Growth hormone deficiency/insufficiency	Various tests to rule out the endocrine status

Contd.

Contd.

Fertility and pregnancy related issues	• Specific risks during pregnancy include cardiac insufficiency, premature labor, fetal growth retardation, miscarriage and transmission of transfusion related infections to fetus • Pre-pregnancy counseling is essential after a careful evaluation of comorbidities, medications and assessing the risks involved	Induction of ovulation and spermatogenesis may be required
Osteoporosis	Back pain, body pain and fractures	Bone mineral density (DEXA scan), calcium and vitamin D supplementation, bisphosphonates and hormone replacement therapy
Cardiac complications	Palpitation, exercise intolerance, exertional dyspnea and pedal edema General management: Management appropriate transfusion (target hemoglobin 9–10.5 g/dL) proper iron chelation, managing endocrine abnormalities and diuretics Beta blockers can be added in stabilized patients	12 lead ECG and echocardiography (for chamber dimensions, ejection fraction, pulmonary arterial pressures and Doppler analysis) Cardiac MRI can be done wherever feasible
Liver problems	Hemosiderosis or viral hepatitis	Liver biopsy is gold standard test. T2* MRI scan is a noninvasive alternative
Infections	Viral infections (hepatitis B, C, HIV), post-splenectomy infections (pneumococcus, meningococcus and *H. influenzae*) due to iron overload (*Yersinia enterocolitica* and others)	Viral hepatitis markers screen should be done every 6 months. Treatment with antivirals may be required
Splenectomy related complications	Opportunistic infections, thrombophilia and pulmonary hypertension	Presplenectomy vaccinations for pneumococcal and *H influenzae* is must. Penicillin prophylaxis postsplenectomy to be started
Psychological and lifestyle related issues	Very common in these children due to chronic illness	Counseling of child and family

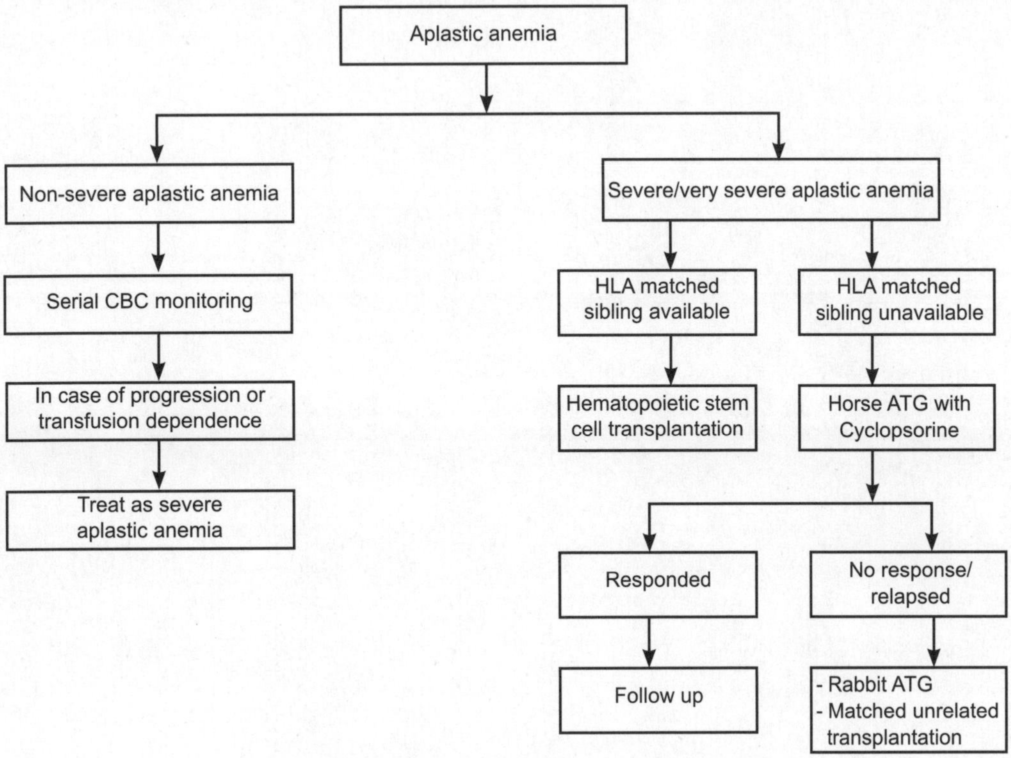

Figure 5.7.3: Approach to aplastic anemia

Acknowledgement

Dr Anupam Sachdeva, Director Pediatric Hematology Oncology and Bone Marrow Transplantation, Institute For Child Health, Sir Ganga Ram Hospital, New Delhi

SUGGESTED READING

1. Cappellini MD, Cohen A, Eleftheriou A, Piga A, Porter J, Taher A. Guidelines for the clinical management of thalassemia, 2nd revised edition. Nicosia; Thalassemia International Federation, 2008.
2. Chandra J. Megaloblastic Anemia: Back in Focus. Indian J Pediatr 2010;77(7):795-99.
3. Cines DB, Bussel JB. How I treat idiopathic thrombocytopenic purpura (ITP)? Blood 2005;106:2244-51.
4. McLean E, de Benoist B, Allen LH. Review of the magnitude of folate and vitamin B12 deficiencies worldwide. Food and Nutrition Bulletin 2008; 29(2):S38-51.
5. Scheinberg P, Young NS. How I treat acquired aplastic anemia? Blood 2012;120(6):1185-96.
6. Stabbler SP. Vitamin B12 deficiency. N Engl J Med 2013;368:149-60.

Rheumatological Problems

5.8

Surjit Singh, Ankur Kumar

INTRODUCTION

Rheumatologic disorders are a group of chronic diseases characterized by the presence of chronic inflammation affecting the musculoskeletal system, blood vessels and other tissues of the body. While some of these are benign and self-limiting, others may have a chronic relapsing and remitting course. At times, these can be fatal. These diseases may present for the first time in adolescence (e.g. lupus and enthesitis related arthritis). Often these are a continuum of conditions presenting early in childhood (e.g. juvenile idiopathic arthritis; see Table 5.8.1).

Table 5.8.1: Common rheumatologic diseases of adolescents
1. Systemic lupus erythematosus (SLE) and Antiphospholipid antibody syndrome (APS)
2. Juvenile dermatomyositis (JDMS)
3. Juvenile idiopathic arthritis (JIA)
4. Enthesitis related arthritis (ERA) and Psoriatic arthritis
5. Localized and Systemic Scleroderma
6. Rheumatic fever and Rheumatic heart diseases
7. Vasculitis (Anti-neutrophil cytoplasmic antibody [ANCA] associated vasculitis, Takayasu arteritis, Polyarteritis nodosa [PAN])
8. Sarcoidosis

HISTORY TAKING

A good clinical history helps in arriving at a diagnosis. Majority of these disorders are more common in girls, the exception being enthesitis related arthritis (ERA).

- Patients usually present with seemingly non-specific complaints of aches and pain and easy fatigability.
- Other common complaints are fever, joint swelling and/or restriction of joint movements.
- Symptoms related to systemic involvement include dyspnea on exertion, palpitation, edema, decreased urine output, hematuria, oral/genital ulceration, skin rashes and photosensitivity.
- Cold sensitivity of peripheries leading to blue fingers is always ominous.
- Headache, seizures, psychosis and neurological deficits may be the presenting features of lupus.
- Ophthalmological complaints like redness of eyes and decreased visual acuity should never be ignored as these are pointers towards an accompanying uveitis.
- A clinical approach to history taking is given in Table 5.8.2.

PHYSICAL EXAMINATION

Table 5.8.3 describes the salient clinical features to be checked during a clinical examination.

INVESTIGATIONS

For Inflammation

1. **Erythrocyte Sedimentation Rate (ESR):** Simple and inexpensive test; insensitive and poorly related to time course of inflammation; very high ESR (>100 mm/hr) is very suggestive of an underlying rheumatological disorder; useful for monitoring inflammatory rheumatic diseases.
2. **C-Reactive Protein (CRP):** CRP has several advantages over ESR; rises rapidly (within 4 hours) and decreases quickly after inflammation subsides; correlates better with inflammation and disease activity.
3. **Hemogram:** Chronic inflammation is usually associated with a normocytic, normochromic anemia, polymorphonuclear leucocytosis and thrombocytosis; low or falling platelet count may suggest SLE, drug toxicity or development of macrophage activation syndrome.
4. **Immunological Investigations:** Autoantibodies are immunoglobulins that react against autologous intracellular antigens (e.g. antinuclear antibodies and anticytoplasmic antibodies), cell surface antigens (e.g. against HLA molecules) or extracellular antigens (e.g. lupus anticoagulant).
5. **Rheumatoid Factor (RF):** Positive in 1-5 % of normal population; positive in only 10% of polyarticular JIA; signifies an aggressive disease course.

Table 5.8.2: Clinical history related to rheumatologic diseases

Chief complaint related to	*Analysis of the history*
Joint pains and swelling	Early morning pain with stiffness that improves with movement suggests inflammation. Night pain may point towards an underlying malignancy. Joint swelling and restriction of movement suggest arthritis. Pattern of joint involvement provides important clues to the diagnosis: • Spine and hip joint involvement is common in spondyloarthropathy. • Distal interphalangeal joint involvement is typical of psoriatic arthritis. • Migratory polyarthritis is seen in rheumatic fever.
Fever	Patients may present as pyrexia of unknown origin. Fever may be the initial presentation of vasculitides. Quotidian pattern of fever is typical of systemic JIA (sJIA). Fever may often be the initial presentation of disease in children with sJIA.
Weakness	Proximal muscle weakness with neck flexor involvement is usually the presenting feature of inflammatory myopathy. Pharyngeal muscle involvement is usually indicative of severe disease in juvenile dermatomyositis. Lupus can present with neurological deficits; peripheral neuropathy can be seen in polyarteritis nodosa (PAN), systemic lupus erythematosus (SLE) and ANCA associated vasculitis.
Skin	Butterfly/ malar rash of lupus is photosensitive, maculopapular and typically involves nose and cheeks and spares the nasolabial folds (Figure 5.8.1). Heliotrope rash and Gottron papules (Figure 5.8.2) are pathognomonic of juvenile dermatomyositis (JDMS); facial rash of JDMS does not spare nasolabial folds. Localized scleroderma is characterized by an area of induration surrounded by erythema or a bluish hue; later there can be indurated, hypopigmented or hyperpigmented lesions. Erythema nodosum is characterized by nodular, erythematous, painful lesions on anterior surfaces of legs in pretibial area; such lesions may be seen sarcoidosis, lupus, and Behcet disease. Raynaud's phenomenon (RP) is characterized by blanching, cyanosis and erythema; it can induced by cold exposure and/or emotional stress; associated with scleroderma, lupus, and mixed connective tissue disease; may, at times, be primary (Raynaud disease). Vasculitic ulcers are seen as punched out lesions typically over toes; may be associated with lupus or PAN (Figure 5.8.3). Erythema marginatum presents as transient non-pruritic, erythematous, macular lesions with a serpiginous border and pale center, seen on trunk and extremities – pathognomonic of acute rheumatic fever.
Cardiovascular system (CVS) and chest	Wegener granulomatosis may present with hemoptysis, persistent cough, and a nasal discharge; a saddle nose deformity may develop later due to involvement nasal cartilage. Hypertension may be seen in several rheumatological disorders (e.g. SLE, PAN, Takayasu arteritis, Wegener's granulomatosis). Dyspnea on exertion/palpitation may suggest valvular lesions of rheumatic heart disease or an underlying myocarditis (related to lupus or vasculitides).
Renal	Periorbital puffiness, decreased urine output and hematuria are always suggestive of a serious underlying disorder and may be presenting features of lupus or ANCA associated vasculitides.
Eye	ERA is associated with acute iridocyclitis presenting as an acute red eye. Early onset oligoarthritis seen in young girls is associated with an asymptomatic chronic uveitis which can be picked up only on slit lamp microscopy.
Central nervous system (CNS)	Seizures and neurological deficits may suggest an underlying vasculitic disorder, lupus (especially if associated with antiphospholipid antibodies or sarcoidosis; Chorea and emotional lability is typical of rheumatic fever.

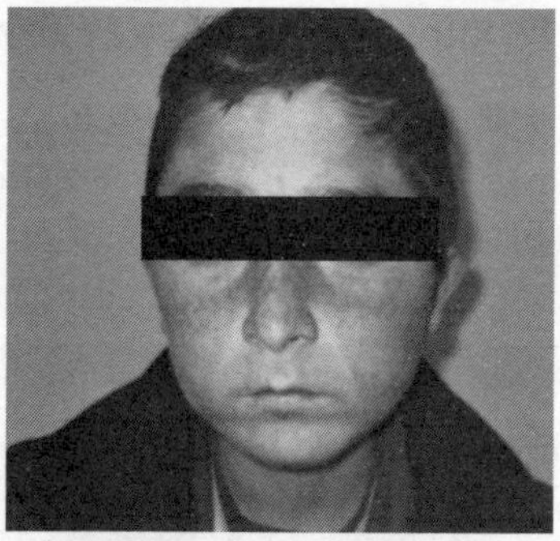

Figure 5.8.1: Classic photosensitive lupus malar rash. Note the distinct sparing of nasolabial folds

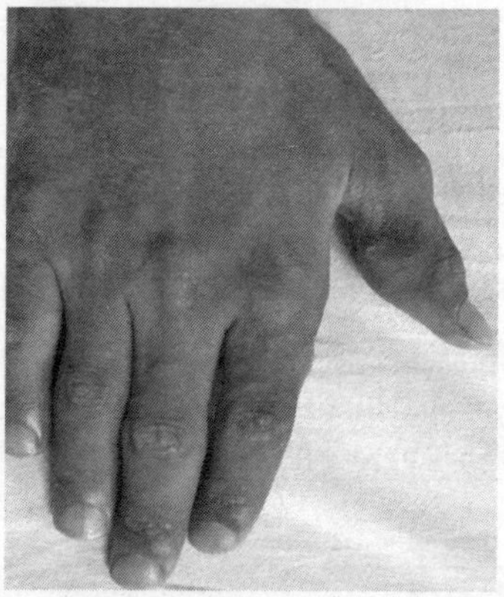

Figure 5.8.2: Gottron papules over proximal and distal interphalangeal joints in an 11-year-old with juvenile dermatomyositis. Also visible over the thumb is calcinosis with extrusion of calcium crystals

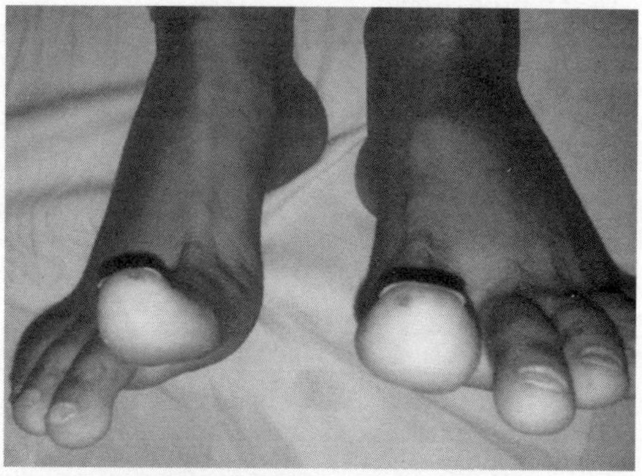

Figure 5.8.3: Vasculitic ulcers at tip of digits of lower limb

6. **Antistreptolysin O (ASO):** ASO is an antibody response to streptolysin, a toxin of group A beta hemolytic streptococcus; appears 1 week after infection, peaks at 3-5 weeks and wanes off after 6-8 weeks; upper limit of normal is 230 IU/ml (5-10 years of age) and 242 IU/ml (11-15 years of age)
7. **Antinuclear Antibody (ANA):** Positive in SLE and several other rheumatologic disorders; seen in 60% of oligoarticular JIA patients, especially in those with uveitis; for detection of ANA it is important to perform immunofluorescence rather than an ELISA test.
8. **Antineutrophil Cytoplasmic Antibody (ANCA):** Usually seen in patients with vasculitis; directed against

Table 5.8.3: Relevant findings on physical examination

Musculoskeletal system	An inflamed joint is usually swollen, tender and warm; loss of depressions around the joint (e.g. knee) suggest joint swelling. Fixed posture of joint may either suggest inflammation or deforming arthritis. Synovial thickening around the joint can be appreciated by gentle palpation with thumb and forefinger; patellar tap is useful to detect fluid in knee joint. Enthesitis (i.e. inflammation at sites of tendon, ligament, or joint capsule attachment to bone) is typical of ERA. Range of motion at joints can be assessed by active and passive movements; it may be impaired because of joint inflammation or deformity; to assess range of motion of lumbar spine "Modified Schober test" is used (Figure 5.8.4 and 5.8.5). This test is done by marking the lumbosacral junction by joining the dimple of Venus. Then two points are marked, one 5 cm below and second 10 cm above lumbosacral junction. Patient is asked to flex with knees straight and the increase in distance is measured. Less than 6 cm increase is abnormal.
Eye	Uveitis may be associated with asymmetry of pupil size and poor response to light; for detection of chronic asymptomatic uveitis, slit lamp microscopy is essential.
Oral cavity	Oral ulcers may be seen in lupus (in which these are painless) and Behcet disease.
Capillaroscopy	Using a hand held magnifier/ low power microscope, changes in nail fold capillaries can be made out in several conditions (e.g. JDMS, scleroderma).
Blood Pressure	Should be measured in all patients.
Systemic Examination	
CVS	To look for evidence of myocarditis, pericarditis, dilated cardiomyopathy and valvular pathology. Loud P2 suggests pulmonary hypertension.
Chest	Serositis in form of pleural effusion (seen in lupus). Evidence of aspiration pneumonia (may be seen in inflammatory myopathy).
CNS	Assessment of muscle power is important in patients with inflammatory myopathy; neck flexor weakness is virtually pathognomonic of inflammatory myopathy. Pharyngeal weakness should be assessed by gag reflex. For respiratory muscle involvement, single breath count should be used.
Abdomen	Hepatosplenomegaly in case of sJIA and lupus. Arterial bruits in Takayasu arteritis.

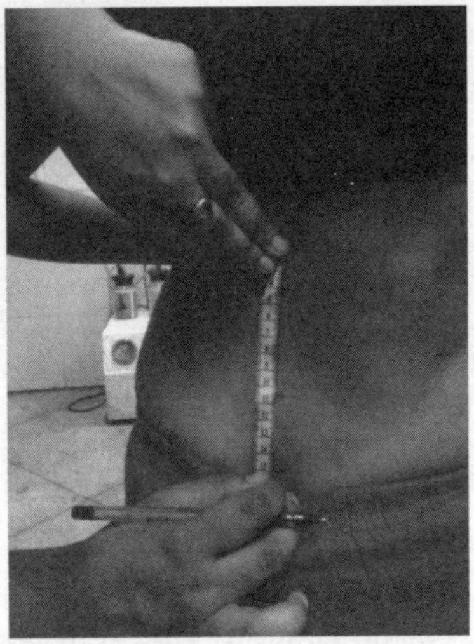

Figure 5.8.4: Demonstration of Modified Schober test in a 12-year-old with suspected enthesitis related arthritis. Marks are first put 10 cm above and 5 cm below lumbosacral junction and the child is then asked to bend forward

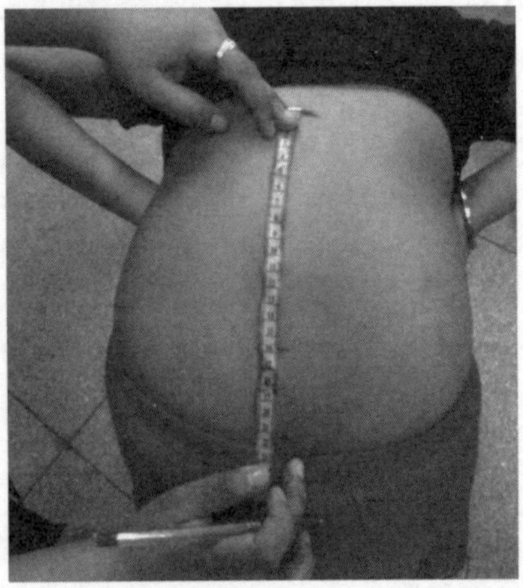

Figure 5.8.5: Demonstration of Modified Schober test. An increase of 6 cm or more is considered normal

antiproteinase3 (c-ANCA) and antimyeloperoxidase (p-ANCA); c-ANCA specific for Wegener granulomatosis; p-ANCA ma y be associated with many diseases such as microscopic PAN, Churg-Strauss syndrome, SLE, idiopathic rapidly progressive cresentic glomerulonephritis, ulcerative colitis, rheumatoid arthritis and in autoimmune liver disease.

9. **Complement:** Levels of C3 and C4 rise in most inflammatory conditions, but in diseases associated with complement activation (like SLE), levels fall due to consumption and correlate with disease activity.

COMMON RHEUMATOLOGIC DISEASES IN ADOLESCENTS

Detailed description of all rheumatologic disorders is beyond the scope of this chapter. Hence the three most common conditions presenting in adolescent age group are discussed below.

Idiopathic Inflammatory Myopathies

The salient clinical features of idiopathic inflammatory myopathies are given in Box 5.8.1. The details of management of idiopathic inflammatory myopathies are detailed in Table 5.8.4.

Box 5.8.1: Idiopathic inflammatory myopathies

Juvenile Dermatomyositis (JDMS):

1. Symmetric proximal weakness
2. Skin changes (Heliotrope rash and Gottron papules)
3. Elevation of muscle enzymes: creatine kinase (CPK), aspartate aminotransferase (AST), lactate dehydrogenase (LDH), and aldolase
4. Electromyographic (EMG) changes of myopathy and denervation
5. Necrosis and inflammation on muscle biopsy.

3/5–probable diagnosis and 4/5–definite myositis. Diagnosis of dermatomyositis requires presence of cutaneous changes. Magnetic resonance imaging (MRI) has now supplanted the requirement for performing muscle biopsy in these patients.

Juvenile Polymyositis

Idiopathic myositis without skin rash is very uncommon in children. JDMS and juvenile polymyositis are managed similarly.

Table 5.8.4: Management of inflammatory myopathies

Drugs	*Remarks*
Prednisolone	2 mg/kg/ day; improvement seen over 6-8 weeks; gradually tapered and stopped over several months
Methylprednisolone	Initial treatment in the presence of dysphagia, dysphonia, pulmonary disease, or suspected gastrointestinal vasculopathy
Methotrexate	Started from beginning along with steroids
Cyclophosphamide, Azathioprine, IVIG, Anti-TNF-α therapy (Etanercept)	In severe cases not responding to above treatment

Systemic Lupus Erythematosus (SLE)

SLICC criteria (2012) used for the diagnosis includes 11 clinical and 6 immunological criteria.

Presence of 4 criteria (at least 1 clinical and 1 immunologic) establishes the diagnosis. Lupus nephritis (biopsy-proven) with positive ANA or anti–double-stranded DNA also satisfies the diagnosis. Table 5.8.5 lists the various drugs used in the management of SLE in adolescents.

Table 5.8.5: Management of SLE	
Drug	***Remarks***
Hydroxychloroquine	In all cases @5-6 mg/kg/day
Prednisolone	For nephritis > class 2, cytopenias and CNS lupus
Methylprednisolone	Severe cytopenias and initial management of lupus class 3 and 4, CNS lupus
Cyclophosphamide	For nephritis class 3 and 4
Mycophenolate mofetil (MMF)	Alternate to cyclophosphamide

Juvenile Idiopathic Arthritis (JIA)

Box 5.8.2 highlights the diagnostic criteria use for the diagnosis of JIA in adolescents.

For Oligoarticular Disease

- Non-steroidal anti-inflammatory drugs (NSAIDs) [naproxen (15-20 mg/kg/day)] for 4-6 weeks with/without intraarticular triamcinolone injection.
- Disease modifying anti-rheumatic drugs (DMARDs), mostly methotrexate in nonresponsive cases.
- If still no response, TNF inhibitors (etanercept/infliximab/adalimumab) are used.

For Polyarticular Disease

- Methotrexate is started, and is usually given subcutaneously every week.
- Initial dose is 15-20 mg/m^2/week. As the full effects of methotrexate may not be discernible till 6-8 weeks, bridge therapy with steroids and/or biological agents is often necessary for symptomatic relief.
- Failure of this therapy to achieve remission warrants addition of biological agents like TNF-α inhibitors (e.g. etanercept, infliximab, adalimumab), IL-1 inhibitors (e.g. anakirna), or IL-6 inhibitors (e.g. tocilizumab).

For Systemic Disease (sJIA)

Steroids are the initial treatment of choice.

- Duration of therapy depends on severity of disease and degree of inflammation.

Box 5.8.2: Juvenile Idiopathic Arthritis (JIA)
• Onset of arthritis before the age of 16 year and duration of disease ≥6 week.
• ILAR (International League of Associations for Rheumatology) has given classification criteria for JIA which is most widely used.

- If there is inadequate response, biological agents in the form of IL-1 and IL-6 inhibitors are used. Anti-TNF therapy is not very useful in sJIA.

Enthesitis Related Arthritis (ERA) and Juvenile Ankylosing Spondylitis (JAS)

- Initial therapy is usually based on NSAIDs (e.g. naproxen, indomethacin) and intra-articular triamcinolone.
- If symptoms persist one can start sulfasalazine.
- While methotrexate may be appropriate for peripheral arthritis, it is usually not effective for spondyloarthropathy. TNF-α inhibitors (e.g. adalimumab, infliximab, and etanercept) may need to be used early for axial involvement.
- Uveitis in association with rheumatologic disorders can usually be managed with mydriatics and topical steroids.
- Systemic glucocorticoids and other immunosuppressive drugs (e.g. methotrexate, azathioprine, mycophenolate mofetil) are required in patients with more recalcitrant disease. Anti-TNF-α therapy (with adalimumab and infliximab, but not etanercept) is required in a subset of patients who do not respond to conventional treatment.

LEARNING POINTS

1. A significant proportion of adolescents with underlying rheumatological disorders may present with seemingly nonspecific signs and symptoms and hence their diagnosis may be delayed. A high index of suspicion is necessary to diagnose these illnesses early.
2. A good clinical history and a meticulously performed clinical examination are crucial.
3. Laboratory investigations should be selected carefully and interpreted in the context of the clinical problem.
4. Effective treatment is now available for most rheumatological disorders.
5. Prognosis of these disorders has markedly improved with availability of effective DMARDs and newly introduced biological agents.
6. For best results a multidisciplinary team approach is necessary.

SUGGESTED READING

1. Gewitz MH, Baltimore RS, Tani LY, Sable CA, Shulman ST, Carapetis J, *et al.* Revision of the Jones Criteria for the

Diagnosis of Acute Rheumatic Fever in the Era of Doppler Echocardiography A Scientific Statement From the American Heart Association. Circulation 2015;131(20):1806-18.

2. Kliegman RM, Stanton BM, St Jeme J, Schor NF, Eds. Nelson Textbook of Pediatrics. 20th edition. Philadelphia; Elsevier 2015; 153-69.
3. Kumar RK, Tandon R. Rheumatic fever & rheumatic heart disease: The last 50 years. Indian J Med Res 2013;137(4):643-58.
4. Lawry GV. Fam's Musculoskeletal Examination and Joint Injection Techniques, 2nd edition. Philadelphia; Elsevier 2010.
5. Petri M, Orbai AM, Alarcon GS. Derivation and Validation of Systemic Lupus International Collaborating Clinics Classification Criteria for Systemic Lupus Erythematosus. Arthritis Rheum 2012;64(8):2677-86.
6. Petty RE. Textbook of Pediatric Rheumatology. 7th edition. Philadelphia; Elsevier 2016.
7. Shet A, Kaplan EL. Clinical use of and interpretation of group A streptococcal antibody tests: a practical approach for the pediatrician or primary care physician. Pediatr Infect Dis J 2002;21:420-26.
8. Singh S. Pediatric Rheumatology. 2nd edition. New Delhi: Peepee Publishers; 2015.

5.9

Surgical Problems

Devendra K Gupta, Shilpa Sharma

INTRODUCTION

Surgical conditions in adolescents are peculiar in having common causes and presenting as emergency conditions to clinicians of various specialties (Table 5.9.1). Most are related to the change in growth pattern, hormonal effects on internal organs, body habitus, personal hygiene etc. Change in diet habits can cause appendicitis, or low intake of iodine is associated with thyroid problems. Rallison *et al.* reported 3.7% thyroid disorders and 1.8% thyroid nodules in adolescent school children. Parotid gland infections are related to poor oral hygiene and change in oral microbial flora. Genitourinary emergencies are also commonly seen with gonadal abnormalities. Often the adolescent is unable to understand the difference between the physiological changes at puberty and the initial mild pain associated with pathological conditions. Hence by the time the pain is severe the condition becomes an acute emergency situation.

HISTORY TAKING

The exact time and nature of onset of symptoms should be taken from the patient him/herself, if the condition is not very acute. The usual symptoms include swelling, pain, vomiting, lump abdomen and fever. The progress of the symptoms, the relation with any event, relation to bowel and bladder habits and response to any medication should be carefully elicited. Any history of trauma, medication, worm infestation or allergy should be noted. Any history of similar illness in past or any chronic illness should be noted.

Table 5.9.1: Surgical conditions in adolescence

Head and Neck Swellings	Parotid gland swelling and pleomorphic salivary adenoma Thyroid Swelling–Goiter, papillary carcinoma
Acute Surgical Abdominal Conditions	Appendicitis is the most common cause of pain abdomen. It may present as an acute onset or delayed presentation with lump formation or perforation.
Genitourinary Emergencies	Testicular torsion Ovarian torsion Acute epididymo-orchitis Paraphimosis and balanoposthitis when the prepuce is tight

CLINICAL EXAMINATION

For surgical conditions, the main crux of diagnosis lies on careful clinical examination. A general physical examination for consciousness, built, nutrition, organomegaly and lymphadenopathy is done. Any swelling is inspected and then palpated for tenderness, site, shape, surface, consistency, fluctuation, overlying skin, mobility, fixity to underlying structures and draining lymph nodes. The abdomen is carefully palpated for any lesion or organomegaly, tenderness, guarding or rigidity. The hernia sites and gonads in males are examined for any hidden pathology.

INVESTIGATIONS

The routine investigations include a complete hemogram, total and differential counts, liver and renal functions and microscopic urine examination for sugar, albumin and any pus cells.

In case there is a swelling or any abdominal symptoms, an ultrasound examination may help to locate the organ of origin of symptoms. Only in very rare occasions does the need of other investigations like CT scan, renogram or MRI arise.

MANAGEMENT PROTOCOL

If the child is hemodynamically stable, symptomatic treatment is instituted till the diagnosis is reached. In infective or inflammatory lesions, a course of antibiotics may help. Most surgical lesions in adolescence would need a surgical intervention in case there is no response to conservative management.

The common surgical conditions in adolescents are outlined in Tables 5.9.2 to 5.9.5.

Table 5.9.2: Surgical conditions of head and neck in adolescence–parotid gland

Etiology	*Presenting symptoms*	*Clinical examination*	*Investigations*	*Management*
1. Congenital lesions with late presentation due to cosmetic reasons: Hemangiomas Lymphatic malformations (25%). 2. Acquired Inflammatory, Infectious Disorders: • Bacterial suupurative adenitis • Viral sialoadenitis 3. Autoimmune 4. Traumatic 5. Neoplastic: >50% mucoepidermoid carcinoma, acinic cell carcinoma, adenoid cystic carcinoma, rhabdomyosarcoma.	Acute onset of pain or sudden increase in size may suggest an inflammatory lesion. Associated skin changes, overlying erythema support the diagnosis. Exacerbation of symptoms during eating may suggest ductal obstruction. The malignant lesions are usually associated with enlarged lymph nodes. Painless mass and skin changes may be seen in certain chronic granulomatous disorders and atypical mycobacterial infetions.	Bimanual palpation should be done with one gloved finger in the mouth. Palpation of the duct and inspection of the major salivary gland ductal openings for purulent discharge or stenosis. The distribution of the facial nerve is examined for any involvement due to the lesion	A plain radiograph can visualize 80-90% of submandibular and 60% of parotid calculi. There may be parenchymal calcification. Ultrasonography to delineate the mass–solid/cystic nature; provide guidance for fine needle aspiration cytology (FNAC)/ biopsy. Contrast enhanced computed tomography if malignancy is suspected.	Infection: Attention to hydration and appropriate antibiotics. Surgery and/or appropriate referrals for malignancy.

Table 5.9.3: Surgical conditions of head and neck in adolescence – thyroid gland

Etiology	*Presenting symptoms*	*Clinical examination*	*Investigations*	*Management*
Endemic goiter–Iodine deficiency Simple colloid goiter–Puberty Autoimmune–Chronic lymphocytic thyroiditis (Hashimoto thyroiditis, HT) The peak age of onset-first two decades of life in early to mid puberty 55-65% of all euthyroid goiters and almost all cases of thyroiditis are HT Papillary carcinoma (see Box 5.9.1)	Higher risk of Hashimoto thyroiditis with chromosomal abnormalities such as Turner syndrome, Klinefelter syndrome & Down syndrome Goiter with or without symptoms of thyroid dysfunction	Multinodular goiter Hashimoto thyroiditis Asymptomatic, solitary thyroid nodule is a thyroid adenoma, thyroid carcinoma or a thyroid cyst	TSH and thyroid antibody levels Thyroid hormone (T4) if the TSH level is abnormal Ultrasound and radionuclear scans: for single palpable nodule or irregular enlargement Fine-needle aspiration biopsy	Thyroid hormone supplement Surgery

Table 5.9.4: Acute surgical abdominal conditions

	Presenting symptoms	*Clinical examination*	*Investigations*	*Management*
Appendicitis	M: F ratio - 3:2. Pain abdomen (periumbilical), anorexia, vomiting, indigestion, alteration in the bowel habits, fever, lump formation or perforation Retrocolic appendicitis – flank pain Pelvic appendicitis – prominent urinary symptoms, diarrhea or tenesmus	Localized tenderness at the McBurney point Palpable mass in the right iliac fossa Guarding and rigidity may be present If appendix has perforated and caused generalized peritonitis: sluggish or absent bowel sounds, signs of shock (tachycardia, cold-clammy skin, dry mucosa and oliguria)	Ultrasound by an experienced radiologist is useful Demonstration of free fluid and noncompressible appendix, which is more than 7 mm in diameter and presence of appendicolith are suggestive of appendicitis	Surgical/laparoscopic appendicectomy Conservative management

Table 5.9.5: Genitourinary emergencies

	Presenting symptoms	*Clinical examination*	*Investigations*	*Management*
Testicular torsion	Sudden scrotal pain, swelling, and discoloration, nausea, vomiting	Tender, swollen testicle. Elevation of the affected testicle does not improve the pain (negative Prehn sign). No transillumination. Absent cremasteric reflex. Scrotal edema, reactive hydrocele.	A scrotal color Doppler ultrasound (or testicular blood flow scan with technetium-99m) can demonstrate reduced or absent vascular flow.	Surgical correction and testicular fixation.
Acute epididymo-orchitis	Gradual/acute pain, swelling in the epididymis/scrotum, fever, chills, nausea, urinary frequency, dysuria, pyuria, bacteriuria, oligo-azoospermia, and/or positive urethral cultures.	Tenderness. Cremasteric reflex is intact. Prehn sign is positive. Associated prostatitis, septicemia, or genitourinary tuberculosis. Idiopathic epididymo-orchitis may result from exercise or trauma-induced reflux of sterile urine through the vas deferens leading to chemical irritation. Infectious causes include viruses (mumps, varicella, influenza, coxsackievirus, Epstein-Barr virus) and bacteria (*Mycobacterium tuberculosis*).	Idiopathic or resulting from infection by *Chlamydia trachomatis, Neisseria gonorrhoeae,* urinary tract infection, orchitis, testicular tumor, urologic surgery (or instrumentation).	Appropriate antibiotics are necessary. Bed rest with cold compresses over the area of swelling/pain, scrotal elevation, analgesics, and anti-inflammatory medications and anti-tubercular treatment. Complications include epididymal abscess, infarction and atrophy; testicular atrophy increases risk for testicular cancer. If inflammation persists over 14 days, consider a testicular tumor.
Paraphimosis	Severe pain and swelling of the glans and prepuce.	A tight prepuce can lead to phimosis with fibrosis as the age increases. If the condition persists till adolescence, there is formation of Balanitis Xerotica Obliterans (BXO). An attempt at retracting the prepuce and failure to pull it back can lead to paraphimosis.	No investigation required.	Warm pack and forced reduction after applying local xylocaine jelly. Emergency slitting of the tight ring; later circumcision.
Balanoposthitis (inflammation of the foreskin and glans in an uncircumcised male)	In one third of the patients, a specific cause may not be established even after clinical examination and microbiologic and serologic tests. Ulceration and deep erosion are seen in patients with advanced disease, often in association with fungal infections and in individuals who are immunocompromised.	It may be caused by bacterial or fungal infection. It often results from a poorly retractile foreskin and poor hygiene that leads to colonization and overgrowth. Candidal infection appears to be the most common cause of disease accounting for 30% of the causative organisms, followed by beta-hemolytic streptococci accounting for 13%. Other organisms include bacteroides and Gardnerella.	Potassium hydroxide slide preparation allows for the rapid visualization of the candidal hyphae and culture often isolates candidal species and helps to direct proper treatment.	Clearing the acute infection and improved hygiene. Circumcision Topical antibiotics (metronidazole cream) and antifungals (clotrimazole cream) or low-potency steroid creams for contact dermatitides often clears the lesion. Proper hygiene with frequent washing and drying of the prepuce is preventive.

Contd.

Contd.

Ovarian torsion	Acute onset lower abdominal pain and vomiting. Presentation 9 to 12.5 years. Torsion may cause symptoms related to venous engorgement before arterial blood supply is compromised.	Most cases of torsion occur in ovaries containing masses, such as functional cysts, dermoid cyst and neoplasms. Torsion is reportedly more common on the right side (3:2). Most cysts are follicular or luteal. Their timing with menarche is due to increased hormonal stimulation.	Ultrasound: Echogenic pelvic mass with nonvisualization of the ipsilateral ovary or an adnexal mass. Presence of vascular flow does not rule out torsion. A dual blood supply from ovarian and uterine arteries provides persistent arterial blood flow.	Laparoscopy or laparotomy. Detorsion with or without cystectomy

Box 5.9.1: Papillary carcinoma

- Most common form of well-differentiated thyroid cancer.
- Predisposing factors: Past irradiation to head, neck or chest; exposure to nuclear fallout; family history of thyroid cancer (MEN).
- Appears as an irregular solid/cystic mass or nodule in normal thyroid.
- May be overtly or minimally invasive.
- More frequent than follicular carcinoma in young population.
- Life expectancy is related to age, being good in children with localized disease. Prognosis is better in females. Survival rate is around 95%.
- About 11% present with metastases outside the neck and mediastinum. Occult cervical lymph node metastases are common. Metastases are most common in the neck lymph nodes and lung, bone, brain, liver, and other sites. Metastasis is related to the primary tumor size. Metastases are rare with microscopic occult papillary carcinoma.
- Surgery is the definitive management of papillary thyroid cancer. Approximately 4-6 weeks after surgical thyroid removal, patients may have radioiodine therapy to detect and destroy any metastasis and residual tissue in the thyroid.

LEARNING POINTS

- Most common benign parotid lesion in adolescence is pleomorphic adenoma.
- A multinodular goiter is almost invariably caused by Hashimoto thyroiditis.
- Papillary carcinoma is the most common form of well-differentiated thyroid cancer.
- Appendicitis is the most common surgical emergency in adolescents.
- Elevation of the affected testicle does not improve the pain in torsion testes (negative Prehn sign), while it relieves the pain in epididymo-orchitis (positive Prehn sign).
- Torsion is a known complication of ovarian cysts and ovarian neoplasms in adolescents and children.
- Balanoposthitis is defined as inflammation of the foreskin and glans in an uncircumcised male. It may be caused by bacterial or fungal infection.

SUGGESTED READING

1. Muirhead S. Diagnostic approach to goitre in children. Paediatr Child Health 2001;6:195-99.
2. Poonai N, Poonai C, Lim R, Lynch T. Pediatric ovarian torsion: Case series and review of the literature Can J Surg 2013;56:103-08.
3. Rallison ML, Dobyns BM, Meikle AW, Bishop M, Lyon JL, Stevens W. Natural history of thyroid abnormalities: Prevalence, incidence, and regression of thyroid diseases in adolescents and young adults. Am J Med 1991;91:363-70.

Ophthalmic Problems

6.1

Quresh B Maskati

INTRODUCTION

This chapter does not review every eye problem that could be possibly encountered by the adolescent. The problems covered are those that can be encountered by any clinician dealing with adolescents, so that they can decide which problem can be treated by them and which definitely require referral to an ophthalmologist.

Due to lack of awareness of pre-school visual screening even in large cities and a complete lack of infrastructure facilities in the rural areas, refractive errors that are present since early childhood are often detected only in the adolescent age group.

Also the patient may have visited an ophthalmologist and he/she merely seeks reassurance that they are on the right track. Hence it is important for clinicians to have a passing knowledge of common eye problems in adolescents (Table 6.1.1).

HISTORY TAKING

Detailed history taking for the onset and duration of symptoms will help in making a correct diagnosis.

Refractive Errors

Many adolescents neglect their eye symptoms especially refractive errors as they do not like wearing spectacles and often deterioration in academic performance may be the first clue to refractive error. Routine visual screening should be done as part of well adolescent monitoring in adolescent health. However, several times refractive errors in one or both eyes may manifest for the first time only in this age group.

- Children with history of refractive error, especially myopia in one or both parents and those with symptoms of asthenopia (eye strain) or difficulty in seeing distant or near objects should be sent for an eye examination when detected.
- Most times, the adolescent may present with inability to view distance or near objects clearly. Occasionally they may complain of headaches or eye strain. Uncommonly, uncorrected refractive errors could act as trigger factors for migraine; hence migraine in an adolescent should raise a suspicion of uncorrected refractive errors.

Eye Strain

Several teenagers typically complain of headaches around the time of examinations, forcing stressed out parents to desperately seek appointments with the nearest ophthalmologist. These are usually tension headaches. Good reading habits help to reduce eye strain (Box 6.1.1).

Table 6.1.1: Common ophthalmic problems in adolescence

Refractive errors	Can be congenital or appearing in childhood; but are missed due to lack of visual screening at appropriate age
Squint	Myth that the operation can only be done when child is grown up
Conjunctivitis	Allergic variety is seen predominantly in this age group alone
Keratoconus	Starts manifesting in early to middle teens and can progress till the age of 40-45 years
Stevens-Johnson syndrome	Can occur at any age
Ocular trauma	Common due to aggression and violence and risk taking behavior at this age
Primary pigmentary degeneration (PPD), formerly called 'Retinitis pigmentosa (RP)'	Causes night-blindness–Becomes symptomatic only in this age
Cataracts	Untreated congenital, traumatic or metabolic
Tumors	Uveal tumors, superficial lesions like nevi and dermoids

Box 6.1.1: Good reading habits to reduce eye strain
Encourage to sit up and read, rather than reading lying down.
Read in good light.
Wake up early morning and study on fresh eyes rather than late into the night, when the eyes and body are already tired.
Take frequent breaks of 20 to 30 seconds every half an hour.
Gently close eyes or look into the distance at frequent intervals.

Squint

Most children with squint will have no complaints. However, a history of low self-esteem can often be elicited.

Conjunctivitis

In epidemic conjunctivitis there is history of red, watery eyes. The discharge is usually scanty, unless secondary bacterial infection occurs, when it may become mucopurulent. Occasionally these epidemic cases cause subconjunctival hemorrhages, which will take 2 to 3 weeks to disappear completely.

Allergic conjunctivitis can be seasonal (vernal or spring catarrh) or perennial or occur at any time of the year.

Keratoconus

If an adolescent is not happy with quality of vision even with spectacles, suspect keratoconus (Box 6.1.2 and Figure 6.1.1). In moderate to advanced cases, the quantity of vision may also drop in spite of wearing spectacles.

Box 6.1.2: Keratoconus
This corneal degeneration typically becomes symptomatic in the adolescent age group.
Usually binocular, occurring more commonly in girls.
The cause is multifactorial, probably due to genetic mutations.
The cornea becomes conical–affects quality of vision (distortion) and quantity of vision (drop in best corrected visual acuity).
The adolescent is not happy with quality of vision even with changing spectacles.
Only 20% progress. All the rest can be managed without surgical procedures with various types of contact lenses.
It may be difficult for a non-ophthalmologist to diagnose by clinical examination. Ophthalmologists see the cone shape well with a slit lamp biomicroscope (Figure 6.1.1).

Other Disorders

In Stevens-Johnson syndrome there would be history of treatment with antibiotics, anti-inflammatory medications, anti-malarials and other drugs. Cataracts in adolescent age group are not very common (see Box 6.1.3).

CLINICAL EXAMINATION

Refractive Errors

All adolescent clinics should have the Snellen distance viewing chart; it is handy and inexpensive. The patient is

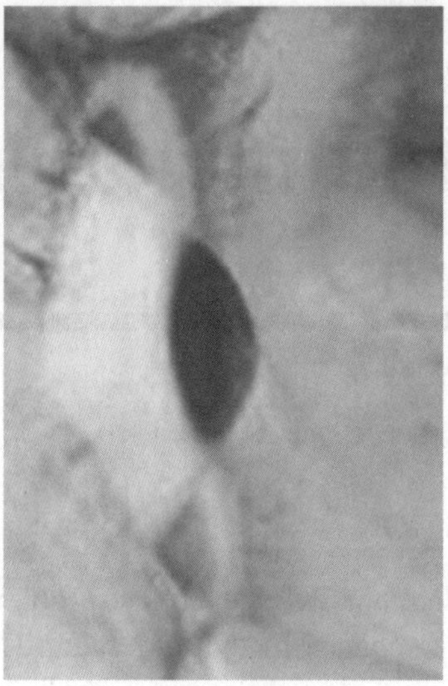

Figure 6.1.1: Keratoconus

asked to read the chart from a distance of approximately 6 metres firmly closing one eye at a time. If there is failure to read up to the last line with each eye and the patient is symptomatic or if there is a difference of more than 2 lines between the 2 eyes, the adolescent needs an ophthalmic referral (Table 6.1.2).

Squint

A large angle squint can be made out by simple torch light examination. The "cover-uncover" test is easy to perform to detect the smallest of squints. Simply ask the patient to focus on a distant object and cover one eye with the 4 fingers of the hand, pointing downwards. Move the hand quickly to the other eye and back again to the first one. If there is no squint, there will be no movement of either eye when covered or uncovered, while the opposite is true in an adolescent with a squint (Table 6.1.3).

Stevens-Johnson Syndrome

The acute stage ocular features are conjunctival eruptions, lid ulcerations, mucopurulent conjunctivitis, and secondary corneal ulceration. Late complications include adhesions between lids and conjunctiva/cornea (symblepharon formation) and dry eyes.

Conjunctivitis

For detailed descriptions of different forms of conjunctivitis, please see Table 6.1.4 and Figures 6.1.2A and B and 6.1.3A and B.

INVESTIGATIONS

A clinician should perform basic clinical examination as outlined above and if any abnormality is detected refer to ophthalmologist for further investigations.

Box 6.1.3: Cataracts in adolescents
Common causes include metabolic disturbances e.g. diabetes, hypoparathyroidism.
It may be secondary to ocular disease, e.g. trauma, PPD/RP, long-standing or recurrent uveitis, retinal detachment, aniridia, keratoconus, dislocation or subluxation of lens in certain syndromes, such as Marfan or Weil-Marchesani syndrome.
If the cataract is not dense or involving the whole lens or if the patient has not developed amblyopia, cataract surgery during adolescence does not carry any additional risk and has a good prognosis.
It is handled similar to an adult age-related cataract, with the same formulae used to calculate the power of the IOL to be inserted.
The surgical technique used, i.e. phacoemulsification with insertion of a foldable IOL is also the same as in adults.

Table 6.1.2: Refractive errors

Type	*Treatment*	*Comments*
Myopia	Corrected by use of concave spectacle lenses Contact lenses in adolescents mature enough to take care of lenses and hygiene; >15 years of age	Overuse of contact lenses could cause complications in the short or long-term Myth–Constant use of contact lenses prevent the myopia from progressing
	Adolescents > 18 years whose myopia has not progressed from the past one year may be considered for LASIK (Laser Assisted In-situ Keratomileusis) surgery	All adolescents are not suitable candidates for LASIK as the cornea cannot be thinned beyond a point in the interest of safety
Hypermetropia (less common in adolescents)	Corrected by use of convex spectacle lenses or appropriate contact lenses	Usually decreases with age as the eyeball grows in length or may remain constant, but seldom increases as the teen grows older
Astigmatism: Myopic, hypermetropic or mixed	Corrected with a 'cylinder', i.e. a number in the spectacle frame, which is present in only a particular direction, called 'axis' and not in the entire spectacle glass In case the teen has myopia or hypermetropia in addition to astigmatism, the spectacle lens will be a fusion of the spherical number with the cylinder	Does not increase or decrease, as the child grows older. It can be corrected with spectacles, contact lenses or by LASIK

Table 6.1.3: Squint in adolescents

Disorder	*Treatment*	*Comments*
Squint or strabismus: Paralytic (non-comitant) and non-paralytic (comitant)	Most non-paralytic squints manifest in early childhood, usually following a fever or a prolonged illness causing general debility. Many parents bring their children only in the adolescent age group for evaluation of squint. A squint present since early childhood has usually caused irreversible amblyopia and loss of binocular vision. Surgical correction achieves excellent cosmetic results but does not restore vision or improve binocularity if operated late, such as in adolescence.	In all adolescents, surgery is offered to completely correct the squint and offer excellent cosmesis. It is a myth that in the absence of binocular vision the surgical success is only temporary and the squint recurs! It does restore self-esteem and especially for girls reduces dowry at time of marriage.
Traumatic paralytic squint e.g. blows out fracture of the floor of the orbit or as a result of head injury.	The ophthalmologist usually waits for a minimum of six months for spontaneous recovery to occur, before attempting surgical correction.	However, each case of trauma is unique and this dictum may not hold true in all cases.

Table 6.1.4: Conjunctivitis

Type of conjunctivitis	*Clinical features*	*Management*
Epidemic conjunctivitis, usually viral	Watery discharge, red eye with or without conjunctival hemorrhages	Clean hands, avoid spread to others, simple broad spectrum antibiotic drops to prevent secondary bacterial infection
Bacterial conjunctivitis	Muco-purulent discharge with red eye	Frequent topical antibiotics
Allergic conjunctivitis	Multiple papillae on bulbar conjunctiva around limbus or on palpebral conjunctiva (Figures 6.1.2 and 6.1.3)	Mast cell inhibitor eye drops twice a day; in severe cases, a short course of topical steroids

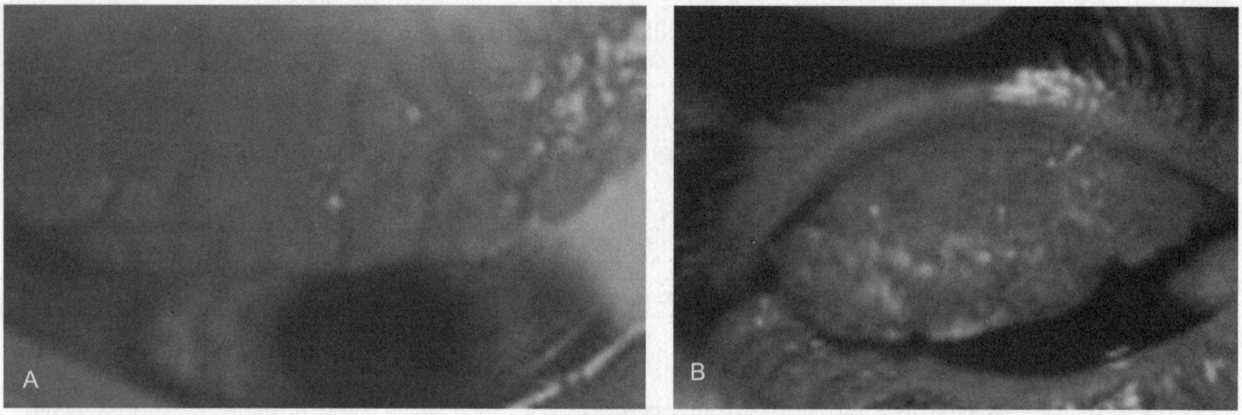

Figure 6.1.2A and B: Giant or cobblestone papillae on tarsal conjunctiva–Palpebral allergic conjunctivitis

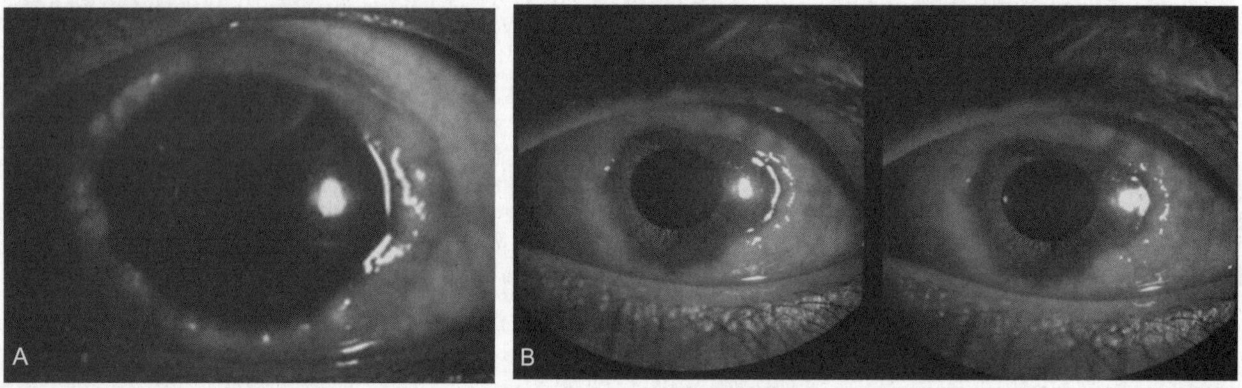

Figure 6.1.3A and B: Confluent papillae at limbus–Bulbar allergic conjunctivitis

MANAGEMENT

Refractive Errors

These should be corrected with spectacles or in older adolescents with contact lenses or LASIK (Laser Assisted In-situ Keratomileusis) surgery (see Table 6.1.2).

For a Child Coming with Headache During Examination

The child is examined for a refractive error, a very minor error of plus or minus quarter dioptre may be found. The child is given spectacles to wear. This may work as placebo therapy, but should be discontinued after the period of stress, e.g. examinations are over, as the headache magically disappears by then. During the examination period, it is better to counsel the adolescent in correct studying habits, to reduce eye strain (see Table 6.1.2).

Keratoconus

Most patients can be managed without surgical procedures. In early stages it is well corrected with spectacles. Initially, the patient may require change of spectacle glasses. However, as the cone progresses, the cornea thins and the quality and quantity of vision may not improve sufficiently with spectacle glasses alone. Various contact lenses can then be tried, e.g. hard lenses, rigid gas permeable (RGP) lenses, semi-soft lenses and scleral lenses. Some patients may do well with "piggy back" lenses, i.e. a soft contact lens worn first with an RGP lens over it.

If these do not help and the cone is progressing, then surgical methods will be needed. The progression can be halted by collagen cross linkage (CXL) procedure with over 95% success rate. In advanced cases, a keratoplasty will be necessary to restore vision (see Box 6.1.2).

Stevens-Johnson Syndrome

Aggressive treatment in the early phase with topical antibiotics and copious use of lubricants and breaking of early adhesions using the piston of a tuberculin syringe coated with an eye ointment is essential to prevent late complications. In spite of this, a majority of the patients will develop keratoconjunctivitis sicca or dry eye, with corneal opacities and symblepharon.

Ocular Trauma

Adolescents have high incidence of both mechanical and chemical trauma (Figures 6.1.4, 6.1.5 and 6.1.6). This

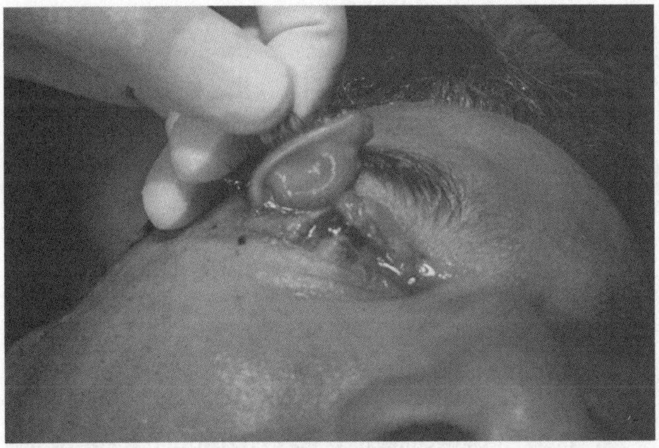

Figure 6.1.4: Upper eyelid avulsion due to road accident

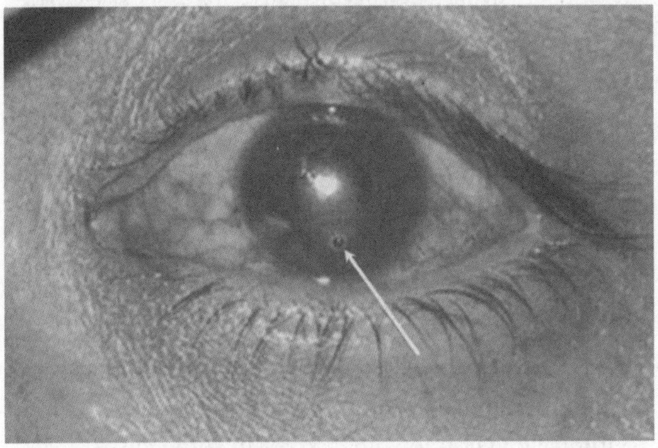

Figure 6.1.5: Corneal foreign body (white arrow)

is an ophthalmic emergency and after first aid in clinic should be immediately referred to an ophthalmologist in a hospital set up to salvage the eyes (Table 6.1.5).

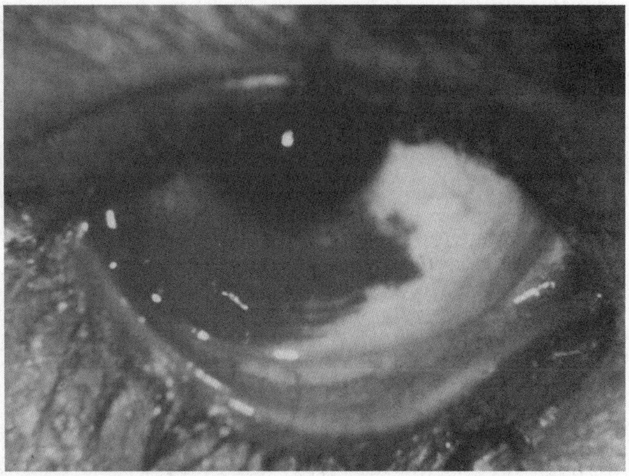

Figure 6.1.6: Sub-conjunctival hemorrhage due to injury

Other Eye Problems

Other eye problems that can present in an adolescent include ambyopia and primary pigmentary degeneration. These are detailed in Table 6.1.6.

LEARNING POINTS

- Distance reading chart should be kept in every clinic to quickly check for refractive errors.
- Any physician can check for even small degrees of squint without any equipment in his/her clinic. All squints can be corrected by surgery, at any age Squint surgery is a permanent solution to restore cosmesis.

Table 6.1.5: Ocular trauma in adolescents

Type	*Etiology*	*Management*
Mechanical trauma: Intraocular foreign body (IOFB)	Sharp toys, such as scissors and knives are often left unattended around the house, which young adolescents may pick up and injure themselves accidentally.	Immediate referral to salvage the eyes. Corneal lacerations or partial thickness corneal tears—Firm patching. A full thickness corneal tear or a penetrating injury requires surgery. MRI should not be done when a metallic IOFB is suspected; it will shift causing further damage. The eye surgeon will do a B-scan ultrasonography or slit lamp biomicroscope examination.
Chemical burns	Acids and alkalis are often used in 'crimes of passion' to disfigure a former lover and may end up causing irreversible blindness. This results in loss of stem cells, present at the limbus. The prognosis is dependent on the number of clock hours of limbal ischemia. Better results with new treatments now such as fetal amniotic membrane, stem cell transplants and artificial cornea (keratoprosthesis).	Ophthalmic emergency: Prompt first aid and urgent referral. Eye should be washed copiously with water or normal saline or Ringers solution to remove as much of the chemical as possible. The eyelids should be everted so that the palpebral conjunctiva can be washed as well. Lime (calcium hydroxide): Attempt physical removal of the lime particles with a forceps. Topical ascorbate eye drops (ampoule of injection vitamin C broken and dispensed in eye dropper bottle) instilled hourly for the first 48 hours and then put in reducing doses for up to two weeks.

Table 6.1.6: Miscellaneous eye problems in adolescents

Disorder	*Treatment*	*Comments*
Amblyopia–"lazy eye"	Can be corrected <5 years age. Adolescent age is too late for reversal of amblyopia. If detected in adolescent age correcting the squint or giving the correct spectacle number will not improve the vision in the amblyopic eye.	The teenager and more importantly the parents need to be counseled to accept the defective vision in the lazy eye and avoid indulging in needless and often expensive doctor shopping. The adolescent does not have to restrict his/her visual activities, such as reading, studying, and TV or computer usage. She/he needs no patching of the good eye or visual stimulation exercises for the lazy eye.
Primary pigmentary degeneration (PPD) or Retinitis pigmentosa (RP)	Various treatments can be tried: • Attempts to increase blood supply to the retina by medical and surgical means. • Vitamin supplements, antioxidant therapy. • Hyperbaric oxygen. • Genetic therapy may hold some promise in the future. • Under research is implantation of a silicon chip into the retina.	Congenital PPD may present in the adolescent age. It may remain stationary for years or progress gradually leading to complete blindness in the third to fifth decade.

- Adolescents with refractive errors should be taught correct reading and computer viewing habits, to prevent eye strain.
- LASIK or laser removal of numbers should only be done in adolescents above the age of 18 years with a stable refraction for minimum of one year prior.
- Adolescents with amblyopia should be counselled to accept their poor vision in one eye.
- Adolescents with obvious squints should be operated upon for cosmetic purposes as surgery improves self-esteem and prevents late development of inferiority complex.
- Keratoconus can be managed depending on severity with glasses, contact lenses and as a last resort, surgery, with excellent visual prognosis.
- Steroids should be very sparingly used in allergic conjunctivitis, now that there are several other topical non-steroid drops that are effective in a large number of such cases.
- Patients with mechanical or chemical trauma need immediate referral to a competent ophthalmologist or centre. Visual prognosis in seemingly bad cases has also improved due to modern methods of management, including stem cell transplants.
- Adolescents with cataracts, who are not amblyopic, pose no special problems for surgery.
- Primary pigmentary degeneration still has no specific treatment at present. Low vision aids may help improve vision to some extent in some cases.

SUGGESTED READING

1. Duke-Elder S. System of Ophthalmology, Vol V, Ophthalmic Optics and Refraction. London; Henry Kimpton 1970; 255-88.
2. Duke-Elder S. System of Ophthalmology, Vol VI, Ocular Motility and Strabismus. London; Henry Kimpton 1973; 421-31.
3. Harley RD. Pediatric Ophthalmology. Toronto, WB Saunders Co 1975;353-54.
4. Maskati Q, Chapter 12.2 Ophthalmology. In: Bhave SY, Ed. Adolescent Health Case Scenarios, New Delhi; Byword Books Pvt Ltd 2011;374-80.
5. Maskati QB, Maskati BT, Sadarangani D. Chemical Burns of the Eye. In: Shukla B, Natarajan S, Eds, Management of Ocular Trauma. New Delhi; CBS Publishers and Distributors 2005;263-69.
6. Vasavada AR. Intraocular lens implantation. In: Dutta LC, Ed. Modern Ophthalmology. New Delhi; Jaypee Brothers Medical Publishers Pvt. Ltd 1994; 367-73.

Ear, Nose and Throat Problems

6.2

Divya Prabhat

INTRODUCTION

Adolescents seek the advice of the family doctor or ear, nose and throat (ENT) specialists for common problems like discharge from the ear, bleeding from nostrils, headache, recurrent sneezing and/or allergic rhinorrhea which are the common problems they face during their growing phase of adolescence with interface with their day-to-day activities.

HISTORY TAKING AND PRESENTING SYMPTOMS

Otitis Externa

The characteristic clinical features of otitis externa are as follows (see Box 6.2.1 and Table 6.2.1):

- Itching in the canal is severe.
- Pain is intense.
- Deafness due to the blocked canal.
- Ear discharge is blackish or brownish.
- Tinnitus may be present.

Mastoiditis

The characteristic clinical features of mastoiditis are as follows (see Table 6.2.2):

- Scanty ear discharge.
- Foul odor.
- Post-aural pain and headache.

Table 6.2.2 shows differences between otitis externa and mastoiditis.

Box 6.2.1: Otitis externa
Otitis externa primarily occurs in the external auditory canal or it may be a manifestation of a generalized skin condition.
The incidence is high in those suffering from excessive negative middle ear pressure which causes discomfort inducing the sufferer to probe the ears to relieve it and thus traumatizing the canal skin.
The outer third of the ear canal is cartilaginous, while inner two-thirds is bony and this junction is the site for injuries following using ear buds.
Secondary infection complicates the course.

Otitis Media

The state of the middle ear cleft in the adolescent depends on the attacks of respiratory tract infections during childhood (as the eustachian tube is short, wide and horizontal). In many the infections resolve but in a few adolescents it leaves behind a legacy of mucosal disease; intratympanic negative middle ear pressure and perforation of the tympanic membrane which affect their development of subsequent chronic suppurative otitis media later in life.

Table 6.2.3 shows the characteristic features of the various types of otitis media.

- History of instrumentation—match sticks, hair pin, exposure to heat, humidity and swimming, inherent tendency to eczema, excessive wax formation.
- The tubo-tympanic variety manifests as copious, non-foul smelling mucoid discharge. The ear drum shows a central perforation involving the pars tensa and the mucosa is clean and healthy pink in color.
- Attico-antral variety manifests as scanty and foul smelling discharge. The ear drum shows a small perforation in the pars flaccida with the pars tensa being normal.
- In the safe type there is a preceding history of respiratory tract infection.
- Pain is severe and aggravated by movement of the jaw.
- Ear discharge is purulent and blood stained; and may be profuse.
- Deafness if the lumen is blocked due to a furuncle, debris or edema.
- Trismus following limitation of movement of temporo-mandibular joint.
- Itching.
- There also may be complaints pertaining to academic performance being affected.
- In attico-antral disease (unsafe) there would be complaints of foul smelling ear discharge but not associated with respiratory infections.
- There also may be complaints of headache or vertigo.

Table 6.2.1: Types of otitis externa

Type	*Clinical signs and symptoms*	*Treatment*
Viral *Herpes simplex*	With or without facial nerve palsy (Ramsay Hunt syndrome).	No specific treatment. Keep ear dry.
Herpes zoster	Crop of small vesicles which dries up after a few days to a week.	
Bullous myringitis	Blebs on the tympanic membrane and the deep meatal skin. Purplish due to hemorrhagic effusion filling the vesicles. Differential diagnosis–In otitis media the complete drum is inflamed.	Analgesics to relieve the severe pain. The ears are kept dry and antibiotics have no influence on the course of the disease. Bleb incision is of no use and may cause secondary infection.
Fungal infection	*Candida albicans* and *Aspergillus niger* are common pathogens. Greyish white debris. Wet blotting paper appearance. Diabetes and immunocompromised host + Humidity–due to swimming or bath. Prolonged use of antibiotic ear drops–Infection.	Remove epithelial debris, as fungi thrive on them. Ear drops 2% salicylic acid in spirit, 1% clotrimazole or antifungal antibiotics like nystatin. Antibiotics–secondary infection. Analgesics and antipruritic agents. Treatment is continued for a week after the condition has apparently cleared up clinically.
Reactive otitis externa	Eczematous reaction due to infection, allergy or antibiotic ear drops, e.g. neomycin.	Ear kept dry. Local application of steroids and antihistaminics
Seborrheic dermatitis (Dandruff)	Scaling in the external auditory canal, postauricular sulcus and below the lobe of the pinna.	Regular removal of debris from the canal. Washing hair with a shampoo for keeping the dandruff under control. Steroid-antibiotic ear drops.
Neurodermatitis	Underlying psychosomatic disturbance makes the condition difficult to clear up. Constant scratching leads to lichenification or secondary infection of the skin causing a diffuse otitis externa.	Clearing up of secondary infections and attempting to alleviate irritation with topical hydrocortisone cream. A course of anti-histamincs to reduce itching and congestion of the canal. In severe cases it may be necessary to bandage the ears to prevent scratching. Due attention must be paid to the psychological aspects.

Table 6.2.2: Features of otitis externa and mastoiditis

Features	*Otitis externa*	*Mastoiditis*
History of water entering the ear trauma/ instrumentation/deafness common	Symptoms of discharge	
Respiratory tract infection	Absent	Common
Pinna position	Normal	Displaced forwards, downwards and outwards
Mastoid tenderness	Absent	Present
Pinna movement	Painful	No pain
Post-aural groove	Normal	Obliterated
External canal	Stenosed and edematous	Normal
Tympanic membrane	Normal	Congested or perforated
Post-aural lymph node	Enlarged	Not palpable
X-ray mastoids	Normal	Haziness or destruction of air cells seen

Sinusitis

The characteristic clinical features of sinusitis are as follows (Box 6.2.2):

- Headache, malaise and fever.
- Loss of normal vocal resonance.
- Pain around the various sinuses.
- Referred pain in the ear.
- Nasal discharge.
- Nose block.

Nasal Polyp

See Box 6.2.3 and Table 6.2.4 for detailed description about nasal polyps and the distinctive features of antrochoanal and ethmoid polyps. Figures 6.2.1, 6.2.2 and 6.2.3 demonstrate anatomy of the antrochoanal and ethmoid polyps.

- Nasal block is unilateral with antrochoanal polyp and bilateral with ethmoidal polyps.
- Headache may be a constant complaint in either case.

Table 6.2.3: Features differentiating various types of otitis externa		
Features	***Safe ear***	***Unsafe ear***
Type of disease	Tubo-tympanic	Attico-antral
Perforation site	Central	Attic
Granulations	Absent	Common
Discharge	Copious, mucoid and non-foul smelling	Scanty, purulent and foul smelling
Bleeding	Never	Sometimes
Respiratory tract infection	Increase in the amount of discharge	Not affected
Audiogram	Conductive hearing loss	Mixed hearing loss
X-ray mastoid	Sclerotic	Sclerotic with destruction
Complications (Fatal)	Nil	Common

Box 6.2.2: Sinusitis

All sinuses are fully developed by puberty; the frontal sinus by 15 years age

Maxillary sinusitis is the most common in this age group as the floor is at a lower level than ostia with poor drainage and proximity to the teeth

Infecting agent: Viral, bacterial (tuberculosis) and fungal

Predisposing factors: Poor general health, spread from rhinitis, pharyngeal and dental infections, swimming and diving, trauma (contusions fractures), foreign body and barotrauma

Investigations

1. Bacteriological examination is required if the sinusitis does not respond to antibiotic treatment
2. Radiology: Water's and Caldwell's view of the paranasal sinuses may show:
   - Mucosal thickening
   - Opacity of sinuses or
   - An air-fluid level
3. CT scan to see the osteo-meatal complex
4. MRI: In case of suspected angiofibroma (differentiate from antrochoanal polyp)
5. Diagnostic antral puncture
6. Nasal sinus endoscopy

Management

Acute sinusitis: This may respond to medical treatment

Chronic sinusitis requires surgery:

- Correction of a deviated septum
- Antral puncture
- Functional endoscopic sinus surgery

Box 6.2.3: Nasal polyps

Polyp is prolapsed edematous respiratory mucosa, which may result from vascular derangements in the mucosa or from mechanical obstruction.

The mechanism appears to be an area of simple edema, then the stroma becomes filled with intercellular fluid, the edematous mucosa becomes polypoid:

If not arrested at this stage it enlarges to come down into the nasal cavity acquiring a pedicle and being called a polyp (Figure. 6.2.1).

Serum immunoglobulins IgA especially and IgE are present in greater amounts in the polypus fluids than as would be expected.

However there is a significant role of allergy and also infections in the nose and sinuses which commonly co-exists in ethmoidal nasal polyposis.

Table 6.2.4: Differences between polyps	
Antrochoanal polyp	***Ethmoidal polyp***
Single	Multiple
Unilateral	Bilateral
Infective origin	Allergic
From maxillary sinus	Ethmoid sinus
Triradiate polyp	Pedunculated polyp
Grows posteriorly	Anteriorly
More in adolescents	More in elderly
Surgery only treatment	Antihistamines/steroids first
Recurrences rare	Common
Functional endoscopic sinus surgery (FESS)/Caldwell Luc	Polypectomy with FESS

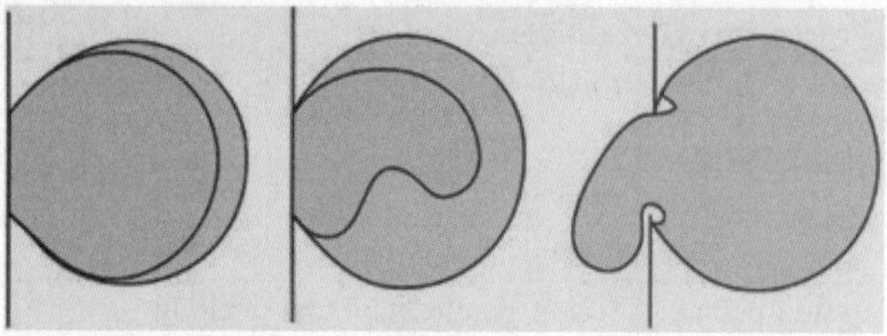

Figure 6.2.1: Bilateral multiple polyps, hanging downwards

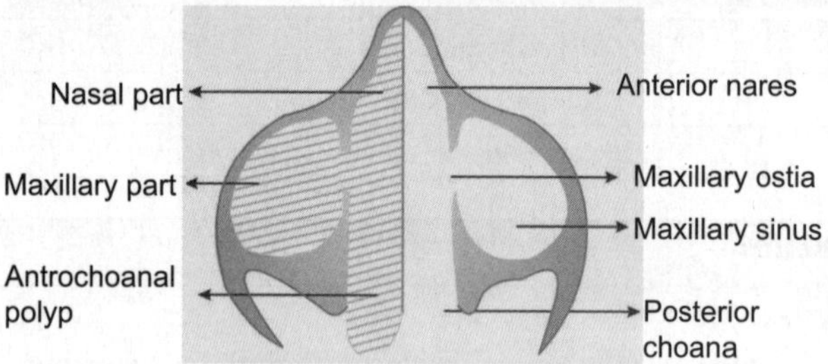

Figure 6.2.2: Antrochoanal polyp

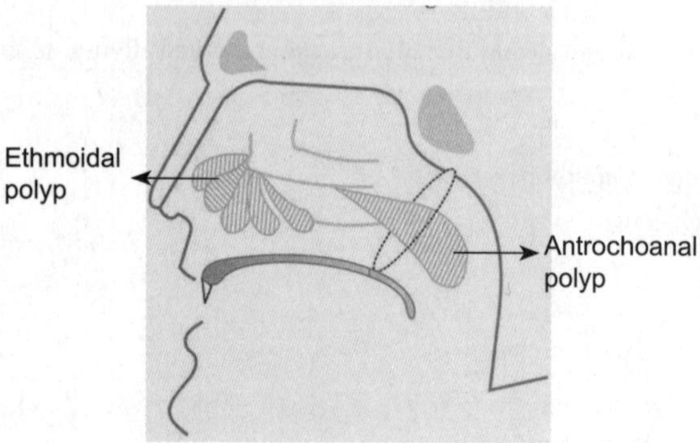

Figure 6.2.3: Ethmoidal polyp and antrochoanal polyp

- In case of superadded infections there would be purulent discharge.

CLINICAL EXAMINATION

Otitis Externa

The characteristic clinical features of otitis externa are as follows:

- Pain is present with ear discharge.
- Movement of the pinna is very painful.
- Canal edema is diagnostic.

Mastoiditis

The characteristic clinical features of mastoiditis are as follows:

- Mastoiditis occurs with attico-antral disease when the infection crosses the confines of the middle ear cleft.
- Central perforations occurring with tubo-tympanic diseases do not lead to mastoiditis.
- Specific diagnostic signs as position of the pinna and tenderness over the mastoid bone.

Otitis Media

The characteristic clinical features of otitis media are as follows:

- The external canal appears congested, edematous and stenosed.
- Pain occurs on movement of the pinna.
- Discharge may be present.
- Trismus.

Sinusitis

The characteristic clinical features of sinusitis are as follows:

- Flushing of the cheek with swelling in case of maxillary sinusitis and involving the upper eyelid in frontal sinusitis.
- Tenderness is elicited at the canine fossa in maxillary sinusitis and above the medial canthus in frontal sinusitis.
- Anterior rhinoscopy reveals redness and mucosal congestion.
- Pus may be seen trickling from the middle meatus area.
- Posterior rhinoscopy may also reveal pus from the middle meatus area.

Nasal Polyp

The characteristic clinical features of nasal polyps are as follows:

- Antrochoanal polyps are always unilateral, however on post-rhinoscopy the choanal part can be seen (as is the largest part).
- Ethmoidal polyps are always bilateral and multiple in number.
- There may be extensive nasal discharge on account of being allergic in origin.

MANAGEMENT

Otitis Externa

- **Glycerin icthammol (10%)**—With glycerin pack is placed into external canal. Glycerin reduces the edema by its hygroscopic action and icthammol acts as an antiseptic.
- **Heat application**—It is helpful in reducing the pain and inflammation.
- **Antibiotics**—They are given only in cases of marked edema or when local lymph nodes are palpable.
- **Analgesics**—To reduce pain.
- **Incision and drainage**—Under aseptic conditions in furunculosis, in cases of failure of relief from pain.

- **Diabetes**—It should be ruled out in patients having recurrent attacks of otitis externa.

Mastoiditis

- Requires intravenous antibiotics and drainage in case of abscess formation.

Otitis Media

- Treatment of the upper respiratory infection.
- Aural toilet—It is performed meticulously under direct vision, preferably suction and irrigation done under the operating microscope.
- Boro-spirit ear drops—Ear drops are advised only during active discharge.
- Foci of infection—These are treated medically or surgically, e.g. tonsillitis, sinusitis etc.
- Removal of polypi or granulation tissue—If present in the middle ear.
- Chemical cautery using 50% trichloroacetic acid for smaller perforations (<65% area if tympanic membrane).
- Myringoplasty or tympanoplasty may be required for a persisting perforation.

Sinusitis

- Antibiotics—Erythromycin, amoxicillin, azithromycin, sparfloxicillin, etc. can be given.
- Local decongestants are used, which do not interfere with the ciliary functions, i.e. ephedrine, zylometazoline nose drops or sprays are used.
- Analgesics and anti-inflammatory drugs such as paracetamol, diclofenac, nimesulide etc. are commonly used for relief of headache and pain.
- Antihistaminics such as terfenadine, chlorpheniramine loratidine, levocetrizine or fexofenadine are used.
- Steam inhalation–For clearing out the secretions. Tincture benzoin or menthol provide symptomatic relief and promote sinus drainage. Figure 6.2.4 shows the drainage direction of major sinuses.

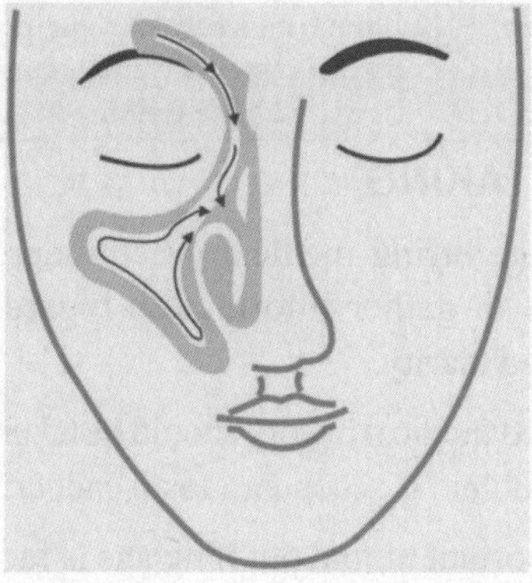

Figure 6.2.4: Drainage direction of mucociliary clearance towards the natural ostia

Nasal Polyp

- Antrochoanal polyp need to be removed surgically.
- Nasal endoscopy is done to remove the polyp or Caldwell Luc operation is performed.
- Ethmoidal polyps are treated with antihistaminics and steroid nasal sprays.
- Those not responding to medical treatment are managed surgically by nasal sinus endoscopy techniques.

LEARNING POINTS

1. ENT problems are quite common in adolescent age group.
2. Sinusitis is the most common cause for absence from school.
3. Otitis media affects hearing and can also cause intracranial complications.
4. Nasal polyps usually require surgical intervention for removal of the polyps.
5. Untreated childhood allergic rhinitis leads to adulthood asthma.

SUGGESTED READING

1. Ballantyne J, Groves J. Scott-Brown's Diseases of the Ear, Nose and Throat; 5th edition. Vol 2, The Ear. London; Butterworth and Co. Ltd 1979;104-12.
2. Bluestone CD, Simons JP, Healy GB. Bluestone and Stool's Pediatric Otolaryngology, 5th edition. McGraw Hill; 2013.
3. Cutler J, Duncavage JA, Matheny K, Cross JL, Miman MC, Oh CK. *et al.* Results of Caldwell-Luc after failed endoscopic middle meatus antrostomy in patients with chronic sinusitis. Laryngoscope 2003:113(12):2148-50.
4. Graham J, Scadding G, Bull P, Eds. Pediatric ENT. Verlag, Berlin, Heidelberg; 2007.
5. Hathiram BT, Grewal DS. Ent Ear-Nose-Throat Simplified. Mumbai; Bhalani Book Depot 2003;12:103-11.
6. Hussain SM, Ed. Logan Turner's Diseases of Ear, Nose and Throat, Head and Neck Surgery,11th ed. CRC Press, 2015.
7. Kothari S, *et al.* Imaging of the Paranasal sinuses. Mumbai; AOI Mumbai Branch 2001;48-62.
8. Prabhat D. Practical ENT, 10th edition. Mumbai; The National Book Depot; 2015.
9. Rosenfeld RM, Culpepper L, Doyle KJ, *et al.* Natural history of untreated otitis media. Laryngoscope 2003;113:1645-57.
10. Stammberger H. Functional endoscopic sinus surgery (FESS) by Karl Storz; 1989.

Voice Problems

6.3

Nehal Kothari

INTRODUCTION

Voice is a powerful tool. In adolescence, it plays a very important role in building one's identity and forming peer relationships. Like fingerprints and DNA, every voice has its unique characteristics. We communicate emotions and expressions with our voice. Hence, appropriate care and timely management of voice disorders is vital.

The vocal cords in the larynx vibrate to produce sound. If one of the vocal cords is not working the right way, the result will be voice problems.

Before puberty, both male and female children have approximately the same pitch and larynx is approximately of the same size. At puberty, male larynx undergoes a greater magnitude change in comparison to female larynx. Larynx descends down in neck. Alongside development of secondary sex characteristics, there is a growth spurt in phonatory, respiratory and resonance structures. As a result, male voice drops down in pitch significantly (close to one octave) whereas female voice drops only by few notes. Hence, male voice at and post-puberty is considerably low pitched and female voice is high pitched.

Voice disorders include the problems of pitch, loudness, resonance and/or quality that distracts the listeners from what is being said. These disorders may also cause pain or discomfort while speaking.

Voice disorders common during adolescence are mainly the following:

1. Secondary to physiological and/or structural changes of the larynx (Table 6.3.1).
2. Endocrine/hormonal changes: Endocrine disorders can have a major impact on the pitch of the voice. It can make the voice extremely low pitched or high pitched (Table 6.3.2).
3. Secondary to abuse or misuse (Table 6.3.3).
4. Miscellaneous causes (Table 6.3.3).

Table 6.3.1: Voice problems secondary to puberty–Physiological and/or structural changes

Puberphonia	If an adult male who has completed puberty, still presents with high pitched voice, it is known as puberphonia. These patients face several social challenges and stigma. Owing to high pitched and feminine voice they are considered effeminate and inadequate. They are often teased and face difficulty in interviews and peer relationships. People often misjudge them as female speaker especially when they are not in front of them for e.g. while talking on phone.
Androphonia	This is characterized by abnormally low pitched voice in females. It can be less than 100 Hz and sounds like a male voice. Similar to puberphonia patients, these patients also face several difficulties and stigma in social interactions.

Table 6.3.2: Voice problems due to endocrine dysfunction

Hypo-function of pituitary gland, tumors of pituitary gland, Addison disease	Hormonal imbalance can result in continued high pitched voice in adolescent male. It can at times result in deepening of voice in females.
Thyroid dysfunction	Hypothyroidism can result in hoarse and at times low pitched voice. Hyperthyroidism can result in breathy voice with decreased loudness.
Pre-menstrual voice changes	Some girls complain of reduced pitch range and vocal fatigue prior to menses. This is especially important for adolescent girls who are training in singing.

HISTORY TAKING

- For the referring medical practitioner, it would be relevant to gather information regarding patient's voice and clarity.
- A detailed medical history should be taken if suspecting voice problem is secondary to an endocrine disorder.
- It is important to find out if he/she is facing difficulty in being understood by others and if any pitch breaks are reported by the patient.

Table 6.3.3: Voice disorders	
Vocal abuse and misuse	Vocal abuse is any behavior or occurrence that strains or injures the vocal cords. This may include excessive talking, inhaling irritants, smoking, screaming, or yelling. Frequent vocal abuse and misuse can damage the vocal folds and cause temporary or permanent changes in vocal function, voice quality, and possible loss of voice.
Vocal nodules and polyps	They are common benign growths that develop on the vocal cords. Mature nodules are similar to "calluses" and develop on both vocal folds. Polyps tend to be more fluid filled than nodules. Typical symptoms noted for nodules and polyps are hoarseness, vocal fatigue and effortful voice. Both are caused secondary to vocal abuse and misuse. Other factors that may also increase the likelihood of development of these pathologies are smoking, alcohol use, and allergies, exposure to noxious chemicals and or frequent laryngitis and upper respiratory tract infections.
Others	Other pathologies (though less common in this age group) such as vocal cyst, sulcus, hemorrhage (varices) have also been noted secondary to vocal abuse and misuse in adolescents.

- In case of voice abuse, ask questions regarding onset of voice change and if the patient abuses his/her voice frequently.

CLINICAL EXAMINATION

- Physical examination (palpate for nodularity or adenopathy).
- Signs of thyroid dysfunction and other endocrine disorders.

INVESTIGATIONS

- Appropriate blood and relevant medical investigations for systemic diseases, e.g. thyroid function tests and thyroid scan should be done.
- Laryngoscopy/stroboscopy.

The patient should be first referred to a laryngologist for endoscopy or stroboscopy to assess structure, function and degree of impairment of the laryngeal structures and their function. This also helps to rule out any other pathology in the larynx and vocal cords.

MANAGEMENT PROTOCOL

Voice disorders require a qualified speech language pathologist (SLP) trained in management of voice disorders. If not treated in time the voice quality may be permanently affected. Speech therapy has to be carried out for an appropriate amount of time till results are seen.

- Puberphonia patients are helped to facilitate low pitch voice. On an average, typically it takes 3-4 sessions to achieve the appropriate pitch and few more sessions to facilitate carry over in daily conversations.
- In females the pitch can be raised via voice surgery and voice rehabilitation.
- Voice training for adolescent patients undergoing singing training can also significantly improve their vocal performance and help them understand their pitch range.
- Primary treatment for hormonal imbalance should be hormonal therapy.
- For vocal nodules, the voice therapy (speech therapy) is almost always recommended as the first line of treatment. Therapy focuses on relaxation and strengthening exercises and incorporation of vocal hygiene.
- For patients with polyp, depending on the degree of severity laryngologist may refer for speech therapy along with medications or they may recommend surgery.
- In case of tumor, appropriate surgery should be done when indicated. In many cases, post-surgery voice function may get altered. In such cases, relaxation voice therapy can significantly aid in improving and maintaining the voice quality.

LEARNING POINTS

- In adolescence, voice plays a very important role in building one's identity and forming peer relationships.
- Puberphonia and androphonia are important voice problems that are associated with pubertal changes and can have an adverse effect on their self-esteem unless treated in time.
- Changes in quality and pitch of voice, hoarseness and voice fatigue are indications that endoscopic evaluation of the function of the vocal cords is done and other pathologies are ruled out.
- The mainstay of management for voice disorders are voice therapy from a qualified speech language pathologist (SLP).

SUGGESTED READING

1. Anderson T, Sataloff RT. The power of voice therapy. Ear Nose Throat J 2002;81(7):433-34.

2. Boone DR. Dismissal criteria in voice therapy. J Speech Hear Disord 1974;39(2):133-39.
3. Carroll LM. The Role of the Voice Specialist in Nonmedical Management of Benign Voice Disorders. In: Rubin J, Sataloff RT, Korovin GS, Eds. Diagnosis and Treatment of Voice Disorders, 3rd edition. San Diego, CA; Plural Publishing, 2005.
4. Colton RH, Casper JK. Understanding voice problems. A physiological perspective for diagnosis and treatment. Baltimore MD: Lippincott Williams and Wikins, 1996.
5. McCrory E. Voice therapy outcomes in vocal fold nodules: A retrospective audit. Int J Lang Commun Disord 2001; 36 Suppl:19-24.
6. Murry T, Woodson GE. A comparison of three methods for the management of vocal fold nodules. J Voice 1992;6:271-76.
7. Pedersen M, Beranova A, Moller S. Dysphonia: Medical treatment and a medical voice hygiene advice approach. A prospective randomised pilot study. Eur Arch Otorhinolaryngol 2003;261(6):312-15.
8. Smith E, Verdolini K, Gray S, Nichols S, Lemke J, Barkmeier J, *et al.* Effect of voice disorders on quality of life. J Med Speech Lang Path 1996;4:223-44.
9. Strobovideoscopy: http://www.asha.org/policy/RP1998-00132/Accessed on 26/8/2015.
10. Voice Rehabilitation: http://www.asha.org/policy/TR2005-00147/ Accessed on 26/8/2015.

Dermatological Problems

6.4

Jayakar Thomas, Parimalam Kumar

INTRODUCTION

Any small blemish on the skin causes great concern to the adolescent. The adolescent feels that he or she is being looked at with social dislike. This is essentially because adolescents are establishing a sense of autonomy by scrutinizing, modifying, or rejecting their parents' values and instead comparing and identifying with the standards of their peer group. The 'internal struggle' between being dependent and independent at the same time, results invariably in non-compliance of treatment.

To sell beauty products the cosmetic industry highlights the skin blemishes like acne and promotes the lightening of the skin. This adds to the negative body image adolescents develop during puberty. A clear healthy skin adds to the self-esteem of an adolescent. Hence the treatment of skin lesion is not just a medical problem but also involves a lot of psychological counseling including referral to mental health specialists if the adolescent has depression caused by the skin problem.

For the above reasons, as in any other specialty, history taking, examination, laboratory examination and treatment carry a specific adolescent friendly pattern. All adolescents must be told about confidentiality as they are reluctant to discuss sensitive and personal information. Physicians must elicit history in a caring and respectful manner with non-judgmental questions that may include factors related to their hobby, home, studies, job and other activities. Special attention must be paid while inquiring about the drug history, sexuality and emotional status, e.g. depression. Doctor must have an easy going, relaxed and unhurried approach. While focusing on the area of chief complaint, attention must also be paid to other findings including, the stage of secondary sexual development. In case of examination of the skin of the covered parts, it is always advisable to give an overview of the examination prior to disrobing, respecting the privacy and modesty of the patient for both girls and boys. This chapter does not cover all the skin lesions but only those that are important to adolescent mind as a compelling problem. In most cases lifestyle modification holds the key.

HISTORY TAKING

Skin lesions in an adolescent are very much dependent on his/her diet, lifestyle, sleep habits , cosmetics used etc. which vary greatly from time to time depending on the developmental stage of adolescence and mood swings and proprieties at that time.

Hence for any skin lesion it is very important to take a very detailed history.

Acne: It is important to take detailed history of multiple factors like exposure to acnegenic mineral oils and dioxin, drugs like lithium, hydantoin and systemic corticosteroids, endocrine factors (androgens) (see Box 6.4.1).

Emotional stress (school, social problems), pressure on skin by leaning face on hands, are known to exacerbate acne. A psychological assessment should be done as acne can badly affect the psyche of the adolescent due to a negative body image.

Body odor or bromhidrosis is a common phenomenon in post-pubertal adolescents who present with particularly offensive body odor that most commonly originates from the axillary region (see Box 6.4.2).

Dark axillae are a very disturbing and cosmetically unacceptable problem especially in adolescent girls. These girls are so desperate and seek advice mainly due to very restrictive wardrobe options. The causes are very many like atopic dermatitis, freckles, nevi, fungal infections, and erythrasma. However the main cause often is due to acanthosis nigricans (AN) (see Box 6.4.3). High glycemic diet, lack of physical exercise and a 'dirty' appearance of the axillae are hallmarks of personal history.

Cosmetically concerning pigmentation can affect anyone; this condition is more prevalent among Asians. Pigmentation can affect any part of the body including the face, hands and neck. These open and exposed areas are of great concern to adolescents (see Box 6.4.4).

Box 6.4.1: Acne vulgaris

Acne is a common chronic inflammation of the pilosebaceous units that affects many adolescents during puberty.

As psychological disturbance is so high and manifests as depression, it should be diagnosed early and proper counseling given at appropriate time.

Asymptomatic, small, skin colored papules and few pustules appear peri-menarche and disappear with pigmentation and scarring.

Acne starts at the age of 10 to 17 years in females and 14 to 19 in males, but it may appear first at 25 years.

It is usually more severe in males than females, but may persist in women till the age of 35.

Acne is associated with increased oiliness of the facial skin with premenstrual flair.

Acne can be genetic.

The skin eruptions primarily appear on the face, upper back and/or chest and manifest as comedones, papules, nodules, cysts, or papulopustules, often but not always, followed by pitted or hypertrophic scars.

The disease is graded as:

- Grade 1: Predominantly comedones
- Grade 2: Predominantly papules
- Grade 3: Predominantly pustules
- Grade 4: Predominantly cysts and nodules

Acne conglobata is associated with systemic disturbance in grade 4 acne and spill over to trunk.

Box 6.4.2: Bromhidrosis or body odor

This is a chronic condition in which excessive odor, usually an unpleasant one, emanates from the skin and can substantially impair a person's quality of life.

The odor has been described as pungent, rancid, musty, or sour in character.

Apocrine bromhidrosis: Most common, bacterial decomposition yields ammonia and short-chain fatty acids, with their characteristic strong odors.

Eccrine bromhidrosis: Eccrine sweat softens keratin and bacterial degradation of the keratin yields a foul smell. It may also result from underlying metabolic or endogenous causes. Ingestion of some foods, including garlic, onion, curry, alcohol and certain drugs (e.g. penicillin and bromides) may be responsible for the odor.

When a treatment method is chosen, it is important to consider the cultural implications and the degree of impairment in quality of life, as well as the patient's expectations and goals of treatment.

Box 6.4.3: Acanthosis nigricans (AN)

Commonly seen in obese adolescents more so in girls.

It is a very disturbing and cosmetically unacceptable problem.

The definitive cause for AN has not yet been ascertained.

It is associated with insulin resistance (IR) and polycystic ovary syndrome (PCOS).

Final outcome of AN varies depending on the cause of AN.

There is no specific treatment except to improve cosmetic appearance and include topical retinoids, dermabrasion, laser therapy and oral dietary fish oil supplementation.

Lifestyle changes such as healthy eating habits and regular physical exercises have good outcome.

Treatment of associated metabolic syndrome and/or PCOS.

Box 6.4.4: Hyperpigmentation and melasma

Pigmentation is the result of either of two occurrences:

- An abnormally high concentration of melanocytes produce melanin; or
- When melanocytes are hyperactive e.g. lentigo/lentigenes, stain, nevus, a tan, freckles, solar lentigos (i.e., sun spots, age spots) and under-eye dark circles.

Melasma: Often known as the 'pregnancy mask', melasma is caused by hormonal changes due to pregnancy and is characterized by splotchy, pigmented areas usually on the face except the eye area.

Various causes of hyperpigmentation:

- Overexposure to the sun
- Heredity
- Picking at the skin
- Hormonal changes
- Certain medications such as antibiotics, hormone treatments and anti-seizure drugs
- Inflammation and skin injuries such as acne vulgaris

Facial pigmentation is very distressing to adolescents as it affects their self-esteem.

CLINICAL EXAMINATION

The skin lesions in *Acne* include the following: (see Figures 6.4.1 and 6.4.2).

1. Comedone
2. Papules
3. Nodules, nodulo-ulcerative lesions, or cysts 2 to 5 cm in diameter.
4. Scars, atrophic depressed or hypertrophic scars.
5. Seborrhea of the face and scalp is often present.

In *body odor* the skin appears normal, except when bromhidrosis is associated with concomitant skin conditions such as erythrasma (Figure 6.4.3), in which case a sharply marginated erythematous macular rash is seen, or trichomycosis axillaris (caused by *Corynebacterium tenuis*, in which case concretions are visible on the hairs in the affected area (Figure 6.4.4). Individuals with eccrine bromhidrosis caused by bacterial degradation of keratin

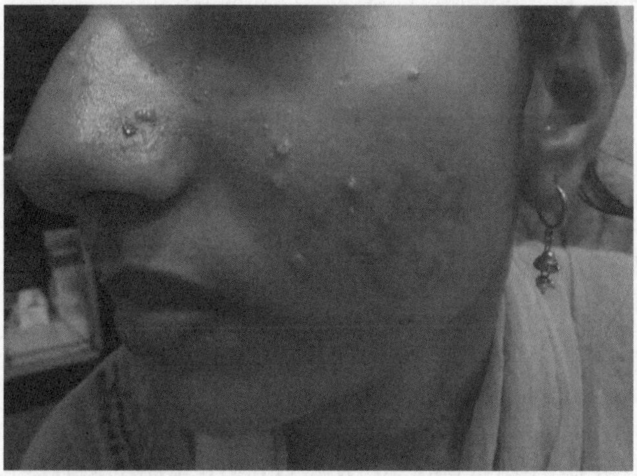

Figure 6.4.1: Grade I acne vulgaris

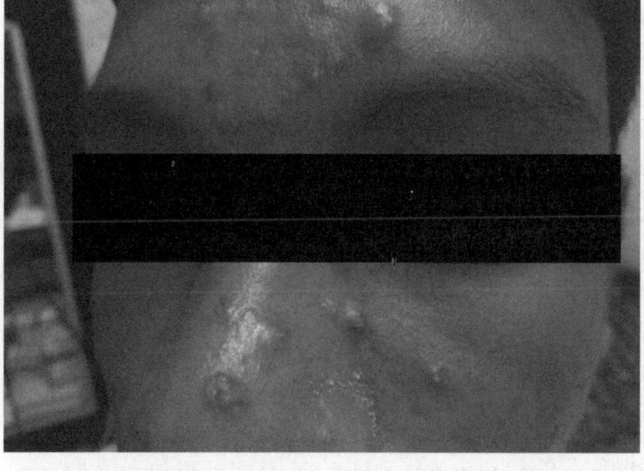

Figure 6.4.2: Grade IV nodulocystic acne

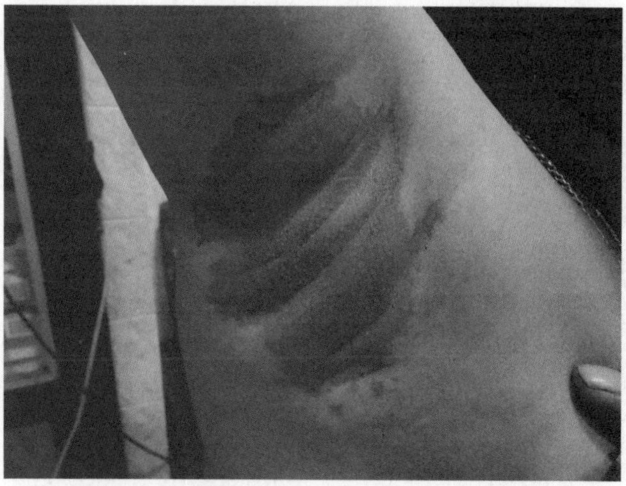

Figure 6.4.3: Erythrasma caused by *Corynebacterium minutissimum*

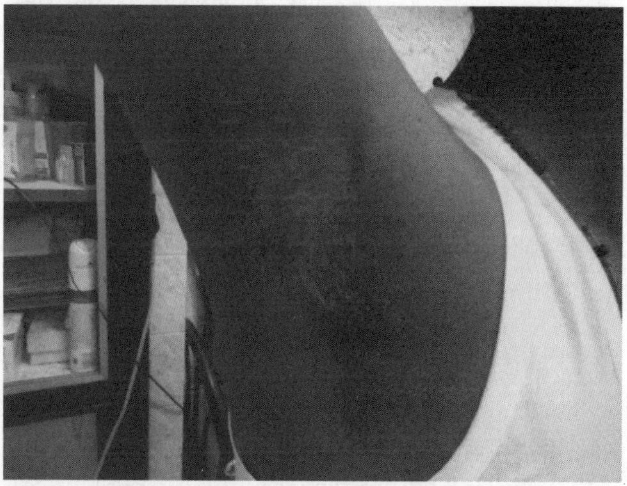

Figure 6.4.4: Trichomycosis axillaris caused by *Corynebacterium minutissimum*

may have maceration and a thick mat of moist keratin on examination. This finding is most common on the plantar and intertriginous surfaces.

In *Acanthosis nigricans (AN)* the skin appears dark, thick and velvety (Figures 6.4.5 and 6.4.6). Apart from the dark axillae, the neck is also involved. Malignant AN is diagnosed if the face, palms and soles show similar velvetiness.

Hyperpigmentation due to an abnormally high concentration of melanocytes or due to melanin hyperactivity can involve sun-exposed areas especially face (Figure 6.4.7). Melasma causes brown to gray-brown patches on face (Figure 6.4.8).

INVESTIGATIONS

There are no specific investigations for *acne* unless there is an endocrine abnormality or as part of treatment protocol.

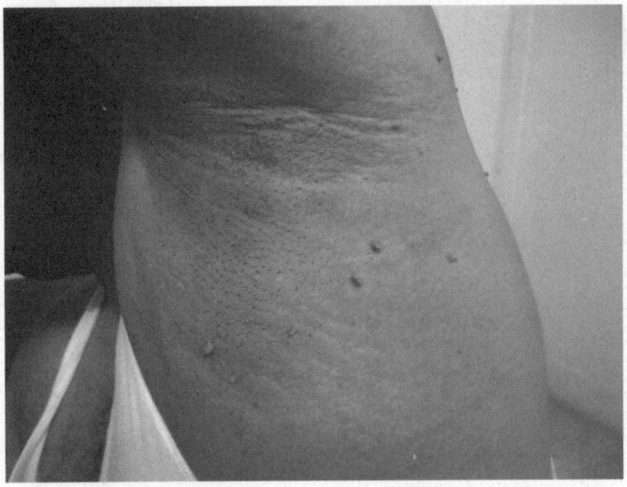

Figure 6.4.5: Acanthosis nigricans with velvety appearance over axilla

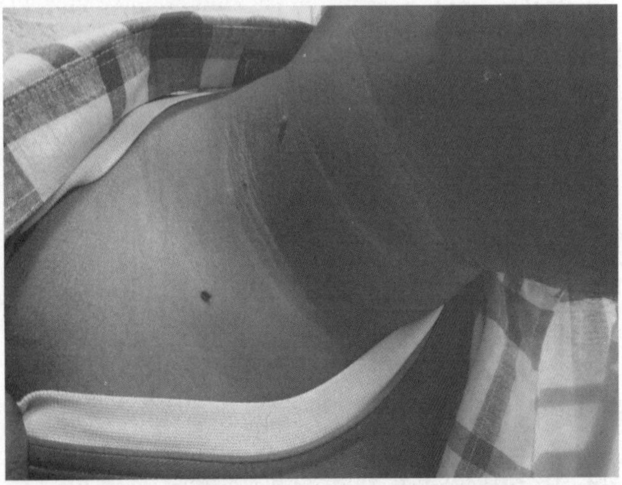

Figure 6.4.6: Acanthosis nigricans over neck

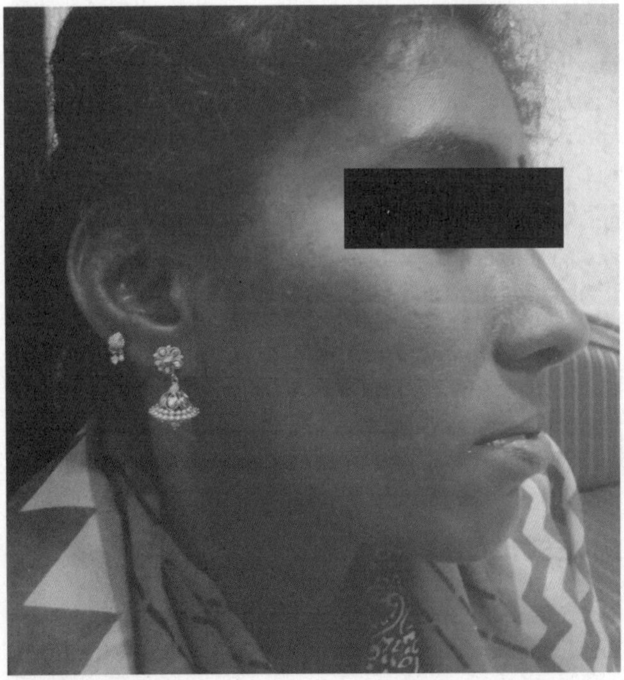

Figure 6.4.7: Facial pigmentation in an adolescent girl due to overexposure to sunlight

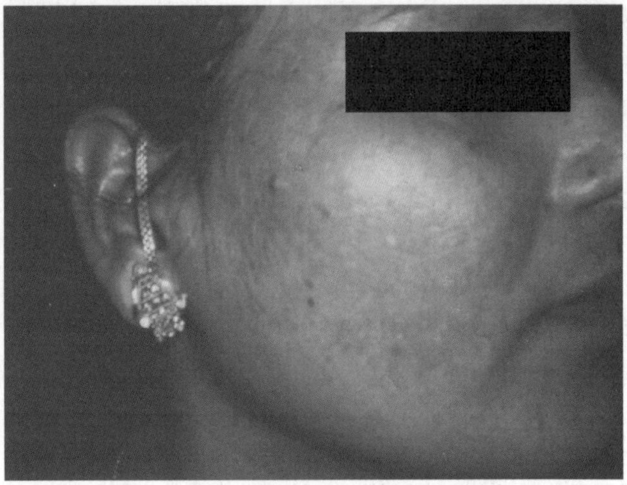

Figure 6.4.8: Melasma in an adolescent girl

Laboratory studies in cases of *body odor* are not at all productive. Biochemical studies such as examination for inborn errors of metabolism have proven to be non-contributory.

Laboratory investigations for *dark axillae–acanthosis nigricans* should be directed towards detection of insulin resistance and polycystic ovary syndrome (PCOS).

There are no specialized investigations for *hyperpigmentation/melasma*. Serum cortisol levels might help in ruling out Addisonian pigmentation.

MANAGEMENT

Table 6.4.1 details the management of common skin problems such as mild and severe forms of acne, body odor and hyperpigmentation in adolescents. Box 6.4.3 describes the management options for acanthosis nigricans.

PROBLEMS PECULIAR TO ADOLESCENT AGE GROUP DUE TO PEER PRESSURE

These come under unclassified skin disorders due to cultural practices.

Clinicians should warn teens about the various fashions that can harm them. This comes under preventive counseling and anticipatory guidance which should be given in the adolescent wellness clinics.

Tattoo

A tattoo is a permanent mark or design made on your skin with pigments inserted through pricks into the skin's top layer. Typically, the tattoo artist uses a hand-held machine that acts much like a sewing machine, with one or more needles piercing the skin repeatedly. With every puncture, the needles insert tiny ink droplets (see Figures 6.4.9 and 6.4.10). Table 6.4.2 lists the common complications of body piercing and their management.

Table 6.4.1: Management of common skin problems in adolescents

Lesion	*Treatment*	*Comments*
Mild acne (comedones and papules)	1. Topical antibiotics (clindamycin, erythromycin). 2. Benzoyl peroxide gels (2%, 5%). 3. Topical tretinoin 0.01% gel. 4. Intermittent courses of oral antibiotics (azithromycin/tetracycline/doxycycline).	Acne associated with puberty is a transient phase but causes psychological distress.
Severe forms (pustules, nodules, and cysts)	1. Oral tetracyclines added to the above/minocycline, 50 to 100 mg b.i.d., for instance; could be tapered to 50 mg/day. 2. In females only, severe acne can be controlled with high doses of oral estrogens combined with progesterone. 3. Oral isotretinoin is highly effective for cystic acne.	As retinoids are teratogenic, counseling is of paramount importance. Careful monitoring of the blood is necessary during therapy, especially in patients with elevated blood triglycerides before therapy is begun.
Body odor	1. Measures to enhance drying and limit maceration–local hygiene, antiperspirants, and deodorants including aluminium chloride, topical antibiotics. 2. Iontophoresis, which disrupts sweat production–eccrine bromhidrosis. 3. Treatment of coexisting skin conditions, such as intertrigo, erythrasma, and trichomycosis axillaris, is important. 4. Regular shaving of axillary hair to prevent the accumulation of sweat and bacteria on the hair shafts. 5. Electrolysis might also be considered for hair removal to minimize bacterial growth.	For patients who desire more long-lasting treatment–lasers and surgical reduction of sweat glands: 1. Q-switched Nd:YAG laser (1064 nm). 2. Botulinum toxin A to decrease sweat production by denervating eccrine sweat glands. 3. Surgical reduction in the number of apocrine glands.
Hyperpigmentation/melasma	1. With a customized skin care regimen, one can minimize the appearance of hyperpigmentation. 2. Using sunscreen with at least an SPF of 15. 3. Alpha hydroxy acids (AHAs). 4. First-line treatment of melasma is a triple combination topical therapy, including hydroquinone, retinoid cream, and corticosteroids. 5. Other excellent Kojic acid and vitamin C.	Second line treatment includes peels either alone or in combination with topical medications. Laser targeting cutaneous pigment may be used in cases that fail medical topical therapy.

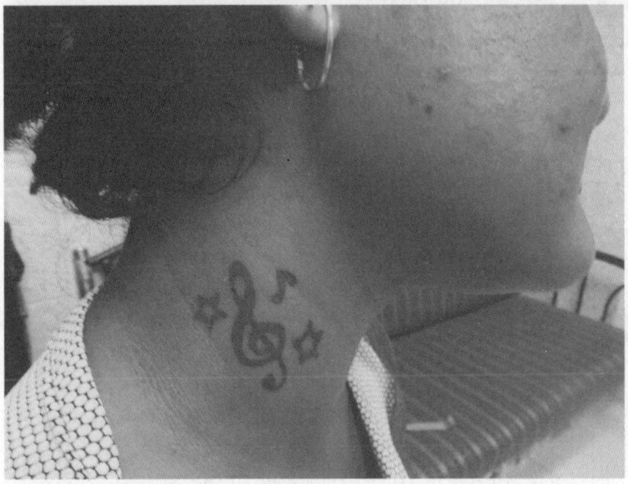

Figure 6.4.9: Depiction of tattoo in an adolescent female

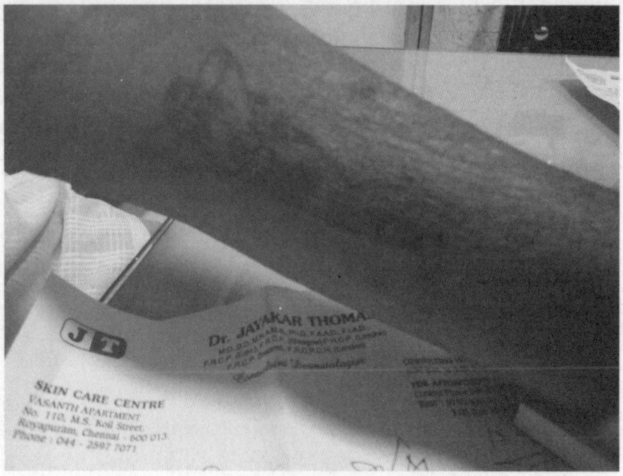

Figure 6.4.10: Depiction of tattoo in an adolescent male

Body Piercing

This means a piercing or puncture made in your body by a needle. After that, a piece of jewelry is inserted into the puncture. The most popular pierced body parts seem to be the ears, the nostrils, and the belly button.

Ear piercing (karna vedha) is Hindu religious custom practiced extensively in India. While some believe that the pierced ears help ward off evil, others pierce their ears for purely aesthetic reasons (Figure 6.4.11). Table 6.4.2 lists the common complications following body piercing and their management.

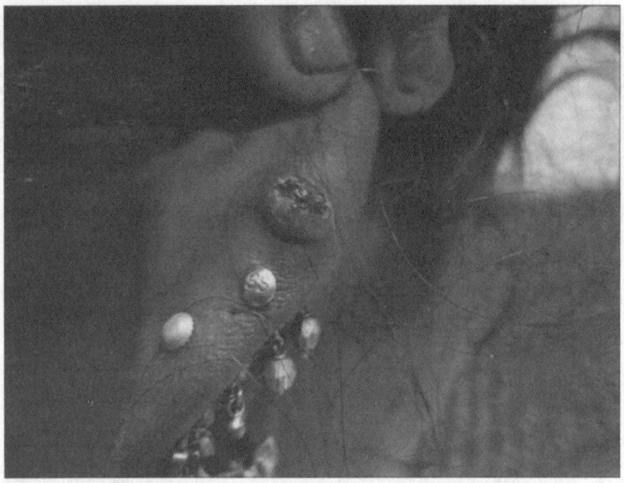

Figure 6.4.11: Pyogenic granuloma arising at the ear-boring site

Hair Coloring

Current fashion demands different types of hair coloring that includes highlighting and using unusual colors as well. Young women as well as men are changing color of their hair more often than ever. Table 6.4.2 lists the common complications following hair coloring and their management.

Wearing Cheap Costume Jewelry

Teens often wear a lot of costume jewelry which is either made of plastic or cheap metal. The various medical complications that follow the wearing of cheap jewelry and their management are provided in Table 6.4.2.

LEARNING POINTS

1. Treating dermatological problems in adolescents may require psychological counseling in addition to standard medical treatment.
2. Many dermatological disorders in adolescence have an endocrine basis.
3. Major dermatological concerns for adolescents include acne, body odor, acne nigricans and hyperpigmentation.
4. In addition some dermatological concerns are due to tattooing, body piercing and wearing imitation jewelry due to adolescent's fascinations to these fashions.
5. Most dermatological drugs appear to be safe for adolescents with the exception of oral retinoids used in the management of acne.

Table 6.4.2: Complications of adolescent fashions

Procedure	*Complications*	*Treatment*
Tattoos	Tattoos breach the skin, which means that skin infections, cellulitis and other complications such as granuloma and keloids can occur. • *Blood borne diseases:* If the equipment used to create the tattoo is contaminated with infected blood, one can contract various blood borne diseases—including tetanus, hepatitis B and hepatitis C. • *Allergic reactions*: Tattoo dyes—especially red, green, yellow and blue dyes—can cause allergic skin reactions, such as an itchy rash at the tattoo site. This can occur even years after you get the tattoo. • *MRI complications:* Rarely, tattoos or permanent makeup might cause swelling or burning in the affected areas during magnetic resonance imaging (MRI) examination.	There is no treatment for removal of tattoo except excision and laser surgery.
Piercing	Chronic infection/pyogenic granuloma, uncontrollable or prolonged bleeding, scarring, hepatitis B and C and tetanus infections, skin allergies to the jewelry that is used. Keloid is a rare complication.	Strict aseptic precautions will prevent complication. Intralesional steroid and Laser are treatment options for keloid.
Hair coloring	Irritant and allergic reactions leading to eczemas and infections. The commonly used chemical is paraphenylene diamine that causes dark pigmentation on the face due to photosensitivity. Hair shaft damage also occurs and this results in hair breakage and hair fall. The undesired effect is even worse when manipulations such as curling or straightening of hair are indulged in.	Systemic anti-histamines along with topical or systemic corticosteroids in selected cases. Best is to avoid such procedures in future.
Wearing cheap costume jewelry	This can lead to irritation, contact dermatitis or eczema. It can also cause acute or chronic fungal or bacterial infection. Allergy to the metal may also occur.	Antihistamines and judicious use of topical corticosteroids.

SUGGESTED READING

1. Chan A, Kung S. Hair Colorant Technology Advances Further. Personal Care 2006;11-16.
2. Grimes PE. Melasma. Etiologic and therapeutic considerations. Arch Dermatol 1995;131(12):1453-57.
3. Laumann AE, Derick AJ. Tattoos and body piercings in the United States: A national data set. J Amer Acad Dermatol 2006;55(3):413-21.
4. Leyden JJ, McGinley KJ, Holzle E, Labows JN, Kligman AM. The microbiology of the human axilla and its relationship to axillary odor. J Invest Dermatol 1981;77(5):413-16.
5. Nguyen TT, Keil MF, Russell DL, *et al*. Relation of acanthosis nigricans to hyperinsulinemia and insulin sensitivity in overweight African American and white children. J Pediatr 2001;138(4):474-80.
6. Ortonne JP, Passeron T. Melanin pigmentary disorders: Treatment update. Dermatol Clin 2005;23(2):209-26.
7. Schmidt RM, *et al*. Tattooing in adolescents and young adults. http://www.uptodate.com/home. Accessed July 29, 2015.
8. Sherertz EF. Improved acanthosis nigricans with lipodystrophic diabetes during dietary fish oil supplementation. Arch Dermatol 1988;124(7):1094-96.
9. Thomas J, Sindhu BR. Pyogenic granuloma at ear piercing site: Report of a case. Indian Dermatol Online J 2014;5:347.
10. Thomas J. Acanthosis Nigricans. In: Thomas J. Ed. Pediatric Dermatology Ward Rounds, 1st ed. New Delhi: Jaypee Brothers 2007;5-6.
11. Thomas J. Common Dermatological Problems in Adolescents. In: Bhave SY, Nair MKC, Parthasarathy A, Menon PSN, Eds. Textbook of Adolescent Medicine. 1st ed. New Delhi: Jaypee Brothers Medical Publishers 2006;554-76.

6.5

Dental Problems

Ashish Kakar, Subik Nagi

INTRODUCTION

The aim of this chapter is to make all clinicians dealing with adolescents aware that whatever problem the adolescents have come to the clinician with, it would be important to do a good examination of the oral cavity. This is all the more important because unlike in the West, a routine wellness checkup with the dentist is not the norm in our country. Physicians on finding oral health problems should teach and educate the adolescents about these issues and instill in them knowledge as to how to avoid certain problems and also encourage them to pay a visit to the dental specialist.

As quoted by William Shakespeare, "The eyes are the window to your soul"; so can be said for "oral health" of an adolescent to be a reliable indicator of overall wellbeing. Oral anomalies discovered during an oral examination can predict certain systemic disorders related to them, those which could be missed during the general health check up alone. It is essential that physicians who work with adolescents are aware of different possible conditions of the oral cavity (see Tables 6.5.1 and 6.5.2).

Table 6.5.1: Common dental problems

Etiology	*Conditions*
Congenital	Tongue tie and high frenum attachment Dental anomalies like fusion of teeth/taurodontism/concrescence Mesiodens Peg laterals
Traumatic	Fractured teeth Ecchymosis Laceration Bleeding Swelling Inflammation
Infection	*Herpes simplex* type 1
Inflammation	Gingival inflammation
Developmental	Crowding Ugly duckling stage Crossbite
Lifestyle	Staining due to tobacco Attrition/erosion
Pathological	Sinus tract Necrosed tooth Swelling
Miscellaneous	Sensitivity Worn fillings Exposed tooth roots Dry mouth Temporomandibular joint disorders (TMJD) Halitosis Wisdom tooth eruption pain Ectopic eruption Gingival recession

HISTORY TAKING

The following questions should be asked to understand the dental hygiene followed and the lifestyle of the adolescent. This should also be used as an opportunity to educate the adolescent for good dental care.

1. Brushing habits
2. Consumption of tobacco products
3. Sugar and sticky sweets consumption
4. In between meals snacking
5. Type of food
6. Any pain or discomfort felt in mouth
7. Any bleeding from gums
8. Oral habits

CLINICAL EXAMINATION

While performing a general examination a physician can broadly check for anomalies in the oral cavity by using a simple light source and retracting instruments. Physician should look out for the following conditions–black spots indicating caries, plaque and calculus deposition, bleeding on probing, mobile teeth, crowded teeth, missing teeth, left over root stumps, presence of sinus tract, gingival enlargement, abnormal positioning of teeth, gingival color (normal color is coral pink), any lesions or ulcers on the oral mucosa, fibrous bands on the buccal mucosa and mouth opening.

For descriptions of various conditions refer to Table 6.5.2 and Figures 6.5.1 to 6.5.13.

Table 6.5.2: Diagnosis and management of various dental problems		
Conditions	***Description and interpretation***	***Management***
Mesiodens (Figure 6.5.1)	Extra tooth between central incisors generally conical shaped	Extraction and realignment of gap
Diastema (Figure 6.5.2)	Spacing between teeth	Space closure
Crowding (Figure 6.5.3)	Due to lack of space in arch, teeth overlap each other	Orthodontic intervention
Fluorosis (Figure 6.5.4)	Developmental disturbance of dental enamel caused by the consumption of excess fluoride during tooth development	Tooth bleaching, micro-abrasion, conservative composite restorations or porcelain veneers
Presence of stains (Figure 6.5.5)	Coffee/tea stains, smoking induced patterns of stains	Oral prophylaxis
Ugly duckling stage (Figure 6.5.6)	Self-correcting anomaly	No treatment required
Cross bite (Figure 6.5.7)	Negative overjet	Correct as soon as it is detected by removable orthodontic appliances or fixed mechanotherapy
Gingivitis	Inflammation involving only the gingival tissues next to the tooth. Microscopically it is characterized by presence of inflammatory exudate and edema, some destruction of collagenous gingival fibres, and ulceration and proliferation of the epithelium facing the tooth.	Removal of etiology
Enamel hypoplasia	Disturbance of ameloblastic function during amelogenesis. Enamel is hard but thin and deficient	Esthetic rehabilitation like composite restoration or porcelain veneers
Trauma leading to tooth fracture (Figures 6.5.8A and B)	Traumatic injury	Tooth reconstruction, pulpal treatment also if required
Presence of rampant caries (Figure 6.5.9)	Dental neglect, more than 10 carious lesions in a year	Diet modification and treatment of condition
Tongue tie and high frenum attachment (Figure 6.5.10)	High frenum attachment causes lisping and also leads to midline diastema	Frenectomy by surgical blade, electrocautery and lasers
Presence of a sinus tract (Figure 6.5.11)	Seen in cases of periapical abscess	Self resolving after etiology is cured
Black necrosed tooth (Figure 6.5.12)	Pulpal degeneration, non-vital tooth	Pulp therapy followed by prosthetic rehabilitation for esthetics
Generalized attrition/erosion (Figures 6.5.13 A and B)	Caused by gastroesophageal reflux disease (GERD), bruxism, excessive brushing, deep bite	Mouth guard or splints for bruxism Management of etiology
Dental anomalies like fusion of teeth, taurodontism or concrescence	Congenital anomalies	Retention or extraction
Herpes simplex type 1	Acquired viral infection	Medications for pain and numbing; specific antiviral agents

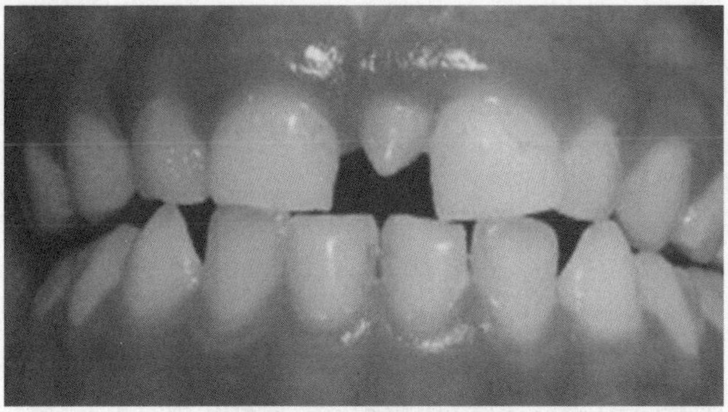

Figure 6.5.1: Mesiodens

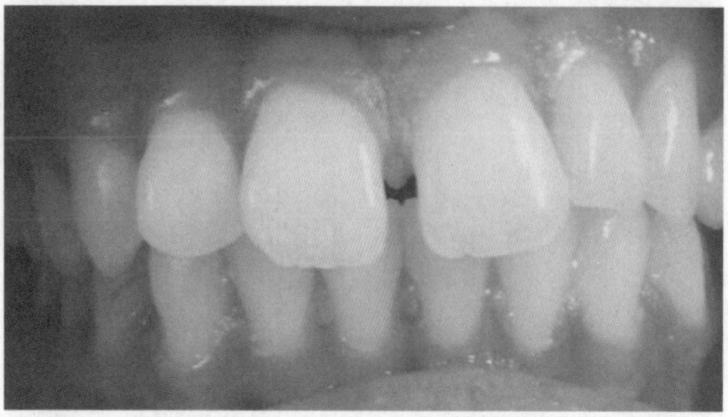

Figure 6.5.2: Midline diastema

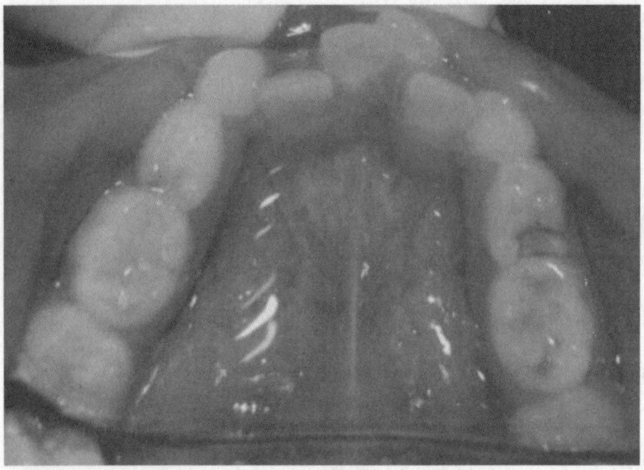

Figure 6.5.3: Crowding

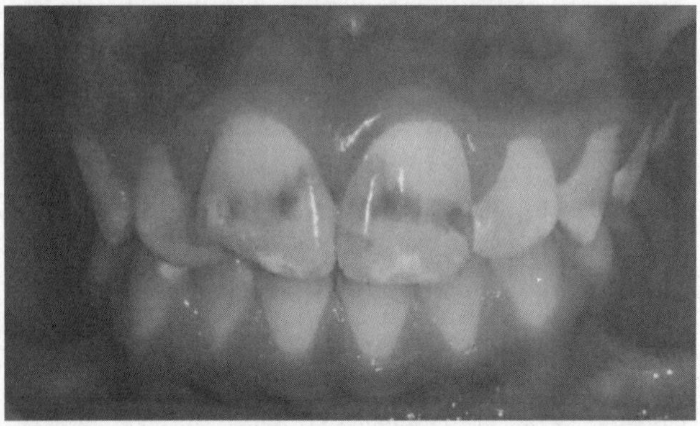

Figure 6.5.4: Dental fluorosis

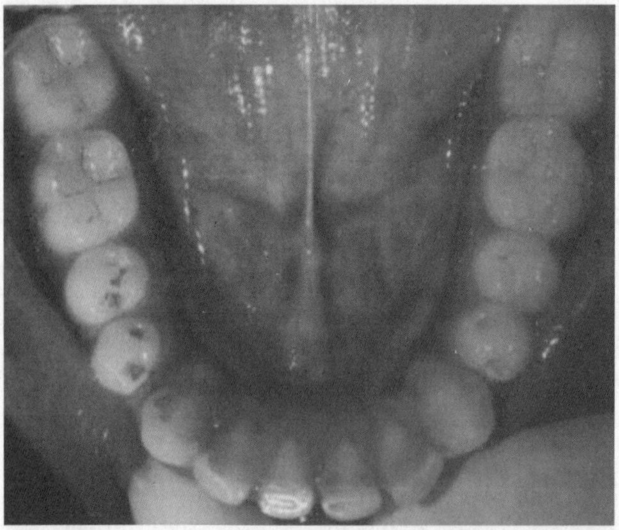

Figure 6.5.5: Stains on teeth

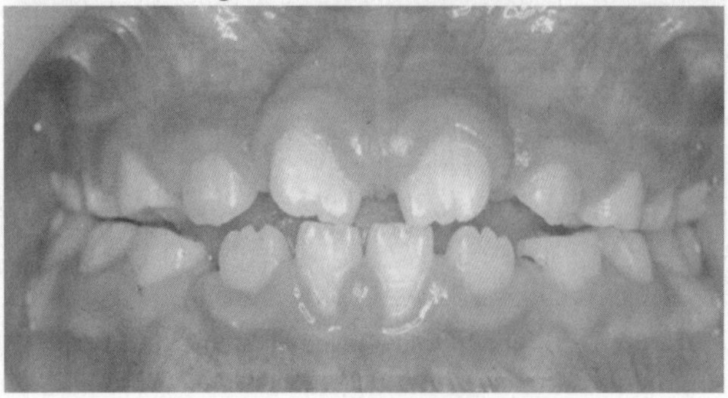

Figure 6.5.6: Ugly duckling stage

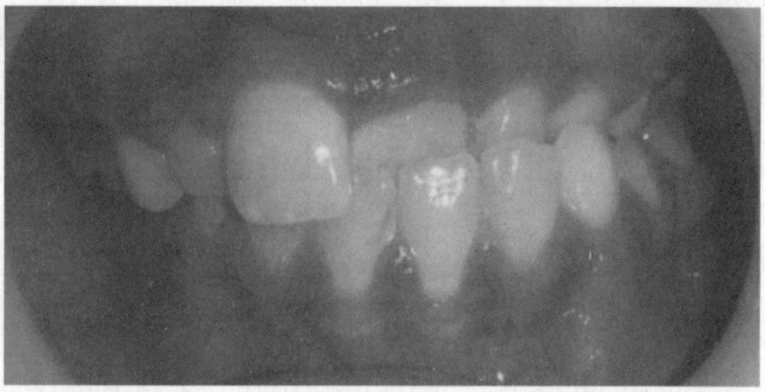

Figure 6.5.7: Cross bite

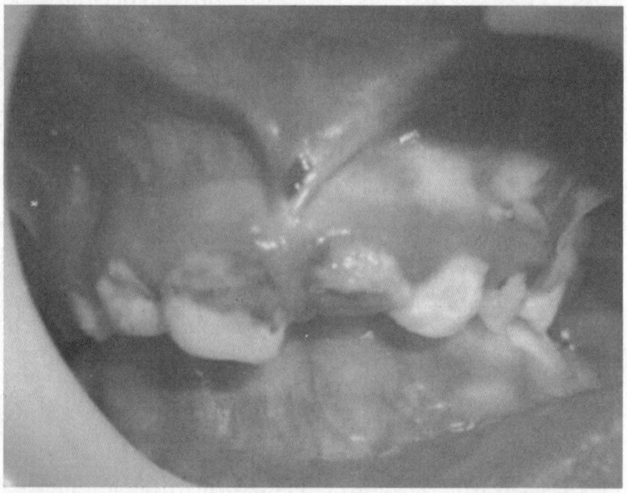

A

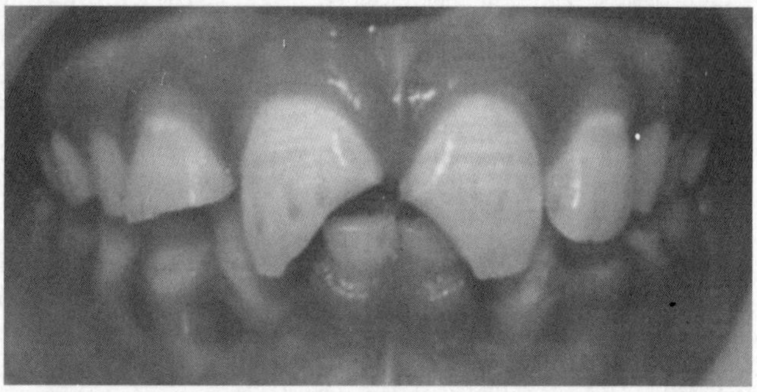

B

Figure 6.5.8A and B: Trauma leading to tooth fracture

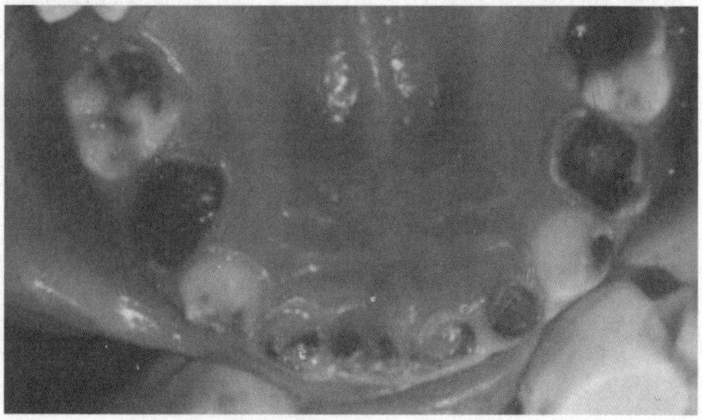

Figure 6.5.9: Rampant caries

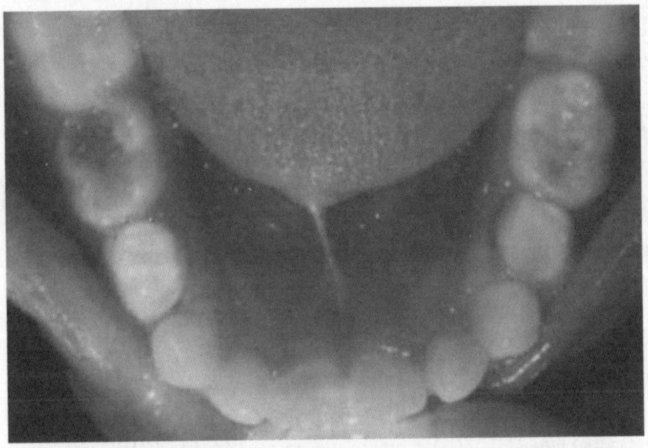

Figure 6.5.10: Tongue tie and high frenum

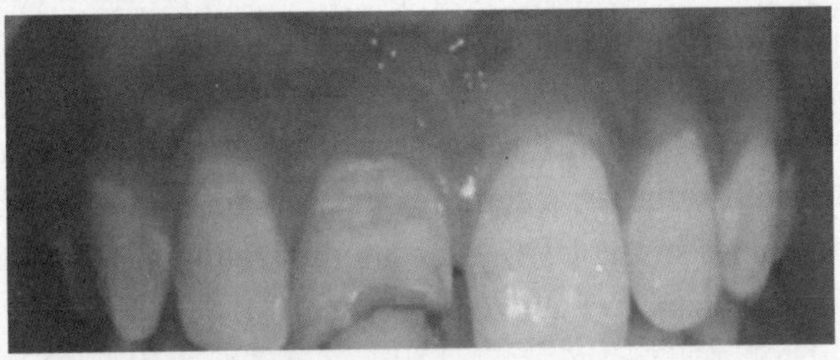

Figure 6.5.11: Sinus tract

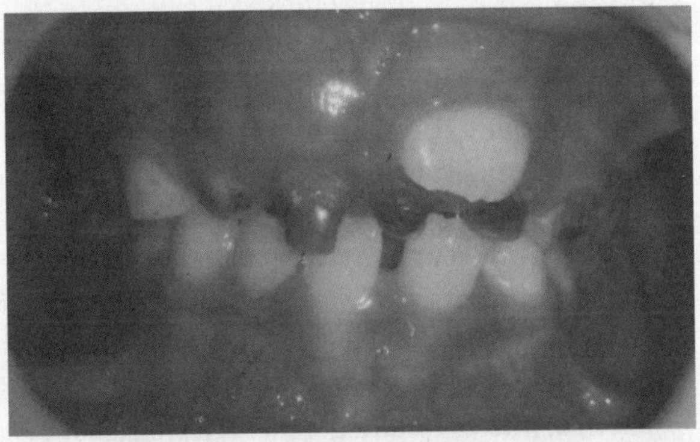

Figure 6.5.12: Black necrosed tooth

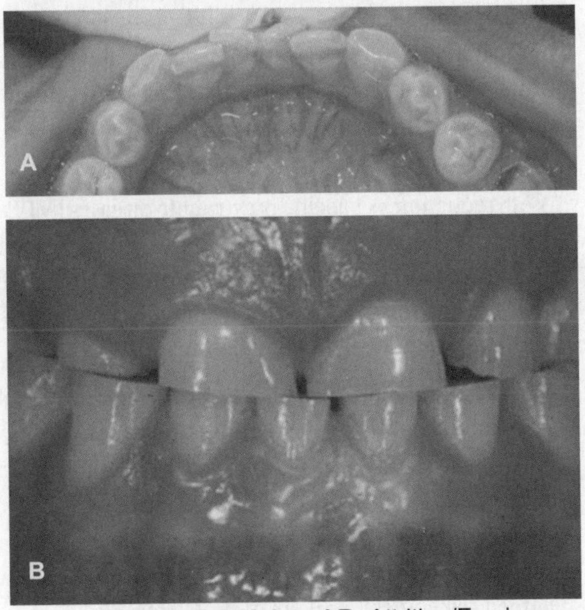

Figures 6.5.13 A and B: Attrition/Erosion

MANAGEMENT

It is advisable for the physician to refer the patient to the dental surgeon if any abnormality or any discomfort is found in the oral cavity of the patient. For management of various conditions please refer to Table 6.5.2.

LEARNING POINTS

1. Crowding of teeth suggest inadequate space for teeth in the arch; orthodontic intervention is necessary in such cases.
2. Dental neglect: Willful failure of parents or guardian to seek and follow through the treatment necessary to ensure a level of oral health essential for adequate function and freedom from pain and infection.
3. Unhealthy oral habits could be observed as staining on teeth for tobacco stains, keratinization of lips and smokers palate in smokers. Adolescent should be educated about the adverse affects of such habits and inspired to quit the habit.
4. Any mark of traumatic injury should be questioned in an open ended question manner, so as to come to a conclusion about the cause of trauma. It is advisable to be patient and let the adolescents speak themselves.
5. Bad breathe (halitosis) and bleeding gums are also due to calculus and plaque accumulated on the teeth adjacent to the gums.
6. Any missing teeth inside the oral cavity should be thoroughly evaluated as it could lead to shift in occlusion.
7. If any problem is found to be significant, refer the patient to a dental surgeon.

SUGGESTED READING

1. Braham RL, Morris ME. Textbook of Pediatric Dentistry, 2nd ed. New Delhi: CBS Publishers and Distributors; 1990.
2. Casamassimo PS, McTigue DJ, Fields HW Nowak AJ. Pediatric dentistry infancy through adolescence, 5th ed. St. Louis: Saunders; 2013.
3. Finn SB. Clinical Pedodontics, 4th ed. Philadelphia: WR Saunders Company; 2003.
4. Graber TM, Swain BF. Orthodontics current principles and technique. Ed. Saint Louis: CV Mosby Company; 1985.
5. Mathewson RJ, Primosch RE. Fundamentals of Pediatric Dentistry, 3rd ed. North Kimberly: Quintessence Publishing Co; 1995.
6. McDonalds RE, Avery DR, Dean JA. Dentistry for the child and adolescent, 9th ed. Missouri Elsevier; 2011.
7. Sim JM. Minor tooth movement in children, 2nd ed. Saint Louis: CV Mosby Company; 1977.
8. Stewart RE, Barber TK, Troutman KC, Wei SHY. Pediatric Dentistry. Scientific foundations and clinical practice. St Louis: CV Mosby Company; 1982.
9. Wei SHY. Pediatric Dentistry Total Patient Care. Philadelphia: Lea and Febiger; 1988.

Adolescent Immunization 7.1

A Parthasarathy, Swati Y Bhave

INTRODUCTION

Adequate immunization is one of the most important preventive health services that can be provided for adolescents. Adolescents present unique challenges for immunization because of their lifestyle and other social issues, while they also offer special opportunities, such as mass vaccination in educational institutions. The recommendations for the immunization of adolescents are to improve vaccination coverage among them and also to ensure a routine visit of adolescents to health care providers for other preventive services and health counseling. Every visit of an adolescent should be an opportunity to take history of vaccination.

In clinical practice, several questions by parents on adolescent vaccines need to be answered. Most parents are aware of childhood vaccine schedules and these get administered in the well-baby visit. In India we still do not have the concept of well adolescent monitoring. In USA there is a well adolescent visit scheduled at 11-12 years age where ACIP (Advisory Committee on Immunization Practices) recommends four vaccines in a single visit: One dose of quadrivalent meningococcal conjugate vaccine, one dose of human papilloma virus (HPV) vaccine, one dose of Tetanus, diphtheria, acellular pertussis (Tdap) vaccine; every one above age of 6 months should get a flu vaccine shot every year.

In India since 1985, tetanus toxoid (TT) is the only adolescent vaccine in the National Immunization Program. The twin objectives of adolescent immunization in India are: administration of age specific boosters e.g. for 10-12 years age group for those immunized with appropriate childhood vaccines; administration of newly recommended vaccines like Tdap/HPV; administration of epidemic response vaccines like Japanese encephalitis (JE) in endemic regions as well as combined seasonal and swine flu vaccine following pandemic recommendations. The Indian Academy of Pediatrics (IAP) has recommended several newer vaccines for adolescents viz. Td/Tdap (Tetanus and diphtheria/Tetanus, diphtheria and acellular pertussis), MMR (mumps, measles and rubella) varicella, HPV etc. (Figure 7.1.1). One can also refer to the universally accepted vaccine schedules of Center for Disease Control (CDC), USA for 0-18 age group (Figure 7.1.2). There is also a parent friendly version from 7-18 years which patients find easy to understand (Figure 7.1.3). Since 10-24 years is labeled as young people by WHO, physicians should also be aware of vaccinations recommended for these ages in the CDC adult immunization schedule for ages 19 years and above (Figure 7.1.4).

IMMUNOLOGICAL CONSIDERATIONS OF ADOLESCENT VACCINATION

- In the past in the non-vaccine era, most adolescents acquired natural immunity to common infections in childhood. After the well-established childhood immunizations in most countries there is a change in patterns of immunity over a period of time. For example, mothers who were immunized with measles vaccine as infants now bear children and their lower titers of measles antibodies are transferred across the placenta. Infants resulting from such pregnancies may well lose acquired antibody protection earlier than infants whose mothers had wild measles (and who passed higher titers of antibody across the placenta), thus making them both susceptible to measles infection earlier and hence now need measles vaccine at an earlier age of around 9 months.
- With reduction in Vaccine preventable diseases (VPDs), there is no continuous stimulation of antibodies with natural infections as in the past. Hence many adolescents will have waning antibodies to the vaccines given in childhood and would require booster doses.
- With a large number of new vaccines becoming available, population-based age-specific sero-epidemiological surveillance studies are important in developing control strategies for some diseases for the foreseeable future. Such surveys are, however, not without their problems—for instance many vaccine-preventable diseases lack agreed serological markers of protection.

Age ▶ Vaccine ▼	Birth	6 wk	10 wk	14 wk	18 wk	6 mo	9 mo	12 mo	15 mo	18 mo	19-23 mo	2-3 Yr	4-6 Yr	7-10Yr	11-12 Yr	13-18Yr
BCG	BCG															
Hep B	Hep B1	Hep B2						Hep B3								
Polio	OPV 0	IPV1	IPV2	IPV3		OPV1	OPV2		IPV B1				OPV3			
DTP		DTP 1	DTP 2	DTP 3						DTP B1			DTP B2			
Tdap															Tdap	
Hib		Hib 1	Hib 2	Hib 3					Hib-booster							
Pneumococcal		PCV 1	PCV 2	PCV 3				PCV -booster							PCV	
PPSV23														PPSV		
Rotavirus		RV 1	RV 2	RV 3												
MMR							MMR 1			MMR 2						
Varicella										VAR 1			VAR 2			
Hep A										Hep A1 & Hep A2						
Typhoid							Typhoid CV (TCV)					Booster				
Influenza												Influenza (yearly)				
HPV															HPV	
Meningococcal														Meningococcal		
Cholera													Cholera 1 & 2			
JE												Japanese Encephalitis				
Rabies										Rabies (Pre-EP & PEP)						

Figure 7.1.1: Recommended schedule for vaccination: The Indian Academy of Pediatrics (IAP)

Vaccine	Birth	1 mo	2 mos	4 mos	6 mos	9 mos	12 mos	15 mos	18 mos	19–23 mos	2-3 yrs	4-6 yrs	7-10 yrs	11-12 yrs	13–15 yrs	16–18 yrs
Hepatitis B[1] (HepB)	1st dose	←2nd dose→					←3rd dose→									
Rotavirus[2] (RV) RV1 (2-dose series); RV5 (3-dose series)			1st dose	2nd dose	See footnote 2											
Diphtheria, tetanus, & acellular pertussis[3] (DTaP: <7 yrs)			1st dose	2nd dose	3rd dose			←4th dose→				5th dose				
Tetanus, diphtheria, & acellular pertussis[4] (Tdap: ≥7 yrs)														(Tdap)		
Haemophilus influenzae type b[5] (Hib)			1st dose	2nd dose	See footnote 5		←3rd or 4th dose, See footnote 5→									
Pneumococcal conjugate[6] (PCV13)			1st dose	2nd dose	3rd dose		←4th dose→									
Pneumococcal polysaccharide[6] (PPSV23)																
Inactivated poliovirus[7] (IPV: <18 yrs)			1st dose	2nd dose			←3rd dose→					4th dose				
Influenza[8] (IIV; LAIV) 2 doses for some: See footnote 8							Annual vaccination (IIV only) 1 or 2 doses				Annual vaccination (LAIV or IIV) 1 or 2 doses			Annual vaccination (LAIV or IIV) 1 dose only		
Measles, mumps, rubella[9] (MMR)					See footnote 9		←1st dose→					2nd dose				
Varicella[10] (VAR)							←1st dose→					2nd dose				
Hepatitis A[11] (HepA)							←2-dose series, See footnote 11→									
Human papillomavirus[12] (HPV2: females only; HPV4: males and females)														(3-dose series)		
Meningococcal[13] (Hib-MenCY ≥ 6 weeks; MenACWY-D ≥9 mos; MenACWY-CRM ≥ 2 mos)							See footnote 13							1st dose		Booster

Range of recommended ages for all children

Range of recommended ages for catch-up immunization

Range of recommended ages for certain high-risk groups

Range of recommended ages during which catch-up is encouraged and for certain high-risk groups

Not routinely recommended

This schedule includes recommendations in effect as of January 1, 2015. Any dose not administered at the recommended age should be administered at a subsequent visit, when indicated and feasible. The use of a combination vaccine generally is preferred over separate injections of its equivalent component vaccines. Vaccination providers should consult the relevant Advisory Committee on Immunization Practices (ACIP) statement for detailed recommendations, available online at http://www.cdc.gov/vaccines/hcp/acip-recs/index.html. Clinically significant adverse events that follow vaccination should be reported to the Vaccine Adverse Event Reporting System (VAERS) online (http://www.vaers.hhs.gov) or by telephone (800-822-7967). Suspected cases of vaccine-preventable diseases should be reported to the state or local health department. Additional information, including precautions and contraindications for vaccination, is available from CDC online (http://www.cdc.gov/vaccines/recs/vac-admin/contraindications.htm) or by telephone (800-CDC-INFO [800-232-4636]).

This schedule is approved by the Advisory Committee on Immunization Practices (http//www.cdc.gov/vaccines/acip), the American Academy of Pediatrics (http://www.aap.org), the American Academy of Family Physicians (http://www.aafp.org), and the American College of Obstetricians and Gynecologists (http://www.acog.org).

Figure 7.1.2: Recommended immunization schedule for persons aged 0 through 18 years–United States, 2015
(FOR THOSE WHO FALL BEHIND OR START LATE, SEE THE CATCH-UP SCHEDULE [Figure 7.1.3])
These recommendations must be read with the footnotes that follow. For those who fall behind or start late, provide catch-up vaccination at the earliest opportunity as indicated by the green bars in Figure 7.1.3.
To determine minimum intervals between doses, see the catch-up schedule (Figure 7.1.3). School entry and adolescent vaccine age groups are shaded.

Footnotes — Recommended immunization schedule for persons aged 0 through 18 years—United States, 2015

For further guidance on the use of the vaccines mentioned below, see: http://www.cdc.gov/vaccines/hcp/acip-recs/index.html.
For vaccine recommendations for persons 19 years of age and older, see the Adult Immunization Schedule.

Additional information

- For contraindications and precautions to use of a vaccine and for additional information regarding that vaccine, vaccination providers should consult the relevant ACIP statement available online at http://www.cdc.gov/vaccines/hcp/acip-recs/index.html.
- For purposes of calculating intervals between doses, 4 weeks = 28 days. Intervals of 4 months or greater are determined by calendar months.
- Vaccine doses administered 4 days or less before the minimum interval are considered valid. Doses of any vaccine administered ≥5 days earlier than the minimum interval or minimum age should not be counted as valid doses and should be repeated as age-appropriate. The repeat dose should be spaced after the invalid dose by the recommended minimum interval. For further details, see *MMWR, General Recommendations on Immunization and Reports* / Vol. 60 / No. 2; Table 1. *Recommended and minimum ages and intervals between vaccine doses* available online at http://www.cdc.gov/mmwr/pdf/rr/rr6002.pdf.
- Information on travel vaccine requirements and recommendations is available at http://wwwnc.cdc.gov/travel/destinations/list.
- For vaccination of persons with primary and secondary immunodeficiencies, see Table 13, *"Vaccination of persons with primary and secondary immunodeficiencies,"* in *General Recommendations on Immunization* (ACIP), available at http://www.cdc.gov/mmwr/pdf/rr/rr6002.pdf.; and American Academy of Pediatrics. "Immunization in Special Clinical Circumstances," in Pickering LK, Baker CJ, Kimberlin DW, Long SS eds. *Red Book: 2012 report of the Committee on Infectious Diseases. 29th ed.* Elk Grove Village, IL: American Academy of Pediatrics.

1. Hepatitis B (HepB) vaccine. (Minimum age: birth)

Routine vaccination:

At birth:

- Administer monovalent HepB vaccine to all newborns before hospital discharge.
- For infants born to hepatitis B surface antigen (HBsAg)-positive mothers, administer HepB vaccine and 0.5 mL of hepatitis B immune globulin (HBIG) within 12 hours of birth. These infants should be tested for HBsAg and antibody to HBsAg (anti-HBs) 1 to 2 months after completion of the HepB series at age 9 through 18 months (preferably at the next well-child visit).
- If mother's HBsAg status is unknown, within 12 hours of birth administer HepB vaccine regardless of birth weight. For infants weighing less than 2,000 grams, administer HBIG in addition to HepB vaccine within 12 hours of birth. Determine mother's HBsAg status as soon as possible and, if mother is HBsAg-positive, also administer HBIG for infants weighing 2,000 grams or more as soon as possible, but no later than age 7 days.

Doses following the birth dose:

- The second dose should be administered at age 1 or 2 months. Monovalent HepB vaccine should be used for doses administered before age 6 weeks.
- Infants who did not receive a birth dose should receive 3 doses of a HepB-containing vaccine on a schedule of 0, 1 to 2 months, and 6 months starting as soon as feasible. See Figure 2.
- Administer the second dose 1 to 2 months after the first dose (minimum interval of 4 weeks), administer the third dose at least 8 weeks after the second dose AND at least 16 weeks after the **first** dose. The final (third or fourth) dose in the HepB vaccine series should be administered **no earlier than age 24 weeks**.
- Administration of a total of 4 doses of HepB vaccine is permitted when a combination vaccine containing HepB is administered after the birth dose.

Catch-up vaccination:

- Unvaccinated persons should complete a 3-dose series.
- A 2-dose series (doses separated by at least 4 months) of adult formulation Recombivax HB is licensed for use in children aged 11 through 15 years.
- For other catch-up guidance, see Figure 2.

2. Rotavirus (RV) vaccines. (Minimum age: 6 weeks for both RV1 [Rotarix] and RV5 [RotaTeq])

Routine vaccination:

Administer a series of RV vaccine to all infants as follows:

1. If Rotarix is used, administer a 2-dose series at 2 and 4 months of age.
2. If RotaTeq is used, administer a 3-dose series at ages 2, 4, and 6 months.
3. If any dose in the series was RotaTeq or vaccine product is unknown for any dose in the series, a total of 3 doses of RV vaccine should be administered.

Catch-up vaccination:

- The maximum age for the first dose in the series is 14 weeks, 6 days; vaccination should not be initiated for infants aged 15 weeks, 0 days or older.
- The maximum age for the final dose in the series is 8 months, 0 days.
- For other catch-up guidance, see Figure 2.

3. Diphtheria and tetanus toxoids and acellular pertussis (DTaP) vaccine. (Minimum age: 6 weeks. Exception: DTaP-IPV [Kinrix]: 4 years)

Routine vaccination:

- Administer a 5-dose series of DTaP vaccine at ages 2, 4, 6, 15 through 18 months, and 4 through 6 years. The fourth dose may be administered as early as age 12 months, provided at least 6 months have elapsed since the third dose. However, the fourth dose of DTaP need not be repeated if it was administered at least 4 months after the third dose of DTaP.

3. Diphtheria and tetanus toxoids and acellular pertussis (DTaP) vaccine (cont'd)

Catch-up vaccination:

- The fifth dose of DTaP vaccine is not necessary if the fourth dose was administered at age 4 years or older.
- For other catch-up guidance, see Figure 2.

4. Tetanus and diphtheria toxoids and acellular pertussis (Tdap) vaccine. (Minimum age: 10 years for both Boostrix and Adacel)

Routine vaccination:

- Administer 1 dose of Tdap vaccine to all adolescents aged 11 through 12 years.
- Tdap may be administered regardless of the interval since the last tetanus and diphtheria toxoid-containing vaccine.
- Administer 1 dose of Tdap vaccine to pregnant adolescents during each pregnancy (preferred during 27 through 36 weeks' gestation) regardless of time since prior Td or Tdap vaccination.

Catch-up vaccination:

- Persons aged 7 years and older who are not fully immunized with DTaP vaccine should receive Tdap vaccine as 1 dose (preferably the first) in the catch-up series; if additional doses are needed, use Td vaccine. For children 7 through 10 years who receive a dose of Tdap as part of the catch-up series, an adolescent Tdap vaccine dose at age 11 through 12 years should NOT be administered. Td should be administered instead 10 years after the Tdap dose.
- Persons aged 11 through 18 years who have not received Tdap vaccine should receive a dose followed by tetanus and diphtheria toxoid (Td) booster doses every 10 years thereafter.
- Inadvertent doses of DTaP vaccine:
  - If administered inadvertently to a child aged 7 through 10 years may count as part of the catch-up series. This dose may count as the adolescent Tdap dose, or the child can later receive a Tdap booster dose at age 11 through 12 years.
  - If administered inadvertently to an adolescent aged 11 through 18 years, the dose should be counted as the adolescent Tdap booster.
- For other catch-up guidance, see Figure 2.

5. *Haemophilus influenzae* type b (Hib) conjugate vaccine. (Minimum age: 6 weeks for PRP-T [ACTHIB, DTaP-IPV/Hib (Pentacel) and Hib-MenCY (MenHibrix)], PRP-OMP [PedvaxHIB or COMVAX], 12 months for PRP-T [Hiberix])

Routine vaccination:

- Administer a 2- or 3-dose Hib vaccine primary series and a booster dose (dose 3 or 4 depending on vaccine used in primary series) at age 12 through 15 months to complete a full Hib vaccine series.
- The primary series with ActHIB, MenHibrix, or Pentacel consists of 3 doses and should be administered at 2, 4, and 6 months of age. The primary series with PedvaxHib or COMVAX consists of 2 doses and should be administered at 2 and 4 months of age; a dose at age 6 months is not indicated.
- One booster dose (dose 3 or 4 depending on vaccine used in primary series) of any Hib vaccine should be administered at age 12 through 15 months. An exception is Hiberix vaccine. Hiberix should only be used for the booster (final) dose in children aged 12 months through 4 years who have received at least 1 prior dose of Hib-containing vaccine.
- For recommendations on the use of MenHibrix in patients at increased risk for meningococcal disease, please refer to the meningococcal vaccine footnotes and also to *MMWR* February 28, 2014 / 63(RR01);1-13, available at http://www.cdc.gov/mmwr/PDF/rr/rr6301.pdf.

For further guidance on the use of the vaccines mentioned below, see: http://www.cdc.gov/vaccines/hcp/acip-recs/index.html.

5. ***Haemophilus influenzae* type b (Hib) conjugate vaccine (cont'd)**

Catch-up vaccination:

- If dose 1 was administered at ages 12 through 14 months, administer a second (final) dose at least 8 weeks after dose 1, regardless of Hib vaccine used in the primary series.
- If both doses were PRP-OMP (PedvaxHIB or COMVAX), and were administered before the first birthday, the third (and final) dose should be administered at age 12 through 59 months and at least 8 weeks after the second dose.
- If the first dose was administered at age 7 through 11 months, administer the second dose at least 4 weeks later and a third (and final) dose at age 12 through 15 months or 8 weeks after second dose, whichever is later.
- If first dose is administered before the first birthday and second dose administered at younger than 15 months, a third (and final) dose should be given 8 weeks later.
- For unvaccinated children aged 15 months or older, administer only 1 dose.
- For other catch-up guidance, see Figure 2. For catch-up guidance related to MenHibrix, please see the meningococcal vaccine footnotes and also *MMWR* February 28, 2014 / 63(RR01);1-13, available at http://www.cdc.gov/mmwr/PDF/rr/rr6301.pdf.

Vaccination of persons with high-risk conditions:

- Children aged 12 through 59 months who are at increased risk for Hib disease, including chemotherapy recipients and those with anatomic or functional asplenia (including sickle cell disease), human immunodeficiency virus (HIV) infection, immunoglobulin deficiency, or early component complement deficiency, who have received either no doses or only 1 dose of Hib vaccine before 12 months of age, should receive 2 additional doses of Hib vaccine 8 weeks apart; children who received 2 or more doses of Hib vaccine before 12 months of age should receive 1 additional dose.
- For patients younger than 5 years of age undergoing chemotherapy or radiation treatment who received a Hib vaccine dose(s) within 14 days of starting therapy or during therapy, repeat the dose(s) at least 3 months following therapy completion.
- Recipients of hematopoietic stem cell transplant (HSCT) should be revaccinated with a 3-dose regimen of Hib vaccine starting 6 to 12 months after successful transplant, regardless of vaccination history; doses should be administered at least 4 weeks apart.
- A single dose of any Hib-containing vaccine should be administered to unimmunized* children and adolescents 15 months of age and older undergoing an elective splenectomy; if possible, vaccine should be administered at least 14 days before procedure.
- Hib vaccine is not routinely recommended for patients 5 years or older. However, 1 dose of Hib vaccine should be administered to unimmunized* persons aged 5 years or older who have anatomic or functional asplenia (including sickle cell disease) and unvaccinated persons 5 through 18 years of age with human immunodeficiency virus (HIV) infection.

** Patients who have not received a primary series and booster dose or at least 1 dose of Hib vaccine after 14 months of age are considered unimmunized.*

6. **Pneumococcal vaccines. (Minimum age: 6 weeks for PCV13, 2 years for PPSV23)**

Routine vaccination with PCV13:

- Administer a 4-dose series of PCV13 vaccine at ages 2, 4, and 6 months and at age 12 through 15 months.
- For children aged 14 through 59 months who have received an age-appropriate series of 7-valent PCV (PCV7), administer a single supplemental dose of 13-valent PCV (PCV13).

Catch-up vaccination with PCV13:

- Administer 1 dose of PCV13 to all healthy children aged 24 through 59 months who are not completely vaccinated for their age.
- For other catch-up guidance, see Figure 2.

Vaccination of persons with high-risk conditions with PCV13 and PPSV23:

- All recommended PCV13 doses should be administered prior to PPSV23 vaccination if possible.
- For children 2 through 5 years of age with any of the following conditions: chronic heart disease (particularly cyanotic congenital heart disease and cardiac failure); chronic lung disease (including asthma if treated with high-dose oral corticosteroid therapy); diabetes mellitus; cerebrospinal fluid leak; cochlear implant; sickle cell disease and other hemoglobinopathies; anatomic or functional asplenia; HIV infection; chronic renal failure; nephrotic syndrome; diseases associated with treatment with immunosuppressive drugs or radiation therapy, including malignant neoplasms, leukemias, lymphomas, and Hodgkin's disease; solid organ transplantation; or congenital immunodeficiency:
  1. Administer 1 dose of PCV13 if any incomplete schedule of 3 doses of PCV (PCV7 and/or PCV13) were received previously.
  2. Administer 2 doses of PCV13 at least 8 weeks apart if unvaccinated or any incomplete schedule of fewer than 3 doses of PCV (PCV7 and/or PCV13) were received previously.
  3. Administer 1 supplemental dose of PCV13 if 4 doses of PCV7 or other age-appropriate complete PCV7 series was received previously.
  4. The minimum interval between doses of PCV (PCV7 or PCV13) is 8 weeks.
  5. For children with no history of PPSV23 vaccination, administer PPSV23 at least 8 weeks after the most recent dose of PCV13.

6. **Pneumococcal vaccines (cont'd)**

- For children aged 6 through 18 years who have cerebrospinal fluid leak; cochlear implant; sickle cell disease and other hemoglobinopathies; anatomic or functional asplenia; congenital or acquired immunodeficiencies; HIV infection; chronic renal failure; nephrotic syndrome; diseases associated with treatment with immunosuppressive drugs or radiation therapy, including malignant neoplasms, leukemias, lymphomas, and Hodgkin's disease; generalized malignancy; solid organ transplantation; or multiple myeloma:
  1. If neither PCV13 nor PPSV23 has been received previously, administer 1 dose of PCV13 now and 1 dose of PPSV23 at least 8 weeks later.
  2. If PCV13 has been received previously but PPSV23 has not, administer 1 dose of PPSV23 at least 8 weeks after the most recent dose of PCV13.
  3. If PPSV23 has been received but PCV13 has not, administer 1 dose of PCV13 at least 8 weeks after the most recent dose of PPSV23.
- For children aged 6 through 18 years with chronic heart disease (particularly cyanotic congenital heart disease and cardiac failure), chronic lung disease (including asthma if treated with high-dose oral corticosteroid therapy), diabetes mellitus, alcoholism, or chronic liver disease, who have not received PPSV23, administer 1 dose of PPSV23. If PCV13 has been received previously, then PPSV23 should be administered at least 8 weeks after any prior PCV13 dose.
- A single revaccination with PPSV23 should be administered 5 years after the first dose to children with sickle cell disease or other hemoglobinopathies; anatomic or functional asplenia; congenital or acquired immunodeficiencies; HIV infection; chronic renal failure; nephrotic syndrome; diseases associated with treatment with immunosuppressive drugs or radiation therapy, including malignant neoplasms, leukemias, lymphomas, and Hodgkin's disease; generalized malignancy; solid organ transplantation; or multiple myeloma.

7. **Inactivated poliovirus vaccine (IPV). (Minimum age: 6 weeks)**

Routine vaccination:

- Administer a 4-dose series of IPV at ages 2, 4, 6 through 18 months, and 4 through 6 years. The final dose in the series should be administered on or after the fourth birthday and at least 6 months after the previous dose.

Catch-up vaccination:

- In the first 6 months of life, minimum age and minimum intervals are only recommended if the person is at risk of imminent exposure to circulating poliovirus (i.e., travel to a polio-endemic region or during an outbreak).
- If 4 or more doses are administered before age 4 years, an additional dose should be administered at age 4 through 6 years and at least 6 months after the previous dose.
- A fourth dose is not necessary if the third dose was administered at age 4 years or older and at least 6 months after the previous dose.
- If both OPV and IPV were administered as part of a series, a total of 4 doses should be administered, regardless of the child's current age. IPV is not routinely recommended for U.S. residents aged 18 years or older.
- For other catch-up guidance, see Figure 2.

8. **Influenza vaccines. (Minimum age: 6 months for inactivated influenza vaccine [IIV], 2 years for live, attenuated influenza vaccine [LAIV])**

Routine vaccination:

- Administer influenza vaccine annually to all children beginning at age 6 months. For most healthy, nonpregnant persons aged 2 through 49 years, either LAIV or IIV may be used. However, LAIV should NOT be administered to some persons, including 1) persons who have experienced severe allergic reactions to LAIV, any of its components, or to a previous dose of any other influenza vaccine; 2) children 2 through 17 years receiving aspirin or aspirin-containing products; 3) persons who are allergic to eggs; 4) pregnant women; 5) immunosuppressed persons; 6) children 2 through 4 years of age with asthma or who had wheezing in the past 12 months; or 7) persons who have taken influenza antiviral medications in the previous 48 hours. For all other contraindications and precautions to use of LAIV, see *MMWR* August 15, 2014 / 63(32);691-697 [40 pages] available at http://www.cdc.gov/mmwr/pdf/wk/mm6332.pdf.

For children aged 6 months through 8 years:

- For the 2014-15 season, administer 2 doses (separated by at least 4 weeks) to children who are receiving influenza vaccine for the first time. Some children in this age group who have been vaccinated previously will also need 2 doses. For additional guidance, follow dosing guidelines in the 2014-15 ACIP influenza vaccine recommendations, *MMWR* August 15, 2014 / 63(32);691-697 [40 pages] available at http://www.cdc.gov/mmwr/pdf/wk/mm6332.pdf.
- For the 2015–16 season, follow dosing guidelines in the 2015 ACIP influenza vaccine recommendations.

For persons aged 9 years and older:

- Administer 1 dose.

For further guidance on the use of the vaccines mentioned below, see: http://www.cdc.gov/vaccines/hcp/acip-recs/index.html.

9. Measles, mumps, and rubella (MMR) vaccine. (Minimum age: 12 months for routine vaccination)

Routine vaccination:

- Administer a 2-dose series of MMR vaccine at ages 12 through 15 months and 4 through 6 years. The second dose may be administered before age 4 years, provided at least 4 weeks have elapsed since the first dose.
- Administer 1 dose of MMR vaccine to infants aged 6 through 11 months before departure from the United States for international travel. These children should be revaccinated with 2 doses of MMR vaccine, the first at age 12 through 15 months (12 months if the child remains in an area where disease risk is high), and the second dose at least 4 weeks later.
- Administer 2 doses of MMR vaccine to children aged 12 months and older before departure from the United States for international travel. The first dose should be administered on or after age 12 months and the second dose at least 4 weeks later.

Catch-up vaccination:

- Ensure that all school-aged children and adolescents have had 2 doses of MMR vaccine; the minimum interval between the 2 doses is 4 weeks.

10. Varicella (VAR) vaccine. (Minimum age: 12 months)

Routine vaccination:

- Administer a 2-dose series of VAR vaccine at ages 12 through 15 months and 4 through 6 years. The second dose may be administered before age 4 years, provided at least 3 months have elapsed since the first dose. If the second dose was administered at least 4 weeks after the first dose, it can be accepted as valid.

Catch-up vaccination:

- Ensure that all persons aged 7 through 18 years without evidence of immunity (see *MMWR* 2007 / 56 [No. RR-4], available at http://www.cdc.gov/mmwr/pdf/rr/rr5604.pdf) have 2 doses of varicella vaccine. For children aged 7 through 12 years, the recommended minimum interval between doses is 3 months (if the second dose was administered at least 4 weeks after the first dose, it can be accepted as valid); for persons aged 13 years and older, the minimum interval between doses is 4 weeks.

11. Hepatitis A (HepA) vaccine. (Minimum age: 12 months)

Routine vaccination:

- Initiate the 2-dose HepA vaccine series at 12 through 23 months; separate the 2 doses by 6 to 18 months.
- Children who have received 1 dose of HepA vaccine before age 24 months should receive a second dose 6 to 18 months after the first dose.
- For any person aged 2 years and older who has not already received the HepA vaccine series, 2 doses of HepA vaccine separated by 6 to 18 months may be administered if immunity against hepatitis A virus infection is desired.

Catch-up vaccination:

- The minimum interval between the two doses is 6 months.

Special populations:

- Administer 2 doses of HepA vaccine at least 6 months apart to previously unvaccinated persons who live in areas where vaccination programs target older children, or who are at increased risk for infection. This includes persons traveling to or working in countries that have high or intermediate endemicity of infection; men having sex with men; users of injection and non-injection illicit drugs; persons who work with HAV-infected primates or with HAV in a research laboratory; persons with clotting-factor disorders; persons with chronic liver disease; and persons who anticipate close personal contact (e.g., household or regular babysitting) with an international adoptee during the first 60 days after arrival in the United States from a country with high or intermediate endemicity. The first dose should be administered as soon as the adoption is planned, ideally 2 or more weeks before the arrival of the adoptee.

12. Human papillomavirus (HPV) vaccines. (Minimum age: 9 years for HPV2 [Cervarix] and HPV4 [Gardasil])

Routine vaccination:

- Administer a 3-dose series of HPV vaccine on a schedule of 0, 1-2, and 6 months to all adolescents aged 11 through 12 years. Either HPV4 or HPV2 may be used for females, and only HPV4 may be used for males.
- The vaccine series may be started at age 9 years.
- Administer the second dose 1 to 2 months after the first dose (minimum interval of 4 weeks); administer the third dose 24 weeks after the first dose and 16 weeks after the second dose (minimum interval of 12 weeks).

Catch-up vaccination:

- Administer the vaccine series to females (either HPV2 or HPV4) and males (HPV4) at age 13 through 18 years if not previously vaccinated.
- Use recommended routine dosing intervals (see Routine vaccination above) for vaccine series catch-up.

13. Meningococcal conjugate vaccines. (Minimum age: 6 weeks for Hib-MenCY [MenHibrix], 9 months for MenACWY-D [Menactra], 2 months for MenACWY-CRM [Menveo])

Routine vaccination:

- Administer a single dose of Menactra or Menveo vaccine at age 11 through 12 years, with a booster dose at age 16 years.
- Adolescents aged 11 through 18 years with human immunodeficiency virus (HIV) infection should receive a 2-dose primary series of Menactra or Menveo with at least 8 weeks between doses.
- For children aged 2 months through 18 years with high-risk conditions, see below.

Catch-up vaccination:

- Administer Menactra or Menveo vaccine at age 13 through 18 years if not previously vaccinated.
- If the first dose is administered at age 13 through 15 years, a booster dose should be administered at age 16 through 18 years with a minimum interval of at least 8 weeks between doses.
- If the first dose is administered at age 16 years or older, a booster dose is not needed.
- For other catch-up guidance, see Figure 2.

Vaccination of persons with high-risk conditions and other persons at increased risk of disease:

- Children with anatomic or functional asplenia (including sickle cell disease):
  1. Menveo
     - o *Children who initiate vaccination at 8 weeks through 6 months:* Administer doses at 2, 4, 6, and 12 months of age.
     - o *Unvaccinated children 7 through 23 months:* Administer 2 doses, with the second dose at least 12 weeks after the first dose AND after the first birthday.
     - o *Children 24 months and older who have not received a complete series:* Administer 2 primary doses at least 8 weeks apart.
  2. MenHibrix
     - o *Children 6 weeks through 18 months:* Administer doses at 2, 4, 6, and 12 through 15 months of age.
     - o If the first dose of MenHibrix is given at or after 12 months of age, a total of 2 doses should be given at least 8 weeks apart to ensure protection against serogroups C and Y meningococcal disease.
  3. Menactra
     - o *Children 24 months and older who have not received a complete series:* Administer 2 primary doses at least 8 weeks apart. If Menactra is administered to a child with asplenia (including sickle cell disease), do not administer Menactra until 2 years of age and at least 4 weeks after the completion of all PCV13 doses.
- Children with persistent complement component deficiency:
  1. Menveo
     - o *Children who initiate vaccination at 8 weeks through 6 months:* Administer doses at 2, 4, 6, and 12 months of age.
     - o *Unvaccinated children 7 through 23 months:* Administer 2 doses, with the second dose at least 12 weeks after the first dose AND after the first birthday.
     - o *Children 24 months and older who have not received a complete series:* Administer 2 primary doses at least 8 weeks apart.
  2. MenHibrix
     - o *Children 6 weeks through 18 months:* Administer doses at 2, 4, 6, and 12 through 15 months of age.
     - o If the first dose of MenHibrix is given at or after 12 months of age, a total of 2 doses should be given at least 8 weeks apart to ensure protection against serogroups C and Y meningococcal disease.
  3. Menactra
     - o *Children 9 through 23 months:* Administer 2 primary doses at least 12 weeks apart.
     - o *Children 24 months and older who have not received a complete series:* Administer 2 primary doses at least 8 weeks apart.
- For children who travel to or reside in countries in which meningococcal disease is hyperendemic or epidemic, including countries in the African meningitis belt or the Hajj, administer an age-appropriate formulation and series of Menactra or Menveo for protection against serogroups A and W meningococcal disease. Prior receipt of MenHibrix is not sufficient for children traveling to the meningitis belt or the Hajj because it does not contain serogroups A or W.
- For children at risk during a community outbreak attributable to a vaccine serogroup, administer or complete an age- and formulation-appropriate series of MenHibrix, Menactra, or Menveo.
- For booster doses among persons with high-risk conditions, refer to *MMWR* 2013 / 62(RR02);1-22, available at http://www.cdc.gov/mmwr/preview/mmwrhtml/rr6202a1.htm.

For other catch-up recommendations for these persons, and complete information on use of meningococcal vaccines, including guidance related to vaccination of persons at increased risk of infection, see MMWR March 22, 2013 / 62(RR02);1-22, available at http://www.cdc.gov/mmwr/pdf/rr/rr6202.pdf.

CS 244083-B

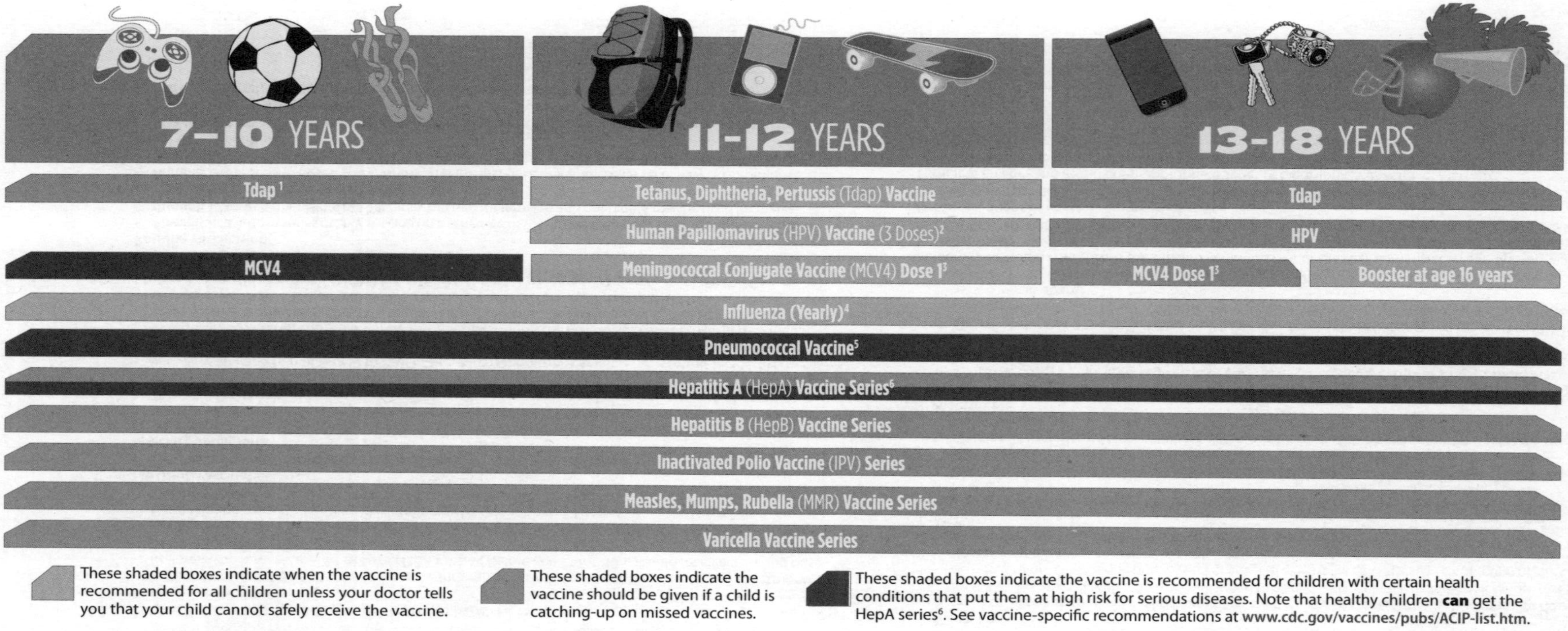

FOOTNOTES

[1] Tdap vaccine is recommended at age 11 or 12 to protect against tetanus, diphtheria and pertussis. If your child has not received any or all of the DTaP vaccine series, or if you don't know if your child has received these shots, your child needs a single dose of Tdap when they are 7 -10 years old. Talk to your child's health care provider to find out if they need additional catch-up vaccines.

[2] All 11 or 12 year olds – both girls *and* boys – should receive 3 doses of HPV vaccine to protect against HPV-related disease. The full HPV vaccine series should be given as recommended for best protection.

[3] Meningococcal conjugate vaccine (MCV) is recommended at age 11 or 12. A booster shot is recommended at age 16. Teens who received MCV for the first time at age 13 through 15 years will need a one-time booster dose between the ages of 16 and 18 years. If your teenager missed getting the vaccine altogether, ask their health care provider about getting it now, especially if your teenager is about to move into a college dorm or military barracks.

[4] Everyone 6 months of age and older—including preteens and teens—should get a flu vaccine every year. Children under the age of 9 years may require more than one dose. Talk to your child's health care provider to find out if they need more than one dose.

[5] Pneumococcal Conjugate Vaccine (PCV13) and Pneumococcal Polysaccharide Vaccine (PPSV23) are recommended for some children 6 through 18 years old with certain medical conditions that place them at high risk. Talk to your healthcare provider about pneumococcal vaccines and what factors may place your child at high risk for pneumococcal disease.

[6] Hepatitis A vaccination is recommended for older children with certain medical conditions that place them at high risk. HepA vaccine is licensed, safe, and effective for all children of all ages. Even if your child is not at high risk, you may decide you want your child protected against HepA. Talk to your healthcare provider about HepA vaccine and what factors may place your child at high risk for HepA.

For more information, call toll free 1-800-CDC-INFO (1-800-232-4636) or visit http://www.cdc.gov/vaccines/teens

U.S. Department of Health and Human Services
Centers for Disease Control and Prevention

American Academy of Pediatrics
DEDICATED TO THE HEALTH OF ALL CHILDREN™

AMERICAN ACADEMY OF FAMILY PHYSICIANS
STRONG MEDICINE FOR AMERICA

Figure 7.1.3: 2015 recommended immunizations for children from 7 through 18 years old

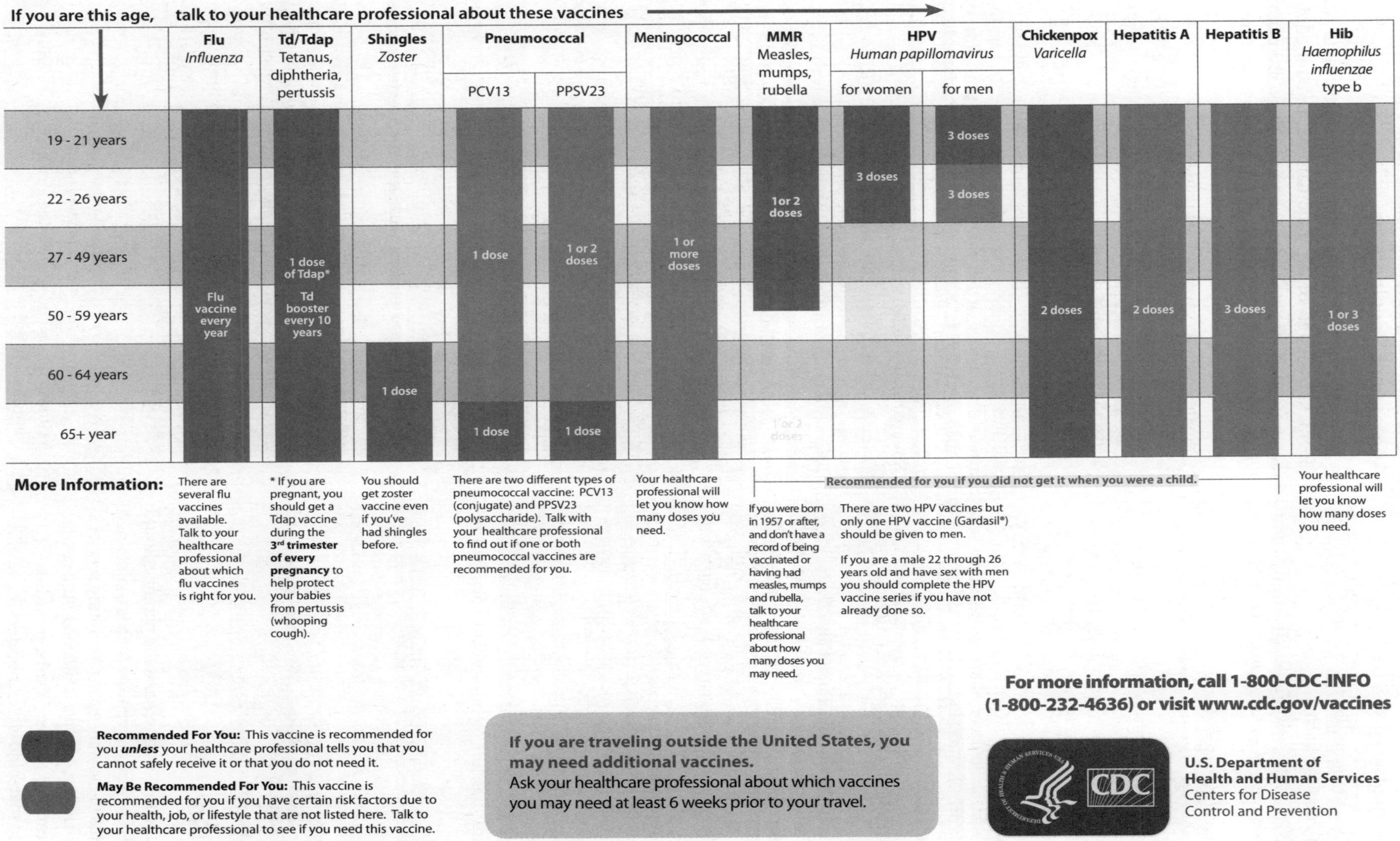

Figure 7.1.4: 2015 recommended immunizations for adults: By age

- There are many reasons why immunization in adolescent is important (Box 7.1.1).

Box 7.1.1: Reasons for adolescent immunization
To Boost Immunity that is Waning
• To increase the duration of effective protection derived from the vaccines already given earlier in life, especially in the absence of "natural" boosting (of primary immunization) from exposure to the particular disease. • This strategy mimics to some extent the boosting effect of infectious agents in the prevaccine era. • The goal is to protect adolescents from the dreaded complications of childhood vaccine preventable diseases (VPDs) when they occur during adolescence. Whereas chickenpox during childhood is considered as a harmless self-limiting infection, it can result in severe complications and may even add to mortality figures in adolescents between 10-18 years of age. • Epidemiologic shift of childhood VPDs to adolescents e.g. measles, mumps, pertussis, diphtheria etc.
Catch-Up Vaccination
• For those adolescents who were not immunized/partially immunized during their childhood e.g. MMR, Hep A, Hep B, Varicella vaccines.
To Accelerate Disease Control or Elimination Efforts
• Disease control initiatives frequently encompass immunizing across a wide age range, including adolescents, with the aim of increasing herd immunity, interrupting transmission or catching-up on cohorts missed in the past. E.g. measles elimination in certain countries has targeted individuals from 9 months to 14 years.
To Counter a Specific Risk
• Adolescents may adapt lifestyles like tattooing piercing and sexual experimentation which has increased risk, for instance from hepatitis B virus. • Travel represents a special need as adolescent enjoy traveling to exotic places. Special efforts may be appropriate to immunize them before they enter the risk period.

There are many barriers to adolescent vaccinations (Box 7.1.2).

Box 7.1.2: Barriers to vaccination in adolescents
Principal barriers that have prevented vaccines from wide administration to date (and are likely to remain impediments in the future) are:
1. The lack of awareness by parents.
2. The cost of the interventions.
3. The lack of suitable infrastructure to reach the target.

HISTORY TAKING

At the first contact with the adolescent the parents should be asked to get the vaccination record which is maintained by most pediatricians in the well-baby monitoring services.

- This will give an idea of what childhood vaccines are missed so that "catch-up vaccines" can be given (Box 7.1.1).
- It will also help to decide which boosters are needed.

Important Aspects to Remember for Adolescent Vaccinations

A physician should educate himself and have upto date recent knowledge of all vaccinations and schedules recommended by professional bodies. There are certain issues which are different in adolescent age group (Box 7.1.3). It should be ensured that the clinic has adequate setup to vaccinate an adolescent (Box 7.1.4).

Box 7.1.3: Points to remember when advising vaccinations to adolescents
Scheduling vaccinations
Flexibility in scheduling vaccinations is an important factor for improving vaccination coverage among adolescents. The combination vaccines or simultaneous administration of several vaccines may be indicated for adolescents, but the providers need to be flexible in determining which vaccines are to be administered during the initial visit and which to be administered on return visits.
Simultaneous administration of vaccines
Extensive clinical experience and experimental evidence from studies of infants and children have strengthened the scientific basis for administering certain vaccines simultaneously. Although specific studies have not been conducted regarding the simultaneous administration of all vaccines recommended for routine use in adolescents, no evidence has established that this practice is unsafe or ineffective.
Well adolescent visit
All indicated vaccinations should be administered at the scheduled immunization visit for adolescents who are 11 to 12 years of age. However, some adolescents may require multiple (i.e. four or more) vaccinations and the provider may choose not to administer all indicated vaccines during the same visit.

Box 7.1.4: Tips to remember while immunizing adolescents
• Explain all about the vaccine and possible side effects of the vaccine
• Take an informed consent
• Never vaccinate a reluctant adolescent. Ask him/her to come back again
• Adolescents are more susceptible to vasovagal syncopal attacks after any pricks. (Take special precautions while giving HPV vaccine. It is best to give in lying down position and observe for 10-15 minutes before allowing them to leave the clinic.)
• Ensure in history taking that the female adoelscent is not pregnant
• Follow all safe injection practices
• Ensure proper storage of all vaccinations
• Ensure you have all drugs and equipment available to treat any adverse reactions after immunizations
• Maintain a good adolescent vaccination record card as is done for pediatrics

Detailed History of Any Adverse Reactions to Immunizations Should be Noted

- Unlike children, adolescents are aware of the possibility of experiencing negative effects from vaccines. While infants have not been taught that injections hurt, adolescents know this very well.
- When subjected to mass vaccination in a school setting, emotions may run high with fainting and other dramatic hysterical reactions. Staff-patient communication therefore becomes important so that the issue of relative risk can be explained.
- While giving HPV vaccine which is known to cause syncopal attack in some girls, it is important to get detailed history of past syncopal attacks, giddiness or dizziness specially after blood collection or injections.

Rule Out Pregnancy

- Certain live vaccines e.g. live attenuated measles, mumps, rubella, varicella and yellow fever can theoretically damage the fetus. Hence it is very important to ensure that the adolescent girl is not pregnant.
- It is possible that girls coming for vaccination may be unaware that they are in the early stage pregnancy. Others may be reluctant to admit to the pregnancy (which may result in their exclusion from school) and therefore go ahead with vaccination, perhaps despite being warned of the danger.

Special Situations

1. Prescribing Vaccines for Travel

Adolescents can largely be treated on the same basis as adults regarding immunization for travel, taking into account previous exposure, vaccination history and medical conditions. However, many adolescents undertake travel of a more adventurous "back-packing" style, which may expose them to greater risks than other visitors to particular countries (Table 7.1.1).

2. Vaccine for Adolescents Staying in Hostel

- The mandatory vaccines are chickenpox, hepatitis A, typhoid and MMR in view of epidemic nature of these diseases and serious life threatening complications.
- IAP now recommends including rabies vaccination also in 3 doses for pre-exposure prophylaxis in view of the impending threat of bites by stray dogs.

PHYSICAL EXAMINATION

A complete physical examination should be performed before giving any vaccination to rule out any medical condition that needs treatment.

- One should avoid giving vaccinations if the adolescent is febrile, ill looking or not in a mood to take vaccinations, but persuade them to come back when better and more amenable.
- Reminder calls should be made to ensure that the vaccination is not missed.

VACCINATIONS IMPORTANT IN ADOLESCENT AGE GROUP

The Indian Academy of Pediatrics Committee of Immunization also updates the IAP recommended schedule every year (Figure 7.1.1).

Each year, the Advisory Committee on Immunization Practices (ACIP) in USA publishes immunization schedules for person's age (birth through 18 years) and also adult vaccination above 19 years of age. (Figures 7.1.2 and 7.1.3). These are also approved by the Advisory Committee on Immunization Practices (ACIP), the American Academy of Pediatrics (AAP), the American Academy of Family Physicians (AAFP) and the American College of Obstetricians and Gynecologists (ACOG). Summary of various vaccines recommended for adolescents is given in Table 7.1.2.

Table 7.1.1: Travel related adolescent vaccines

Vaccine	*Place of travel*	*Dose recommended*
Meningococcal Vaccine	USA/UK/endemic areas Saudi Arabia and Africa #	2 doses 4-8 weeks apart
Yellow Fever Vaccine	Yellow fever endemic zones**	10 days before travel
Oral Cholera Vaccine	Endemic area or area with an outbreak	2 doses 1 week apart
Japanese Encephalitis (JE) Vaccine	Endemic areas for JE	Single dose up to 15 years
Rabies Vaccine (Pre-exposure Prophylaxis)	For adolescents going on trekking	0,7, 28 days

- # Quadrivalent vaccine for those traveling to the USA and Bivalent (A+C) or Quadrivalent for those traveling to the UK.
- ** Mandatory for all travelers to yellow fever endemic zones as per international health regulations.
- The list of endemic countries can be obtained at http://wwwn.cdc.gov/travel yellow Book ch4, Yellow Fever.aspx currently available only at select government controlled centers in India.
- For more information on travelers vaccination, visit http://wwwnc.cdc.qov/travel/default.as:

Reproduced with permission from Hand Book on Adolescent and Adult Immunization; Eds A. Parthasarathy, Alok Gupta, 2014 Jaypee Brothers Medical Publishers (P) Ltd, New Delhi, pp 67-68.

Table 7.1.2: Various types of vaccines for adolescents

Vaccine	*Comments*
Measles	A one-time measles campaign ("catch-up") targeting children 9 months to 14 years of age. Secondary and tertiary education institutions may offer an extra dose in late teens to avoid outbreaks among students.
Pneumococcal	Revaccination is recommended for high risk for provided first dose >5 years ago.
Hepatitis B	• Non-protective level < 10 μ IU/100 ml. • Males having sex with males. • Travelers to endemic countries. • Those injecting recreational drugs. • Tattooing and piercing.
Poliomyelitis	Booster doses are not required for the adolescent living in endemic countries—natural boosting with wild virus is likely to be a continual process that maintains immunity. WHO recommends that one additional dose of polio vaccine should be offered to previously vaccinated persons traveling from industrialized countries to endemic areas. For unvaccinated travelers and those with no previously documented polio vaccination, a full course should be offered.
Yellow Fever	WHO recommends that travelers to endemic areas should have an up-to-date dose of yellow fever vaccine to meet international health regulations. Adolescents may be included in yellow fever outbreak control immunization.
Hepatitis A	High endemic areas. Travel to endemic countries. Outbreaks. Chronic liver disease.
Typhoid	WHO recommends school age children in endemic areas with drug resistant typhoid. Oral Ty21a or with injectable Vi vaccine. Traveling to endemic area should be immunized.
Japanese Encephalitis	Booster doses are not usually given beyond ten years of age. *Adolescents traveling to endemic areas should be immunized.*

Human Papilloma Virus (HPV) Vaccine

The bivalent and quadrivalent vaccines have been available in India for last many years (for schedules see Figures 7.1.1 and 7.1.2). Now there is a newer 9-valent HPV vaccine—hpv9 which is available abroad. The 9-valent vaccine protects against the same four HPV types in the quadrivalent vaccine and five additional types. These additional types cause about 10% of HPV-associated cancers, including about 15% of cervical cancers. The 9-valent vaccine cause slightly more reactions—primarily swelling and redness—where the injection was given but there are no major side effects. The protective levels have been shown to be good in a follow-up of 4 years so far for hpv 9, and 8-10 years for both hpv 2 and hpv 4.

Should One Wait for hpv9 Availability?

- ACIP recommends that for those who are eligible for vaccination start the HPV vaccine series with whatever vaccine is available from their health care professional. Do not wait for the newer vaccine.
- For females, any HPV vaccine may be used to complete the series.
- For males, either quadrivalent or 9-valent HPV vaccine may be used to complete the series.

Recent recommendations about HPV vaccine (Box 7.1.5).

Box 7.1.5: New ACIP recommendations for HPV vaccination
Effective March 27, 2015
9vHPV, 4vHPV, or 2vHPV for routine vaccination of females 11 or 12 years* (can be given at starting 9 years) of age and females through 26 years of age who have not been vaccinated previously or who have not completed the 3-dose series.
9vHPV or 4vHPV for routine vaccination of males 11 or 12 years* of age and males through 21 years of age who have not been vaccinated previously or who have not completed the 3-dose series.
9vHPV or 4vHPV vaccination for men who have sex with men and immunocompromised men (including those with HIV infection) through age 26 years if not vaccinated previously.
* *Syndicated and print schedules do not yet reflect this change. This recommendation will be incorporated in the immunization schedules that will be published in February 2016.*

Tetanus, Diphtheria and Pertussis Vaccines

The recent concepts and recommendations for the administration of tetanus toxoid (TT), tetanus and diphtheria (Td) and tetanus, diphtheria and acellular pertussis (Tdap) are given in Box 7.1.6.

Box 7.1.6: Recent concepts and recommendations for TT/Td/Tdap vaccines
Repeated TT injections following trivial injuries may result in: • Reduced immunogenicity • Hypersensitivity • Hemolytic anemia • Amyloidosis • Increased risk of hemorrhagic disease of the newborn
Td is now WHO recommended immunogen for antenatal boosters and for wound prophylaxis for all ages including adolescents due to: (a) Occurrence of diphtheria in adolescents and adults in some regions of the world due to epidemiological shift (b) Waning immunity to the diphtheria component resulting in more severe disease during adolescence and even adulthood with fatal complications like myocarditis
Children and adolescents should receive 7 doses of TT (5 doses as DTPw/DTPa at 6,10 and 14 weeks, first booster at 18 months followed by booster at 5 years and 2 doses as Tdap/Td at 10 and 20 years respectively)
Pregnant woman After 7 doses of TT an adequately immunized pregnant woman needs only a single booster dose of Td during first pregnancy and once in 3 years for subsequent pregnancy
For Wound Prophylaxis • Td is recommended
Tdap vaccine This protects against tetanus, diphtheria and pertussis. In common language called "adult DPT" • ACIP recommendation: A single dose is recommended at well adolescent visit at 11-12 years of age • Adolescents 11-18 years who have completed childhood immunization of diphtheria, tetanus and pertussis (DPT/DTaP) a single booster dose is recommended instead of Td • Adults above 19 years who have not received Tdap should receive one single dose • Td can be used for booster every 10 years thereafter

Meningococcal Vaccine

The recent concepts and recommendations regarding the administration of meningococcal vaccine in adolescents are given in Box 7.1.7.

Box 7.1.7: Recent concepts and recommendations for meningococcal vaccine
Available Meningococcal Poly Saccharide Vaccine (MPSV) MCV: Meningococcal Conjugate Vaccine (MCV) Quadrivalent (Sero Groups A,C, W135 & Y) and Bivalent (A&C) Monovalent B sero group
ACIP 2015 recommends routine vaccination of quadrivalent meningococcal conjugate vaccine MenACWY to certain groups of people who are increased risk of meningococcal disease (MD): a. Persons who have persistent complement component deficiencies; b. Persons who have anatomic or functional asplenia; c. Microbiologists who are routinely exposed to Neisseria meningitis; d. Persons identified to be at increased risk because of MD outbreaks attributable to sero group A,C,W or Y : military recruits, first year college students living in residence halls; e. Persons who travel to or reside in areas where MD is hyperendemic or endemic.
Meningococcal B vaccine is recommended only above the age of 10 years for the same indications as above and persons at risk for getting Meningococcal B disease. It is not recommended to persons who travel to or reside in areas where MD is hyperendemic or endemic because serotype B does not cause MD in these countries.
IAP Policy is Meningococcal Vaccine for travelling adolescents seeking job/proceeding for higher studies in meningococcal disease endemic countries and adolescents in the high risk group (chronic heart and lung disease, leukemia, HIV/AIDS, diabetes mellitus, etc.) only and NOT for routine immunization.

LEARNING POINTS

1. Adequate immunization is one of the most important preventive health services that can be provided for adolescents.
2. Every visit of an adolescent should be an opportunity to take history of vaccination.
3. Adolescents present unique challenges for immunization because of their lifestyle and other social issues, while they also offer special opportunities, such as mass vaccination in educational institutions.
4. Reasons for adolescent immunization are many: to boost immunity that is waning, as catch-up vaccination for missed vaccinations in childhood; to accelerate disease control or elimination of vaccine preventable diseases and efforts to counter a specific risk that is related to their lifestyle.
5. Physicians should follow standard recommendations and schedules that are made by professional organizations.

Acknowledgements

1. IAP for permission reproduce the IAP Pediatric and Adolescent Immunization schedules 2014 (Figure 7.1.1) from the IAP Guide Book on Immunization Edition 2013-14 published on behalf of IAP CoI 2011-13 (IAP Committee on Immunization) and IAP ACVIP (IAP Advisory Committee on Vaccines and Immunization Practices) 2013-14.
2. CDC and ACIP schedules (Figures 7.1.2, 7.1.3 and 7.1.4) images found in the Public Health Image Library (PHIL) are royalty-free and available for personal, professional and educational use in electronic or print media, with appropriate citation. URL http://www.cdc.gov/Other/imagereuse.html accessed on 27th September 2015.

SUGGESTED READING

1. Bhave SY, Parthasarathy A, Yadav S (Eds.). Ready reckoner for immunization neonate to adult. New Delhi; Jaypee Brothers Medical Publishers Pvt Ltd.; 2010.
2. HPV Vaccine URL http://www.cdc.gov/vaccines/who/teens/for-hcp-tipsheet-hpv.html accessed on 28th Sep 2015.
3. http//redbook.solutions.aap.org/Communization schdules.aspx accessed on 29 Aug 2015.
4. IAP website for guidelines on immunization www.iapindia.org accessed on 29 Aug 2015.
5. Parthasarathy A, Gupta A (Eds). Hand Book on Adolescent and Adult Immunization. New Delhi; Jaypee Brothers Medical Publishers Pvt. Ltd. 2014; 60-68.
6. Petrosky E, Bocchini Jr JA, Hariri S, Chesson H, Curtis CR, Saraiya M, *et al.* Use of 9-Valent Human Papillomavirus (HPV) Vaccine: Updated HPV Vaccination Recommendations of the Advisory Committee on Immunization Practices. Morbidity and Mortality Weekly Report (MWR) 2015;64(11):300-04.
7. Siddiqui M, Bhave SY (Eds.) FAQS on HPV Infection and its prevention. Cancer Foundation of India; 2009; Reprinted 2010.
8. www.cdc.gov/vaccines/schedules/index.html accessed on 29 Aug 2015.

Sports Participation 7.2.1

Dilip R Patel, Devika Malhotra

INTRODUCTION

Studies have shown that adolescents who participate in sports have a reduced risk of depression, are more successful at school, are more successful at maintaining healthy relationships with others, and more likely to maintain an active lifestyle as adults, thus, improving overall health. In this chapter, we briefly discuss various issues that are important for adolescent sports participation and also appropriately clearing athletes for sports participation based on sports classification.

FITNESS FOR SPORTS PARTICIPATION

A careful medical history and physical examination are the cornerstones of effective clinical practice. The frequency, format, contents, and usefulness of a physical fitness preparticipation evaluation in predicting and preventing morbidity and mortality related to sport participation have not been validated by any long-term systematic research. Studies suggest that between 0.3% and 1.3% of the athletes are disqualified from participation based on sports physical findings and between 3.2% and 13.9% of all athletes require further evaluation. Athletes should receive a formal evaluation annually, preferably 6 to 8 weeks before the sports season or event to allow for adequate rehabilitation of most injuries that may be found and to allow for further medical evaluation of any other problems identified (see Box 7.2.1.1).

Box 7.2.1.1: Physical fitness evaluation

This evaluation is best done in an office setting by an athlete's primary care physician.

This allows for continuity of care and exploration of a wider range of health-related issues in a confidential manner.

It is not a substitute for a general annual or preventive health visit.

The main goals are to:

- Assess the general health of the athlete.
- Identify any health condition that may predispose the athlete to increased risk for injury or illness.
- Match the athlete with the sport best suited for him or her depending on physical health, cognitive abilities, and athletic abilities.

HISTORY TAKING

A comprehensive medical history obtained from the athlete and parents is the most important aspect of the evaluation and can identify about 75% of the potential concerns associated with sports participation. Data can be obtained from various sources, including the athlete, parents or guardians, previous medical records, and school records. Standard questionnaires may be used for initial screening. Key elements to be explored in the history are summarized in Table 7.2.1.1.

The medical history should identify any known medical conditions (such as asthma, epilepsy, diabetes mellitus, hepatitis, high blood pressure, congenital heart disease, arrhythmias, coagulation disorders, one functional kidney, one functional or anatomical eye, juvenile rheumatoid arthritis, spondylolysis, anorexia nervosa, pregnancy, depression, attention-deficit/hyperactivity disorder, and others). Such knowledge will allow for proper management of these conditions in the athlete to ensure safe and continued sport participation.

Musculoskeletal Conditions

Gather history regarding previous or current musculoskeletal problems so that they can be clearly identified and treated to result in minimal interference with the athlete's sports performance and participation. If there is a positive history for previous musculoskeletal injury, further inquiry is warranted regarding the nature of this injury, what treatment occurred, whether full recovery occurred, and if the athlete is engaged in overtraining. If the athlete is allowed to return to sports without full rehabilitation, risks for additional injury are increased. In addition, it is important to rule out other causes of musculoskeletal pain or injury, such as neoplasm or infection.

Cardiovascular Disorders

A careful assessment of cardiac disorders is critical to identify not only previously diagnosed conditions but also

Table 7.2.1.1: Key elements of physical fitness evaluation history

Past history	Major trauma (musculoskeletal, head and neck, chest and abdomen) Major surgeries (spine, cardiac, abdomen and genitourinary) Chronic disease Heat-related illness
Medications	Therapeutic medications Nutritional supplements Over-the-counter medications
Allergies	Environmental allergy Drug allergy Food allergy History of anaphylactic reactions Exercise-induced allergic or anaphylactic reactions
Nutritional	Dietary habits Attempts to manipulate weight Recent weight loss or gain
Neurologic	Details of head and neck trauma Symptoms of concussion History of seizures Exercise-related headaches
Pulmonary	Exercise-related difficulty breathing Chronic-exercise related cough Persistent wheezing
Cardiovascular	Family history of sudden cardiac death prior to age 50 Family history of known heart disease Exertional chest discomfort, pain, pressure and tightness Exertional syncope or near-syncope Excessive unexplained dyspnea or fatigue Previous evaluation–ECG, echocardiogram, exercise stress test and visit with cardiologist
Health risk behaviors	Pathogenic weight control High-risk sexual practices Abuse of illicit drugs Use of performance-enhancing agents
Others	Recent febrile illness Undue fatigue Hearing problems Vision problems Eye trauma and surgery Missing paired organ Musculoskeletal injuries Immunization status Menstrual history in females

previously unrecognized conditions in order to allow an athlete to participate in sports. Cardiovascular screening seeks to find those at increased risk for exercise-induced sudden cardiac death. A cardiac cause represents 75% of sudden death in adolescent and young adult athletes. The etiology of sudden cardiac death is often due to structural (i.e. hypertrophic cardiomyopathy, coronary artery anomalies, aortic stenosis, aortic rupture in Marfan syndrome, congenital heart disease, etc.) and electrical abnormalities of the heart (i.e. long QT syndrome, Wolff-Parkinson-White syndrome, Brugada syndrome, ion channel disorders, etc.). Sometimes it can also be related to drug and stimulant use. The majority of the time, these abnormalities go undetected because they often are asymptomatic under normal conditions without physiologic stress. For this reason, a thorough evaluation including obtaining a personal and family history of each athlete is critical.

Medications

The physical fitness evaluation should include identifying what medication(s) the athlete is taking, in addition to the athlete and parents being aware of and understanding potential adverse effects of these drugs. Sports officials should be made aware of these medications as determined by the physician and the athlete as well as the parents or guardians. The athlete should understand if the drug has a negative effect on sports performance. For example, beta blockers prevent optimal increase in heart rate in response to physical activity. If the athlete is not in compliance with recommended medication, sports performance may be reduced, such as in the individual with poorly controlled diabetes mellitus who experiences diabetic reactions.

Non-prescription drugs can lead to problems, as noted with the increased risk for heat illness when taking anti-histamine medication, trauma-induced bleeding in the athlete taking aspirin (acetyl salicylic acid), or abdominal pain and bleeding from non-steroidal anti-inflammatory drugs (NSAIDs).

Other important medical conditions in history taking and their implications are outlined in Tables 7.2.1.2 and 7.2.1.3, Boxes 7.2.1.2 and 7.2.1.3.

Table 7.2.1.2: Important medical conditions and implications for adolescent athlete

Medical conditions	*Importance*	*Implications*
Heat Disorders	A past history of heat-related illness is a risk factor for recurrent heat-related illness.	Preventive measures (i.e. adequate hydration) to be implemented.
Asthma	Asthma can have direct effects on the quality of life and if not adequately treated can adversely impact the athlete's sports performance.	Adequate management and control ensures that adolescent can enjoy the benefits of full and unrestricted participation in sports.
Allergies	Allergic history including both environmental and drug allergies that may interfere with sports performance is essential. A history of exercise induced allergic reaction or anaphylactic reaction should be ascertained. Some athletes are also known to have exercise induced urticarial reactions.	An epinephrine injection kit should always be available for emergency treatment of anaphylactic reactions for those athletes with a positive history.
Febrile Illness	A history of recent febrile illness is important to consider. An upper respiratory tract infection or febrile illness may interfere with optimal performance.	However, a more serious threat is the uncommon development of myocarditis that may be the result of a viral illness leading to potentially lethal cardiac arrhythmias and sudden death.
Ophthalmologic Conditions	Obtain a history of visual acuity, eye symptoms, and history of eye surgery.	Clearance for sports is dependent on normal or corrected normal visual acuity. Complex eye conditions will require evaluation and clearance by an ophthalmologist. Some eye conditions including retinal disorders can limit participation in certain sports.
Surgical History	Obtain history of major surgeries, such as surgery of spine, chest, and abdomen, as well as cardiac surgery for congenital heart disease.	Athlete and family should be aware of if the athlete has fully recovered and has been cleared by the surgeon for some or all levels of exertion. Current cardiac health should be understood, as well as what risks continue for physical activity at all levels.

Table 7.2.1.3: Special issues in female athlete

Issues	*Comments*
Menstrual and Gynecologic History	Menarche (age of menses onset), date of the last menstrual period, presence of menstrual problems such as amenorrhea (primary or secondary), dysfunctional uterine bleeding and dysmenorrhea.
Female Athlete Triad–Highly Competitive Sports	1. Menstrual abnormality. 2. Disordered eating behaviors. 3. Osteopenia.
Sexual Abuse and Harassment	This may be present in a variety of ways including: • Salacious comments or suggestions. • Ridiculing of ability. • Written threats with or without lewd jokes, unsolicited attention, sexual bullying and others.

Box 7.2.1.2: Diet and weight control practices

Competitive athletes may use a variety of weight control and dietary methods in futile attempts to allow improved sports performance, especially in sports that have classification based on athlete's body weight.

These measures may not only fail to aid the athlete's performance but may be harmful as well.

Thus, it is important to ask about these practices which may include irregular nutrition intake, fad diets, ignoring overall nutrition, or symptoms of eating disorders.

It is also important to ask about recent changes in weight.

Box 7.2.1.3: Immunizations

Any time an adolescent is seen, one should ask about immunization status (see Chapter 7.1 Adolescent Immunization for more details).

Tetanus and Hepatitis B immunity are especially important in the context of sport participation where bleeding injuries take place.

The status of all other immunizations should be reviewed.

This will help to prevent and control a variety of outbreaks with vaccine preventable diseases, such as influenza, Hepatitis A and measles.

The physical fitness evaluation is sometimes the only time some adolescents see a primary care physician and thus, provision of immunizations is critical.

CLINICAL EXAMINATION

A thorough physical examination is part of the physical fitness evaluation with special focus on cardiovascular, neurologic, and musculoskeletal components. The physical examination of athletes is conducted in the same manner as any complete head-to-toe physical examination. Box 7.2.1.4 highlights the importance of evaluating the sexual maturity rating (SMR) or Tanner staging of an athlete (Refer to Section 2.1 for more details).

Box 7.2.1.4: The sexual maturity rating (SMR) or Tanner stage of an athlete

SMR of all adolescent athletes should be done to help identify those with delayed, normal, or precocious puberty.

It should be noted that athletes of the same weight but different SMR maturity are not of equal strength, since muscle is stronger than adipose tissue.

Thus, an individual with an SMR of 4 to 5 is typically stronger than the obese individual with an SMR of 2 to 3.

INVESTIGATIONS

There are no screening laboratory tests or imaging studies that are routinely recommended as part of the physical fitness evaluation. A careful medical history with focused physical examination determines if specific testing is needed for sports clearance or for evaluation of identified potential problems.

At the elite level of national and international participation, major sport governing bodies have lately endorsed the recommendation for obtaining a 12-lead electrocardiogram as part of cardiovascular screening of young athletes. Interpretation of ECGs in athletes should be done by those familiar with reading such ECGs so as to be able to appropriately discern normal exercise related changes from truly abnormal findings.

QUALIFYING ATHLETES FOR SPORT PARTICIPATION

The athlete should be matched with appropriate sport based on the athlete's preference for sport, any limitations found on fitness evaluation and the physical demands and nature of a given sport.

Based on the initial history and physical examination, a determination is made to either clear the athlete for unrestricted sport participation or limited participation or to restrict participation until further evaluation is done (Box 7.2.1.5).

Box 7.2.1.5: Appropriate matching of an adolescent athlete with a sport

This is influenced by multiple factors and a decision must be made on an individual basis.

Following questions may guide the decision to qualify athlete for sports:

1. What is the overall health status and fitness level of the athlete?
2. Is the desired activity a contact or non-contact sport?
3. What are the static or dynamic demands of the chosen sport?
4. What is the competition level of the athlete and his or her position?
5. What is the Sexual Maturity Rating or Tanner stage of the teen athlete?
6. Do the athlete and the parents/guardians understand the risks involved based on the desired sport and identified conditions of the athlete (e.g. epilepsy, diabetes mellitus, single kidney and single eye)?
7. Are the athlete and family willing to change the sport if necessary based on results of the physical fitness evaluation?
8. Does the athlete's medical condition, if any, place him or her or others at increased risk for injury or illness?
9. Is it possible to allow limited participation?
10. Is it possible to modify the rules and conduct of the sport to accommodate the special needs of the athlete?

Sport-related concussion deserve a special mention in the context of clearing adolescent athletes for participation because of long-term complications from repeated concussions. Although a detailed discussion is out of scope for this chapter the concussion guidelines have been widely disseminated and can be accessed from multiple online sources including the following: http://bjsm.bmj.com/content/47/5/250.full.pdf+html.

Only a brief summary of evaluation for physical fitness is presented in this chapter and all physicians who evaluate athletes for sport participation should be thoroughly familiar with current consensus guidelines presented in the Preparticipation Physical Evaluation Monograph (see full reference under "Suggested Reading").

LEARNING POINTS

- Fitness for sports participation evaluation provides and important opportunity for adolescent health assessment.
- History alone can identify 75% of potential concerns for fitness evaluation.
- Physical examination should particularly focus on cardiovascular, neurological and musculoskeletal systems.
- No routine laboratory investigations are indicated.
- An electrocardiogram is recommended by some guidelines and endorsed by some sports governing bodies.
- The qualifying process involves matching the adolescent athlete to appropriate sport.
- The primary objectives according to the preparticipation physical evaluation published by the American Academy of Pediatrics include identifying conditions that may be life-threatening, disabling, or predispose to injury or illness.

SUGGESTED READING

1. American Academy of Pediatrics. Preparticipation Physical Evaluation Monograph, 3rd edition, Elk Grove Village: American Academy of Pediatrics, 2012.
2. Maron BJ, Thompson PD, Ackerman MJ, Balady G, Berger S, Cohen D, *et al.* Recommendations and considerations related to pre-participation screening for cardiovascular abnormalities in competitive athletes: 2007 update: A scientific statement from the American Heart Association Council on Nutrition, Physical Activity, and Metabolism: Endorsed by the American College of Cardiology Foundation. American Heart Association Council on Nutrition, Physical Activity, and Metabolism. Circulation 2007;115(12):1643-55.
3. McCrory P, Meeuwisse WH, Aubry M, *et al.* Consensus statement on concussion in sport: The 4th International Conference on Concussion in Sport. British Journal of Sports Medicine 2013;47:250-58.
4. Patel DR, Luckstead EF. Update on cardiovascular screening: Can we prevent sudden cardiac death in adolescent athletes? Adolescent Medicine State of the Art Reviews 2013; 24(1):225-41.

Musculoskeletal Sports Injuries

7.2.2

Dilip R Patel, Sonia Joychan

INTRODUCTION

Unique features associated with adolescents should be considered when assessing musculoskeletal sports injuries. The differences between the mature and skeletally immature athlete influence sporting injuries seen in adolescents. Factors that should be taken into account include somatic growth, presence of growth cartilage, properties and characteristics of bone, and the mindset of the adolescent. The increased weight and load associated with growth spurts increase the risk and severity of injuries.

Growth cartilage is present at the epiphyseal plate, articular cartilage, and apophysis (insertion site of major tendons). Injuries to these areas are exclusive to the adolescent age group. The growth cartilage is particularly susceptible to overuse injuries, which can occur as a result of repetitive macro- or microtrauma. Overuse injuries are secondary to recurring musculoskeletal stress that is greater than the tissue can absorb. In addition, in skeletally immature athletes, ligaments and tendons tend to be stronger than bone. Thus, the risk of apophyseal tendon or bone avulsions is increased compared to ligamentous injuries.

Apart from the physical effects, the emotional impact of an injury should not be undermined. Pressure to continue playing may result in a delay in seeking medical attention, and negative emotions may further impact rehabilitation.

When treating an adolescent, it is important to remember that the size of the individual poorly correlates with skeletal maturity, and one should always maintain a high index of suspicion for injuries specific to the adolescent age group. Table 7.2.2.1 shows injuries commonly associated with the various sports.

HISTORY TAKING AND CLINICAL PRESENTATION

Shoulder Injuries

- Stress injury to proximal humeral epiphysis is common.
- Typical presentation is that of gradual onset of shoulder or proximal arm pain associated with throwing.
- There may be an associated increase in amount or intensity of throwing.
- The average duration of symptoms ranges from 7 to 8 months.
- Often, the symptoms are mild, lasting for several weeks to months, and there is pressure to continue to play, thus, there is a delay in seeking medical help.

Overuse Injury of the Elbow

- Most common presentation is with pain on the medial aspect of the elbow; some athletes also have forearm pain.
- The pain is aggravated by the throwing activity, and there is deterioration in performance. Initially, this pain resolves with rest but recurs with resumption of throwing.

Overuse Injury of the Wrist

- Gymnasts may present with recurrent or chronic wrist pain.
- The pain is aggravated by movements, especially stressing the wrist in dorsiflexion.
- Bilateral wrist pain has been reported in up to 30% of gymnasts.
- Associated discomfort and forearm pain are also common.
- In female gymnasts, floor exercises and vault are most often associated with wrist pain; whereas in male gymnasts, floor exercises and pommel horse are most often associated.
- There may be localized tenderness and prominence of the distal radius physis.

Ankle injury

- The history taking should include questions about the mechanism of injury, history of previous ankle injury and the degree of pain and swelling which has developed.
- It is helpful to ask about the foot position at the time of injury and whether the athlete can now bear weight.
- The athlete may have rolled or fell on a stretched ankle–often noted in soccer injuries.

Table 7.2.2.1: High risk sports and associated injuries

Injury	*Type of sports*	*Age*	*Comments*	*Etiology*
Shoulder: Proximal humeral physis stress injury	Baseball Cricket Gymnastics Racquet sports Swimming Volleyball	11-16 years, peak–14 years	Common during rapid growth. 80% in proximal humeral physis. Physis closes by 17 years (19-22 years).	Overhead throwing, subjects the physis to significant amount of stress, leading to microtrauma, throwing-related pain. Epiphysiolysis of the proximal humerus is classically described as the "little leaguer's shoulder", because of its original description in little league pitchers.
Elbow: Overuse injuries	Racquet sports–Tennis, Badminton Throwing sports–Pitcher in baseball, bowling in cricket Gymnastics	12 -15 years	Secondary ossification centers around elbow fuse between 14 and 17 years of age.	Subject the elbow to significant stress resulting in overuse injuries. During throwing there is stress to medial structures from stretching, and lateral and posterior structures from impaction.
Wrist: Stress injury to distal radial physis	High level competitive gymnastics	More common in female gymnasts, 12-14 years: 25-80%	Growth plate of the distal radius is particularly susceptible to stress injury. Closes by 15 years in girls and by 17 years in boys.	Wrist joint excessive, repetitive loading activity, especially in a dorsiflexed position. This may result in a number of injuries causing wrist pain.
Ankle sprains	American football Baseball Basketball Dance Gymnastics Hockey Rugby Running Soccer Volleyball	Older–Skeletally mature athlete 10-28%. In the skeletally immature athlete the ligaments are usually stronger than the bone.	*High risk factors:* Previous ankle injury with limited recovery, Limited flexibility of the Achilles tendon, Increased ligamentous laxity in general, and Possibly increased height and/or weight. Eversion (turning the joint out) and dorsiflexion (upward motion) of the foot can disrupt the deltoid ligament and also the syndesmotic ligament.	Inversion (turning the joint in or under) with plantar flexion (downward motion) of the foot, which leads to the sprain of the lateral ankle ligamentous group. Suddenly decelerating, landing from a jump, and/or suddenly changing direction. External rotation can lead to a "high" ankle sprain or disruption of the syndesmotic ligament–most severe type of sprain. Greater incidence of bone injury with disruption of the deltoid and the tibiofibular ligaments.

- Others state that it feels as though they stepped off a curb or stepped into a hole.

Worrisome History in Ankle Injuries

- Popping or snapping sensation or feeling at the time of injury.
- Rapid onset of swelling.
- Pain lasting more than 4 hours after injury.

CLINICAL EXAMINATION

Shoulder Joint: Stress Injury to Proximal Humeral Physis

- Tenderness over the lateral aspect of the proximal humerus is the most common finding on examination, and may be present in almost 70% of athletes.
- A few athletes may have weakness of external rotators of shoulder.
- Usually, the active and passive range of motions of shoulder is normal, until later in the course, when a relative decrease of internal rotation develops.
- While clinical examination is helpful, it is insufficient to provide a definite diagnosis. Imaging studies is needed to confirm suspicions.

Elbow Joint: Overuse Injuries

- There is generally no swelling or limitation of motion.
- Tenderness can be localized over the medial collateral ligament.

- Tenderness over the medial epicondyle.
- If the ulnar nerve is involved, there may be paresthesias in the ulnar nerve distribution.
- Ulnar nerve involvement will give positive Tinel sign.
- There may be tenderness along the ulnar nerve at elbow.

Ankle Joint: Ankle Sprains

- Being a hinge joint, the primary movements of the ankle include dorsiflexion (upward motion) and plantar flexion (downward motion).
- Eversion (outward motion) and inversion (inward motion) occur at the subtalar joint.
- Ligaments provide stability to the ankle.
- Examination should include evaluation for the pain, swelling, deformity and ecchymosis.
- The vascular integrity of the injured ankle should be assessed as well.
- There can be minimal swelling if ice was immediately applied.
- Ecchymosis is a common yet nonspecific and often delayed finding.
- It is helpful to locate the specific area of tenderness and which ligaments are involved.
- The anterior talofibular ligament is palpated 2 to 3 fingerbreadths anterior and slightly inferior to the lateral malleolus.
- The calcaneofibular ligament is palpated 1 to 2 fingerbreadths inferior to the lateral malleolus. However, significant ankle swelling makes this examination very difficult. The range of motion at the ankle joint (with and without resistance) is also important to evaluate (See Table 7.2.2.2 for details).

INVESTIGATIONS

Table 7.2.2.3 provides the details of the various diagnostic imaging procedures done for shoulder, elbow, wrist and ankle injuries. Box 7.2.2.1 provides the salient features of radiology of the wrist whereas Box 7.2.2.2 highlights those of ankle joint.

Table 7.2.2.2: Special tests for examination of ankle sprain

The anterior drawer test	Used to evaluate the integrity of the anterior talofibular ligament. With the foot in the neutral position, one hand is just above the ankle (holding the leg steady) while the other examiner's hand is around the heel, seeking to move the heel forward. Slight movement represents a +1, moderate movement +2, and marked movement is a +3. A positive sign is reflected by increase forward motion of the foot compared to the other foot.
Inversion stress test	Useful to assess sprain of the calcaneofibular ligament, with or without associated injury to the anterior talofibular ligament. With one hand over the lower leg just above the ankle, the examiner steadies the leg. With the other hand, the examiner turns the foot inwards (inversion). This is compared to the uninjured ankle. With sprain of the calcaneofibular ligament, there is increased pain and/or laxity depending upon the degree of tear.
The squeeze test	Used to assess for syndesmotic injury. The examiner places the hand 6 inches below the knee with thumbs on the fibula and fingers on the medial aspect of the tibia. Then he squeezes the tibia and fibula at the same time. If pain is produced, it suggests syndesmotic injury.

Table 7.2.2.3: Diagnostic imaging

Injury	*X-ray*	*Diagnostic findings*	*Other modalities*
Shoulder: Stress injury to proximal humeral physis	Shoulder in external and internal rotation, as well as anteroposterior (AP) and lateral views should be obtained. Comparison views of the opposite shoulder should also be obtained	Widening of the proximal physis Physis fragmentation Calcification of physis Sclerosis of physis Demineralization of physis	MRI is indicated if tear of tendons is suspected or injury to the glenoid labrum is suspected
Elbow: Overuse injuries	Normal in early stages	Untreated late conditions–Hypertrophy and fragmentation of the medial condylar apophysis and widening of the space between the apophysis and the metaphysis of the humerus	MRI is needed in some cases to confirm diagnosis. MRI is also useful in staging osteochondritis dissecans of capitellum.
Wrist: Stress injury to distal radial physis	AP and lateral views Normal in early cases	Widening of the distal radial physis Beaking of the physis Cystic changes in the metaphysis Indistinct appearance of the physis	MRI is needed in some cases which shows damage to the physis and to the distal bony metaphysis as well. MRI is useful in confirming tear of triangular fibrocartilage complex.
Ankle: Sprains and fractures	AP, lateral and mortise views	To rule out growth plate injuries and fractures. X-ray in eversion sprains to assess syndesmotic injury	CT scans for evaluation of possible occult fractures and further assessment of intra-articular fractures noted on radiographs

Box 7.2.2.1: Radiology of the wrist
Ulnar variance on the AP view of the wrist refers to the length of the distal ulna relative to that of the distal radius.
In positive ulnar variance, the length of the distal ulna exceeds that of the distal radius by 1 mm or more.
The opposite is true of negative ulnar variance.
Normally, ulnar variance is negative before skeletal maturity, when it is generally neutral.
In mature gymnasts, a higher prevalence of positive ulnar variance has been reported, attributed to various factors such as overgrowth of the distal ulnar physis, growth arrest of the distal radial physis, or genetic predisposition.

Box 7.2.2.2: Radiology of the ankle
Stress films are not recommended by most experts when dealing with acute ankle injuries in teenagers.
Some experts suggest stress films are helpful for chronic ankle instability and before surgical repair of ligaments.
A foot series is recommended for an inability to bear weight and/or pain over the mid-foot (anterior process of the calcaneus, base of the fifth metatarsal, navicular, cuboid, cuneiforms).

The Ottawa Rules and Recommendations for Ankle X-rays

- Pain in the area of the malleoli.
- Inability to bear weight right after the injury.
- Unable to take 4 steps while being examined.
- Other localized bony tenderness.

MANAGEMENT

After initial evaluation in the primary care setting, appropriate orthopedic consultation should be sought for proper management of these injuries.

Knee injuries are often seen in active athletes (see Tables 7.2.2.4 and 7.2.2.5). Box 7.2.2.3 discusses ankle sprains whereas Box 7.2.2.4 details the evaluation of sacroiliac joint pain.

BACK PAIN IN ADOLESCENTS

Pain in the back can be seen in adolescents due to a variety of causes including sports injuries and adolescent specific diseases like Scheuermann disease. Back pain also can be referred pain from a variety of lesions (Tables 7.2.2.6 and 7.2.2.7). Some common conditions are discussed in Table 7.2.2.8.

HISTORY TAKING AND CLINICAL PRESENTATION OF BACK PAIN

Scheuermann Disease (Juvenile Disk Disease)

- Chronic or recurrent thoracic back pain, present

Table 7.2.2.4: Knee problems commonly seen in adolescents
Juvenile Osteochondritis Dissecans (JOCD)
Significant cause of knee pain in both athletes and non-athletes.
10-15 years age, highly active athlete, more in females; 10-20% bilateral.
Lateral aspect of the medial condyle of the femur is the most common site.
Closed or open and either stable or unstable.
Delamination and localized necrosis of the subchondral bone, with or without the involvement of the overlying articular cartilage.
Etiology: Repetitive microtrauma, local bone vascular insufficiency, abnormal ossification, inflammation and genetic predisposition.
Can be incidental radiographic finding or come with symptoms.
Aching and gradual onset of knee pain of several days to weeks' duration typically located over anterior knee, worse during activity; intermittent knee swelling following a practice or game session; locking or catching of the knee.
Examination: May have mild effusion or limitation of motion of the knee.
Early stages with the articular cartilage over the femoral condyle still intact–signs are nonspecific.
Late stages–articular cartilage eroded; fragment may separate and become an intra-articular loose body; tenderness, effusion and locking.
Diagnostic Imaging: X-ray AP lateral and tunnel views–well-demarcated radiolucent area.
MRI indicated if there is significant edema, hemarthrosis and marked discomfort and inability to bear weight without pain. Also useful in determining the stability of the lesion, and to monitor healing post therapy.
Non-surgical treatment: Stable lesions with open physis–Spontaneous healing often seen. Restriction of activities and symptomatic treatment of pain. Immobilization–divided opinion.
Lower rates of healing–closed or closing physis.
Full sport participation can be resumed once the athlete is pain free and there is healing seen on X-ray.
Prognosis is excellent in younger patients.
Surgical intervention: Unstable/advanced lesion, patients approaching skeletal maturity.
Weight bearing and activity modifications are continued in all cases until imaging and clinical confirmation of healing has occurred and the athlete is completely asymptomatic.

Table 7.2.2.5: Idiopathic anterior knee pain (AKP) or patellofemoral pain in young athletes
The diagnosis of idiopathic anterior knee pain is made after excluding all other known causes of knee pain.
Intense physical activity overloading the patellofemoral mechanism in young active athletes; more common in females. Several weeks of pain and severity can affect the sports performance.
The pain is nonspecific, poorly localized.
Typically gradual in onset, unilateral or bilateral.
Associated with a history of recent increase in physical activity.
Aggravated after prolonged sitting, going up and coming downstairs, and squatting. Sensations of the knee catching, locking or giving away.
Swelling is not a typical finding and its presence should prompt a search for specific underlying cause.
Examination: Decreased flexibility of the hamstrings and quadriceps. With palm of the hand over the patella, a crepitus may be felt with movement of the knee in flexion and extension. Pain may also be elicited or exacerbated when the quadriceps is contracted and the examiner holds the patella down preventing its upward movement. Tenderness may be elicited by palpating and exerting pressure on the articular margins of the patella while displacing it medially or laterally.
Also examine for presence of gait abnormality, increased lumbar lordosis, asymmetry of hips or lower extremities, hyperpronated feet, and atrophy and weakness of the quadriceps muscles by comparing to the normal side to rule out other pathological causes.
X-rays if signs and symptoms not consistent with AKP. AP standing, true lateral and a patella axial view in low flexion. Abnormal tilt of the patella may be associated with maltracking.
In most cases X-rays are normal.
Conservative treatment: Rest local ice, short-term avoid prolonged sitting, squatting, climbing up or going down stairs, and full arc knee extension exercises. Cycling and swimming recommended.
AKP is a benign self-limiting condition that resolves over few months–2 years. Complete rest and immobilization not recommended; continue sports.

Box 7.2.2.3: Indications for orthopedic consult: Ankle sprains

- Athletes with medial ligament or syndesmotic injuries
- Associated injuries, especially when a fracture is suspected

If the athlete with an uncomplicated lateral ankle sprain is not improved within two weeks of the PRICE treatment

Box 7.2.2.4: Sacroiliac joint (SIJ) pain

SIJ is a diarthrodial joint with minimal movements in the transverse or longitudinal planes not exceeding 2 to 3 degrees.

Affected in rowing and cross-country skiing.

Clinical presentation: Pain may be in the lower back, buttocks, posterior thighs, or pelvis.

Tenderness may be localized over the SIJ, and pain may be elicited or exacerbated with some provocative movements of hip and SI joint.

The diagnosis is based primarily on history and examination findings.

Imaging studies may be indicated to exclude other causes of pain.

Plain radiographs are initial study of choice in most cases.

Treatment: Chronic pain may be difficult to treat. In addition to relative rest, modification of activities, and use of pain medications as needed.

Various other treatment modalities: Manual or manipulative treatment, prolotherapy, intra-articular injections of local anesthetics and corticosteroids, and radiofrequency neurotomy.

Significant chronic pain should be referred to experts with experience in treating SIJ pain and dysfunction.

Table 7.2.2.6: Intrinsic causes of back pain in adolescents	
Acute pain	Acute fractures of the thoracolumbar spine Acute musculotendinous strains and sprains Acute pain Acute spondylolysis Disk herniation Muscle contusions
Chronic/insidious or recurrent pain	Benign and malignant tumors of the spine or cord Diskitis and vertebral osteomyelitis Facet joint syndrome Hypermobility syndrome Idiopathic juvenile osteoporosis Lumbar spondylolysis and spondylolisthesis Lumbarization or sacralization Postural Psychosomatic Sacroiliac joint pain Scheuermann disease Spine bifida occulta

Table 7.2.2.7: Extrinsic causes of back pain in adolescents	
Referred pain	Abdominal or pelvic neoplasms Acute appendicitis Pancreatitis Pyelonephritis Renal stones Urinary tract infection Pelvic inflammatory disease Pelvis osteomyelitis with or without abscess
Systemic disease	Leukemia Inflammatory bowel disease Spondyloarthropathy Ankylosing spondylitis Rheumatoid arthritis Metabolic diseases Neuromuscular disease Myopathy

Table 7.2.2.8: Some common conditions

Disease	*Characteristics*
Thoracic Scheuermann disease (juvenile disk disease) Males >females 10-15 years 4-10%	Most common cause of back pain fixed kyphotic deformity of the spine >45°. The normal range of thoracic spine curvature in the sagittal plane 20-40°.
Lumbar spondylolysis Common sports injury 50% Mean age 15 to 16 years	Stress fracture of the pars interarticularis (isthmic type). Most lesions bilateral (80%) and affect L5 (95%). A higher incidence is seen in ballet dancers, gymnasts, competitive cheerleaders, football linemen, weight lifters, wrestlers, divers, volleyball players and fast bowlers in cricket. Repetitive axial loading and rotation, especially in an extended lumbar spine, is the most important contributing mechanism leading to fatigue fracture of the pars interarticularis.
Spondylolisthesis Isthmic spondylolisthesis is the most common type seen in adolescent athletes	Anterior slippage of a vertebra over the one just below it, most commonly L5 over S1. Common complication of bilateral spondylolytic lesions.
Disk herniation Male : Female equal Not very common	Most commonly affected levels are L4-L5 and L5-S1. Weight lifting, gymnastics, wrestling, and collision sports are high-risk sports for disk herniation.

for several weeks to months before progressive kyphosis develops. Occasionally, the pain is of sudden onset.

- Some may present only with poor posture and kyphotic deformity. Most have pain located between the scapulae that is aggravated by physical activity, prolonged sitting, standing and forward flexion.
- Pain tends to diminish as the adolescent approaches skeletal maturity.
- The severity of pain and progressive worsening of the kyphosis have poor correlation.

Adolescent Idiopathic Scoliosis (AIS)

- Adolescent idiopathic scoliosis can be asymptomatic.
- Pain and deformity may become apparent with larger curves and with progression of the curve.

Spondylolysis

- Many are asymptomatic and may or may not progress to symptomatic lesions.
- Insidious onset, recurrent, activity-associated, low back pain.

- Sudden onset pain has also been reported in competitive cheerleaders and gymnasts with acute spondylolysis. The pain is localized to the lower back, nonradiating, and dull aching to sharp. Pain is also reported in the buttocks and posterior thighs.
- Generally, patients do not have any neurological symptoms or signs.
- Decreased flexibility of the hamstrings and lumbodorsal muscles and fascia is seen in may be the only and/or initial presenting sign.
- Increased lumbar lordosis and a relative weakness of the abdominal muscles are also common findings.
- Lower back pain can be reproduced or exacerbated by one-leg hyperextension movement of the lumbosacral spine.

Spondylolisthesis

- Gradual onset, aching pain in the lower back, buttocks, or posterior thighs.
- The pain is aggravated with physical activity, especially those involving repeated flexion, extension, and rotation. In some cases, spondylolisthesis is asymptomatic.
- Patient often assumes a characteristic posture while standing or walking with increased hip and knee flexion or crouched posture (known as the Phalen-Dickson sign).

Disc Herniation

- Sudden onset pain related to a particular activity.
- They may also present with insidious onset, intermittent activity-related pain of several weeks to months duration.
- A clear history of acute trauma is elicited in only 40%–50% of patients.
- Sports-related presentations can be secondary to either acute or overuse injury.
- The most common presenting symptoms are back and leg pain and stiffness that are exacerbated by activity.
- The pain may or may not radiate to the legs.

CLINICAL EXAMINATION

Scheuermann Disease (Juvenile Disk Disease)

- Kyphotic deformity is evident in the forward-bending position (Adam's test; see details under AIS).
- In addition to kyphosis of the thoracic spine, patients also have decreased flexibility of the hamstrings and exacerbated lumbar lordosis.
- The kyphosis should be differentiated from adolescent postural round back that disappears when the athlete hyperextends the back while prone.

Adolescent Idiopathic Scoliosis (AIS)

- The spine should be examined at all preventive visits during the adolescent years, typically once a year.
- Measure leg length (from the anterior superior iliac spine to the medial malleolus) to rule out leg length inequality.
- The Adam's test is a useful screening and diagnostic maneuver to identify scoliosis and kyphosis. Have the standing patient bend forward as far as he or she can, with both upper extremities extended and palms held together hanging down. The examiner should inspect for asymmetry of the spine. The presence of a thoracic hump in this position indicates scoliosis. Lateral observation of the patient in the forward bend position should also be performed, assessing for kyphosis.
- It is important to determine the sexual maturity rating of the patient. Curve progression is a function of gender, remaining skeletal maturity at the time of diagnosis, and the magnitude of the curve at the time of diagnosis.

Spondylolisthesis

- On examination, there is hamstring tightness (80% of patients) and exacerbated lumbar lordosis, and a step-off over the lumbar spine may be palpated.
- Lumbar radicular symptoms are rare but may be present in high-grade spondylolisthesis. Lower limb strength, sensation, and reflexes should be tested.

Disk Herniation

- Generally, neurological signs are absent in most children and adolescents.
- Pain is also exacerbated by coughing, sneezing, or sitting.
- In some athletes, lumbar radicular signs may be elicited.
- Most patients have limitation of lumbosacral spine movement, and mild scoliosis may be detected in some patients.
- A positive straight leg raise test is the most common finding and is present in almost all patients.

- Hamstring tightness is common and may be an early sign of disk herniation.

Once history taking and clinical examination is done one must decide on further management (Table 7.2.2.9).

INVESTIGATIONS

X-rays should reveal the diagnosis and monitoring in most of the cases. In cases where X-rays are normal MRI should be done to get more detailed views or diagnosis (Table 7.2.2.10).

MANAGEMENT

After initial evaluation in the primary care setting, sports medicine or orthopedic consultation should be sought for further management.

LEARNING POINTS

- Somatic growth, presence of growth cartilage, properties and characteristics of bone, and emotional factors influence the type of sports-related injuries that adolescents are susceptible to.
- Adolescents are more likely to be treated for overuse injuries than younger children.
- Early recognition and treatment of overuse injuries are necessary to prevent further complications.
- Collaboration with parents, the adolescent, and the coach to avoid overuse injuries is the best form of prevention.

Acknowledgement

Authors acknowledge Dr Meveshni Govender, MD, Instructor in the Department of Pediatric and Adolescent

Table 7.2.2.9: Approach to back pain

When to consider underlying significant cause:	*When to seek orthopedic surgical consultation:*
Associated neurological signs	Acute back pain with neurological symptoms and signs
Associated systemic symptoms and signs	Acute disk herniation with neurological signs
Continuous or constant pain	Apophyseal fractures
Pain at rest	Diskitis and osteomyelitis
Pain lasting 2 or more months	Fractures of thoracolumbar spine
Pain that wakes the patient up from sleep	High-grade spondylolisthesis
Severe progressive pain	Scheuermann kyphosis
	Scoliosis of 20 degree or more in during peak growth
	Significant scoliosis, progressive curve, atypical scoliosis
	Spondylolysis not responding to conservative treatment
	Tumors of spine and cord

Table 7.2.2.10: Diagnostic imaging for back pain

Lumbar spondylolysis	*Scheuermann disease*	*Idiopathic scoliosis*	*Spondylolisthesis*	*Disk herniation*
X-ray AP and lateral and oblique view of LS spine: In the oblique view the stress fracture is seen as "Scotty dog" with a collar appearance. It may take 1-2 weeks to develop. Associated congenital anomalies e.g. spina bifida occulta, and spondylolisthesis. *MRI:* Early or acute lesions, delineating the anatomic nature of the pars defect, and detecting any spinal or soft tissue pathology.	*X-ray:* Vertebral endplate irregularities. Narrowing of the intervertebral disk space. Anterior wedging and decreased height of the vertebrae. Schmorl nodes (protrusion of nucleus pulposus into the vertebral body anteriorly). The apex of the kyphotic deformity is usually located at the level of T7-T8.	*X-ray:* Cobb method is used to measure the curvature; lateral curvature of the spine > 10°. Periodic radiographic evaluation is indicated based on the initial degree and risk of progression of the scoliosis.	*X-ray Lateral LS spine:* The severity of lesion is graded I to IV, based on radiographic findings of percentage of slippage of the superior vertebra over the inferior. *MRI:* If neurological symptoms or signs; to evaluate for other causes such as disk herniation in conjunction with spondylolisthesis.	*X-ray* may appear to be normal. *MRI* is the study of choice to detect disk herniation and any neurological compromise. It must be correlated with clinical findings because many individuals have abnormalities on MRI that are of no clinical significance.

Medicine, Western Michigan University Homer Stryker MD School of Medicine for her valuable contributions to this chapter.

SUGGESTED READING

1. Crowther M. Elbow pain in pediatrics. Curr Rev Musculoskelet Med 2009;2:83-87.
2. Gorman McNerney ML, Arendt EA. Anterior knee pain in the active and athletic adolescent. Curr Sports Med Rep 2013;12:404-10.
3. Gurd DP. Back pain in the young athlete. Sports Med Arthrosc 2011;19(1):7-16.
4. Kerssemakers SP, Fotiadou AN, de Jonge MC, Karantanas AH, Maas M. Sport injuries in the paediatric and adolescent patient: A growing problem. Pediatr Radiol 2009;39:471-84.
5. Mariscalco MW, Saluan P. Upper extremity injuries in the adolescent athlete. Sports Med Arthrosc 2011;19:17-26.
6. Patel DR, Baker RJ. Musculoskeletal Injuries in Sports. Prim Care Clin Off Pract 2006;33:545-79.
7. Patel DR, Greydanus DE, Baker RJ, eds. Pediatric Practice: Sports Medicine. New York: McGraw Hill Medical, 2009.
8. Sciascia A, Kibler WB. The pediatric overhead athlete: What is the real problem? Clin J Sport Med 2006;16:471-77.
9. Shanley E, Thigpen C. Throwing injuries in the adolescent athlete. Int. J. Sports Phys Ther 2013;8, 630-40.
10. Stracciolini A, Casciano R, Levey Friedman H, Meehan WP, Michel LJ. Pediatric sports injuries: An age comparison of children versus adolescents. Am J Sports Med 2012;41: 1922-29.

Environmental Issues

7.3

Ruth A Etzel, Swati Y Bhave

INTRODUCTION

During much of the 20th century, when it was routine for doctors to make house calls, doctors could observe the home environment of a child or adolescent. Making house calls is no longer part of standard practice. Today's physicians, therefore, must ask questions to find out about the home environment and other places where the adolescent lives or spends leisure time. Questions about these environments are basic to a comprehensive health history. The answers can help physicians to understand an adolescent's physical surroundings and to offer appropriate guidance to prevent some and mitigate other possibly hazardous exposures. Questions can be incorporated into adolescent health supervision visits and visits for illnesses with known environmental causes. Questions about the environment also are appropriate when symptoms are unusual, persistent, or when multiple people in the home (or school) have similar symptoms.

Keeping these caveats in mind, this chapter reviews important areas in an adolescent's environmental history and provides advice that may prevent or mitigate exposures. Because there are many items in the complete history, it is unlikely that busy practitioners will have the time to ask about everything. At minimum, it seems prudent to suggest that physicians inquire about the age and condition of the home, second hand smoke exposure, exposure to ultraviolet radiation, and the adolescent's occupation. Other questions may be asked depending on the situations of individual patients taking into account factors, such as socioeconomic status, geographic location, and known hazards in the community (Box 7.3.1).

Box 7.3.1: Health supervision visits

When a clinician suspects an adolescent is having symptoms related to environmental factors, it is ideal to have a health supervision visit to see his/her home and surroundings. However this is neither practical nor feasible in most cases. Time constraints are also a common challenge for all practitioners.

Hence we must learn to take a detailed environmental history in our clinics. Environmental health history screening forms have been developed to facilitate the history-taking process.

The following are basic areas of questioning about the adolescent's environment:

1. Physical surroundings.
2. Tobacco smoke exposure and tobacco use by adolescents and household members.
3. Water sources.
4. Sun and other exposure to ultraviolet radiation (UVR).
5. Exposures resulting from adolescent jobs and hobby activities.

HISTORY TAKING

Presenting Symptoms

Presenting symptoms of environmental related illness can be non-specific. That is why it is important to consider environmental etiologies in the differential diagnosis.

- Diarrhea may be caused by exposure to pesticides, arsenic, or infectious agents.
- Wheezing and coughing may result from exposure to second hand tobacco smoke. It is the most common toxicant associated with respiratory diseases such as asthma and recurrent lower and upper airway disease.
- Recurrent abdominal pain, constipation, irritability, developmental delay, seizures, or unexplained coma may result from lead poisoning.
- Headaches may be caused by acute and chronic exposure to carbon monoxide (CO) from improperly vented heating sources, formaldehyde, or chemicals used on the job.

It is important to take a detailed history because environmental causes of illness may not always be apparent (Box 7.3.2).

Environmental History

A detailed environmental history may give clues to the diagnosis. It is possible that the presenting symptoms can be linked to environmental factors (Tables 7.3.1 to 7.3.5 and Boxes 7.3.3 to 7.3.6).

Box 7.3.2: Environmental causes of illness may not always be apparent

Because most environmental illnesses present as common medical problems or have nonspecific symptoms, the diagnosis may be missed unless a history of exposure is obtained. This is especially important if the illness is atypical or unresponsive to treatment.

The following questions may provide information about whether an illness is related to the environment:

- Do symptoms subside or worsen in a particular location (e.g. home, school, or certain room)?
- Do symptoms subside or worsen during a particular time? At a particular time of day? On weekdays or weekends? During a particular week or season?
- Do symptoms worsen during a particular activity? While the adolescent is outside, or engaging in hobby activities, such as working with arts and crafts?
- Are siblings or other adolescents experiencing similar symptoms?
- What are parents' thoughts about why symptoms are occurring?

Table 7.3.1: Environmental history taking

PHYSICAL SURROUNDINGS	
At home	*Questions to ask*
Adolescents spend much of their time indoors—in their own home or in relatives' or friends' homes. These spaces may contain environmental hazards.	• Is it a house, apartment, or temporary shelter? • What are the age and condition of the home? Is it damp or visibly moldy? • What type of heating/air system does the home have? • Where and how are chemicals and pesticides stored?
Building environments Adolescents may live in or spend a lot of time in other buildings. Depending on the type of structure, different risks will be likely.	• What type of building environments does the adolescent live in or spend time in? • What are the age and condition of the buildings? • Are they dusty or damp? • Does the environment smell musty or moldy?
Heating air system at home Wood stoves emit respiratory irritants (nitrogen dioxide [NO_2], respirable particulates, and polycyclic aromatic hydrocarbons), especially when they are not properly vented and maintained. Wood stoves and other fuel-burning appliances may be sources of carbon monoxide (CO).	• What fuel do you use at home? • Do you use biogas? • Do you use wood stoves? • If yes, are they properly vented and maintained? • Are your AC units regularly cleaned and serviced?
Tobacco exposure Exposure to second hand smoke (SHS) places adolescents at risk of significant morbidity. Physicians should discuss the hazards of tobacco use with teenagers. Even if they are not using tobacco, teenagers should be asked about SHS exposure, because they may be exposed by family or friends who smoke.	• Do any of your friends smoke? • Do any of your family members smoke? • Are you often exposed to SHS? • Are you aware of hazards of SHS? • Do other family members of your household use tobacco? • Is the home smoke free? • Do you use tobacco, or other chewable products? • Do you go to hookah bars? Do you smoke or use electronic cigarettes? • Are you aware of all the hazards of smoking? • Are you interested in quitting?
Pesticides and other chemicals These can cause acute poisoning and death as well as subacute and chronic poisoning.	• Are pesticides applied to the home or garden? • Where are these stored? • Are they kept safely out of reach? • Are they kept in the original containers? • If stored in other containers, are they labeled as dangerous? • Are they kept in containers that previously contained edible items like sugary drinks?
Exposure to sun and Ultraviolet (UV) rays	• How many hours a day are you exposed to sun and UV rays? • Do you take any precautions to protect yourself?
Jobs and hobbies can expose to hazards	• Do you have a job? • What is your work environment like? • What are your hobbies?

Table 7.3.2: Environmental history taking	
AT SCHOOL	
At school	*Questions to ask*
Adolescents spend one-third of their day in school. Many hazards found in school environments are similar to those in homes. Adolescents with certain disabilities may be at more risk for toxic exposures. Visually impaired adolescents working close to a project or adolescents with asthma may be affected by fumes.	• What are the age and condition of the school? • Do you have any disabilities or are you specially challenged?
Arts and Crafts Felt-tip markers (containing aromatic hydrocarbons) and oil-based paints present hazards. Emotionally disturbed adolescents may abuse art materials, endangering themselves and others.	• What arts and crafts activities do you take part in? • What material do you use or handle? • Do you follow safety precautions while dealing with hazardous material in school?

Table 7.3.3: Environmental history taking	
IN THE COMMUNITY	
Issues	*Questions*
Toxic hazards may exist in the community. Sources of exposure include polluted lakes and streams, industrial plants, and uncontrolled hazardous waste sites, such as waste storage and treatment facilities, landfills, former industrial sites, military facilities, waste recycling facilities, and unsanctioned waste water discharge. Low-income communities and ethnic minority communities are more likely to face toxic hazards.	• Is there a source of pollution in your community? • Do you live downwind from a lead smelter or any lead associated factories or workshops? • Are you living on or near agricultural land where they use pesticides? • Are you living near e-waste recycling and have a chance of exposure to lead and cadmium?
Water Sources	• Do you use tap water? Well water? • Do you use any purifier or filtration at home for drinking water? • What about at school? • Are you careful about the water you drink?

Table 7.3.4: Examples of adolescent job-related exposures
• Blood-borne pathogens in clinics/hospitals
• Cleaning agents in restaurants and schools
• Pesticides in agricultural work, and when buildings are sprayed
• Isocyanates (pulmonary sensitizers) during auto body repair or roofing with newer forms of roofing materials
• Benzene when pumping petrol
• Lead from radiators in auto body repair and from paint. Also from backyard cottage industries (e.g. battery recycling)
• Asbestos in auto brake repair, renovation/demolition of old buildings
• Solvents in T-shirt screening
• Second hand smoke in restaurant jobs
• Heat in dishwashing and outdoor work in the summer or in hot climates
• Asthma-exacerbating wood dusts in shop and furniture making
• Welding fumes resulting in eye exposures
• Cosmetology chemicals and dyes
• Tetanus and other biological/infectious hazards in farming (hypersensitivity pneumonitis) and veterinary clinics
• Noise from operating equipment. Noise-induced hearing loss in agriculture and factory work
• Nicotine in harvest of tobacco (green tobacco sickness)
• Workplace contaminants may be transported to the home on clothes, shoes and skin surfaces
• Pesticides from agricultural work

(Table adapted from *Pediatric Environmental Health*, 3rd Edition. Etzel, RA (Editor). Elk Grove Village, IL: American Academy of Pediatrics, 2012)

Table 7.3.5: Recommendations to parents for prevention of environment related illness

Issues	*Recommendations*
Heating systems	• Properly maintain and clean heating systems. • Discourage use of wood-burning appliances when children have asthma or other chronic respiratory conditions.
Pest control Integrated pest management (IPM). This is an approach that integrates chemical and nonchemical methods to provide the least toxic alternative for pest controls. IPM uses regular monitoring (rather than predetermined chemical applications) to determine whether and when treatments are needed.	• Encourage families to use the least toxic options for pest control. • If chemicals are used, store them in original labeled containers and never in containers such as soft drink or juice bottles.
Tobacco exposure	• Ask about smoking at every clinical encounter and offer smokers at least a brief (1- to 3-minute) intervention at each visit. • Advise parents to quit and offer help in doing so. • Educate parents about the associations between SHS and an adolescent's illness may help them to quit. • Inform them that an adolescent is more likely to begin smoking if parents smoke. • Whether or not parents choose to quit, advise them to introduce and enforce strict no-smoking bans in the home.
Parental home occupation Adolescent's job details. An occupational history may be obtained when information about family composition and the family history is obtained.	• At home, do not allow adolescents in rooms where parents work with toxic matter. • Advise adolescents who work with toxic substances to shower, if possible, and change clothes and shoes before leaving work.
Sun and other exposure to ultraviolet radiation (UVR) About one quarter of a person's exposure to the sun occurs before 18 years of age. Early exposure to UVR increases skin cancer risk.	• Advise parents and adolescents to cover up with clothing and hats. • Time adolescents' activities to avoid peak sun exposure. • Use sunscreen and reapply frequently and wear sunglasses.

Box 7.3.3: Exposure–Hobbies and recreation

- Hobby activity may pose a risk to adolescents.
- Adolescents may be especially at risk of huffing (inhaling) if glue is present in their environments, resulting in easy access.
- Art materials contain toxicants such as lead used in solder, pottery glazes, or stained glass.
- Environmental exposures include UV radiation with outdoor play without using adequate protection.
- Second hand smoke may be found in restaurants and bars.

Box 7.3.4: Specialized concept of environmental history–GREEN PAGE

The Green Page is an example of an environmental history.

The Green Page has about 50 fields for recording information about the adolescent, the built and ambient environments, the characteristics of the community and other data.

The environmental history is both a tool (set of questions) and an opportunity for interaction.

Green Page – A tool for:

- Identifying and assessing adolescents' exposure to environmental threats in the different places where they spend time: home, school, playground or even the work place or small cottage industry;
- Responding with the right therapeutic and preventive measures–as only a good knowledge of potential sources of exposure will guide an appropriate medical diagnosis and treatment; and
- An opportunity for interaction with the adolescent and his/her family, and with others.

The environmental history may motivate:

- Enquiring of colleagues about similar cases or observations;
- Contacting professionals who may have information on the situation observed; and
- Informing the responsible authorities about situations observed.

(Table from World Health Organization. http://www.who.int/ceh/capacity/paedenvhistory/en/)

Box 7.3.5: Mold and dampness

- Homes that have flooded or that have leaky plumbing or roofs may have mold growth.
- A damp or musty smell indicates the presence of mold.
- Ineffective and unused ventilation contributes to mold or dampness.
- Mold can cause allergies; it can cause asthma and trigger asthma attacks.

Recommendations:

- Water leaks and other sources of water intrusion should be repaired, and all reservoirs of mold should be removed.
- Mold present on hard surfaces can be wiped clean.
- Dry cleaning may be attempted for visible mold growth on clothing.
- Permeable and semi-permeable materials, such as upholstered furniture and carpeting, should be discarded if there is mold growth.
- Mold is ubiquitous, and the expectation of creating an entirely "mold-free" environment is unrealistic.
- However, a healthy environment is dry and free of visible mold growth.

Box 7.3.6: Arsenic exposure

Arsenic is naturally high in water in some areas of the world, including West Bengal, India.

In addition to its natural presence in water, arsenic is also produced by a variety of activities, such as smelting and coal burning.

After 20 or more years of exposure to high arsenic levels in drinking water, arsenic causes bladder, kidney, lung and skin cancers.

Neurologic effects, cardiovascular and pulmonary diseases, skin lesions and diabetes are also associated with arsenic exposure from drinking water.

See Table 7.3.4 for examples of job-related exposures.

The environmental history is not a new idea. But in view of the recent research that has given better insight into the effect of environmental risk, and greater awareness of these issues, the questions in history taking are more specific and detailed so that the recording is done in a more systemic manner. The World Health Organization (WHO) has come up with the concept of a "Green Page" for clinicians to take the environmental history. The data collection form is green, to make it clearly visible within the clinical records (which are still kept in paper form in most primary health care centers). This format is being tested by WHO with selected health care providers (Box 7.3.4).

CLINICAL EXAMINATION

Once aware of the environment of the adolescent, the physician will be in a better position to correlate the symptoms of the patient with environmental factors.

It is not possible to review all the symptoms of environmental illness in this short chapter. But some common ones are listed below.

Lead poisoning: The symptoms may include headaches, recurrent abdominal pain, and loss of appetite, constipation, clumsiness, irritability, developmental delay, vomiting, seizures, or unexplained coma.

Allergy and asthma: Symptoms of asthma include cough and wheeze and exercise limitation. Asthma symptoms may be accompanied by evidence of atopy.

Nose bleeds or hemoptysis should prompt an investigation for mold in the home (Box 7.3.5).

Arsenic poisoning: Symptoms of chronic arsenic poisoning can include generalized fatigue and malaise. Skin changes include eczematoid eruptions, hyperkeratosis, and dyspigmentation. Alopecia may also occur (Box 7.3.6).

CLINICAL INVESTIGATIONS

Investigations for Some Common Problems are Listed Below:

- Adolescents who are working with lead (for example, in battery recycling) should have a blood lead test.
- If exposure to arsenic is a concern, urine arsenic should be measured because the half-life of arsenic in blood is short. The diagnostic test of choice is estimation of arsenic in a 24-hour urine collection.
- When the substance itself cannot be measured, end-organ effects of exposure may be measured (e.g. hepatocellular enzymes following solvent exposure).

MANAGEMENT

Management should be focused on educating the parents and adolescent to remove the sources of exposure in their environment. For adolescents who present with allergy and respiratory symptoms the management is to avoid the exposure to respiratory allergens or irritants, e.g. keep the home free of second hand tobacco smoke and remove sources of dampness and molds from the home and places where the adolescent spends a lot of time.

If levels of lead in the adolescent's blood are confirmed to be higher than 45 µg/dl, chelation therapy may be indicated. If diagnosis of arsenic poisoning is made following a 24-hour urine collection, chelation therapy may be indicated. Chelation therapy should be undertaken only in consultation with a toxicologist.

Parent education is extremely important for prevention of environmental illnesses in children and adolescents (Table 7.3.5).

When giving recommendations to parents it is important to keep in mind that families may face important challenges in modifying their home environments.

- For example, families may not know the age of the home or may be unable to answer questions about possible home exposures.
- When offering advice, physicians should recognize that recommendations may be difficult or impossible to implement because of factors such as cost or lack of influence on a landlord.
- There may be discomfort with "raising a fuss" as in delicate situations when a wife is advised to ask a husband to stop smoking inside the home.
- Additionally, recommendations may not be followed, because families' cultural beliefs and practices may differ from those of the physician.

LEARNING POINTS

- Environmental factors can lead to a variety of health problems.
- The symptoms can mimic other diseases.
- A detailed environmental history will give clue to the diagnosis and prevent the physician from missing the opportunity to prevent environmental disease.

SUGGESTED READING

1. American Academy of Pediatrics Council on Environmental Health. Pediatric Environmental Health, 3rd Edition. Etzel, RA (Editor). Elk Grove Village, IL: American Academy of Pediatrics, 2012.
2. Agency for Toxic Substances and Disease Registry, Case Studies in Environmental Medicine http://www.atsdr.cdc.gov/csem/exphistory/ehcover_page.html http://www.atsdr.cdc.gov/HEC/CSEM/pediatric/docs/pediatric.pdf
3. Balk SJ, Forman JA, Johnson CL, Roberts JR. Safeguarding kids from environmental hazards. Contemp Pediatr 2007; 64-81.
4. Landrigan PJ and Etzel RA (Editors). Textbook of Children's Environmental Health. New York: Oxford University Press, 2014.
5. World Health Organization. The pediatric environmental history. Recording children's exposure to environmental health threats: A "green page" in the medical record. http://www.who.int/ceh/capacity/paedenvhistory/en/

Media Impact

7.4

Samir H Dalwai, Gitanjali Pillai

INTRODUCTION

The impact of media on the psychosocial development of adolescents is well recognized and is the subject of study as well as speculation across the world. Media violence on television particularly is pervasive and uniquely accessible. Violence on screen, especially by role models, ends up glamorizing sadistic, brutal behavior. It is estimated that if television viewing happens for three to four hours every day on an average, over years the impact is immense! (Table 7.4.1). The fact that television is watched at home often with the family gives it an insidious, unrecognized acceptance as the 'norm' or to get subtly imbibed as 'culture'.

Table 7.4.1: Effects of media on adolescent health
• Substance abuse
• Eating disorders
• Physical violence
• Mood and anxiety disorders
• Personality disorders
• Pornography
• Sexual disorders, unwanted pregnancies, sexually transmitted diseases (STDs)
• Sleep disorders
• Social crimes/truancies
• Communalism/racism

Media can adversely affect an adolescent brain as it is still under development; and adolescent health (Box 7.4.1).

Box 7.4.1: Cortical plasticity, media and behavior

Neuroplasticity indicates changes in synapses and neural pathways due to changes in environment, emotion, experiences and behavior.

Number of hours spent watching television (TV) has:

- Positive correlation with grey matter density in prefrontal and primary visual cortex
- Negative correlation with grey-to-white matter density in the prefrontal cortex and verbal intelligence quotient (IQ)
- Reinforcement of activity in the medial prefrontal cortex which is associated with attention control

Habitual multi-tasking can lead to symptoms of attention deficit hyperactivity disorder (ADHD).

HISTORY TAKING

A detailed history should be taken to elicit symptoms of internet addiction (Table 7.4.2).

Table 7.4.2: Symptoms of internet addiction
History taken from the adolescent
• Prefers to stay online longer than intended
• Neglects household chores to spend more time online
• Prefers media indulgence rather than social interactions with peers
• Prefers to make friends online than in real life
• Poor school grades due to the time and distraction of online activities
• Keeps checking social networking sites/e-mail/chat forums
• Develops anxiety if the internet connection fails
• Avoids discussing online activities or behavior
• Loss of sleep due to late nights spent online
• Complaints of feeling lonely, depressed or nervous if offline
• Assessment of co-morbid conditions: Altered eating habits, use of laxatives, diet pills, binge eating
• History of recent sexual activity, pregnancy, use of condoms, masturbation, venereal disease, homosexual concerns, body image concerns
History obtained from the parent
• Decline in academic performance
• Feels tired and sleepy during the day
• Diminished interest in activities
• Poor socialization with peers
• Avoids discussing about internet usage
• Avoids family activities or outings
Information from the siblings/friends/school
• Truancy/absenteeism
• Frequent quarrels with peers
• School teachers' complaints
• Breaking the rules/law
• Stealing
• Trespassing
• Lying
• Forging
• Engaging in promiscuity, eve teasing, drugs, smoking

Since a lot of co-morbidities exist, it is important to take a detailed history regarding these also (Table 7.4.3).

Table 7.4.3: Co-morbid conditions associated with media impact
Eating disorders • Anorexia nervosa • Bulimia nervosa • Obesity
Mood, personality and anxiety disorders • Obsessive compulsive behavior • Histrionic personalities • Paranoia • Anti-social personality • Relationship issues • Depression • Impulse control disorders
Sleep disorders • Insomnia • Hypersomnia
Substance abuse and related disorders • Alcohol • Nicotine • Narcotics
Inappropriate sexual behavior • Promiscuity • Sexually transmitted diseases
Social anxiety disorder • Text messaging addiction
Ophthalmic disorders • Dry eye

With increasing use of the net we need to get familiar with new definitions (Boxes 7.4.2 and 7.4.3).

Box 7.4.2: Important definitions
Internet Addiction or Compulsion: When computer use is repetitive and constant, and the users are unable to resist strong urges to use the computer.
Phantom Vibration: Perception of vibration from a cell phone even when it is not vibrating.
Mobile Phone Compulsion: When a person compulsively uses mobile phones to call people excessively and unnecessarily.
Cyber-sexual Addiction: Compulsive use of websites for cybersex and pornography.
Cyber-relationship Addiction: When a person shows over-involvement in online relationships and reflects a fast-paced generation's idea of equally fast and 'easy' relationships.

Box 7.4.3: Cyber stalking
Cyber Stalking is the use of the internet or other electronic media to harass or stalk an individual, a group, or an organization • Repetitively and regularly checking a previous partner's social media profile or their new relationship • Using a friend's profile to check out or 'stalk' another's profile • Monitoring, identity theft, threats, vandalism • Sending vulgar and defamatory messages or threats, false accusations, slander and libel. • Commenting rudely on other's public statuses (public shaming)

The content of various forms of media affects the adolescent's attitudes and behavior with regard to sexuality, and also affects personal relationships (Table 7.4.4).

Table 7.4.4: Impact of media on relationships and sexual behaviors
Relationship Issues • Adolescent's identities are shaped by how they are perceived online • Parents feel texting makes communicating with their children easier • The amount of 'friends' one has on social media networks, the number of 'likes' one receives may boost one's self image • Accepting friend requests of strangers or mere acquaintances in a race to have more number of friends than someone else on your list.
Sexual Misconduct/Inappropriate Behaviors • Engaging in casual and unprotected intercourse as they see the people they admire on TV • **Histrionic Personality Disorder,** as a result of the current phenomenon known as "sexting" (sending text messages with sexual content) • Advertisements on the use and ease of availability of oral contraceptives misinterpreted by adolescents

Prolonged hours of media exposure also impacts sleep (Table 7.4.5).

Table 7.4.5: Effects of sleep deprivation
Lower academic performance and increased risk of academic failure
Impaired mood
Increased risk of motor vehicle accidents
Computer use in the hour before bed is associated with less restful sleep, higher epworth sleepiness scales and drowsy driving
Frequent use of cell phones around bedtime is associated with difficulties falling asleep or repeated awakenings
Light exposure from various electronic sources may suppress the release of melatonin, thus delaying sleep onset
Playing video games before bed can increase sleep latency

CLINICAL EXAMINATION

A detailed head-to-toe exam is required (Table 7.4.6).

Table 7.4.6: Clinical examination
Look for signs of
• Substance abuse
• Eating disorders
• Mood, anxiety, personality disorder
• Obsessive-compulsive traits/rituals
• Mannerisms
• Injuries from violence

INVESTIGATIONS

Apart from medical testing for co-morbidities it is important to have detailed psychological evaluation (Table 7.4.7).

Table 7.4.7: Standardized psychological testing
Intelligence testing–Important for gauging mental capacity
Achievement testing (Psycho-educational assessment) • Decline in academic performance may point towards learning disability. • Neglect towards academics due to excessive gaming, TV
Projective tests–Reveal hidden emotions and internal conflicts • Rorschach, ink-blot test
Checklists and Rating scales • Child Behaviour Checklist (CBCL) – Measure for identifying problem behavior between 6-18 years. • Conners-Wells' Adolescent Self-Report Scale–Used for ADHD screening. • Vanderbilt ADHD Rating scales for teacher and parent – used for evaluation of ADHD symptoms. • Conners' Rating Scales–Oppositional problems, cognitive problems, hyperactivity. • Beck Depression Inventory (BDI-II)–Used for assessing severity of depression.
Specific Rating Scales • Internet Addiction Test • Chen Internet Addiction Scale • Compulsive Internet Use Scale

COMPREHENSIVE MANAGEMENT

Please refer to Table 7.4.8 and Figure 7.4.1.

Table 7.4.8: Key areas in psychological management
Encouraging interests/social activities • Hobbies • Team sports • Afterschool clubs
Monitoring computer use and setting clear limits • Restrict the use of computers or tablets, mobiles, television • Keep an eye on the child's online activity • Limiting time online
Recognizing underlying problems that increase intensity of addiction • Stress • Anxiety issues • Depression • Substance abuse/addiction • Major life changes (divorce, death of a family member, change of residence or school)
Building coping skills • Providing healthy and appropriate outlets for anxiety/aggression • Cognitive restructuring • Behavior modification • Identifying the ABC's (antecedent, behavior, consequence) • Building and maintaining support systems (family, peers)
Strengthening existing support systems • Setting aside specific time for family and friends • Finding people with common interests (book reading clubs, sports activities) • Support groups for addictive behaviors

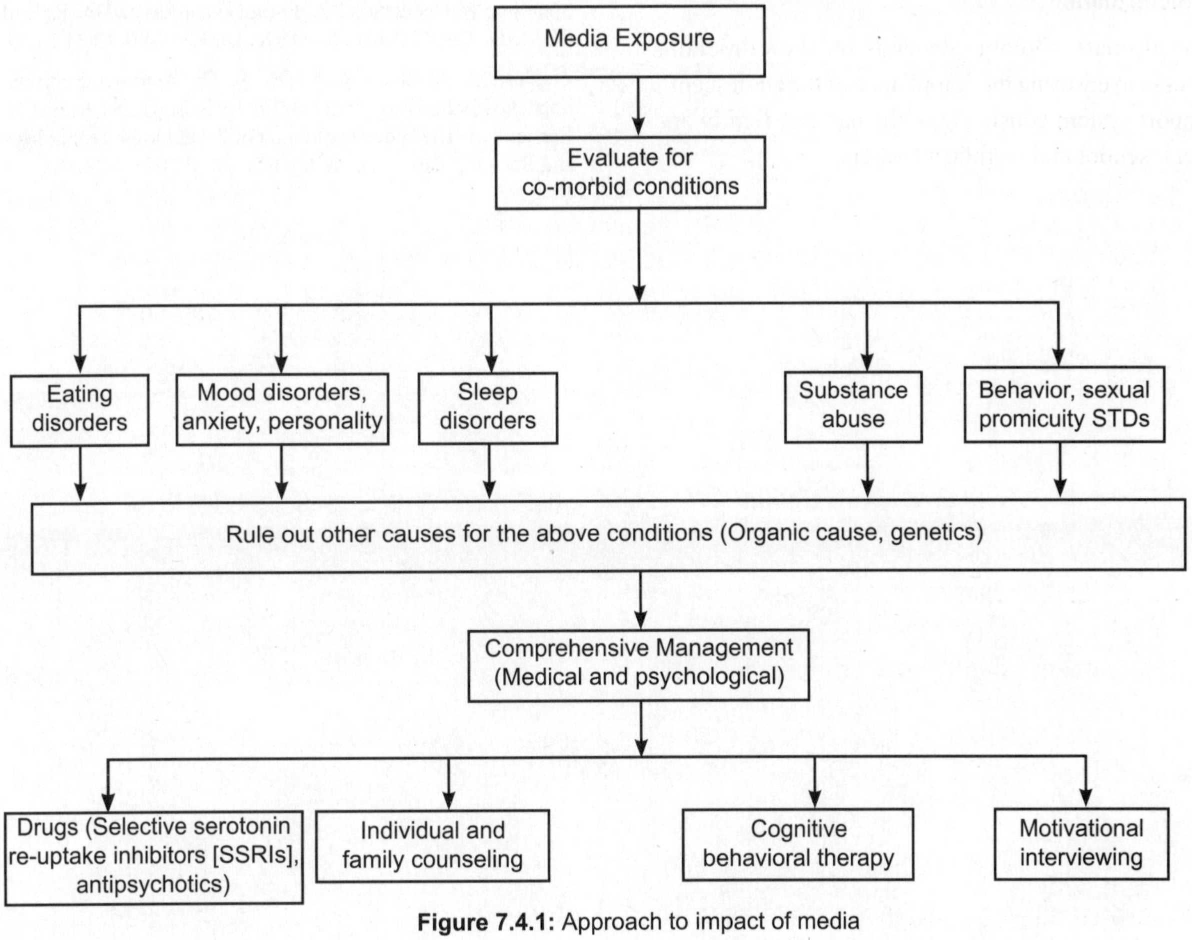

Figure 7.4.1: Approach to impact of media

LEARNING POINTS

1. The pervasiveness of digital media cultures that increasingly characterize an adolescent's life has a significant impact on the highly vulnerable period of development of the adolescent brain and cognition.
2. The rapid growth of technology and its ease of access, coupled with issues like poor media education about the messages that various forms of media delivers complicates the situation further.
3. Co-morbid conditions like substance abuse, eating disorders, anxiety, and mood disorders complicate the presenting concerns and require specific attention and management.
4. Evaluating the socio-cultural environment is as essential for assessment as addressing the presenting concerns.
5. Individual evaluation also helps to form a baseline to track future prognosis and psychotherapeutic planning.
6. The clinician's role includes meticulous assessment of the entire psychosocial profile, the enumeration of co-morbid and aggravating factors, establishment of the management protocol and its fastidious implementation.
7. The ultimate outcome depends on the clinician's success in ensuring the compliance of the adolescent's support system consisting of the parents, family and peers, school and significant others.
8. Comprehensive management with pharmacotherapy, cognitive restructuring, relapse prevention, management of co-existing conditions and family counseling in a meticulous documented manner is key to managing an adolescent with the impact of media.

SUGGESTED READING

1. Cash H, Rae CD, Steel AH, Winkler A. Internet Addiction: A Brief Summary of Research and Practice. Curr Psychiatr Rev 2012;8(4):292-98.
2. Choudhary S, McKinney KA. Digital media, the developing brain and the interpretive plasticity of neuroplasticity. Transcultural Psychiatry 2013;50(2):192-215.
3. Earles KA, Alexander R, Johnson M, Liverpool J, McGhee M. Media influences on children and adolescents: Violence and sex. J Natl Med Assoc 2002; 94(9):797-801.
4. Hershner SD, Chervin RD. Causes and consequences of sleepiness among college students. Nat Sci Sleep 2014;6:73-84.
5. Hogan MJ. Adolescents and media violence: Six crucial issues for practitioners. Adolesc Med Clin 2005;16(2), 249-68. vii.
6. Loh KK, Kanai R. How has the internet reshaped human cognition? Neuroscientist July 13, 2015 pii: 1073858415595005.
7. Rosen LD, Whaling K, Rab S, Carrier LM, Cheever NM. Is Facebook creating "iDisorders"? The link between clinical symptoms of psychiatric disorders and technology use, attitudes and anxiety. Computers in Human Behavior 2013;29:1243-54.
8. Spettigue W, Henderson KA. Eating Disorders and the Role of the Media. Can Child Adolesc Psychiatr Rev 2004;13(1):16-19.
9. Ziegler DA, Mishra J, Gazzaley A. The Acute and chronic impact of technology on our Brain. In: Rosen LD, Cheever N, Carrier LM. The Wiley Handbook of Psychology, Technology and Society; New York; Wiley Blackwell 2015;3-20.

Palliative Care

7.5

Kumar Abhishek, Smriti Rana

INTRODUCTION

Most cases of adolescents requiring palliative care will be handled by the respective specialists. However, sometimes primary care physicians may have to be involved as well. Through this chapter we discuss age-specific physical, emotional, social and spiritual needs experienced by adolescents with disease-related suffering, so as to improve their quality of life.

WHO defines palliative care in children (0-18 years) thus:

Pediatric palliative care is the active total care of child's body, mind and spirit and it also involves giving support to the family (Box 7.5.1).

Box 7.5.1: Children's palliative care

- It starts when illness is first diagnosed, and continues irrespective of the child receiving treatment directed at the disease.
- A child's physical, psychological, and social distress must be evaluated and alleviated by the health providers.
- Effective palliative care requires a multidisciplinary approach which includes the family and makes use of the best available community resources. However it can be successfully implemented even if resources are limited.
- It can be provided in tertiary care centers, in community health centers and even in patients home.
- In India, palliative care services are largely located in big urban cities.

The principles apply to any chronic disorder for pediatric age group (WHO;1998a).

When approaching palliative care in children and adolescents it is imperative that clinicians familiarize themselves with the developmental context of the individual and its impact on the experience of illness. Details of psychosocial development are given in Chapter 2.3.

Varying levels of physical, emotional and psychological maturity bring their unique set of challenges in delivering appropriate palliative care. The anatomical, physiological, psychosocial, sexual and emotional development in an adolescent may stop; be hindered or even reversed due to treatments or the general condition during advanced disease phase. This should be closely considered when dealing with adolescents in palliative care setting.

HISTORY TAKING AND PRESENTATION

Review of literature shows that 89% of patients experience distressing symptoms. More than half of them will experience three or more symptoms (Table 7.5.1).

Table 7.5.1: Most reported symptoms

Fatigue	57–86%
Reduced mobility	76%
Pain	73%
Poor appetite	71%
Dyspnea	6-21%

Neurological Symptoms

These are almost always present in patients with central nervous system tumors. Headaches are more common in patients with solid tumors compared to hematological malignancies.

Pain is the most distressing symptom that is central to palliative care.

The concept of "Total Pain" is central to providing good palliative care. It is a subjective feeling with multidimensional aspects—physical, psychosocial and spiritual. All aspects should be taken into account when treating distress in the patient.

The assessment of pain is subjective and pain in adolescents should be evaluated with tools like numerical rating scale in which "0" means no pain and "10" is the worst imaginable pain. If the subject cannot comprehend this scale, body language, distressed facial expression, sleeping difficulties or medical history as remembered by the patient provide useful indicators.

CLINICAL EXAMINATION

This may identify the cause of the pain but sometimes radiological imaging may be necessary to get more specific details.

MANAGEMENT

Pain may be managed by both drug and non-drug interventions. Drug treatment should take into account the different pharmacokinetics in younger adolescents, while older adolescents may be treated in a similar way as adults. Pain can be treated by analgesics and adjuvant drugs (Table 7.5.2). The doses mentioned are only the starting doses. The dosage will have to be titrated up according to the response. They have no upper limit and the right dose is the dose required to treat the pain adequately.

Opioids are titrated with immediate release formulations. After the daily dose has stabilized, a slow release formulation may be used safely in adolescents. Side effects are constipation, nausea, pruritis, confusion and hallucinations, myoclonus and somnolence.

Adjuvant drugs are used to minimize side effects or to enhance the effects of analgesics. They can also help to relieve pain by elevating mood, reducing anxiety levels (Table 7.5.3).

Clinicians should take all symptoms into consideration and try to control them as best as possible to improve the quality of life.

Non-Drug Interventions

These may be categorized as:

1. Supportive (psychosocial, family-centered care, empathy).
2. Cognitive (Mindfulness-integrated cognitive behavior therapy (MiCBT), visualization, music and games).

Table 7.5.2: Analgesics for palliative care

Medication	*Daily oral dosing schedule*		
	50 kg	*>50 kg*	*18 years*
Non-opioids			
Paracetamol	10–15 mg/kg q 4–6 h	10–15 mg/kg q 4–6 h	1 g q 4–6 h
Ibuprofen	5–10 mg/kg q 6–8 h	5–10 mg/kg q 6–8 h	200–400 mg q 6–8 h
Weak opioids			
Codeine	0.2 mg/kg q 3–4 h	30 mg q 3–4 h	30–60 mg q 3–4 h
Strong opioids			
Hydromorphone	0.06 mg/kg q 3–4 h	2 mg q 3–4 h	2–4 mg q 4–6 h
Methadone	0.2 mg/kg q 4–8 h	5–10 mg q 4–8 h	5–10 mg q 6–12 h
Morphine	0.15–0.3 mg/kg q 4 h	5–10 mg q 4 h	10 mg q 4 h
Oxycodone	0.2 mg/kg q 3–4 h	5–10 mg q 3–4 h	5–15 mg q 4–6 h

kg, kilogram; mg, milligram; q, every; h, hours

Table 7.5.3: Adjuvant drugs

Medication	*Indication*	*Daily oral dosing schedule*	
		<18 years	*18 years*
Antidepressants			
Amitriptyline	Neuropathic pain	0.2–0.5 mg/kg q 24 h	10–25 mg q 8 h
Anticonvulsants			
Carbamazepine	Neuropathic pain	2 mg/kg q 12 h	200 mg q 12 h
Gabapentin	Neuropathic pain	25–35 mg/kg q 8–12 h	300 mg q 24–8 h
Neuroleptics			
Haloperidol	Nausea, delirium, psychosis, agitation	0.01–0.1 mg/kg q 8 h	2–5 mg q 8 h
Benzodiazepines			
Diazepam	Anxiety, muscle spasm myoclonus	0.05–0.01 mg/kg q 4–6 h	2–10 mg q 6–8 h
Midazolam	Invasive procedures	0.3–0.5 mg/kg	
Antihistaminics			
Diphenhydramine	Pruritus, nausea	0.5–1 mg/kg q 4–6 h	25–50 mg q 4–6 h
Psychostimulants			
Methylphenidate	Somnolence	0.1–0.5 mg/kg q 12 h	5–15 mg q 8–12 h

kg, kilogram; mg, milligram; q, every; h, hour

3. Behavioral (breathing techniques; relaxation).
4. Physical therapies (touch, heat or cold applications).
5. Others–External radiotherapy in bone tumors–Ewing sarcoma; osteosarcoma, radioisotopes in patients with cancer in the skeletal structures.

PSYCHOSOCIAL ISSUES

As a result of advanced illness, adolescents may have an abnormal psychosocial development. In addition to delays or disruption of physical development, critical life experiences necessary for achieving normal developmental goals may not happen. The development of personal independence and self-confidence acquired through gradual separation from parents and successful functioning in groups beyond the family such as peers, school, extracurricular activities and employment may be hindered. The impact of advanced illness in adolescence depends upon the stage of development and is different in early, middle or late stages.

- **Early adolescence:** Importance is given to concerns about physical appearance and mobility, privacy and interference with normal relations with peers. In this phase hospitals are experienced as disturbing.
- **Middle adolescence:** Illness is particularly threatening and least well-tolerated. The adolescent experiences a compromised sense of autonomy, interference with attraction of a partner, fear of rejections by peers and social isolation.
- **Late adolescence:** Advanced illness results in absence of work or education, interferes with plans for vocation and relationships, and may lead to unemployment, loss of financial autonomy and self-esteem.

As compared to adults there are different challenges for an adolescent with advanced illness (Box 7.5.2).

Box 7.5.2: Challenges faced by adolescents with advanced illness

- Lack of early maturing responsibilities due to overprotection by parents and learned passivity
- The effects of social rejection where self-esteem is undermined by peer non-acceptance
- Social isolation resulting from difficulty participating in social, athletic, or intellectual activities
- Interrupted education due to reallocation of family finances for treatment
- Lack of sexual outlets in the absence of forming of normal interpersonal relationships, especially those with the opposite sex

There are some special aspects to be kept in mind when communicating with adolescents requiring palliative care (Box 7.5.3).

Box 7.5.3: Special aspects of communication with adolescents requiring palliative care

- It is vital to use correct language and appropriate communication skills, keeping in mind the cognitive and emotional developmental milestones associated with this age group.
- The tendency to treat the adolescent patient as one would a child or a grown-up, or to altogether dismiss the importance of their involvement in deciding the plan of care would be big mistakes.
- A growing sense of role responsibilities, formal-operational thought and a sense of developing a value system mean that the adolescent patient needs to be brought into the decision making process and affiliated conversation with sensitivity and awareness of these aspects.

Though the physician is dealing with the adolescent primarily, he or she must also conduct discussions with the family, to involve them as part of the support unit and also to support the needs of the family members themselves (Box 7.5.4).

Box 7.5.4: Family dynamics–Adolescents requiring palliative care

Families that have healthy dynamics and coping patterns do much better than those families that had dysfunctional dynamics prior to the onset of the health crisis. Dysfunction is exacerbated by an illness and clinicians need to create support networks that may extend outside of the family.

The siblings

- May be unfairly called upon to take on almost parent-like roles themselves, or be asked to stay out of the way while the adults handle the situation.
- Lack of healthy attention on the sibling may lead to behavioral issues, risk-taking, rebellion, withdrawal, isolation and a whole plethora of patterns that may adversely affect the overall life of the sibling.
- All too often, they become invisible in the face of the battle of helping the sick adolescent fight for his or her life. Clinicians must look out for these invisible siblings, drawing and building on the strength of the family unit.

SPIRITUAL ISSUES

The role of professional health caregivers in approaching religion and spirituality with adolescents is controversial. Health care professionals should be trained to discuss these issues with patients of adolescent age group, especially with patients who are hospitalized. Doctors should also be sensitive to those adolescent patients who may not want to discuss spiritual/religious issues in a health care setting.

Spirituality reflects the inner belief system or resources from which one can draw strength, meaning and solace and is often different from religiousness. Most adolescents are capable of abstract religious/spiritual thinking. Religion, spirituality or evolving concepts pertaining to them are important in their lives. Negative beliefs about death and superstitious beliefs appear to be associated with anxiety.

Coping is defined as continuous change in cognitive and behavioral efforts to manage specific external and/or internal demands that are identified as taxing or exceeding the resources of the person. Spirituality may be a positive factor in coping with advanced illness. Understanding both the context and background of the family's spiritual/ religious beliefs, in conjunction with the individual developmental experience of the adolescent in question is vital in helping them cope appropriately.

ETHICAL AND LEGAL ISSUES

Professional health caregivers are confronted with numerous ethical and legal issues when dealing with adolescents with advanced illness.

- Decisions on starting and stopping treatments, symptom control and decisions related to the end-of-life should be addressed. Many professional caregivers of adolescents have recognized that these patients, especially those who are medically experienced, often demonstrate remarkable insight into their illnesses, prospects for survival and preferences for how they wish to spend their remaining time.
- Also, choices about the site of care and dying (home, hospital, or hospice) and providers of palliative care (hospice team, family, and/or others) should be discussed. Adolescents of 14 years and older should be presumed to have the functional competence to make binding medical decisions for themselves, including decisions relating to the discontinuance of life-sustaining therapy and other end-of-life issues. The decision-making process is also complicated by the fact that age 18 is considered the transition from being a minor to a major. Decisions by adolescents less than 18 years must be agreed on by a responsible adult (e.g. parents, legal guardian). However, healthcare teams must make every effort to respect and involve family members in treatment decisions concerning a competent adolescent with an advanced illness. More details of ethical and legal issues are given in Chapter 1.5.

LEARNING POINTS

- The adolescent with advanced illness represents a challenge to the family and professional health caregivers.
- Health caregivers should provide optimal symptom control as well as address the psychosocial aspects of care to ensure that quality of life is compromised as little as possible.
- A multidisciplinary team involving medical and nursing staff, social workers, psychologists and spiritual advisors experienced in working with adolescents, in collaboration with the family as the unit of care, should collaborate in caring for adolescents and their families.
- There is significant need for clinical research in this patient population to develop evidence-based guidelines to improve the care of adolescents in the palliative care setting.

Acknowledgements

For his guidance in writing this chapter: Dr MR Rajagopal, Chairman, Pallium India, Director, TIPS (Trivandrum Institute of Palliative Sciences), WHO Collaborating Center for Training and Policy on Access to Pain Relief.

SUGGESTED READING

1. Hauer JM. A Life with Grace–Caring for Children Who Have Severe Neurological Impairment. Maryland; John Hopkins University Press, 2013.
2. Regnard C, Dean M. A Guide to Symptom Relief in Palliative Care, 6th Edition. London; Radcliffe Publications, 2010.
3. Twycross R. Introducing Palliative Care, 4th Edition. Kerala (India); Publication of Institute of Palliative Medicine Pain and Palliative Care Society, 2013.
4. Watson M. Oxford Handbook of Palliative Care, 2nd Edition. New York; Oxford University Press, 2009.
5. Wolfe J, Hinds P, Sourkes B. Textbook of Interdisciplinary Pediatric Palliative Care: Expert Consult Premium Edition. Philadelphia; Elsevier Publications, 2011.

8.1

Overview of Psychiatric Illnesses

Jay P Shastri, Dimple J Shastri

INTRODUCTION

Many adolescents are suffering from different mental health issues, depression being the most common among them. Studies have concluded that since depression is common, it also results in major morbidity and mortality in adolescents. Mental health issues in adolescents can have a negative impact on their development and also expose them to various risky behaviors such as substance abuse, drop-out from school, teenage pregnancy and delinquent behaviors. Healthy development during this crucial phase of human life cycle can go a long way in developing a resilient individual with positive problem solving capacity. There is growing consensus that healthy development during childhood and adolescence contributes to good mental health and can prevent mental health problems (Box 8.1.1).

Box 8.1.1: Common mental health disorders and difficulties encountered during childhood and the teenage years

- Attention deficit hyperactivity disorder (ADHD)
- Anxiety and a variety of related anxiety disorders ranging from simple phobias to social anxiety, generalized anxiety disorder and post-traumatic stress disorder (PTSD)
- Autism and Asperger syndrome (the Autism Spectrum Disorders, or ASD)
- Behavioral problems; bullying; depression; eating disorders (including anorexia nervosa and bulimia)
- Obsessive compulsive disorders (OCD)
- Psychotic disorders
- Schizophrenia
- Substance abuse

There is no one cause for these disturbances. Reasons are often multiple: genetic, environmental, chromosomal and socio-cultural. Factors like adolescent's temperament, parental health, family relationships and parenting styles are important.

As the other psychiatric disorders are covered in this chapter we will focus mainly on disorders such as adolescent psychosis, anxiety disorders, adolescent bipolar mood disorders and borderline personality traits in adolescents.

HISTORY TAKING

In the diagnosis and planning for treatment of adolescent disorders, the adolescent interview can be a source of insight into the adolescent's thoughts, feelings and behavior. The information collected from an adolescent interview provides the clinician with an understanding of adolescent's perception of the current problems and their willingness to participate in the treatment. Through both the direct observation of the adolescent and the content of the adolescent's response during the interview, the interviewer has the opportunity to gather several types of information (Table 8.1.1).

Table 8.1.1: Interview with adolescent should help
To understand general demeanor of the adolescent
To understand adolescent's general social skills and capacity to relate to others (Through interaction with parents/interviewer)
To evaluate adolescent's coping skills
To evaluate any behavioral or cognitive disturbances
To understand adolescent's perception about self, family and environment
To reconfirm the details provided by the objective data

The adolescent interview is a flexible procedure that is directed by the trained interviewer. By using adolescent's verbal responses and nonverbal behavior as guides, the interviewer can slow the pace of the conversation or redirect the focus of the interview as needed. Process skills are the techniques that interviewers use to guide and direct the interview sequence, build and maintain rapport, and facilitate the resolution of conflict that may occur during the interview.

CLINICAL PRESENTATIONS

Anxiety Disorder or Feeling Anxious

- The feeling of anxiety is generally characterized as diffuse and unpleasant sensations (see Table 8.1.2).
- Anxiety becomes a disorder when the symptoms are severe, long lasting and interfere with normal life. Anxiety disorders can develop gradually over long periods of time or very quickly.
- It could also show some temporal variation where the symptoms appear during certain time or events like examinations.
- These disorders can become disabling and interfere with school, relationships, social activities and work.

Different Types of Anxiety

Post-Traumatic Stress Disorder

Research studies in recent years have confirmed that post-traumatic stress disorder and its inherent comorbidity occurs not only in adult victims of traumatic life events, but in adolescents too.

- Presence of trauma, in case of adolescents along with acute exposure, chronic traumatic events like physical and sexual abuse can also be the cause.
- In adolescents the role of "indirect exposure" could also play an important role.
- Re-experiencing the traumatic events in the form of nightmares or re-enactment.
- Persistent avoidance of stimuli by distracting themselves or motor restlessness or impulsive behavior.
- At times adolescent may exhibit regressive behavior.
- Increased physiological hyper-arousal in the form of sleep disturbances, irritability and poor concentration.
- Adolescents might exhibit a strong survival guilt.

Fears and Phobias

- Unlike adults, adolescent are not required to acknowledge their fears and worries as unreasonable or excessive to make a diagnosis of phobic disorder.
- It is sufficient that the fear causes avoidant behavior that interferes with some aspect of adolescent functioning.
- Heights, loud noises, injections, insects, dogs, and other animals are among the more common fears in adolescent.
- Mild specific phobias are transient and part of normal developmental process.
- With some encouragement and support, most adolescents learn to overcome their fear.

General Anxiety

- Some youngsters feel anxious most of the time for no apparent reason.
- It may be part of their temperament, or it may be part of a pattern of behavior that is shared with other members of the family.
- These adolescents are referred because of somatic complaints, insomnia, social impairments, or comorbid depression and suicidality.
- If the anxiety becomes very severe, it can interfere with the child's ability to go to school, to concentrate and learn, and to be confident with others.

Obsessive Compulsive Disorder

- The obsessive compulsive disorders (OCDs) seen during adult life has most often their origin in early adolescence.
- More than rituals or compulsions seen during adult life, adolescence is more often seen presenting with obsessive ruminations.
- Most common worries they harbor is "something going to happen to their parents or near ones".

Table 8.1.2: Symptoms of anxiety

• Experience of fear	• Rapid heart beat	• Dwelling on fearful possibilities
• Restlessness	• Chest pain or tension	• Problems performing tasks
• Irritability	• Muscle tension	• Frightening images
• Avoidance	• Indigestion or diarrhea	• Thoughts of danger
• Rapid labored breathing	• Dizziness or feeling "light-headed"	• Increased energy
• Sweating or perspiring	• Racing thoughts	• Frustration
• Trembling or "shaking"	• Neglecting responsibilities	• Problems in concentrating
• Weakness	• Impatience	
• Poor memory		

- Adolescents generally respond well to early intervention and are candidates for cognitive behavioral therapy.

Adolescent Psychosis

Among individuals with schizophrenia around 5% have onset of their illness in the adolescent years (Table 8.1.3). Prevalence of psychotic disease increases to a large extent during adolescence. This is a well-known fact even in the absence of large population based studies. Around 0.54% is the prevalence of psychotic disorders seen in age group of 13 to 19 years. The prevalence shows an increasing trend with 0.9 per 10,000 at age 13 to 17.6 per 10,000 at age 18 years.

Table 8.1.3: Adolescent psychosis
Diagnosis is based on the presence of following three characteristic symptoms: • Thought and perceptual disorders (Hallucinations/Delusions) • Disorganized behavior • Negative symptomatology (Anhedonia, social withdrawal and blank affect)
Certain clinical features which are characteristics in adolescent psychosis • Generally adolescent psychosis has an insidious onset • Systematic delusions and catatonic symptoms are less seen • Adolescents might have less complex delusions • Paranoid and undifferentiated types are more common • They might have low IQ.

Schizophrenia

- For diagnosis of schizophrenia an adolescent should have symptoms present for atleast 6 months duration. This period can include both prodromal period and periods with active psychotic symptoms, where active psychotic phase should be present at least for a month.
- As compared to adults, the functional deterioration in adolescents encompasses deterioration in self-care, social, educational and occupational domain.
- Treatment of prodrome of psychosis has been a topic of debate for years now and there are no clear guidelines on whether to treat or observe it.
- Schizophrenia needs treatment with anti-psychotic medications, where second generation medications are preferred over first generation on the basis of their better safety profile.

Adolescent Bipolar Disorders

Adolescent bipolar disorders are discussed briefly in Table 8.1.4.

Table 8.1.4: Adolescent bipolar disorders
In adolescent major depressive episodes occur with increasing frequency • More severe depressions among adolescents that is characterized by mood congruent auditory hallucinations and delusions, psychomotor retardation and pervasive anhedonia has been recognized as the syndromes that more often are followed in the future by a period of mania and consequently diagnosis of bipolar disorder.
• Mania in adolescent is a topic of controversy mainly due to lack of consensus among clinicians and researchers. • Accordingly to a recent review of bipolar illness in adolescence, adolescence-onset bipolar illness may be more severe; it may have chronic, non-episodic course and it may present in a mixed, or rapid cycling form that resembles the form seen in the most severely ill adult bipolar patient. • This group of patients is also considered to be treatment resistant.
Adolescents with mania may present with • Infectious elation and interact in an amusing and silly manner. • Their grandiose delusions are generally seen to have age appropriateness (achieving greatness in academics or becoming popular in school) even in the face of impending failure. • They are well-known for their extremely high energy levels; and they may manifest both high risk behaviors with peers and hypersexual episodes far exceeding the comfort level of their peers. • In contract to adolescents with ADHD, manic adolescents are often illogical and are driven to interact incessantly with peers and family members.

Borderline Personality Disorder of Adolescence

Personality disorders have been defined as relatively enduring and pervasively maladaptive patterns of experiences, relationships and coping styles.

Adolescents are involved in fluid developmental processes in which their personalities and bodies are changing at different rates, creating equilibrium changes in their relationship to their family and friends and within themselves.

One of such personality disorders is "Borderline personality". Many consider it a legitimate diagnostic category for adolescent; others regard it as a "waste basket" for those who do not fit into any other category.

Some believe that many adolescents who receive this diagnosis may have a complex form of post-traumatic stress disorder, particularly following chronic child abuse (see Box 8.1.2).

Box 8.1.2: Borderline personality disorder of adolescence

- This is characterized by pervasive pattern of instability of interpersonal relationships, self-image, and affects and marked impulsivity, beginning early and present in a variety of contexts.
- Adolescents with borderline traits would be seen walking in and out of emotional relationships with same or different individuals.
- Their impulsive behavior is mostly directed towards self and would be seen in the form of multiple cuts or burn marks on their hand.
- Their emotional lability would be hard to explain as they would feel comfortable in their depression and uncomfortable while they are not depressed and describes intense periods of crying that may shift into hysterical laughter.
- Their social communications are likely to be strained.
- They might harbor chronic suicidal ideas.
- Their overall academic functioning is on gradual decline in spite of having enough potential.

ASSESSMENT PROCESS

The assessment of adolescent's intellectual and academic functioning probably is the most common reason for referral and investigations. Assessment can be defined as "a process of gathering information used in screening, diagnosing, determining eligibility, program planning and service delivery, and monitoring progress during treatment or intervention". Investigating the adolescent for various other medical and neurological issues remains the key to reach any meaningful diagnosis (see Table 8.1.5).

Regular evaluation along with meaningful investigations is important to understand the progress of any adolescent mental health problem.

Table 8.1.5: Investigations

Tests	*Interpretation*
Blood investigations	To rule of anemia and other biochemical deficiencies
Genetic and chromosomal studies	To diagnose the genetic disorders
Urine for substance abuse	To rule out comorbid substance use
Electroencephalogram (EEG)	To diagnose any seizure disorder
MRI brain	To understand the presence of any neurodevelopmental issues
IQ assessment	To understand child's potential and get overall prognosis
Hearing assessment	Important in learning problems
Visual assessment	Important in learning problems

Clinicians should make caretakers aware that purpose of assessment should not only for getting concessions or certificates that would benefit adolescent academically, but to understand the adolescent and his problems at length so that he or she can be helped to make them healthy individual.

MANAGEMENT

Multidisciplinary team approach is always ideal for handling adolescent mental health issues. Diversity in resources, expertise and other manpower with different socio-cultural background will need different multidisciplinary team models.

Multidisciplinary team consists of psychiatrist, psychologist, social worker, speech therapist, occupational therapist, remedial teacher, adolescent pediatrician, child and adolescent neurologist and primary referring physician (Figure 8.1.1). One can have more members or smaller team depending on the special group

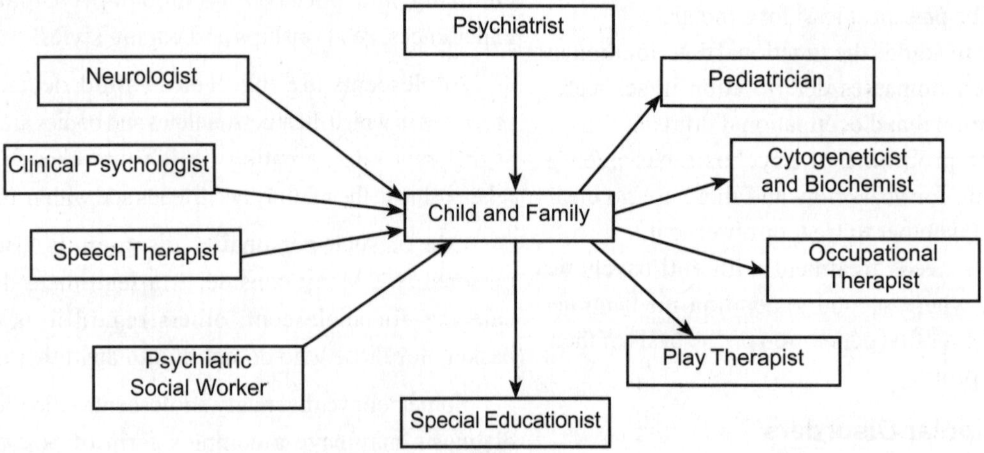

Figure 8.1.1: Multidisciplinary team approach

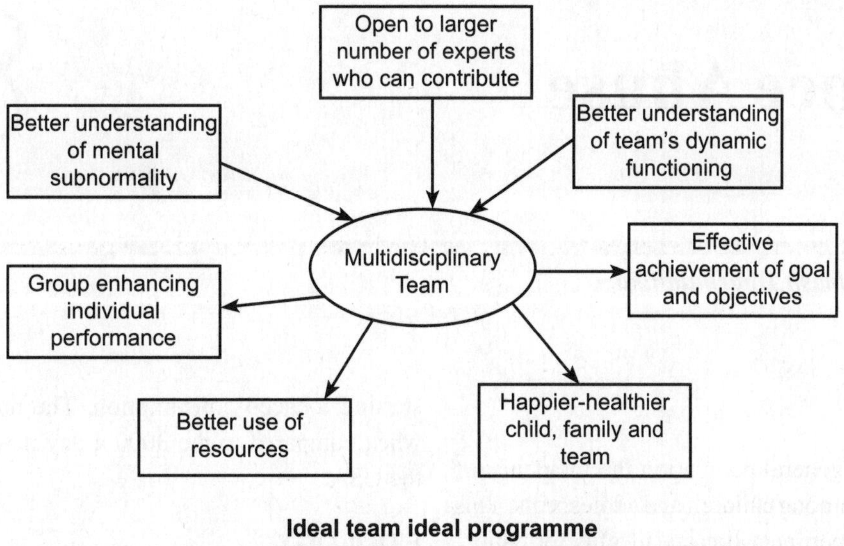

Figure 8.1.2: Goals of the multidisciplinary team

they cater to. Psychotherapy specific to the disorder should always be tried as first line especially when the presentation is not very acute. Involvement of the family remains the key to long-term success of any therapeutic alliance working in the area of adolescent mental health (Figure 8.1.2).

Acknowledgement

We acknowledge the contribution of Dr (Prof) Priyvadan C Shastri for his continuous guidance and support while finalizing this chapter.

LEARNING POINTS

- Like adults adolescents can also experience disturbances in their thoughts, emotions and behavior resulting in impairment of functioning and changes lasting lifelong.
- It is imperative to identify and treat these problems early.
- Challenge would be to change poor help seeking behavior in adolescent and their support group.

SUGGESTED READING

1. Sadock B, Sadock V (Eds). Kaplan and Sadock's Comprehensive Textbook of Psychiatry, 7th edition. Philadelphia; Lippincott Williams and Wilkins; 2000.
2. Sagar R. Child and adolescent mental health: Need for a public health approach. Journal of Mental Health and Human Behavior 2011;16(1):1-4.
3. Sharan P, Sagar R. The Need for National Data on Epidemiology of Child and Adolescent Mental Disorders. J Indian Assoc Child Adolesc Ment Health 2008;4(2):22-27.
4. Walker CE, Roberts MC (Eds). Handbook of clinical child psychology; 3rd edition. New York: John Wiley and Sons 2001;90-111.
5. World Health Organization. Atlas: Child and Adolescent Mental Health Resources–Global Concerns: Implications for the future. Geneva:WHO;2005.

Substance Abuse

8.2

Suyog Jaiswal, Ambrish Dharmadhikari

INTRODUCTION

As compared to the general population the incidence of drug abuse is higher among children and adolescents. This period is a time for experimentation and identity formation. Most children and adolescents develop resilience for coping with life challenges such as educational competitions, parental expectations, loss of a friend or the death of a family member. A complex interaction of biological, behavioral, and environmental factors places certain youths at greater risk than others for substance use disorders. Substance abuse can overwhelm adolescents' ability to cope and can interfere with their ability to learn and mature. In developed countries substance abuse is generally associated with specific lifestyle and culture. Blind imitation of the western culture is bringing problems to our country.

Review of Indian literature shows that 63.6% of patients of substance abuse are <15 years of age. The five most commonly abused drugs in India are heroin, opium, alcohol, cannabis and propoxyphene (see Table 8.2.1). There is an emerging trend of "cocktail" or "combination" of drugs, which are taken simultaneously through injection or taken one after another. Also, sharing of needles is increasing risk of human immunodeficiency virus (HIV) infection. The use of tobacco is another major concern amongst adolescents. In India 20 million children per year and nearly 55,000 children and adolescents per day are starting tobacco consumption. The number is shocking when compared to the 3000 a day new child smokers in the USA.

ETIOLOGY

The complex relationship between personal and community variable, is responsible for adolescent substance use disorder. Important contributing factors include genetic vulnerability, environmental factors and psychological difficulties (i.e., delayed development of milestones, emotional, or cognitive deregulation). Additionally, poor parenting, parental substance use, maltreatment in childhood, child sex abuse and bad role modeling also contribute to the development of the disorder. Cultural and ethnic factors also affect patterns of substance abuse and recovery among adolescents.

The major neurotransmitters of interest in case of substance use disorder are opioid, catecholamine (especially dopamine), and gamma-aminobutyric acid (GABA) systems. The dopaminergic neurons from ventral tegmental area project to the cortical and limbic regions, especially the nucleus accumbens. This pathway is involved in the sensation of reward and is probably the major mediator of the effects of substances. The locus ceruleus, the largest group of adrenergic neurons, probably mediates the effects of the opiates and the opioids. These pathways have collectively been called the brain-reward circuitry.

Table 8.2.1: Commonly used substances for abuse

Category	*Common products*
Tobacco and tobacco products	Smokeless tobacco (*gutka, khaini and pan*), cigarettes, bidis, hukkah
Alcohol	Beer, whisky, rum, vodka, country liquor, *todi*
Cannabis	Bhang, *ganja, charas*, hashish, hash oil, weed, grass, joint
Inhalants	Ink eraser, correction fluid, whitener, glue, petrol
Opioids	Street heroin, pharmaceutical opioids (including propoxyphene, pentazocine, buprenorphine), *apheem, bookie, smack, dodda*
Sedatives	Diazepam, nitrazepam (*Nitra*), alprazolam, flunitrazepam (date rape drug), ketamine (*Vitamin K*), buttons
Stimulants	Methamphetamine, mephedrone (*meow-meow*), methylphenidate, MDMA (3,4-methylenedioxy-methamphetamine, *ecstacy*), cocaine (coke), *speed, speedball* (cocaine with heroin or morphine in the same syringe)

HISTORY TAKING

Current guidelines recommend annual screening of adolescents at every physician visit. Studies show that sick visits and other non-well-child care have higher screen-positive rates than well-child care visits and screening should occur at any visit whenever possible. In the early stages substance abuse can be missed or mistaken for other psychological or psychiatric disorders. It is very important to educate parents, teachers and peers to understand about the adverse effects of substance abuse and learn to pick up signs of substance abuse. Conducting programs in community and schools and colleges for awareness of these flag signs are very important for prevention of substance abuse.

Presence of one or more of the signs below warrants a detailed clinical evaluation of the patient with a differential diagnosis of substance use disorder in mind. The formal evaluation should always include in depth history taking and detailed clinical interview. The clinical interview with the adolescent requires a high degree of empathy, understanding of substance behavior and patience on the clinician's part to form the rapport, therapeutic relationship and get the relevant details for diagnosis and planning management.

Tables 8.2.2 and 8.2.3 describe the flag signs for substance abuse at home, at school/college. Table 8.2.4 details the flag signs for physical and emotional changes due to substance abuse in adolescents.

Table 8.2.2: Flag signs for substance abuse at home
• Loss of interest and involvement in family activities which were previously enjoyed
• Disregard for family rules and discipline
• Avoiding conversations and being distracted
• Withdrawal from responsibilities
• Verbally or even physically abusive towards near ones
• Unexplained changes in appetite (increase or decrease)
• Repetitive loss of money or valuable items from home
• Coming home late or unexplained longer than usual stay outside
• Not revealing his/her whereabouts or hiding whereabouts
• Excuses for unaccepted/changed behavior
• Confined to a room by himself/herself or with friends
• Lying about activities
• Changes in sleep habits
• Finding the following: Cigarette rolling papers, aluminum foil, chilim, small glass vials, injections or needles, remnants of drugs (cannabis etc.)
• Change in peer group, unexplained phone calls suddenly going out of home after a phone call
• Increased need of privacy, locking bathroom or bedroom door for prolonged time

Table 8.2.3: Flag signs for substance abuse at school/college
• Gradual or sudden deterioration in scholastic performance
• Bunking class or being late to school
• Lack of attention in class, drop in attention span or memory
• Sleeping in class
• Not able to complete homework, not completing tasks
• Defiance to authority figures
• Avoiding engaging in sports or extracurricular activities
• Not passing information of parent-teacher meetings to parents, forging signatures on report card

Table 8.2.4: Flag signs for physical and emotional changes due to substance abuse
• Changes friends or loses interest in old friends
• Mood swings and unexplained behavior
• Smell of alcohol, whitener, cannabis in breath or over body
• Being negative, always augmenting, or being paranoid, anxious
• Cannot stand criticism, be rebellious
• Not sharing their personal problems
• Change in mood state from being happy to cranky or dysphoric
• Overly active or tired
• Sudden change in weight
• Remaining unhappy and depressed all the time
• Always demands money in excess of need, or has unexplained excessive amount
• Sloppiness in appearance

The Clinical Assessment

The clinical assessment should include the following details (see Table 8.2.5):

1. Detailed substance use history, including details of previous abstinence and interventions if any.
2. Perceptions of substance-related difficulties, problems, or complications, including social, academic and interpersonal implications.
3. Complete psychiatric and general medical histories, including medication history, medical consequences of substance use.
4. Legal history, including substance-related legal problems, breaking of law and confrontations with law enforcement agencies.
5. Family and social histories, including psychiatric or substance-related disorders in family members, diagnosed/treated or not.

CLINICAL EXAMINATION

It is important to do a general physical and psychiatric examination, including screening for other psychiatric disorders and mental status examination (Table 8.2.6).

Table 8.2.5: Detailed questionnaire for a case of substance abuse
Which substance or substances are being consumed?
What are the routes of consumption?
How did it start and evolve? (Including first use and change in pattern over a period)
How much quantity, frequency?
What is the pattern of consumption? (Solitary or in company)
When was the last time the substance was consumed?
What are other substances that have been consumed and their details? (Current and lifetime)
Are there any episodes of withdrawal, intoxication? (Including frequency, duration and severity)
If IV use, then there was needle or other equipment sharing?
How is substance the procured? (Legal/illegal means, involvement in trafficking)
How much money is spent on the substance? (Including debt, borrowing, stealing)
How much time is spent on procuring, consuming and recovering from the effects of substance?
Are there any complications? (Including medical complications)
What is the impact of the family? (Includes the family view on substance use, approval, support extent, motivation)
What is the impact on academic life? (Absentees, removal, difficulty in studying, etc.)
Has the social life been impacted? (Includes view of society, acceptance, rejection, isolation, support)
Have there been any period or episode of abstinence in the past?
If yes, what were the reasons, methods of abstinence? And factors for relapse?
Has there been any trouble with the law? (With all details)
Is there any interpersonal problems that arose due to substance use? (If yes, details)
Why is he/she presented now? (Reasons for consultation)
What is expectation from treating team?
Was there any previous treatment? (Include all details, durations, inpatient/outpatient, improvement, and compliance, if discontinued why?)
Is there sexual promiscuity? (Number of partners, safe or unsafe sex, knowledge about STDs, orientation)

Table 8.2.6: Examination and investigations	
General physical examination	Look for finger burns, fresh or old marks of laceration over body (especially on the inner side of the forearm), injection marks, septal perforation, redness of eyes, staining of teeth.
Mental status examination	Change in motor behavior (restless, fidgeting, aggressive), change in speech, mood swings, depressed or manic mood, change in thought process, abnormal perception, altered judgment.

In history taking and clinical examination it is also important to assess and evaluate for other comorbid conditions (see Table 8.2.7).

Table 8.2.7: Common comorbidities associated with substance abuse
Conduct disorder
Attention deficit hyperactive disorder
Anxiety disorder
Oppositional defiant disorder
Depressive disorder
Comorbidity is the rule rather than the exception among adolescents in treatment for substance use disorder.

There are high chances of an associated mental disorder in adolescents with substance use disorder and vice versa. The mental disorder may have precipitated the substance abuse. The mental disorder can also get exacerbated due to substance use.

Review of literature shows that persons having a mood or anxiety disorders are highly prone to substance abuse and visa versa. This also holds true for antisocial personality disorder or conduct disorder. The Methods for the Epidemiology of Child and Adolescent mental disorders (MECA) study observed that past 6-month prevalence of comorbid psychiatric disorders with an adolescent substance use disorder was about 76% for any comorbid disorder, 68% for any disruptive behavior disorder, 32% for any mood disorder, and 20% for any anxiety disorder.

INVESTIGATIONS

1. *Laboratory studies:* Like urine for substance, blood level can be ordered to confirm if the patient is taking substance or not. However it is important to collect and examine urine/blood as early as possible for estimation of the substance suspected to be used by the adolescent (Table 8.2.8).
2. The abused substance does not remain in the body system for a very long time. Table 8.2.8 details duration for which the substance may come as positive in urine and blood.

Table 8.2.8: Time period for measuring substance of abuse in urine/blood

Substance of abuse	*Duration for which substance may come positive in urine/blood*
Alcohol	Upto 72 hours
Opioids	Upto 7 days
Cannabinoids	Upto 4 weeks
Amphetamines	Upto 72 hours
Bemzodiazepines	Upto 4 weeks
Cocaine	Upto 96 hours

3. Substance abusing adolescents can also indulge in high risk sexual behavior hence screening for sexually transmitted diseases including HIV testing should be asked for. This is specially important in cases of needle sharing in IV drug users.

MANAGEMENT (WHEN TO INTERVENE AND HOW?)

It is very important to know how to intervene in a case of substance abuse after the assessment is done and the conclusion of problematic substance use is established. The family should be involved in management and decision making about treatment along with the patient. The treatment is directed towards prevention of substance use in the future and addressing the emotional, cognitive, psychiatric factors influencing the substance use in adolescence (see Figure 8.2.1).

The goals of treatment are as follows:

1. Abstinence
2. Harm reduction
3. Improvement of health, social and occupational function
4. Improvement in quality of life

Table 8.2.9 provides the guidelines from the child and adolescent levels of care utilization services (CALOCUS) developed by the American Association of Community Psychiatrists (AACP) and the American Academy of Child and Adolescent Psychiatry (AACAP).

Table 8.2.10 provides an overview of the management.

Table 8.2.9: Child and adolescent levels of care utilization services (CALOCUS)
Level 0: Basic services (prevention)
Level 1: Recovery maintenance (relapse prevention)
Level 2: Outpatient (once per week visits)
Level 3: Intensive outpatient (2 or more visits per week)
Level 4: Intensive integrated services (day treatment, partial hospitalization, wraparound services)
Level 5: Non-secure, 24-hour medically monitored service (group home, residential treatment facility)
Level 6: Secure 24-hour medical management (inpatient psychiatric or highly programmed residential facility)

LEARNING POINTS

1. Many epidemiological surveys and national studies in India have made it evident that substance use is highly prevalent among the adolescent population.

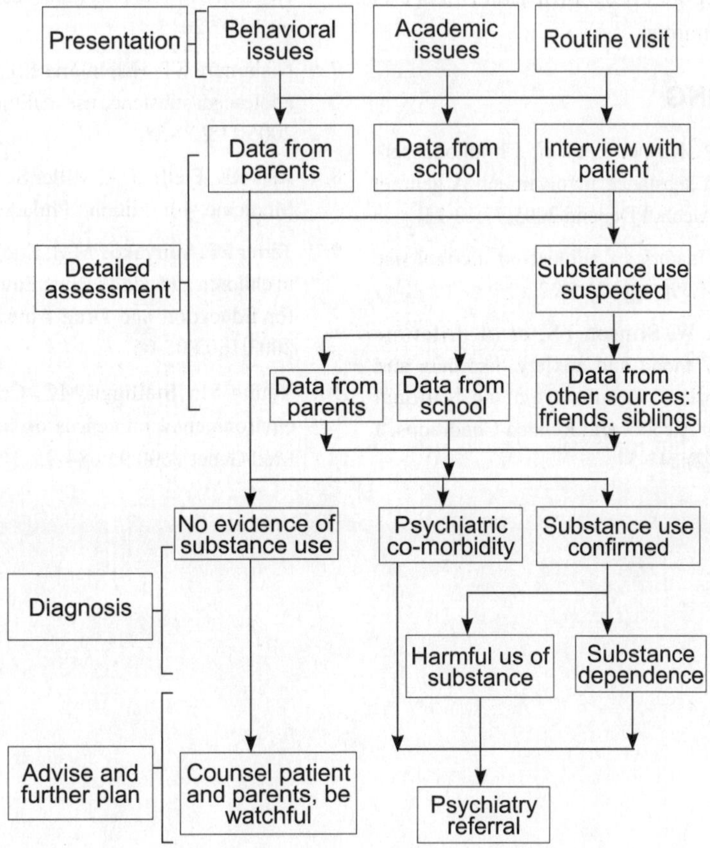

Figure 8.2.1: Assessment of adolescent with substance use disorder

Table 8.2.10: Management overview

Diagnosis	*Harmful use of substance*	*Substance dependence*	*Comorbid psychiatric disorder*
Acute management	Counseling of patient for the need for intervention	• Withdrawal management and detoxification • Anti-craving medications	• Behavioral management • Psychopharmacological intervention • Ensure safety of the patient
Follow-up	• Brief parents about ground situation and address anxieties of caregivers/parents • Psychoeducation of parents/caregivers about substance use disorders, psychiatric comorbidity • Prioritize areas for intervention and design individualized management plan after discussion with patient, parents/caregivers • Motivation enhancement therapy • Substance specific counseling • Family therapy • Cognitive behavioral therapy • Psychopharmacological management if required • Regular follow-up • Be watchful for substance use, changes in behavior		

2. The primary physician, who is usually the first contact can make a significant difference in the prognosis of their patients by identifying problematic substance use as early as possible.
3. Physician dealing with adolescents should be familiar with presenting picture, method of assessment, screening, and available management options.

Acknowledgment

We acknowledge guidance given by Prof Emeritus (Dr) Vihang N Vahia for this chapter.

SUGGESTED READING

1. Clark DB, Cornelius JR, Kirisci L, *et al.* Childhood risk categories for adolescent substance involvement: A general liability typology. Drug Alcohol Depend 2005;77:13-21.
2. Clark DB. The natural history of adolescent alcohol use disorders. Addiction 2004;99(suppl 2):5-22.
3. Conway KP, Compton W, Stinson FS, *et al.* Lifetime comorbidity of DSM-IV mood and anxiety disorders and specific drug use disorders: Results from the National Epidemiologic Survey on Alcohol and Related Conditions. J Clin Psychiatry 2006;67(2):247-57.
4. Deas D, Riggs P, Langenbucher J, *et al.* Adolescents are not adults: Developmental considerations in alcohol users. Alcohol Clin Exp Res 2000;24:232-37.
5. Kandel DB, Johnson JG, Bird HR, *et al.* Psychiatric disorders associated with substance use among children and adolescents: Findings from the Methods for the Epidemiology of Child and Adolescent Mental Disorders (MECA) Study. J Abnorm Child Psychol 1997;25:121-32.
6. Ministry of Women and Child Development, New Delhi. Report: Working group on development of children for eleventh five year plan (2007-2012). http:/wcd.nic.in/ Acsessed on 10/07/2015.
7. Nishimura ST, Hishinuma ES, Else RN, *et al.* Ethnicity and adolescent substance use. Cultur Divers Ethnic Minor Psychol 2005;11:239-58.
8. Ries RK, Fiellin DA, Miller SC, *et al.* Principles of Addiction Medicine, 4th Edition. Philadelphia: Lippincott, 2009.
9. Tarter RE, Vanyukov MM. Etiology of substance use disorder in children and adolescents: Emerging findings from the Center for Education and Drug Abuse Research. Am J Psychiatry 2003;160:805-06.
10. Young SE, Stallings MC, Corley RP, *et al.* Genetic and environmental influences on behavioral disinhibition. Am J Med Genet 2000;96:684-95.

Depression and Prevention of Suicide

8.3

Swati Y Bhave, Himabindu Singh

INTRODUCTION

Adolescents have a very high incidence of depression and are at high risk of suicide due the inherent stresses and strains that occur during this transition from childhood to adulthood (see Box 8.3.1). There are too many changes happening on all fronts–biological, physical, sexual, psychosocial, emotional, academic etc. Adolescents need to be empowered with coping skills and resilience to cope up with this transition. Since depression can adversely affect their development on all fronts, it is very important to pick up the signs and start treatment early (see Box 8.3.2).

A large majority of adolescents who are fortunate to have stable home and school environments with supportive parents and teachers, manage to overcome the various challenges without too much difficulty. But a considerable number, who lack such support systems and are not able to build up their resilience, cannot handle this; and hence depression is one of the most common mental health problems in this age group. Severe depression can lead to suicidal thoughts and many young lives have been lost over very insignificant issues which could have been easily rectified with timely intervention and support.

Box 8.3.1: Factors that can cause depression

Body image issues: Impact of advertisements, media and peer pressure.

Personality: Low self-esteem, self-criticism, poor coping skills (need for life skill education).

Family problems: Domestic violence, abuse of all types, dysfunctional families, divorce of parents, death of loved ones.

Relationships: Broken romantic relationships and friendships.

School and peer problems: Bullying, academic pressures, teacher's partiality.

Genetic/Hereditary/Biological.

Box 8.3.2: Medical causes that can manifest with the symptoms of depression

- *Infections:* Many viral infections and post-viral syndromes
- *Endocrine disorders:* Hypothyroidism
- *Metabolic disorders*
- *Electrolyte dysfunctions*
- *Drugs*: Anti-hypertensives
- Substance abuse
- *Neurological disorders*
- Miscellaneous

It is thus very important for adolescents themselves and the stakeholders dealing with adolescents, be it parents, teachers or clinicians, to understand the various manifestations of adolescent depression and suicidal intentions so that timely interventions can be done. This chapter aims at reviewing the important aspects of these issues in clinical practice.

Mood swings are normal in adolescence as they have a hyperactive limbic system and *feeling low or adolescent blues* are also normal part of growing up. It is very important to distinguish 'adolescent blues' from depression and bipolar disorders (Table 8.3.1). Feeling sad and upset occasionally is a phenomenon that everyone goes through. If the symptoms are severe and last for more than 3-6 weeks; do not seem to have any apparent cause or trigger; come up suddenly and are very different from the adolescent's usual personality; then one must take a note and see that assessment is done by a clinician or mental health professional.

Depression is described based on the severity, duration and type of symptoms.

The Diagnostic and Statistical Manual (DSM) of Mental Disorders criteria are the most often used to diagnose and classify depression.

There are no separate criteria for adolescents. Often the two DSM-IV criteria that are modified for youth are: (i) irritable mood in place of depressed mood in adult, and (ii) failure to attain expected weight gain may replace the weight loss criteria.

DSM-IV primary diagnostic categories involving depression include: (1) major depression, (2) dysthymia (persistent mild depression), and (3) adjustment disorder.

Table 8.3.1: Depression vs feeling 'Blue'		
Features	*Clinical depression*	*Sadness or feeling 'blue'*
Essential difference	A mental illness that needs treatment	Mood swings normal in adolescents. It may be a normal reaction to their transition stage of life.
Symptoms	*Multiple:* Emotional, social, behavioral, cognitive, or somatic dysfunction	*Single:* Mainly sad mood.
Duration	Persists for two to six weeks or more	Brief.
Suicide potential	Very high potential for suicide	Rarely produces suicidal thoughts.
Treatment	Responds to psychotherapy and specific medications	Responds to simple confiding to a good listener. Diverting into a positive activity gives time to bounce back.

Source: Bhave SY, Sovani A. Chapter 20. Adolescence. In: Parthasarathy A, Gupta A, Borker AS, Dharmapalan D (Eds). Partha's Management Protocols in Pediatric and Adolescent Practice. New Delhi: Jaypee Brothers Medical Publishers Pvt Ltd 2016: 417-45.

HISTORY TAKING

A detailed history helps to elicit a lot of signs and symptoms of depression in adolescents (Tables 8.3.1 and 8.3.2).

It is very important to remember that adolescent depression can often be missed. Unlike adults, depressed adolescents may not look sad and in fact may put up a mask of happiness to prevent adults from recognizing their depressed state. It is useful to do a HEADDSSS screening of every adolescent seen in the clinic (for more details see Chapter 1.3) as it gives pointers to the adolescents' state of mind on all aspects of his/her life and may help in diagnosing depression. It is important to analyse the personality of the adolescents as there are many risk factors–low self-esteem, poor coping skills or lack of resilience, impulse control disorders etc. Depression as a syndrome or symptom can co-exist with other mental health issues, the most common being anxiety disorders. Adolescents who are specially challenged or suffering from a psychiatric illness or indulging in substance abuse are also at a higher risk of depression and suicide. Every depressed adolescent should be asked a direct question: *"Have you thought of harming yourself?"* and if the answer is yes, the risk of suicide should be assessed and appropriate referral should be done (see Box 8.3.2).

Table 8.3.2: Symptoms of depression in younger adolescent
• Their emotions are very labile or brittle. They become very irritable and small things annoy them. They may have temper tantrums, keep whining, and may have bouts of crying.
• Because of their behavior they are often rejected by peers or also lose old friends.
• They are very restless–constantly moving or fidgeting or pacing up and down.
• They may become withdrawn; sit at home; do not like company; and become isolated from peers.
• Sleep disturbances are common due to insomnia; they may sleep during daytime.
• Bedwetting may restart in those who had a past history. It may also start in those who never had bedwetting.

Table 8.3.3 describes the salient features of depression in an older adolescent.

Media publicity of an attempted or completed suicide of a peer or a close friend can also have an effect leading to *copycat suicides.*

INVESTIGATIONS

There are screening questionnaires for picking up depressive state of mind e.g. Beckman's inventory for depression. It is important for a clinician to remember that there are certain medical causes for depression leading to suicide and appropriate investigations should be done to rule them out (see Box 8.3.2).

MANAGEMENT

Mild depression can be managed with counseling and psychotherapy. But for moderate and severe depression medications will be required in addition.

Counseling and psychotherapy are required for both the adolescent and his/her family as there are many factors at home which may be the cause of depression.

Medical Treatment

Before deciding the choice of anti-depressants it is important to remember that specific neurotransmitter systems may not be fully developed until adulthood and high levels of hormones during puberty may decrease the effectiveness of anti-depressants.

Selective serotonin-reuptake inhibitors (SSRIs) are best suited to the adolescent age group. This is because the dosages are easy to titrate and adjust; they can be given in once a day schedule and have minimal side effects as compared to other drugs. Due to high risk of fatal

Table 8.3.3: Signs of depression in older adolescents
Increased irritability, emotional outbursts, moodiness, anger, frustration and hostility
Older adolescents often take out their anger on family by being critical, sarcastic and abusive.
They are apprehensive that their family may reject them; hence as a defense mechanism will start showing rejection.
Frequent absences from school and poor school performance
Causing "trouble" at home/school may be a sign of depression.
Poor concentration
Difficulty in concentrating on school work, following conversations or even watching television (TV).
Behavior changes
Restlessness, fidgeting or pacing,
Episodes of crying fear, tension and anxiety
Loss of interest or pleasure
During interaction with others or most activities.
Loss of interest in things which were previously found enjoyable.
Feel discouraged about oneself, and lack of confidence.
Very self-critical
Excessive guilt or inappropriate self-blame.
Low self-esteem.
Unhappiness
Sadness, despair, emptiness, hopelessness, worthlessness and helplessness.
Lack of energy
Fatigue or tired most of the time.
Somatic complaints
There may be many physical symptoms like aches and pains in various parts of the body without any organic cause.
These point towards psychosomatic illness.
Major change in eating and/or sleeping
Too little or too much sleep.
Up all night watching TV; difficulty getting up in the morning; and sleeping during the day.
Loss of appetite or eating too much–leading to weight loss or weight gain.
Alcohol and drug abuse
A way to "medicate" themselves or to escape bad feelings.
Self-injury
Cutting, accident-proneness and driving problems are common.
High risk sexual behavior
Depressed adolescents are more likely to indulge in sexual gratification as a solution to feel happy.

overdosage tricyclic anti-depressants should be avoided in this age group.

SSRI should be started at half the adult dose (e.g. 10 mg of fluoxetine, citalopram, or paroxetine per day) and continued for a week. This helps to tide over the side effects. The dose is then adjusted to equal to 20 mg of fluoxetine. This should then be continued for another 3 weeks. This drug takes four weeks to attain a steady state. Hence dose changes should not be made at a shorter duration. Higher doses than those recommended for adults may have to be given because the metabolism of SSRIs is faster in adolescents. The chance of relapse is high if given for less than 6 months to a year.

Many adolescents are not compliant with the drug treatment as it affects their capacity to study due to a feeling of being zonked out.

Assessing Risk of Suicide and Prevention

The major risks of depression are suicidal thoughts and suicidal attempts (see Box 8.3.3 for details). In every

Box 8.3.3: Suicide	
Suicide is the conscious act of self-induced end of life by an individual who perceives this act as the best solution.	
It is a way out of a problem or crisis that is invariably causing intense suffering.	
Suicide is associated with a feeling of helplessness and unbearable stress, and need for escape.	
Suicide is a permanent solution to a temporary problem and a preventable loss of a young life.	
It is important to look for non-lethal suicidal behavior which is a precursor to suicide.	
Triggers for suicide can be very minor events (from the perception of adults) like being refused a mobile phone, or permission to go for an overnight picnic.	
It may also due to major events such as loss of a loved one, rejection from a romantic relationship, academic failure or performance which is below expected.	
Non-lethal suicide behavior which can be precursor to suicide	
Suicidal ideation	**Suicide threats**
• Thoughts about wishing to kill oneself; making plans; thoughts about the impact of one's suicide on others. • Not all children or young adolescents appreciate that suicide may result in irreversible death. (This should not influence the clinician in judging seriousness of the ideation).	• Utterances made to others that indicate an intent to commit suicide. • May be accompanied by actions. • In a young child/adolescent the most commonly this is a threat to jump out of a window, run into traffic, or to stab himself/herself.
Para-suicide—Non-fatal suicidal acts with non-lethal intent	
The younger the child/adolescent, the less complex and more easily available are methods used to enact suicidal impulses.	

case of suspected or clinically evident depression, it is important to ask a direct question *"Have you ever thought or harming yourself?"*

If the answer is yes, a detailed history should be taken with additional questions as follows:

- *Have you made any plans?*
- *Have you ever made an attempt?*

If you get affirmative answers to any of the above, this means that there is a high risk of a suicide in this adolescent and this should be treated as a psychiatric emergency (Box 8.3.4). The parents should be immediately referred to a psychiatrist. Additional support also should be provided with the help of clinical psychologist and counselors. The adolescent should also be guided to use the suicide helplines. Many suicides have been prevented by the person phoning the helpline when he or she gets thoughts of committing suicide.

Urgent psychiatric admission will be required if there are danger signals (Boxes 8.3.4 and 8.3.5).

Prevention of Suicide by Awareness and Education

Awareness Programs in Schools and Colleges; for Parents and Teachers; and in the Community

- Awareness that depression is a mental illness that can be treated with timely medications and psychotherapy.
- Removing stigma of going to mental health professional for depression.
- Increasing awareness about signs and symptoms about depression and suicidal attempts.
- This can be achieved by teaching adolescent stakeholders and adolescents themselves about the flag signs of depression (Tables 8.3.2 and 8.3.3) and appropriate management to prevent suicide attempts (see Boxes 8.3.3, 8.3.4, 8.3.5 and 8.3.6).

Box 8.3.4: Need for urgent psychiatric referral
If the patient is harboring suicidal feelings or thoughts.
If s/he is indulging in self-harming activities.
If the behavior is dangerous to others: violence, aggression, threats or destruction.
If there is addiction to alcohol or other drugs.
If there are weird or any abnormal behavior which is very very unusual.

Box 8.3.5: Warning signs of suicide
• Preoccupation with death or dying.
• Expressing–*I wish I could end this pain or wish to go to sleep and never wake up.*
• Expressing–*I wish to die suddenly or be killed in an accident.*
• Expressing vague thoughts of suicide or making suicide threats.
• Talking about collection and discussion of information on suicide methods.
• Discussing plans to commit suicide.
• Suddenly start giving away prized possessions.
• Suddenly start making up or asking for forgiveness from people they have hurt or harmed in the past.

Box 8.3.6: Tips for parents, teachers and peers for dealing with warning signs of suicide

Do's	*Don'ts*
• Voice concern and show empathy.	Take it lightly, laugh, ridicule or joke.
• Ask if the person has made a plan.	Challenge or dare the person.
• If you are a teacher or peer, inform parents immediately.	Act shocked.
• Take urgent professional help.	Argue or debate about the moral issues of the proposed action and the reasons for the same.
• Call a doctor.	Give a promise to keep this a secret.
• Go to a psychiatric facility–emergency services.	Assume it is a passing thought and think that the situation will resolve with time on its own.

WHO Life Skill Education Program

This will empower adolescents and help to help to improve communication between parents and adolescents.

LEARNING POINTS

- It is important to distinguish between adolescent blues and mood swings which are normal at this stage.
- Parents and teachers need to be educated to pick up signs of adolescent depression so that timely referral is done and adequate treatment is given.
- Adolescent depression negatively affects their development.
- Severe and chronic depression has high risk of suicide.
- Peer education is useful to help to understand depression of a colleague or friend and the flag signs of depression and suicide so that they can help their peers.

SUGGESTED READING

1. American Psychiatric Association. Diagnostic and Statistical Manual of Mental Disorders, 5th edition (DSM-5). Washington DC; APA, 2013.
2. Bhave SY, Nagpal J. Anxiety and Depression in College Youth; Pediatr Clin N Am 2005;52:97-134.
3. Goldenring JM, Rosen DS. Getting into adolescent heads: An essential update. Contemp Pediatr 2004;21(1):64-90.
4. Gupta RP, Bhave SY. Depression in Adolescents. In: Bhave SY, Ed. Bhave's Textbook of Adolescent Medicine, 1st edition, New Delhi; Jaypee Brothers Medical Publishers Pvt Ltd. 2006;770-78.
5. Hazell P, O'Connell D, Heathcote D, Robertson J, Henry D. Efficacy of tricyclic drugs in treating child and adolescent depression: A meta-analysis. Br Med J 1995;310:897-901.
6. Pataki CS. Mood Disorders and Suicide in Children and Adolescents. In: Sadock BJ, Sadock VA (Eds). Kaplan and Sadock's Comprehensive Textbook of Psychiatry, Vol 2, 7th Edition. Philadelphia; Lippincott Williams and Wilkins 2000; 2740-57.
7. Shastri PC, Shastri J. Chapter 23.6 Adolescent Suicide and Suicide Prevention. In: Bhave SY, Ed. Bhave's Textbook of Adolescent Medicine; 1st edition. New Delhi; Jaypee Brothers Medical Publishers Pvt Ltd 2006;778-82.

8.4

Eating Disorders

Sangeeta Yadav, Kaviya Lakshmipathy

INTRODUCTION

Eating disorders are psychiatric disorders characterized by severe disturbances and distortions in body image with abnormal eating patterns and behaviors. Patients with eating disorders develop abnormal eating habits that threaten their well-being and even their lives. The typical age of onset is adolescence or young adulthood, with peaks at 14–15 years and at 18 years of age. The age of onset of anorexia is a little earlier than bulimia, which has its onset during late adolescence. The onset of puberty has been implicated with the development of these disorders.

Like other psychiatric conditions, these also result from a complex interplay between environmental and biological factors. Adolescents in particular, experience a higher incidence of eating disorders due to their easy susceptibility to the environmental and biological influences. The diagnosis of eating disorders, especially in the initial stages and milder forms, remains a challenge in adolescent age, as they have to be differentiated from normal variations in eating. Eating disorders are the deadliest of all psychological disorders—adolescents with bulimia have the highest risk of suicidal tendency. Various psychiatric conditions such as obsessive-compulsive disorders, depression and anxiety all play a role in the development of these disorders. Dancers, models and athletes have a higher prevalence of eating disorders.

In the past it was mainly seen in females; however currently an increase of these conditions in the male population is noted representing 25% of anorexia and bulimia and almost 40% of binge eaters. In India the exact prevalence is not known. According to some authors, the classic types of eating disorders are rarely seen in India. In 2007, around 1.25% of adolescent females were diagnosed to have one or other type of eating disorders mostly of milder variants e.g. psychogenic vomiting.

The classification of eating disorders is usually done as per the Diagnostic and Statistical Manual of Mental Disorders, edition 5 (DSM-5) as follows:

- The major eating disorders are anorexia nervosa and bulimia nervosa.
- Binge eating disorders, pica and rumination disorders have been added to the DSM-5 classification.
- Other disordered eating behaviors are classified as 'other specified feeding or eating disorders'.

Anorexia Nervosa

Anorexia nervosa (AN) is diagnosed when there is persistent restriction of food intake leading to significantly low body weight along with an intense fear of gaining weight. It should be associated with altered body image, overestimation of body size and shape. Anorexia nervosa is of two subtypes:

- **Restrictive:** Excessive dieting and excessive exercising.
- **Binge purge:** Intermittent overeating and as a compensatory behavior, vomiting or use of laxatives.

Bulimia Nervosa

Bulimia is characterized by recurrent episodes of binge eating followed by compensatory behaviors to prevent weight gain, e.g. self-induced vomiting, use of laxatives, or diuretics. A binge episode is defined as eating a larger amount of food, in a discrete period of time, with a sense of lack of control over eating. According to DSM-5, the episodes of binging and compensatory behaviors should occur at least once a week for 3 months and exclusive of the episodes of anorexia nervosa.

Binge Eating Disorders

This disorder is characterized by occurrence of binge eating episodes as in bulimia but without compensatory behaviors. Binge episodes are characterized by eating more rapidly, eating large amounts of food even when not feeling hungry, feeling uncomfortably full. There is marked distress regarding binging after the episode. These episodes should be present at least once a week for three months.

Pica

It is the persistent eating of non-food substances, inappropriate for the developmental level and cultural practices, for a period of least one month.

Rumination Disorders

It is the repeated regurgitation of food occurring for least one month. Medical conditions causing regurgitation (e.g. gastroesophageal reflux disease) should be ruled out before making a diagnosis of rumination disorder.

Other Specified Feeding or Eating Disorders

Eating behaviors that cause clinically significant distress or complications, but does not fit into the criteria of classic forms of eating disorders, are included in this category.

Examples include:

- Binge eating occurring in a lesser frequency.
- Frequent purging episodes without binge eating.
- Night eating syndrome, in which the patient awakens in the night and eats, even when not feeling hungry.

PATHOPHYSIOLOGY

Biologic and psychosocial factors are implicated in the pathophysiology of eating disorders, but the causes and mechanisms underlying eating disorders remain uncertain even now.

The bio-psychosocial model of eating disorders explains the influence of personality traits, genetics, environmental influences and the hormonal and biochemical changes in the development of these disorders (Figures 8.4.1 and 8.4.2).

Personality Traits

Adolescents diagnosed with eating disorders have low self-esteem, feelings of inadequacy or lack of control in life, fear of becoming fat and being rejected by the peers. Almost all of them are depressed, anxious or angry. They rarely disobey and are usually aloof from others. Patients with anorexia, in particular are perfectionists, achievement-oriented good students and excellent athletes

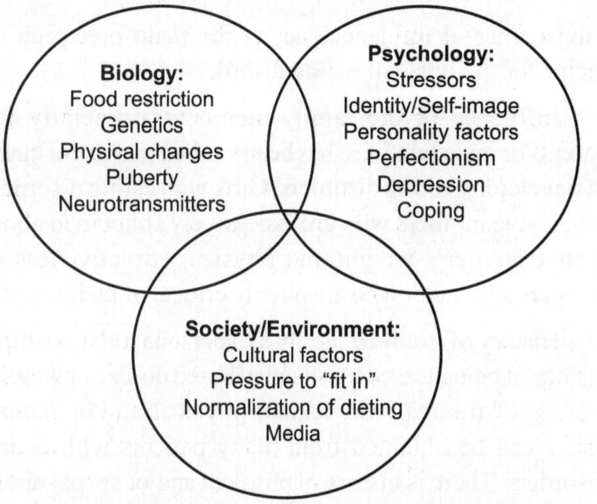

Figure 8.4.1: Factors influencing eating disorders

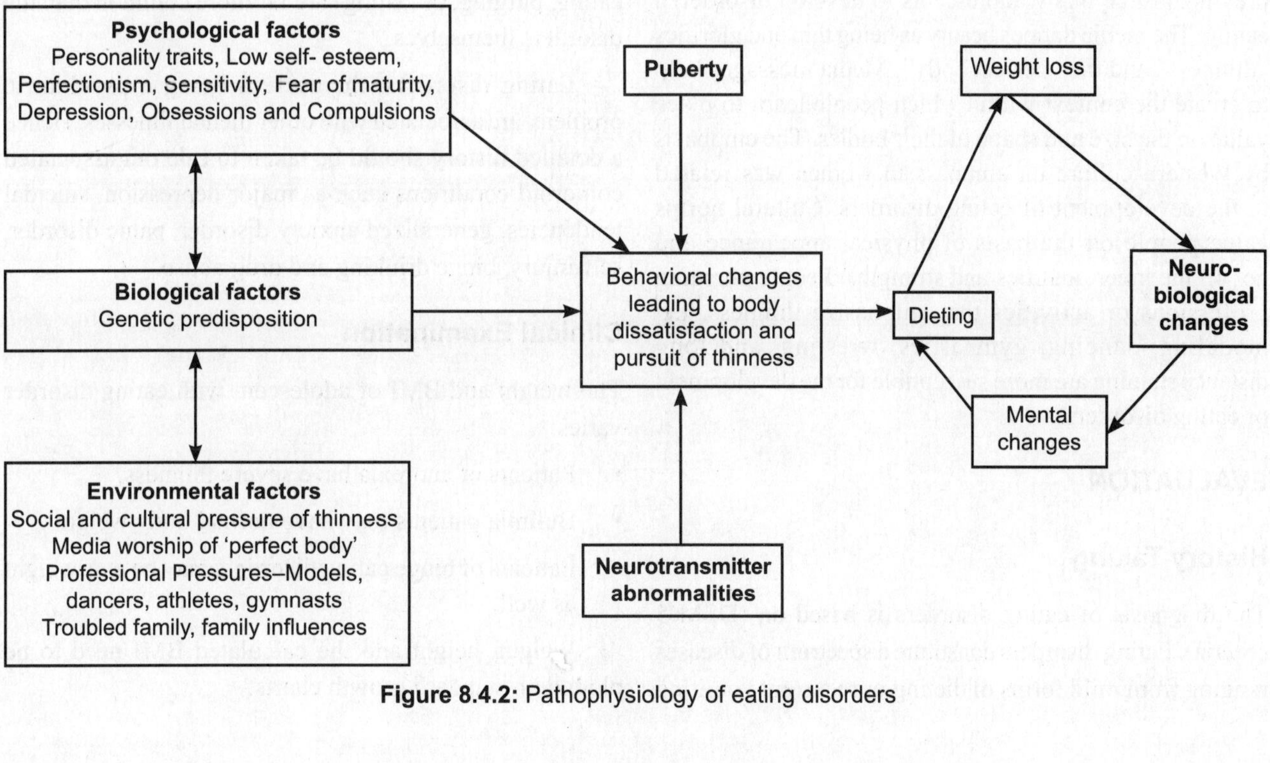

Figure 8.4.2: Pathophysiology of eating disorders

and get involved in competitive careers. Those with bulimia usually have obsessions and compulsions, and have post-traumatic stress disorders.

Genetic Factors

Genetic factors may predispose adolescents to eating disorders. Various studies have shown increased risk among first-degree biological relatives having eating disorders. There is also an increased risk of mood disorders among first-degree relatives of patients with anorexia nervosa, especially in the binge eating/purging type. Twin studies show that concordant rates for monozygotic twins are significantly higher than those for dizygotic twins.

Environmental Factors

Environmental influences act as the main precipitating factor for the onset of eating disorders.

Influence of the family members, especially the parents or male relatives, has been studied as a major cause of developing eating disorders. Girls with eating disorders often have mothers who are excessively concerned about their daughter's weight and physical attractiveness or brothers and father who are overtly critical of their weight.

History of troubled family and personal relationships, history of being teased or ridiculed based on size or weight, history of trauma, and sexual, physical and/or mental abuse can be obtained from many patients with eating disorders. There is history of physical and/or sexual abuse in 60-75% of all bulimia nervosa patients.

Social factors involving the media and cultural pressures force many adolescents to develop disordered eating. The media defines beauty as being thin and glorifies "thinness" and the "perfect body". Media messages help to create the context within which people learn to place value on the size and shape of their bodies. The emphasis by Western culture on slimness in women was related to the development of eating disorders. Cultural norms value people on the basis of physical appearance and not on the inner qualities and strengths. People pursuing professions or activities that emphasize thinness, i.e. modeling, dancing, gymnastics, wresting, and long distance running are more susceptible for the development of eating disorders.

EVALUATION

History Taking

The diagnosis of eating disorders is based on (DSM-5 criteria). Eating disorders constitute a spectrum of diseases ranging from mild forms of dieting or recurrent vomiting to full blown diseases like anorexia nervosa or bulimia nervosa.

Presenting Complaints

1. Eating disorders usually are noticed by parents. It should be suspected in an adolescent who eats only low fat or low carb foods, eats very less quantity of food, and indulges in severe exercise routine. These behaviors may be seen in normal individuals also, but it becomes pathological when associated with body image distortion and when the habits of dieting and exercise become excessively more than normal.
2. Failure to achieve appropriate weight in growing children also should raise a suspicion of eating disorder.
3. Binging behavior or, overeating followed by prolonged periods of starving, applying diet plans very rigidly, feeling guilty after eating foods with high calories, and obsession of studying the food labels for the calorie contents, should also arise suspicion of presence of eating disorders.

Whenever an adolescent is suspected to have an eating disorder few screening questions need to be asked for arriving at the clinical diagnosis and assessing the severity and associated comorbidities present in the patient (Table 8.4.1).

History taking should include direct questions to elicit the diagnostic criteria for eating disorders. Individual symptoms characteristic of each disorder (such as binge eating, purging, or fasting) are far more common than the disorders themselves.

Eating disorders, themselves being a psychiatric problem, are associated with other mental illnesses. Hence a detailed history should be taken to rule out associated comorbid conditions such as major depression, suicidal tendencies, generalized anxiety disorder, panic disorder, self-injury, binge drinking and drug abuse.

Clinical Examination

The weight and BMI of adolescent with eating disorder varies:

- Patients of anorexia have severe thinness.
- Bulimia patients may have normal body weight.
- Patients of binge eating disorders may be overweight as well.

Weight, height and the calculated BMI need to be plotted on standard growth charts.

Table 8.4.1: Screening for eating disorders	
1.	Are you constantly thinking about food?
2.	Is it difficult to concentrate on the daily tasks of studying or work because of food and weight thoughts?
3.	Do you worry about what your last meal is doing to your body?
4.	Do you experience guilt or shame around eating?
5.	Is it difficult for you to eat in public?
6.	Do you count calories every time you eat or drink?
7.	When others tell you that you are too thin, do you still feel fat?
8.	If you see yourself as thin, do you still obsess about your stomach, hips, thighs, or buttocks being too big?
9.	Do you weigh yourself several times daily?
10.	Does the number on your scale determine your mood and outlook, for the day?

Any unrecognized organic illness causing weight loss should be ruled out with a proper history and examination.

Weight loss would be intentional in eating disorders and unintentional in organic conditions. Weight loss might also be due to increased energy needs during growth and exercise.

Adolescents with eating disorders need to be evaluated extensively for the precipitating causes, environmental and family issues, associated illness, complications associated with these disorders.

It is not essential to find all the symptoms and signs in a given patient. The milder varieties of eating disorders may not have any abnormal signs on physical examination. The clinical findings for the classic anorexia and bulimia nervosa are given in the Tables 8.4.2 and 8.4.3.

The major forms of anorexia and bulimia are associated with many medical complications (Table 8.4.4). An adolescent with eating disorder might present for the first time to a physician with any of these complications. The complications result mainly from caloric restriction and purging or use of laxatives.

Investigations

Eating disorder is a clinical diagnosis; hence no definitive diagnostic tests are available for diagnosing them. However, given the multi-organ system effects of starvation, a thorough medical evaluation is warranted. Basic tests include those mentioned in Table 8.4.5. If any organic cause for weight loss is suspected, then additional investigations need to be done.

MANAGEMENT

When intervened in a timely manner, the condition and associated complications can be treated. Hence early recognition and medical risk management in the case of individuals with eating disorders are important.

Table 8.4.2: Signs and symptoms in anorexia nervosa

Symptoms	*Signs*
Restricted food intake of very low calorie foods, scheduled meal plan, no snacks, with excess exercise	Thin, cachectic, scaphoid abdomen, atrophic breasts, loss of muscle and subcutaneous fat
Feels fat with body image distortions	Hypothermia, cold extremities, acrocyanosis and pedal edema
Symptoms like feeling tired and weak due to low metabolism	Dry skin, orange yellow hands, lanugo type hair and scalp hair loss
Dizziness, fainting and palpitations	Bradycardia, hypotension and orthostatic pulse difference
Depression, anxiety and obsessive-compulsive disorder traits	Depressed mood, irritability and anxiety

Table 8.4.3: Clinical findings in bulimia nervosa

Symptoms	*Signs*
Calorie intake is normal to high, binges of high calorie food, frequent dieting with periods of over-eating, and use of purgatives and laxatives	Thin to overweight
Drive for thinness is less than AN, mainly avoids gaining weight	Less hypometabolic state than AN
Self-injurious behavior, depression, and post-traumatic stress disorder traits may be seen	Calluses over knuckles (Russell sign), subconjunctival hemorrhage, erosion of dental enamel, enlarged salivary glands and absent gag
Dizziness, palpitations and fainting	Depression, more likely suicidal than AN
Cramps and diarrhea with laxative use	Increased bowel sounds if recent laxative use

Table 8.4.4: Medical complications in eating disorders

Complications due to purging	*Complications due to caloric restriction*
Fluid and electrolyte imbalance: Hypokalemia, hyponatremia and hypochloremic alkalosis	Sinus bradycardia, T wave inversions, ST segment depression, arrhythmias, and pericardial effusions in severely malnourished
Use of laxatives: Depletion of potassium bicarbonate, causing metabolic acidosis, increased BUN and predisposition to renal stones from dehydration, hyperuricemia, hypocalcemia, hypomagnesemia and chronic dehydration	Delayed gastric emptying, slowed GI motility, constipation, bloating, hypercholesterolemia, abnormal LFT and fatty liver (reversible with weight gain) Re-feeding syndrome
Chronic vomiting causing esophagitis, dental erosions, Mallory-Weiss tears, and rarely esophageal or gastric rupture	Increased BUN, renal stones, and body sodium and potassium depletion (starvation)
Use of ipecac may cause irreversible myocardial damage and a diffuse myositis	Leucopenia, nutritional anemia and thrombocytopenia
With *laxative withdrawal*, may get fluid retention	Euthyroid sick syndrome, amenorrhea and osteopenia

Table 8.4.5: Investigations for evaluating eating disorders

Tests	*Significance*
Complete blood counts	Usually normal; high if dehydration is present
Hemoglobin	Low
Total leukocyte counts	Normal; if high other chronic diseases precipitating anorexic states like SLE to be ruled out
ESR	
Serum electrolytes	Hyponatremia, hypokalemia
Blood gases	Metabolic alkalosis because of vomiting, acidosis if laxatives abused
Renal function tests	Normal; elevated urea if dehydration
Liver function tests	Protein and albumin normal as diet contains more of proteins. Mild elevation of enzymes
ECG	Bradycardia, ST elevation, QT prolongation
Chest X-ray	Osteopenia, in cases of recurrent vomiting, pneumomediastinum due to esophageal tears

Based on the severity of the eating disorder and the associated medical complications, the decision to treat a patient on outpatient basis or after admission as an indoor patient is based on certain criteria (Table 8.4.6).

Management of Adolescents by Themselves

The adolescent's opinion about her/his body shape or image should be enquired for. Patients with anorexia have a feeling of being overweight though they are lean. The adolescent's efforts to get into a lean body shape, dieting habits, exercise routine, body image distortion and indulging in healthy habits of participation in sports etc. to reduce weight need to be enquired in detail.

The adolescents with the disorders will not be willing to accept the fact that they are suffering from a disease and will be reluctant to undergo any treatment as it will result in weight gain. Symptom of the illness may not be recognized by the patients. Thus, they may be ambivalent about accepting the treatment.

Based on the psychological profile and evaluation, the adolescents will require long-term counseling and psychotherapy.

Table 8.4.6: Indication for hospitalization in eating disorders

Anorexia nervosa	*Bulimia nervosa*
<75% ideal body weight, or ongoing weight loss despite intensive management	Syncope
Refusal to eat	Serum potassium concentration <3.2 mEq/L
Body fat <10%	Serum chloride concentration <88 mEq/L
Heart rate <50/min daytime; <45/per min night-time	Esophageal tears
Systolic pressure <90 mm Hg	Cardiac arrhythmias including prolonged QTc
Orthostatic changes in pulse (>20/per min) or BP (>10 mm Hg)	Hypothermia
Temperature <96°F	Intractable vomiting, hematemesis
Arrhythmia	Suicide risk

Modified from: Rome SE, Fisher MM, Kaplan WD, *et al.* Committee on Adolescence. Identifying and Treating Eating Disorders. Pediatrics 2003;111:204-11.

Counseling of Parents

Parents/guardians are the frontline help-seekers. They recognize the symptoms of these disorders and contact the physician. Counseling the family members about the nature of illness and reassuring them that they did not cause the illness is important.

Eating disorders can be treated; but they often require long-term therapy and psychosocial support for the patient. The goal is to stabilize the patient's life and it requires a multidisciplinary team approach which consists of the following:

Primary Physician

- This is the first point of contact with the patient and the relatives and her/his role in management of eating disorders becomes crucial. In addition to establishing the diagnosis she/he has to refer and coordinate with a team. They need to monitor weight, and provide education regarding physical aspects of eating disorders. She/he also needs to diagnose the associated comorbidities or complications, if any, and institute therapy and monitor the progress of the treatment.

Nutritional Specialist

- Provides education, nutrition/dietary plans and options, assess the caloric requirements, and helps in strategizing food related activities.

Mental Health Specialist

- Psychiatrist and counselors have an important role to play in addressing individual and family needs, focus on affective issues, medication management, body image issues and teaching coping skills to the adolescent.

School Personnel

- They assist with reintegrating into more normal functioning.

Family and School Support

- The support of parents and friends is crucial in the proper treatment of these disorders in adolescents.

LEARNING POINTS

1. Eating disorders are one of the most common psychiatric problems faced by adolescents, especially females, though now there is increasing prevalence in males as well.
2. The DSM-5 criteria are used for diagnosing eating disorders.
3. Adolescents have body image issues, which is aggravated by the media and social networks influencing their eating behavior patterns and lifestyle changes. It might start as a simple dieting and progress to a full-blown eating disorder.
4. They are ranked among the ten leading causes of disability among young women, have the highest levels of treatment seeking, inpatient hospitalization, substance abuse, depression, suicide attempts, and mortality of the most common psychiatric syndromes.
5. There are limited studies and data regarding eating disorders in our country. Also, in developing countries like India, mild and non-specific eating disorders are more common such as persistent vomiting, weight loss, amenorrhea rather than anorexia or bulimia. Hence diagnosing them becomes a greater challenge.
6. Treating a patient with eating disorder needs a holistic multidisciplinary approach with the physician playing the central role.

SUGGESTED READING

1. American Psychiatric Association. Diagnostic and Statistical Manual of Mental Disorders, 5th edition (DSM-5). Washington DC; APA, 2013.
2. Gonçalves J, Moreira EA, Trindade E, Fiates GM. Eating disorders in childhood and adolescence. Rev Paul Pediatr 2013;31(1):96-103.
3. Mammen P, Russell S, Russell PS. Prevalence of Eating Disorders and Psychiatric Comorbidity among Children and Adolescents. Indian Pediatr 2007;44:357-59.
4. Nicholls D, Lynn R, Viner R. Childhood eating disorders: British national surveillance study. Br J Psychiatry 2011;198:295-301.
5. Phillips EL, Pratt HD. Eating Disorders in College. Pediatr Clin N Am 2005;52:85-96.
6. Rome SE, Fisher MM, Kaplan WD, *et al.* Committee on Adolescence. Identifying and Treating Eating Disorders. Pediatrics 2003;111:204-11.
7. Upadhyay AA, Misra R, Parchwani DN, Maheria PB. Prevalence and risk factors for eating disorders in Indian adolescent females. Natl J Physiol Pharmacol 2014;4:153-57.

8.5

Autism Spectrum Disorders

Samir H Dalwai, Elyska De Sa

INTRODUCTION

Autism spectrum disorder (ASD) is the new term 'DSM-5' for what was previously known as pervasive developmental disorder (PDD) and includes autism, childhood disintegrative disorder, Asperger syndrome and PDD–not otherwise specified (PDD-NOS). Rett syndrome has been excluded as the gene responsible for it has been identified and specified. ASD may occur with or without genetic, medical, mental, behavioral or other neurodevelopmental disorders including language impairment, attention deficit hyperactivity disorder (ADHD), intellectual impairment. Comprehensive evaluation has four basic objectives (Figure 8.5.1).

HISTORY TAKING

Most adolescents would have received a diagnosis of ASD by the time they reach adolescence. However, some concerns worsen and some new concerns may manifest in adolescence.

The adolescent physician or pediatrician should start with a review of the developmental history, especially birth history, speech, language and communication milestones and social behavior (Table 8.5.1).

CLINICAL EXAMINATION

A thorough clinical examination by the adolescent pediatrician is a must, especially because routine findings may have been missed earlier due to lack of expertise to examine children and/or adolescents with autism. General examination yields a wealth of information and neurological examination needs to be detailed and thorough (Table 8.5.2).

INVESTIGATIONS

Medical tests are needed to rule out comorbid conditions (Table 8.5.3).

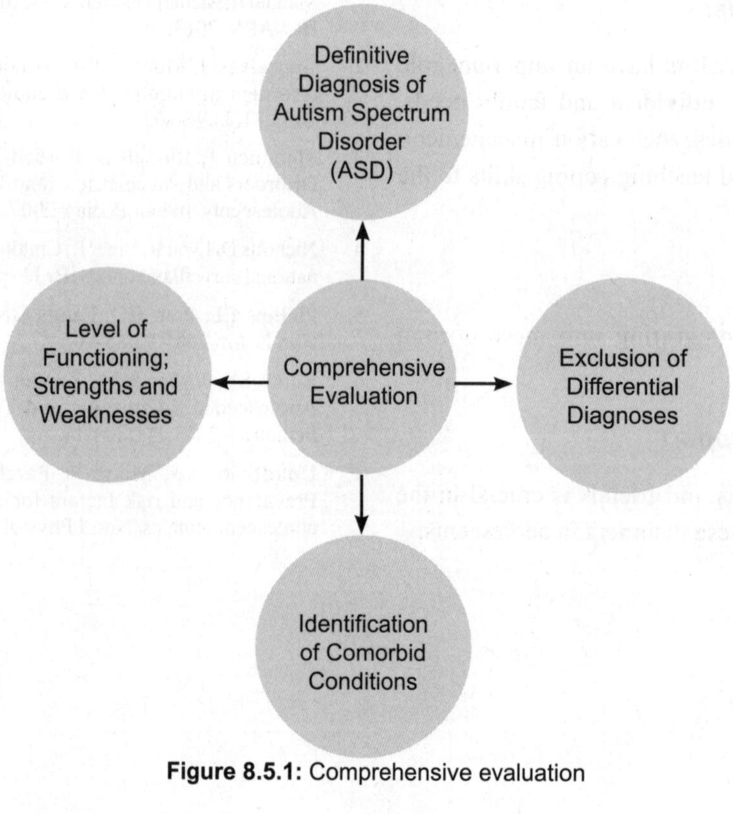

Figure 8.5.1: Comprehensive evaluation

Table 8.5.1: Symptoms of autism in adolescents

Social Communication	• Poor eye contact during conversation • Difficulty expressing themselves verbally or non-verbally • Poor intonation • Difficulty in talking about a range of topics but can speak about a favorite topic • Difficulty in reading non-verbal cues (body language, tone of voice, facial expressions) • Can't follow more than one or two steps of instructions at a time • Has trouble understanding the social rules of friendship and in making friends • Can't wait for their turn in a group conversation • Can't follow the rules of a game • Prefer to spend time on their own, rather than with friends • Poor comprehension of higher language (idioms, puns and proverbs) • Prefer playing with younger children or adults
Social Behavior	• Anxious/overwhelmed to try out something new • Difficulty in adjusting to new situations • Gets upset if routine is changed • Unusual/restricted interests • Unusual obsession with/attachment to objects or toys • Ritualistic behaviors and stereotypic body movements • Repetitive noises (grunts, humming and throat-clearing) • Unusually sensitive and excessively seeking or avoiding sensory stimulation (vibrating objects and deep pressure) • Difficulty in interpreting different sensations (Taste, sounds and smell)
Mood, Affect, Sleep, Eating Disorders	• Difficulty falling asleep, or regularly waking up at night • Depression • Aggressive behavior and poor frustration tolerance • Eating disorders • Tics
Neurological Symptoms	• Seizures • Focal deficits • Vision/audiological problems

Table 8.5.2: Clinical examination

Parameters	***Interpretation***
• Anthropometry (weight, height and head circumference)	A larger than normal head circumference is common in children with autism. Height and weight may be on the higher side which may make behavioral management difficult.
• Dysmorphic features	Various syndromes (mentioned below) can present with an autism like phenotype. Ruling these out is important as other serious medical conditions like cardiac defects, etc. could be associated with it.
• Signs of neurocutaneous syndromes	The association of neurofibromatosis, tuberous sclerosis and autism is well known.
• Signs of self-injury	Rett syndrome. Poor frustration tolerance.
• Fine motor coordination	Motor coordination deficits are seen in many autistic individuals

Table 8.5.3: Medical tests: To rule out comorbid conditions

Genetic evaluation	• Fragile X syndrome • Angelmann syndrome • Tuberous sclerosis • Smitz-Lemli-Opitz syndrome
Metabolic testing	• Phenylketonuria • Biotinidase deficiency • Disorders of purine metabolism • Mitochondrial disorders • Creatine deficiency
Neuroimaging/EEG	• To be done if neurological symptoms/signs are present. Not routinely recommended

Ancillary tests are needed to rule out differentials and/or comorbidities and define strengths and weaknesses (Box 8.5.1).

Box 8.5.1: Ancillary testing

- Vision and hearing assessment
- Speech and language communication assessment
- Sensorimotor and occupational therapy evaluation

DIAGNOSIS

Diagnosis includes the name and severity of the disorder (level 1, 2 or 3) which will depend on the (a) deficit seen in social communication, and (b) the severity of stereotyped repetitive behaviors.

Diagnosis is based on use of DSM-5 criteria (Table 8.5.4).

Degree of severity has to be assessed for further management (Table 8.5.5).

Accompanying or associated conditions that need to be specified in the diagnosis are listed in Table 8.5.6.

Various scales for assessment are depicted in Table 8.5.7.

Table 8.5.4: Diagnostic criteria (DSM-5)—Diagnosis of ASD requires all of the following

Social Communication and Social Interaction: • Persistent deficits in the above • Deficits seen in multiple settings • Must include deficits in all three areas (either currently or by history)	• Social-emotional reciprocity (e.g. failure of back-and-forth conversation; reduced sharing of interests and emotions) • Non-verbal communicative behaviors used for social interaction (e.g. poorly integrated verbal and non-verbal communication; abnormal eye contact or body language; poor understanding of gestures) • Developing, maintaining, and understanding relationships (e.g. difficulty in adjusting behavior to social setting; difficulty making friends; and lack of interest peers)
Behavior, Interests, or **Activities:** • Restricted, repetitive patterns • Must include ≥ 2 of the following (either currently or by history)	• Stereotyped or repetitive movements, use of objects, or speech (e.g, stereotypes, echolalia, ordering toys, etc.) • Insistence on sameness, unwavering adherence to routines, or ritualized patterns of behavior (verbal or non-verbal) • Highly restricted, fixated interests that are abnormal in strength or focus (e.g. preoccupation with certain objects; perseverative interests) • Increased or decreased response to sensory input or unusual interest in sensory aspects of the environment (e.g. adverse response to particular sounds; apparent indifference to temperature; excessive touching/smelling of objects)
• The symptoms must **impair function** (e.g. social, or academic) • The symptoms must be **present in the early developmental period**. However, they may become apparent only after social demands exceed limited capacity; in later life, symptoms may be masked by learned strategies. • The symptoms are not better explained by intellectual disability or global developmental delay.	

Table 8.5.5: Severity level of autism (DSM-5)

• Social communication/ interaction	• **Level 1** ("Requiring support")–Noticeable impairment without support • **Level 2** ("Requiring substantial support")–Marked deficits in communication; impairments apparent even with supports • **Level 3** ("Requiring very substantial support")–Severe impairments in functioning; very limited initiation of social interactions
• Repetitive/ restricted behavior	• **Level 1** ("Requiring support")–Behaviors significantly interfere with function; difficulty switching between activities • **Level 2** ("Requiring substantial support")–Behaviors sufficiently frequent to be obvious to casual observer • **Level 3** ("Requiring very substantial support")–Behaviors markedly interfere with function in all spheres; extreme difficulty coping with change

Table 8.5.6: Associated conditions

Intellectual impairment	To diagnose comorbid autism spectrum disorder and intellectual disability, social communication should be below that expected for general developmental level
Language impairment	E.g. non-verbal single words only, etc.
Medical or genetic conditions	E.g. epilepsy, Rett syndrome, Down syndrome, etc.
Environmental factors	E.g. valproate, fetal alcohol exposure
Another neuro-developmental, mental, or behavioral disorder	E.g. attention deficit hyperactivity disorder, developmental coordination disorder, etc.
Catatonia	

Table 8.5.7: Diagnostic tools for autism

Parental reporting	• The Autism Behavior Checklist (ABC) • Gilliam Autism Rating Scale, 2nd edition (GARS-2) • Autism Diagnostic Interview-Revised (ADI-R)
Direct observation	• The Childhood Autism Rating Scale (CARS) • Autism Diagnostic Observation Schedule-Generic (ADOS-2)

The various differential diagnosis options for autism are given in Box 8.5.2.

Box 8.5.2: Differential diagnosis of autism

- Global Developmental Delay/Intellectual Disability
- Social Communication Disorder
- Hearing Impairment
- Rett Disorder
- Anxiety Disorder
- Obsessive-compulsive Disorder
- Developmental Language Disorder
- Language-based Learning Disability
- Landau-Kleffner Syndrome

Management

Improving the adolescent's skills and enabling her/him to be successfully functionally included in society is the main goal of management. Table 8.5.8 highlights the overview of management.

Table 8.5.8: Overview of management

Focus	Individualized according to the child's age and specific needs
Goals	Maximize functioning, move the child towards independence, and improve the quality of life
Outcome	Although there is no cure for ASD, early diagnosis and early intensive treatment have the potential to affect outcome

The role of the adolescent physician or pediatrician (Figure 8.5.2) signifies a robust balance between day-to-day matters and referral to a specialist for specific concerns. The adolescent needs many different health, educational and social services. The treating physician needs to appropriately plan and document these to develop

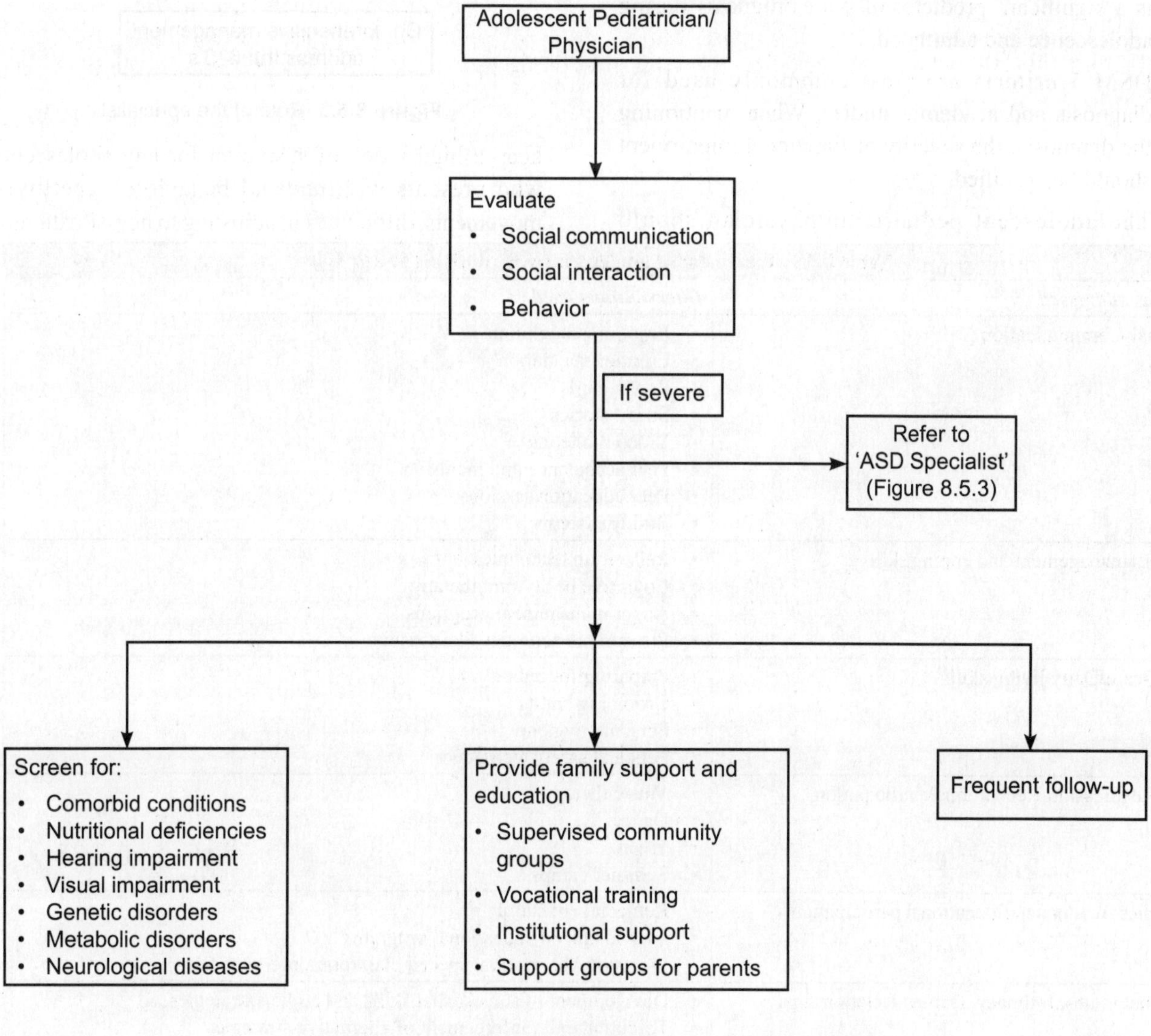

Figure 8.5.2: Role of the adolescent pediatrician or physician

an individualized program for each adolescent, and thereafter coordinate, monitor and evaluate the program on a regular basis.

In addition to the above, there are specific domains that need specialized interventions. Table 8.5.9 lists the six major domains that need to be targeted as part of treatment and Figure 8.5.3 highlights the role of the specialist/ developmental pediatrician.

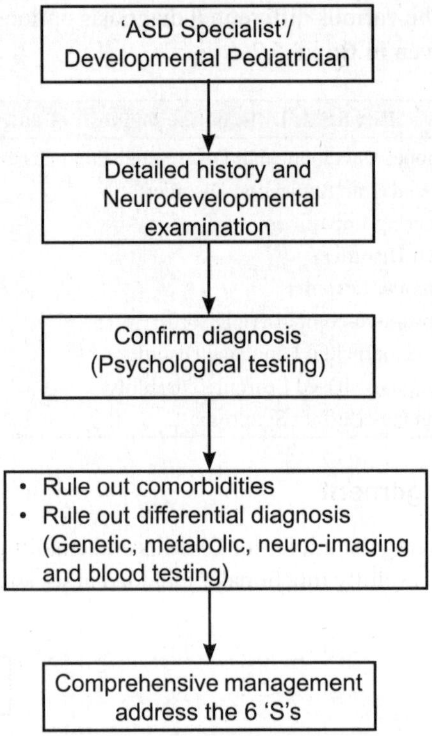

Figure 8.5.3: Role of the specialist

LEARNING POINTS

1. Most adolescents with autism are usually diagnosed in childhood. Early diagnosis and intervention is the key to management of this developmental disorder.
2. If not managed appropriately the adolescent may have severe deficits in social communication (non-verbal as well as verbal) and behavior.
3. Absence of speech development by 5 years of age is a significant predictor of poor prognosis during adolescence and adulthood.
4. DSM-5 criteria are most commonly used for diagnosis and academic studies. When mentioning the diagnosis, the severity of functional impairment should be specified.
5. The adolescent pediatrician/physician should keep a high index of suspicion for any adolescent who presents with unusual behaviors, repetitive movements, difficulties in adjusting to new situations,

Table 8.5.9: Treatment of adolescents with autism (The 6 'S's)

Areas addressed	*Interventions used*
Social-Communication	• Emotion recognition • Emotion regulation • Power cards • Social stories • Video modeling • Peer acceptance and inclusion • Peer education sessions • Buddy systems
Stress management and coping skills	• Relaxation techniques • Cognitive behavioral therapy • Anger management programs • Pleasurable activities like music
Self-care/Daily living skills	• Preparing for puberty • Grooming habits • Personal hygiene • Personal safety techniques
Self-expression/Recreational participation	• Music therapy • Dance • Yoga • Summer camps
Studies Academics/Educational participation	• Remedial education • Individualized educational programs • Inclusion, integration, special classroom interventions
Sexual issues, Intimacy, Dating, Relationships	• Development of sociosexual skills and coping strategies • Teaching and reinforcement of alternative strategies • Aversion therapy–Electric shock, satiation, covert sensitization • Hormonal therapies • Sex education intervention at early age

has restricted limited interests and speech-language-communication impairment.

6. Management needs a comprehensive integrated set-up which should include behavioral modifications, occupational therapy, speech and language interventions, group sessions and customized education programs. The adolescent pediatrician/physician is the conductor of this orchestra.

SUGGESTED READING

1. Autism in the teen years: What to expect, how to help? Interactive Autism Network at Kennedy Krieger Institute. iancommunity.org. Accessed August 28, 2015.
2. Bieberich AA, Morgan SB. Self-regulation and affective expression during play in children with autism or Down syndrome: A short-term longitudinal study. J Autism Dev Disord 2004;34(4):439-48.
3. Institute of social skills training. www.sst-institute.net. Accessed August 28, 2015.
4. Lara J, Bowers K. Expressive Arts: Learning, Growing and Expressing. Autism Asperger's Digest. September/October 2013.
5. Mbarek O, Marouillat S, Martineau J. Association study of the NF1 gene and autistic disorder. Am J Med Genet 1999; 88(6):729-32.
6. Realmuto GM, Ruble LA. Sexual Behaviors in Autism: Problems of Definition and Management. J Autism Dev Disord 1999;29(2):121-27.
7. Taylor JL, Dove D, Veenstra-VanderWeele J, Sathe NA, McPheeters ML, Jerome RN, Warren Z. Interventions for Adolescents and Young Adults with Autism Spectrum Disorders. Comparative Effectiveness Review No. 65: Agency for Healthcare Research and Quality. August 2012.

Academic Underachievement 8.6

Neelkamal S Soares, Mona P Gajre

INTRODUCTION

Academic achievement in adolescents can be due to a variety of causes and is broadly dependent on a complex, interlinked system involving familial, intrinsic potential of the adolescent, and societal factors. Developmental and behavioral disorders are common and impairing in adolescence; often going undiagnosed either due to attribution of the symptoms to other reasons by families or lack of clinician awareness. These disorders have treatment options that allow adolescents to function in their environments, and many treatments involve combinations of medical, psychosocial and educational systems.

Various developmental disorders that may contribute to academic underachievement are listed in Table 8.6.1 and include the following:

Table 8.6.1: Various disorders that can cause academic underachievement

	Onset prevalance	*DSM-5 criteria*	*Classification*	*Comorbidities*
Attention Deficit/ Hyperactivity Disorder (ADHD)	• Prevalence is 5-8%. • 2.5 times more common in boys than girls. • 60-80% continue to carry diagnosis into adulthood.	The symptoms should be present before age 12 years (previously was age 7 years).	• Predominantly inattentive. • Predominantly hyperactive-impulsive. • Combined (with elements of both).	• 35-60% ODD and Conduct disorder. • 25-30% anxiety disorders. • 18-25% depressive disorders. • 15-40% learning disorders. • 20-50% tic disorders. • Untreated ADHD are at greater risk of substance abuse.
Oppositional Defiant Disorder (ODD) and Conduct Disorder (CD)	• ODD 2.6-15.6%; CD 1.8-16.0% boys, and 0.8%-9.2% girls. • ODD often has early childhood onset, remains relatively stable, and about 2/3rd of children ultimately "lose" the diagnosis as they get older. • Earlier onset has poorer prognosis. • Both ODD and CD: Boys>girls; by adolescence ODD is roughly equal in boys and girls.	• Allows co-diagnosis of ODD and CD. • Symptoms such as aggression must be more than one time per week. • For CD, added specifier for children who are lacking in "prosocial" behaviors.	ODD and CD are along a continuum of increasing severity from ODD to CD and in adulthood to Antisocial Personality Disorder (APD).	ODD • 14% anxiety disorder • 9% depressive disorder. • 14% with ADHD. • Increased prevalence of learning disabilities and language disorders. • Suspect substance abuse in treatment non-responders. • CD is invariably being preceded by ODD, but not all ODD proceeds to CD.
Specific Learning Disorders (SLD)	• Prevalence around 5-10%. • SLD-reading accounts for 80% of cases of LD. • Males have higher prevalence than females.	IQ-achievement discrepancy criterion eliminated.	All previous subtypes (dyslexia, dysgraphia, and dyscalculia) are clustered into a single group with specifiers to indicate the difficulty in the core skill of reading, writing and mathematics (math) which are not intended to be mutually exclusive.	• Higher degree of comorbidity among the SLD, e.g. SLD math can occur with SLD reading. • ADHD occurs in about 20-35%, Anxiety Disorder in 10-30%, and Language Disorder in 10-20%.

- Attention Deficit/Hyperactivity Disorder (ADHD)
- Oppositional Defiant Disorder (ODD)
- Conduct Disorder (CD)
- Specific Learning Disorder (SLD)

HISTORY TAKING

- Interviewing the parents and adolescent focuses on symptoms and their impact on educational and social functioning of the adolescent, and previous and current treatments attempted. It also establishes rapport with the family, which is helpful in planning and executing treatment plan.
- Interview of the adolescent together with, and separately from, the parents/caregivers can shed light on the parental expectations of behaviors (Table 8.6.2: Symptoms of ADHD). Often, the adolescent does not perceive his/her behavior as a problem, but his/her perspective yields clues towards bullying or other psychosocial stressors, even possibility of abuse.
- It is also important to obtain data from other situations and sources, and a functional behavior analysis conducted in natural environments (home, school and social settings) can pinpoint triggers and settings where the behaviors exacerbate, and also possible intervention strategies.
- It is important to take family history e.g. ADHD is highly heritable (Table 8.6.2: Symptoms of ADHD).
- History should be taken for associated medical disorders like epilepsy, endocrine disorders, genetic syndromes, neurological or rheumatological conditions so that they can be diligently reviewed and optimally treated.
- History of other psychiatric disorders is also important, as comorbidity is often seen with these disorders.
- For suspected specific learning disorder (SLD) a comprehensive developmental history inclusive of significant birth events such as prematurity and complicated neonatal course may be suggestive of etiologic evidence. A history of global developmental delay especially language or motor coordination issues may be predictive of future academic concerns (Table 8.6.3).
- For ODD and CD, while obtaining history, the level of symptoms and severity, history of any interventions already attempted, family and psychosocial history as well as educational history and performance are essential components (Table 8.6.4: Symptoms of ODD and CD).

Table 8.6.2: Symptoms of ADHD

Symptoms required for diagnosis are: 6 or more in children and younger adolescents, 5 or more in older adolescents and adults, for at least 6 months impacting functioning in at least 2 settings

Type	*Features*
Predominantly inattentive	Not giving close attention to details/making careless mistakes in schoolwork, work, or other activities, difficulty sustaining attention in tasks or play activities. Not listening when spoken to directly. Not following through on instructions or finishing school work, chores, difficulty organizing tasks and activities, losing things, being easily distracted and forgetful.
Predominantly hyperactive/impulsive	Often fidgeting, leaving seat, running about. Difficulty quietly playing, often "on the go". Talking excessively, blurting out answers. Difficulty awaiting turn, and interrupting others.

Table 8.6.3: Specific learning disorder (SLD)

Definition	*Critical components*	*Core deficit*
SLD refers to a heterogeneous group of neurodevelopmental disorders manifested by significant difficulties in the acquisition and use of listening, speaking, reading, writing, reasoning or mathematical abilities despite adequate instruction, cultural difficulties, sensory or emotional problems.	• It is a neurobiological condition. • It is not due to poor instructional practices. • It has demonstrable discrepancy between the individual's intrinsic ability and the actual academic achievement. • The individual has at least average cognition abilities.	• *In reading:* Usually poor phonological awareness, leading to impaired word decoding and slow laborious reading skills. • *In math:* Usually impairments in number sense leading to deficits in memorizing math facts, and inaccurate or slow calculation and math reasoning. • *In writing:* Inefficiency in verbal working memory from phonologic to orthographic memory, leading to inaccuracy in spelling, grammar and punctuation, and clarity or organization of written expression.

Table 8.6.4: Symptoms of ODD and CD		
	Oppositional defiant disorder	***Conduct disorder***
Core Criterion	Pattern of behavior lasting at least six months, with at least four symptoms present.	Repetitive and persistent pattern of behavior in which the basic rights of others, or major age-appropriate societal norms or rules are violated, with at least three symptoms in the past 12 months, and at least one in past six months.
Primary Symptoms	• Often loses temper • Often touchy or easily annoyed • Often angry and resentful • Often argues with adults • Often actively defies or refuses to comply with adults' requests or rules • Often deliberately annoys others • Often blames others for his/her mistakes or misbehavior • Often spiteful or vindictive (twice in previous 6 months)	• Often bullies, threatens, or intimidates others • Often initiates physical fights • Has used a weapon against others • Physically cruel to people • Physically cruel to animals • Confronted a person and stolen their property • Forced someone into sexual activity • Deliberately set fires with intention of causing serious damage • Deliberately destroyed others' property (other than by fire setting) • Broken into someone else's house, building, or car • Lies to obtain goods or favors or to avoid obligations ("cheats" or "cons" others) • Has stolen items without confronting someone (e.g. forgery) • Stays out at night despite parental rules (beginning before age 13) • Run away from home overnight at least twice while living with parents (or once without returning for a lengthy period) • Run away from school (beginning before age 13)
Specifiers	• Mild if only in one setting (e.g. home) • Moderate in two settings • Severe in three or more settings	• Childhood onset (at least one symptoms before 10 years) • Adolescent onset (no symptoms prior to 10 years) • Unspecified onset (not enough information to determine onset age)
Exclusion	• Behaviors occur mainly during course of psychotic, substance use, depressive or bipolar disorder • Criteria for Disruptive Mood Dysregulation Disorder (DMDD) met	• Criteria for anti-social personality disorder met

CLINICAL EXAMINATION

When faced with an adolescent with suspected developmental disorder, it is always important to do a complete medical examination. There are many medical conditions that can present with similar symptoms and need to be ruled out.

- In cases that present with inattention, one needs to rule out epilepsy and hearing loss, while hyperactivity can be side effect of a medication like steroid.
- In case of learning disability, a physical examination is needed to exclude the presence of anemia, thyroid conditions or other systemic illnesses.
- Dysmorphology, neurocutaneous conditions such as neurofibromatosis (NF-1), tuberous sclerosis, genetic syndromes like Turner syndrome, Klinefelter syndrome are to be investigated. Presence of soft neurological findings, balance and coordination issues have been associated with SLD.
- Commonly occurring neurodevelopmental and psychiatric disorders with SLD have to be screened for and treated simultaneously and these include: ADHD, ODD, CD, depressive and anxiety disorders.

A medical examination can give treatment options (identifying cardiac anomaly while considering stimulant treatment), guide towards treatments (thyroid disorders, anemia or lead toxicity) and serial height, weight, blood pressure and pulse need to be monitored.

A neurological examination including cranial nerves, motor coordination, "soft neurological signs" and extraneous movements can point towards other neuropathology that might warrant neuroimaging (not typically indicated in ADHD).

CLINICAL ASSESSMENT

ADHD, ODD and CD

Informal observations of the adolescent's behavior during the clinic visit do not represent natural environment behaviors. To complement history and review of school records, symptom quantification provides more specificity regarding the symptoms and validates presence of symptoms in at least two environments.

Adolescent self-report may be unreliable due to reduced ability for self-awareness and poor impulse control. Detailed questioning has to be done for symptoms of ADHD to see if they are present only at home, outside home–specially in school, or at all settings (Table 8.6.2).

For ODD and CD, there is no requirement (compared to ADHD) that ODD and CD occur in more than one environment; so an adolescent may well exhibit symptoms only at home and not at school.

SLD

SLD is a clinical diagnosis, with no neuroimaging or biomarkers, and although it has an educational manifestation, pediatricians are often called upon to ascertain medical underpinnings or due to associated behavioral problems. While generally presenting in early elementary school, often the diagnosis is delayed till early adolescence when increasing educational challenges make symptoms more pronounced. Academic history from multiple sources such as the adolescent, parents and teachers provides an important clue to the assessment process. Often a history of dropping marks, grade retention or social promotion is present.

- Adolescents with SLD-reading often have slow effortful word reading, difficulty in comprehension of read text and spelling errors.
- Adolescents with SLD-writing show symptoms such as poor written expression, multiple grammatical errors and sloppy handwriting skills.
- Adolescents with SLD-math demonstrate poor number sense, finger counting, and deficits in mastering mathematical concepts.

Handwriting skills should be tested for letter formation, speed, presence of an immature pencil grip and pressure exerted while writing on paper. The adolescent's affect during examination can suggest the emotional status albeit in a clinic based setting.

Finally a synthesis of reports from multiple sources (school, community psychologist and/or tutor) such as cognitive abilities, formal and informal educational tests, visuoperceptual skills assessment in addition to a detailed language assessment helps map the adolescent's strengths and weakness and plan a comprehensive map to tackle the academic, behavioral comorbidities, socio-emotional issues customized to that adolescent's unique environmental demands for implementation in the school or resource room setting.

Instruments for Screening

Standardized instruments collected from parents, teachers and counselors not only help ascertain diagnosis, but can be used to track progress after implementation of interventions.

Broad-based instruments provide an overview of different problem behaviors. Validated specific scales are not diagnostic by themselves but are used to validate clinical information towards the diagnosis (Table 8.6.5).

Table 8.6.5: Various scales for assessment

Name of scale	*Used for*	*Comments*
Achenbach Child Behavior Checklist (Achenbach, 2001)	Broad-based: Many psychiatric disorders	Manual and computerized scoring systems.
Behavior Assessment System for Children (Reynolds and Kamphaus, 2005)	Broad-based: Many psychiatric disorders	Commonly used by educational professionals.
Vanderbilt Rating Scales (Wolraich, 2002)	ADHD	Freely available online.
Conners-3 (Conners, 2008)	ADHD	Available as parent, teacher and self-report.
Conners-Wells' Adolescent Self-Report Scales (CASS-S; Conners and Wells, 1997)	ODD and CD	Self-report by adolescents ages 12 through 17.
The Interview for Antisocial Behavior (IAB; Kazdin and Esveldt-Dawson, 1986)	ODD and CD	Parent interview of different adolescent antisocial behaviors.

It may be necessary to collaborate with the school or private psychologist to conduct psychological tests to rule in or out developmental delay/intellectual disability and specific learning disabilities. These are not essential for a diagnosis but help in educational treatment avenues, but routine neuropsychological test batteries are not recommended.

In the diagnostic process, it is important to rule out ADHD (14% of children with ODD), which confers a worse prognosis on both CD and ODD and is associated with more aggression and a greater range and persistence of problem behaviors, peer rejection and academic underachievement.

INVESTIGATIONS

There is no indication for routine blood or urine tests, unless indicated for medical etiology search when history or examination is suggestive.

Typical medications used in ADHD do not need drug levels measured for efficacy or toxicity.

It is not standard of care to obtain routine electrocardiogram (ECG) while monitoring stimulant or non-stimulant medication in ADHD.

MANAGEMENT

It is important to follow certain protocols in management of these conditions.

Management of ADHD

- Management is primarily through a combination of medication and behavioral options. Stimulants are the primary medication option with few side-effects (see Flowchart 8.6.1).
- Care must be taken with those having pre-existing cardiac conditions due to slight risk of sudden cardiac death.
- In adolescents when substance use is identified, caution must be exercised due to "diversion" (selling or distributing medication or using other than intended medical indication).
- Non-stimulant atomoxetine is slightly less effective than stimulants in controlling ADHD symptoms and takes longer to show effect (3-4 weeks).

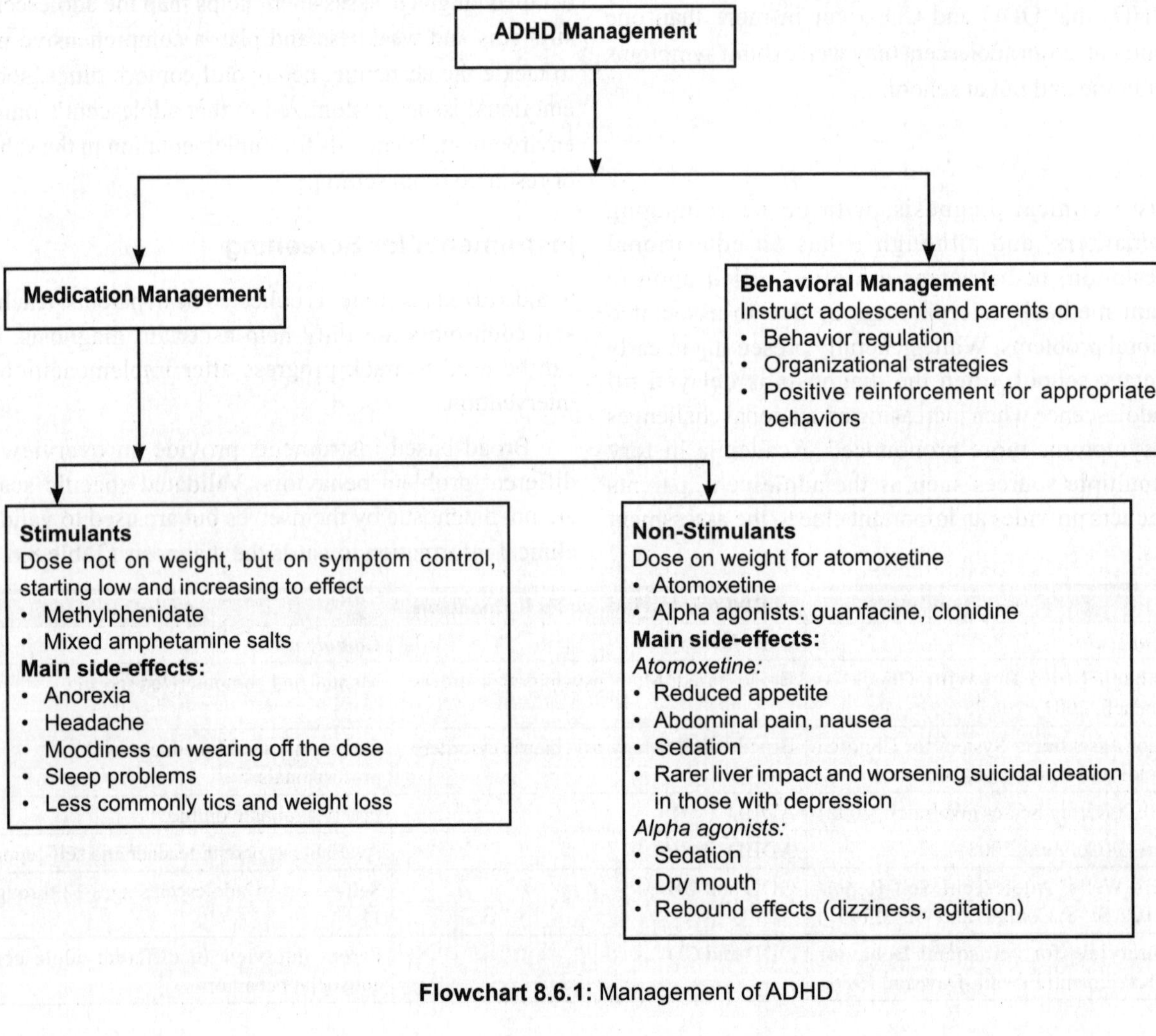

Flowchart 8.6.1: Management of ADHD

- Tricyclic anti-depressants are less used due to higher risk-benefit ratio (compared to stimulants and non-stimulants) of cardiac and anti-cholinergic effects.

Limitations of behavioral strategies include availability of trained professionals and time delay to effect (often several weeks). However, combination of medication management and behavior therapy allows for the use of lower dosages of medications which reduces the risk of adverse effects.

Management of ODD and CD

Treatment of ODD and CD generally is multimodal, combining individual psychotherapy, family psychotherapy, medication therapy, and school-based interventions (see Flowchart 8.6.2).

- Delays in seeking treatment sometimes occur as many parents may feel that the adolescent will "outgrow it" or that ODD and CD are typical "adolescent mood".
- Preventative treatments for ODD (and to some extent CD) can be delivered in schools, outpatient centers and other community locations through collaboration between clinicians and educators (like home visitation to high-risk families).
- Behavioral interventions are either targeted at parents or adolescents, but commonly involve both. Punishment is not recommended as it can worsen the cycle of negativity and model aggression for the adolescent.
- Intensive settings like day-treatment programs or residential facilities are costly with limited evidence regarding efficacy, but are useful in adolescents with CD who cannot be safely treated in a community setting (e.g. fire-setting).
- Involvement of community and other agencies (social services, police and other judicial personnel) may be necessary to provide intensive monitoring and support.
- Medications are not considered a first line of treatment of ODD and CD, except in presence of coexisting disorders, or when psychosocial treatments alone have failed.
- Monitoring is required for lithium and antiepileptics for drug level and target organ function monitoring, and for anti-depressants for depression and/or anxiety.

Management of SLD

While recognized worldwide as a disability, SLD is still to be considered in context of local and regional cultural perspectives. Due to India's rich diversity in language, teaching styles, and curriculum structures, there is concern for the correct identification of SLD with culturally appropriate tests. Additionally the influence of poor socioeconomic status (SES), multilingualism, urban-rural differences in teaching content are significant extrinsic

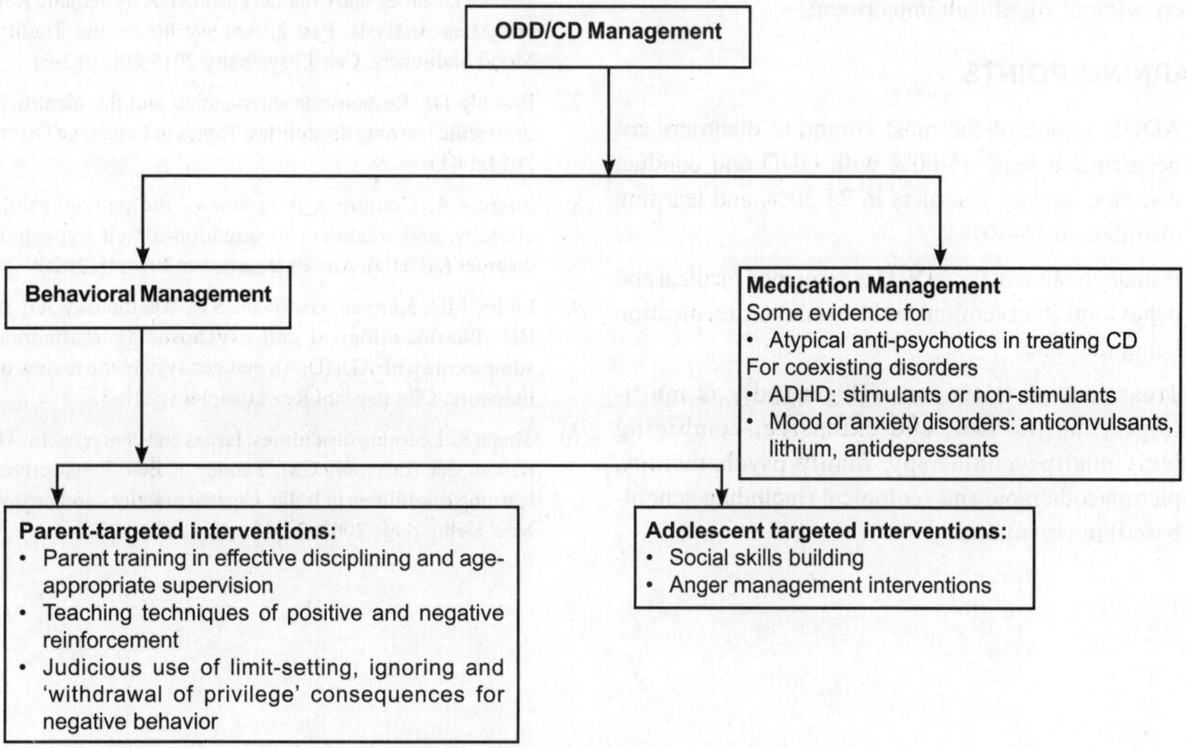

Flowchart 8.6.2: Management of ODD and CD

factors that impact the learning and cannot be overlooked for a correct diagnosis.

Generally there is no medical intervention for SLD; educational techniques include either remediation or accommodation.

- *Remediation strategies:* These aim to correct the underlying impaired cognitive function by phonological skills training using multisensory approach, some examples being Orton Gillingham (OTG) method or Engelmann's Direct Instruction method. Multisensory intervention is most beneficial, via the standard curriculum in school special education services or private tutoring classes.
- *Accommodations or augmentation techniques*: These offer specific assistance to compensate for the adolescent's difficulties by using audiotapes, word processors, extended time, and calculator especially during timed situations such as examinations.

Outcomes

SLD persist lifelong although the manifestations may evolve with time. The transition of an SLD child into adolescence can be stressful if the family and adolescent are unprepared for the change. Options to continue academics via the open schooling process, prevocational and vocational career courses are available. Most adolescents develop their individual learning styles and adults may remain slow readers but able to function in society without significant impairment.

LEARNING POINTS

- ADHD is one of the most comorbid disorders co-occurring at least 35-60% with ODD and conduct disorder, anxiety disorders in 25-30%, and learning disorders in 15-40%.
- Primary treatment for ADHD is combined medical and behavioral interventions, with stimulant medication being first line.
- Treatment of ODD and CD generally is multi-target, multimodal, and extensive, combining individual psychotherapy, family psychotherapy, pharmacotherapy, and ecological (including school-based) interventions.
- Medications are not considered a first line of treatment of ODD and CD, but treat coexisting ADHD, mood or anxiety disorders or complement behavioral strategies in resistant cases.
- Specific learning disorder (SLD) manifestation depends on the educational challenges faced by the individual during his/her academic pursuits.
- Remediation is the cornerstone in the comprehensive management of SLD.

SUGGESTED READING

1. American Psychiatric Association. Diagnostic and statistical manual of mental disorders (5th ed). Washington, DC; 2013.
2. Buitelaar JK, Smeets KC, Herpers P, Scheepers F, Glennon J, Rommelse NN. Conduct disorders. Eur Child Adolesc Psychiatry 2013;22 (Suppl 1):S49-54.
3. Cavendish W. Identification of learning disabilities: Implications of proposed DSM-5 criteria for school-based assessment. J Learn Disabil 2013;46(1):52-57.
4. Frick PJ, Nigg JT. Current issues in the diagnosis of attention deficit hyperactivity disorder, oppositional defiant disorder, and conduct disorder. Annu Rev Clin Psychol 2012;8:77-107.
5. Obioha O, Adesman A. Pearls, perils, and pitfalls in the assessment and treatment of attention-deficit/hyperactivity disorder in adolescents. Curr Opin Pediatr 2014;26(1):119-29.
6. Pringsheim T, Hirsch L, Gardner D, Gorman DA. The Pharmacological Management of Oppositional Behaviour, Conduct Problems, and Aggression in Children and Adolescents With Attention-Deficit Hyperactivity Disorder, Oppositional Defiant Disorder, and Conduct Disorder: A Systematic Review and Meta-Analysis. Part 2: Antipsychotics and Traditional Mood Stabilizers. Can J Psychiatry 2015;60(2):52-61.
7. Reschly DJ. Response to intervention and the identification of specific learning disabilities. Topics in Language Disorders 2014;34(1):39-58.
8. Sharma A, Couture J. A review of the pathophysiology, etiology, and treatment of attention-deficit hyperactivity disorder (ADHD). Ann Pharmacother 2014;48(2):209-25.
9. Sibley MH, Kuriyan AB, Evans SW, Waxmonsky JG, Smith BH. Pharmacological and psychosocial treatments for adolescents with ADHD: An updated systematic review of the literature. Clin Psychol Rev 2014;34(3):218-32.
10. Thapa K. Learning disabilities: Issues and concerns. In: Thapa K, van der Aalsvoort GM, Pandey J, Eds. Perspectives on learning disabilities in India: Current practices and prospects. New Delhi: Sage 2008; 23-47.

Psychometric Assessment 8.7

Anuradha Sovani

INTRODUCTION

Mental health issues are very important aspect of adolescent health. It is important to have scientific evidence to support and/or confirm the clinically suspected diagnosis, as many times parents are in denial or may not be convinced that their adolescent has any mental health issues. A good history taking with both adolescents themselves and the family members, specially parents, would give the clinician a reasonable understanding of the problem that exists. There are standardized structured screening proformas available for screening various issues like anxiety, depression, attention deficit hyperactivity disorder (ADHD), conduct disorders etc. All professionals who work with adolescents—clinicians, pediatricians, psychiatrists, psychologists and social workers, should use these regularly to assess their client, and to record and document their findings.

If any abnormality is found in these screening tests the next step should be to use reliable, valid and standardized psychometric tools which will give more details about the profile that best describes their young client. This gives the health and mental health professional a good understanding of his or her clients, both to understand the areas where they face challenges, and areas of strength which can be built upon. It is important to have scientific evidence to support and/or confirm the clinically suspected diagnosis, as many times parents are in denial or may not be convinced that their adolescent has any mental health issues. This chapter will review some of the state of the art methods and techniques which are used the world over to understand psychological profiles of adolescents.

HISTORY TAKING AND SCREENING

Once a detailed history is taken and the screening tests show that some problem exists, it is necessary to refer to a psychologist for further evaluation and plan of management.

A psychologist has specialized training in administering and interpreting data obtained from tests administered to the young client. Their role in fact begins from choosing these tools from a vast armamentarium available to them. In this process, they have to think carefully about:

1. The age range for which the test can be administered.
2. The conditions for which the test is advised.
3. Whether norms are available for the test in the country where it is being used.
4. Whether they have adequate expertise to administer, score and interpret the test.

VARIOUS STAGES OF PSYCHOMETRIC ASSESSMENT

Initially, what the psychologist needs to do is assess what seems to be the major reason why the client has been referred to them (Table 8.7.1).

Table 8.7.1: Reasons for referral for psychometric assessment

Academic problem	Poor scholastic progress or academic underachievement. Recent falling behind in grades, whereas earlier they were doing fairly well.
Behavior changes	Aggressive behaviors, irritability etc.
Emotional problems	Adolescent depressions are common. Many adolescents also face anxiety symptoms.

Many times the adolescent is not referred for any specific problem but the goal for assessment may simply be to enhance emotional growth and help the adolescent achieve full potential.

Excellent psychological tests are available which can help the psychologist create a clear profile of the adolescent in order to assist the whole team to work with him or her (Table 8.7.2).

PERSONALITY TESTING

One of the important areas for assessment is the area of personality (Table 8.7.2).

These are generally needed in adolescents who require an in depth assessment for the emotional issues that are evidently the root cause of their behavioral problems.

Table 8.7.2: Various psychometric tests

Domain			
PERSONALITY	**Empirical, objective tests** 1. MMPI-The Minnesota Multiphasic Personality Inventory (a) MMPI 2 may be used >18 years (b) MMPI-A is specifically for adolescents 2. MCMI-The Millon Clinical Multiaxial Inventory (MCMI IV used >18 years age) 3. 16PF-The 16 Personality Factors test (can be used with adolescents and adults)	**Projective tests** 1. CAT-Children's Apperception Test (under 12 years) 2. TAT-The Thematic Apperception Test (over 13 years) 3. Rorschach Inkblot Method can be used with adolescents and adults	**Semi-structured tests** 1. Sentence completion 2. Draw a man 3. Word association (All can be used at any age)
INTELLIGENCE	Wechsler series (WISC, WISC III, WISC IV): Wechsler tests have norms from 5 to 15 years 11 months; WISC IV norms extended to 17 years	The Stanford Binet and Kamath Binet (its Indian version): These are tests with age norms, so age can be calculated using a simple conversion formula	Bhatias' battery of intelligence tests Used upto 14 years of age
CAREER COUNSELING	APTITUDE	INTEREST	VALUES
NEURO-PSYCHOLOGICAL Cognitive domain e.g. Memory, Attention, Language, Motor Dexterity, Speed, etc.	NIMHANS Battery, AIIMS Battery in India	Luria Nebraska/Halstead Reitan Batteries in the West	Bender Gestalt Test has separate scoring for children and adults
EMOTIONAL INTELLIGENCE	Meyer Salovey Caruso Emotional Intelligence Test (MSCEIT) can be used with older adolescents and young adults		

Although one can clinically get quite a clear idea, it is always sensible to refer the case to a trained psychologist so that he or she can elicit deep seated issues through the assessment. These pointers can prove very useful later for therapeutic intervention as well. It is particularly useful to send young people for assessment if they are reluctant to respond and very introverted, or if they are defiant. Also, unexplained drops in academics can often be due to personality and emotional issues.

1. Objective Personality Testing

This requires the respondent to read a set of statements and answer in a YES/NO format.

The examples of tools in this domain include:

1. **The Minnesota Multiphasic Personality Inventory, or the MMPI:** This test is now in the second edition (MMPI 2) and there is also a special test constructed for adolescents, which is called the MMPI-A. This test is very useful if one wants to confirm the possibility of some psychopathology, since the test yields a very clear profile.
2. **The Millon Clinical Multiaxial Inventory (MCMI) Which is Now in Its Fourth Edition (MCMI IV):** However, the respondent needs to be 18 years of age in order for this tool to be used, and hence a small portion of the sample seen by us may be given this test. If the youngster seems to have personality disorder traits, and it becomes difficult to pinpoint where exactly the pathology lies, this is a useful test to give.
3. **The 16 Personality Factors Test (16 PF):** This test is now in its fifth edition and is an excellent tool which generates a profile which best describes the personality of the adolescent. This is indeed a very useful tool since unlike the two mentioned above; its use is NOT restricted to troubled populations showing some psychopathology.

2. Projective Personality Testing

1. **The Thematic Apperception Test (TAT)** permits the adolescent to look at a semi-structured stimulus, a pictorial representation of two or more people in some form of interaction. The picture is sufficiently

vague for the adolescent to be able to draw their own conclusions and make a story about what is happening in the picture. All the stories generated are then interpreted by the trained psychologist to draw conclusions about the personality and current concerns of the youngster.

2. **Children's Apperception Test (CAT)** is used for children between 5 and 12 years. The principle is same as the TAT described above, where various pictures are shown and the child asked what they feel looking at the picture. There are various scoring methods used with this test, but most focus on drawing out the key themes that emerge from the client's responses, which in turn tell us more about his or her personality and current emotional concerns.
3. **A Rorschach Inkblot Method** is another popularly used psychological tool, although in many managed care settings in the west its use is on the decline. This test consists of a set of ten cards on which completely unstructured material is present. There is a clear cut scoring system which can help generate a set of scores based on the associations formed by the respondent. The Rorschach can yield a very rich profile of the client's defenses, the degree to which he or she is in touch with reality and the degree to which they may be willing to conform to social norms. It is also interesting to see the way the profile reflects their associative life, their speed of responding to stimuli and the sheer variety of responses they may generate.

INTELLIGENCE TESTING

A very important area of assessment in adolescence is assessment of IQ specially when they are referred for academic under-achievement. Intelligence assessment is also an important tool used in the course of career guidance. There is a wide variety of tests available:

1. **The Wechsler Series (WISC, WISC III, WISC IV):** The WISC IV yields an extremely useful profile covering the various domains along which a person may function, e.g. the verbal comprehension index, the percentual reasoning index, working memory index etc. The earlier versions of the WISC too were useful in their own way since scatter on the subscale scores yielded important performance pointers.
2. **The Stanford Binet and Kamath Binet (Its Indian Version) and the Bhatias' Battery of Intelligence Tests,** are simpler and shorter tools and are often used as backups when detailed testing is not practicable or even possible.

TESTS FOR CAREER COUNSELING

Career testing in adolescence is an important domain. It is possible to base the vocational guidance of a young person on the findings from a battery of psychometric tools geared towards assessing their aptitude, to indicate where exactly their strengths lie, their interests and values.

Occasionally, attitude scales may also be used to clarify how they feel about specific issues.

APTITUDE, INTEREST AND VALUES TESTING

A wide variety of aptitude tests are available and is upto the psychologist to select a particular tool. One of the more widely used tests is the Differential Aptitude Test, which has western as well as Indian norms.

Ability tests are used less often in psychometric evaluation but have a definite role to play in selection of further study domains. Tests such as the TOEFL and the GRE are good examples of this sort of tool.

NEUROPSYCHOLOGICAL TESTS

These are used in adolescents who have a specific cognitive problem, or an organic condition such as epilepsy. They can indeed yield valuable findings in the cognitive domain, e.g. memory, attention, language, as well as motor dexterity, speed, etc.

TESTS FOR EMOTIONAL INTELLIGENCE

In order to gauge the strengths of the young person, one may choose to use tools that assess emotional intelligence (EI), but these tools are still a little controversial. Many different models of EI are posited, e.g. that which speaks of it as an ability, v/s the one which looks upon it more as a personality correlate. However, interesting results can be obtained by administering tests such as the Mayer Salovey Caruso Test of Emotional Intelligence (MSCEIT), in order to assess EQ.

OTHER TESTS

Further one may also explore different strength areas of the adolescent by gauging creativity using tools such as TTCT (Torrance Tests of Creative Thinking) and Remote Associations Test (RAT) and Unusual Uses Test.

RATING SCALES

These are a very useful set of tools. These help to assess problem areas such as anxiety, depression, anger, etc. using rating scales such as respectively for the above three domains:

(a) Hamilton Anxiety Rating Scale (HARS), Speilberger's State Trait Anxiety Inventory (STAI), and Sinha's rating scale, as well as Taylor's Manifest Anxiety Scale (TMAS).

(b) Hamilton Depression Rating Scale (HDRS), Beck Depression Inventory (BDI) and Zung's Depression scale.

(c) State Trait Anger Inventory (STAI) may also be used.

Rating scales may also be useful as research tools to try and establish group differences, test hypotheses etc.

LEARNING POINTS

1. There is a great role of a psychologist in an adolescent clinic as part of the team looking after wellness of the adolescents.
2. They are specially trained to assess the adolescents' strengths and weaknesses in a variety of domains.
3. Psychometric tests help all members of the team to identify the source and extent of the problem. They can thus plan to augment strengths and prop up weaker areas of the young person they are working with.
4. This helps to use the most effective intervention strategies, tailored to the personality of the individual.

SUGGESTED READING

1. Dorfmon WI, Hersen M (2001). Understanding psychological assessment. NY: Kluwer Academic; 2001.
2. Gregory RJ. Psychological Testing: History, Principles, and Applications (Sixth ed.). Boston: Allyn and Bacon; 2011.
3. Murray HA. Thematic Apperception Test manual. Cambridge, MA: Harvard University Press; 1943.
4. Nordin H, Eisemann M, Richter J. MMPI-2 subgroups in a sample of chronic pain patients. Scand J Psychol 2005;46:209-16.
5. Rey JM (Ed.). IACAPAP e-Textbook of Child and Adolescent Mental Health. Geneva. International Association for Child and Adolescent Psychiatry and Allied Professions; 2015.
6. Wechsler D. The Wechsler intelligence scale for children, 4th edition. London: Pearson Assessment; 2004.

9.1 Nuclear Imaging

RD Lele, Vikram R Lele

INTRODUCTION

The four basic questions in the practice of medicine are:

1. What is wrong?
2. What is going to happen?
3. What can be done about it?
4. Is the treatment effective?

Nuclear medicine helps in all four questions. α and β nuclear emissions are used for therapy while γ emissions and positrons are used for diagnostic purposes.

- Nuclear medicine enables quantitative imaging of spatial and temporal distribution of radiolabelled molecules within the living human body including the brain by means of scanning instruments outside the body.
- This provides unique information about regional physiology, biochemistry and metabolism in health and disease even in the pre-symptomatic stage.
- Nuclear magnetic resonance imaging (NMRI) and nuclear magnetic resonance spectroscopy (NMRS) with their chemical orientation, are legitimately part of "nuclear medicine"–the word nuclear was dropped in 1980s due to its scary association with nuclear bombs.
- The development of simultaneous positron emission tomography and magnetic resonance imaging (PET/MRI) in 2010 have brought together all nuclear phenomena for the benefit of patients: regional physiology and tissue chemistry and pH.
- MRI is superior to CT for tissue characterization.
- Nuclear medicine was the first superspecialty to use electronic computers for data acquisition storage qualification, and display in 3 dimensions, using machines like single photon emission computed tomography (SPECT) and positron emission tomography (PET).
- Since 2001 hybrid machines like SPECT-CT and PET-CT now provide simultaneous 3 dimensional information about regional anatomy, regional physiology and biochemistry and metabolism.
- An abnormal function precedes abnormal structure by several weeks. Functional recovery precedes structural recovery by several weeks–these are two important lessons provided by PET/CT.

NUCLEAR DIAGNOSTIC IMAGING

Almost all the organs of the body can be visualized by radioisotopes based on molecular imaging (Table 9.1.1).

- The human body is made up of trillions of cells which are constantly in communication with each of them through recognition molecules.
- Molecular recognition is a fundamental feature of all biological processes encompassing ligand receptors, substrate enzymes and antigen-antibody reactions.
- Imaging specific receptors is a unique capability of nuclear medicine.
- Almost all receptors in the body, especially the brain can now be imaged using different radiopharmaceuticals–benzodiazepine, dopamine, cholinergic and adrenergic, serotonin, cannabinoid, opioid receptors, somatostatin, estrogen, progesterone androgen etc. Table 9.1.2 describes imaging based on molecular recognition.

The scope of nuclear imaging in 10 different body systems for adolescents is outlined in Table 9.1.1.

Many disorders in adolescence such as stress fractures, skeletal infections, neuroendocrine tumors, epilepsy, attention deficit hyperactivity disorder (ADHD) are well studied with nuclear medicine procedures (see Box 9.1.1). Nuclear medicine also has a role to play in certain emergency situations (see Box 9.1.2). It also can help in differentiating various infections especially tuberculosis from cancer (see Box 9.1.3).

Table 9.1.1: Scope of nuclear medicine in adolescent disorders

Nephrourology: (Figure 9.1.1)	• Congenital ureteropelvic junction anomaly • Vesicoureteral reflux and pyelonephritis • Posterior urethral valve • Duplex kidney • Multicystic dysplastic kidney
Gastrointestinal (GI) tract: (Figure 9.1.2)	• GI bleed: Meckel's diverticulum • Gastroesophageal reflux • Pulmonary aspiration • GI protein loss • Colonic transit: Functional fecal retention–chronic constipation • Appendicitis • Inflammatory bowel disease
Liver and Gall-bladder:	• Biliary obstruction and cholecystitis • Biliary leaks
Neurology:	Ictal and interictal epilepsy (drug resistant) SPECT and PET • Extra-temporal-focal cortical dysplasia • Hypoxic ischemic encephalopathy • Traumatic brain injury • Brain tumors
Oncology:	• Neuroblastoma • Wilms' tumor • Neuroendocrine tumors (NETs) • Multiple endocrine neoplasia (MEN) • CNS tumors • Lymphoma, leukemia
Bones:	• Legg-Perthes disease • Osteogenesis imperfecta • Fractures, osteomyelitis, sickle cell bone infarcts • Battered child syndrome • Osteosarcoma • Ewing's sarcoma
Soft tissue:	Rhabdomyosarcoma
Thyroid: (Figure 9.1.3)	• Agenesis • Dyshormonogenesis • Thyroid cancer
Cardiac:	Assessment of shunts • Left to right shunt • Right to left shunt

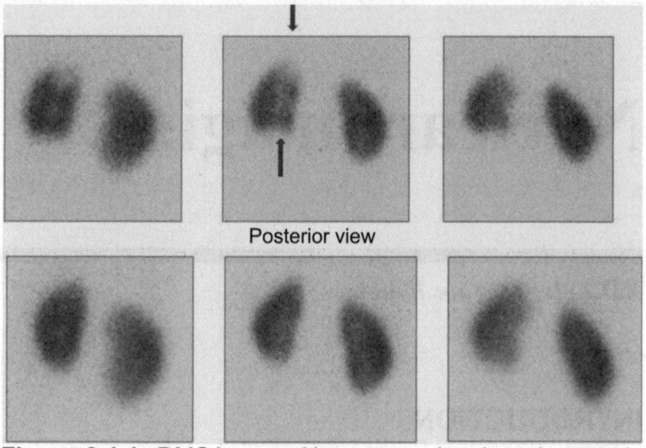

Figure 9.1.1: DMSA scan. Upper row showing photopenic defect in upper and lower poles of left kidney (center image arrows) Follow up at 3 months (lower row) shows resolution of infection (acute pyelonephritis)

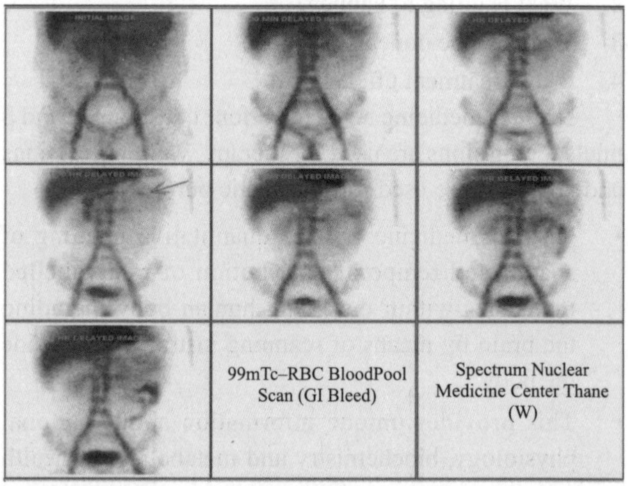

Figure 9.1.2: Labelled red blood cell scan showing normal hepatic and large vessel blood pool. A site of small bowel bleeding is seen in left hypogastric region (arrow) increasing over time

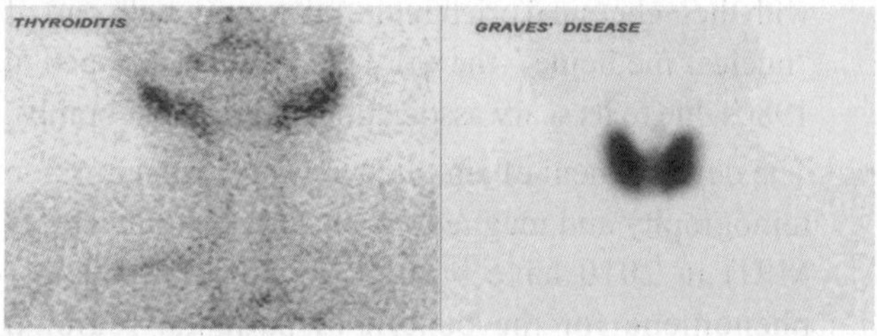

Figure 9.1.3: 99mTc-pertechnetate scans showing absence of uptake in the thyroid gland in thyroiditis (left) and intense uptake in the thyroid in Graves' disease (right) with similar clinical presentation

THERAPEUTIC NUCLEAR MEDICINE

The scope of nuclear medicine has gone beyond being only diagnostic. Table 9.1.3 describes therapeutic uses of nuclear medicine in various disorders.

LEARNING POINTS

- Nuclear medicine has a role to play in both diagnostic and therapeutic medicine with use of radiolabeled molecules.
- It provides unique information about regional physiology, biochemistry and metabolism in health and disease even in the pre-symptomatic stage.
- Nuclear medicine positron emission tomography (PET) and single photon emission computed tomography (SPECT) can be combined with CT and MRI to give simultaneous three dimensional information about regional anatomy, regional physiology, biochemistry and metabolism.

Table 9.1.2: Imaging based on molecular recognition

Imaging cell membrane transporters	***Clinical utility***	
Sodium iodine symporter (NIS)	Thyroid gland with radioiodine or technetium (Tc-99m)	
Sodium potassium Na/K ATPase	Heart with thallium–201	
Sodium hydrogen Na/H antiport	Increased activity in hypertension and diabetes–studied with Na-24	
Calcium channels	Imaging with C-11 nifedipine PET	
Glucose transporters (GLUT 1-3)	Over-expressed in cancer cells Imaging with F18 deoxyglucose–PET	
Amino acid transporters	Over-expressed in malignant gliomas; imaging with F18-Fluoroethyl tyrosine PET, or I-123 iodomethyl tyrosine SPECT	
Serotonin transporters	Imaging with decreased activity in frontal lobes in patients with social phobias or attention deficit hyperactive disorder	
P-Glycoprotein (Pgp) efflux pump	Imaging with Tc-99m MIBI over-expressed in cancer cells which show multiple drugs resistance	
Imaging cell membrane receptors	***Clinical utility***	
Histamine H1 receptors	Imaging with C-11 doxepin PET Increase in epileptic focus helps localization	
Dopamine D1 and D4 receptors	C-11 clozapine	
Dopamine D2 receptors	Imaging with C-11 raclopride or I-123 iodobenzamide (IBZM)	
Benzodiazepine receptors (GABAA)	C-11 flumazenil I-123 iomazenil	
Neurotensin (NT-1) receptors	Imaging with Tc-99 NT-1 for imaging tumors expressing NT-1 Rc	
Somatostatin receptor	Imaging with Tc-99m pentrotide (somatostatin analog)	
Vasoactive intestinal peptide (VIP) receptor	Imaging with Tc-99m VIP	
Serotonin (5HT2) receptors	I-123 iodoketanserin, I-123 iodoethyl LSD C-11 n-methyl spiperone, F-18 setoperone	
B adreno receptors	F-18 carazolol, for imaging heart	
Opioid receptors	C-11 carfentanil, increased activity in epileptic focus in temporal lobe epilepsy	
Radiolabeled peptides	***Imaging utility***	
Tc–Pentetriotide/TC-VIP	Imaging various cancers which over-express receptors for these peptides	
Sigma receptors	F-18 haloperidol, C-11 diprenorphine, C-11 687, 384	
Specific radiolabeled monoclonal antibodies imaging cell surface tumor markers	Tc-99 labeled mAb to carcinoembrogenic antigen (CEA) Alpha-fetoprotein (AFP) Radiolabeled mAb to platelet 2b/3a mAb fibrin	Imaging various cancers which express these markers on their surface e.g colon, breast, liver, lung cancer. Imaging fresh thrombus
Specific radiolabeled monoclonal antibodies (mAb)	***Clinical utility***	
Imaging cell surface tumors markers: Tc-99 labeled mAb to carcinoembryogenic antigen (CEA), Alpha-fetoprotein (AFP)	Imaging various cancers which express these markers on their surface e.g. colon, breast, liver and lung cancer	
Radiolabeled mAb to platelet 2b/3a mAb fibrin	Imaging fresh thrombus	

Box 9.1.1: Nuclear imaging in neuropsychiatric disorders

- Serotonin dysfunction is implicated in a host of neuropsychiatric disorders.
- The ability to quantify serotonin receptor distribution is of great help in studying these disorders and drugs which act on those receptors.
- In Attention Deficit Hyperactivity Disorder (ADHD) methylphenidate responders show increased activity of dopamine transporters in caudate and putamen as shown by Tc-TRODAT imaging.
- A major strength of PET is measurement of *in vivo* physiology.

Box 9.1.2: Nuclear medicine in emergency situations

Some nuclear imaging procedures are required in emergency situations

- Localization of lower gastrointestinal bleeding
- Diagnosis of pulmonary embolism by V/Q scans
- Torsion of testis vs. acute epididymo-orchitis
- Acute cholecystitis
- Rest myocardial perfusion and function imaging in acute coronary syndrome–to establish myocardial infarct and need for admission
- Post-renal transplant determination of rejection vs. acute tubular necrosis

Box 9.1.3: Diagnostic imaging in infections vs cancer

In our country tuberculosis and cancer can co-exist in the same patient which can be distinguished by dual imaging:

- Fluorine-18-fluoro-deoxyglucose (F18-FDG) measures glucose transport.
- 18F-fluoro-ethyl-tyrosine (18F-FET) measures amino acid transport.
- Fluorothymidine (FLT) measures proliferation.

Cancer cells express all three.
Tuberculosis expresses FDG but not FET and FLT.
FDG + ve FLT+ ve = Cancer (Figure 9.1.4).
FDG + ve FLT – ve = Tuberculosis (Figure 9.1.5).
Combination of these scans can also be used for detection of foci of infection in different parts of the body (Figure 9.1.6).

Table 9.1.3: Therapeutic nuclear medicine

Clinical setting	*Isotope used*	*Radiopharmaceutical utility*
Graves' disease	131-Iodine	Single dose cure of thyrotoxicosis
Thyroid cancer	131-Iodine	Effective eradication of systemic metastases
Painful bone metastases	32-P	Effective relief of severe intractable pain in extensive skeletal metastases
Joint pain	81-Strontium 90Y, Erbium, Rhenium, Holmium	Effective relief of joint pains in rheumatoid arthritis, villonodular synovitis, hemophilic arthritis and selected cases of osteoarthritis
Lymphoma	^{131}I-tositumomab	Relapsed and refractory non-Hodgkin lymphoma (NHL)
Somatostatin receptor	90Y-octreotide	Treatment of refractory somatostatin positive tumors
Hepatoma/hepatic metastatis	90Y-spheres	Treatment of hepatoma, colonic cancer metastatis to liver from colon cancer

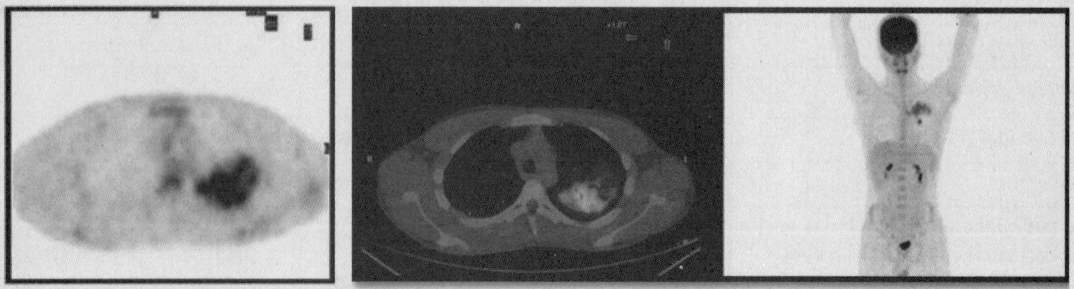

Figure 9.1.4: FDG PET CT images–Showing uptake in the lung lesion

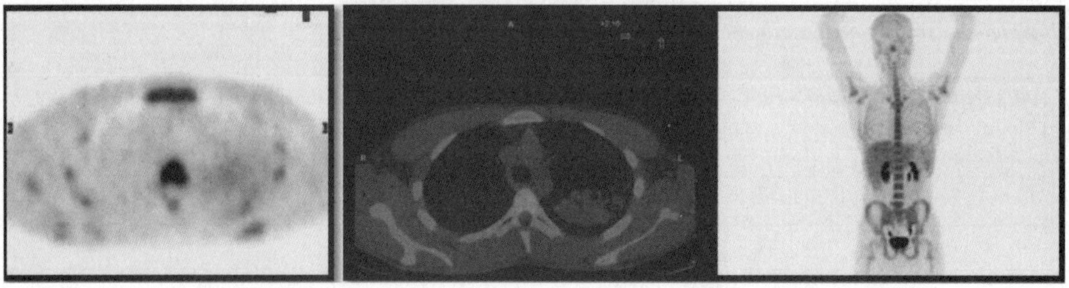

Figure 9.1.5: FLT PET images do not reveal uptake–Diagnosis of tuberculosis

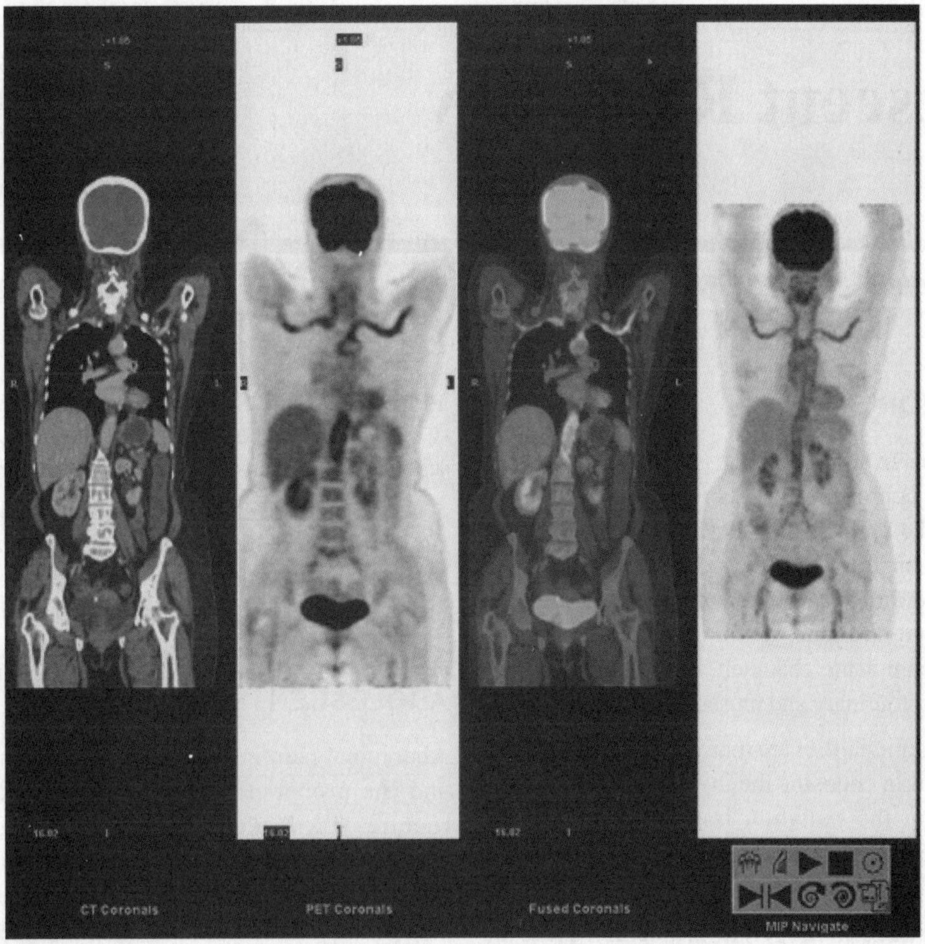

Figure 9.1.6: PET-CT scan with 18F-FDG showing uptake in large arteries (carotids, subclavian, abdominal aorta) in a case of large vessel vasculitis

SUGGESTED READING

1. Treves ST, Ed. Pediatric Nuclear Medicine and Molecular Imaging. New York; Springer Science + Business Media 2014.
2. Veltch TA. Pediatric nuclear medicine, Part II: Common procedures and considerations, J Nucl Med Technol 2000:28(2):69-75.

Adolescent Radiology

9.2

Arun Kumar Gupta, Manisha Jana

INTRODUCTION

Clinical problems in adolescent age group are unique, and the radiological approaches to them also require special consideration. The problems related to the adolescent age group are different from those in adults, and the choice of imaging modalities vary depending on the clinical problem. The common problems in adolescents that may require imaging are acute abdomen, disorders of puberty, renovascular, genitourinary and musculoskeletal disorders.

The imaging modalities are many, and the radiologist should be careful in choosing the investigation modality, keeping in mind the radiation issues and to use the modalities like ultrasonography (US) and magnetic resonance imaging (MRI) wherever feasible.

Adolescent abdominal-pelvic problems should be addressed with US initially, and computed tomography (CT) scan should be used as a problem solving tool, or used when hollow viscus pathology or perforation is suspected.

Musculoskeletal problems require plain radiography first, followed by CT/MRI; and thoracic and sinus pathologies would require CT as ideal second line investigation, after plain radiograph.

APPROACH TO PAIN ABDOMEN IN ADOLESCENTS

Abdominal pain in adolescent may have various causes, and the proper use of appropriate imaging modality requires a knowledge about the imaging modalities (Table 9.2.1) and their appropriateness in a given clinical scenario (Table 9.2.2). The observations on imaging in abdominal pain are listed in Table 9.2.3.

Table 9.2.1: Diagnostic imaging modalities and their utility

Modality	*Advantages*	*Disadvantages*	*Current role*
Plain radiography	• Less costly • Widely available • Detection of gas, calcification and foreign body and skeletal disorders	• Involves exposure to ionizing radiation • Limited information	First line imaging in suspected intestinal obstruction, perforation and renal calculi
Contrast studies	• Good evaluation of gastrointestinal (GI) pathologies, especially subacute obstruction, strictures etc.	• Involves exposure to ionizing radiation • Limited information	Limited utility in suspected intestinal obstruction, and strictures
Ultrasonography (US)	• Cost-effective, widely available • Portable • No ionizing radiation • Good for solid organ evaluation and hemoperitoneum detection	• Operator dependent • Poor evaluation of the bowel pathologies	Most often the first investigation for diagnosis or guiding the next imaging
Computed tomography (CT)	• Cross-sectional study, fast • Multiplanar and 3D imaging • Can detect almost all abdominal pathologies	• Exposure to ionizing radiation • Cost and limited availability • Risk related to iodinated contrast agents	The most useful investigation in surgical acute abdomen
Magnetic resonance imaging (MRI)	• Good soft tissue contrast resolution, multiplanar imaging capability • No ionizing radiation • Good for pelvic pathology evaluation in adolescent females	• Limited availability • Cost • Time consuming	Useful in pregnant adolescents with abdominal pain, having inconclusive US results

Table 9.2.2: Appropriate choice of imaging modalities in abdominal pain	
Clinical scenario	***Ideal imaging modality***
Acute right upper quadrant pain	Ultrasonography (US)
Acute right upper quadrant pain; no fever or leucocytosis US shows only gall stones	CT abdomen with contrast
Acute right lower quadrant pain, fever and leucocytosis (suspected appendicitis) in an adolescent	CT abdomen and pelvis with contrast
Acute right lower quadrant pain, fever and leucocytosis (suspected appendicitis), age less than 14 years or possible pregnancy	US abdomen
Acute non-localized abdominal pain and fever in pregnancy	US abdomen followed by MRI abdomen without contrast
Suspected Crohn's disease, initial evaluation	MR enterography ideal; CT enterography and CT abdomen and pelvis with contrast are other alternatives

Table 9.2.3: Imaging findings in abdominal pain	
Acute appendicitis	• *On ultrasound (US)*: Noncompressible, tubular, blind ending, aperistaltic structure measuring more than 6 mm in diameter (Figure 9.2.1) • Periappendiceal fluid collection or abscess formation • Appendicolith (echogenic focus with distal acoustic shadowing on US, high attenuation on CT) • *On contrast enhanced CT (CECT):* Soft tissue attenuation ring shadow/tubular bling ending structure in right lower quadrant in relation to cecum
Intestinal perforation and peritonitis	• Free gas under diaphragm on plain radiograph • Dilated bowel loops with multiple air fluid levels and air seen within rectum (paralytic ileus) • Free or loculated fluid with debris and septations on US abdomen
Bezoars (Tricho- and phytobezoars)	• Mottled shadow on plain radiograph (Figure 9.2.2) • On barium studies classical mottled appearance is seen due to adherence of barium and extension of barium into the interstitium of hair ball • Highly echogenic arc like structure with dense posterior shadowing on US abdomen
Inflammatory bowel disease–Crohn's disease	• *Classical findings on barium study:* Involvement of terminal ileum and segmental involvement of colon, thickening of mucosal folds, linear and transverse ulcers, rose thorn ulcers, fistulae, strictures and pseudoployps (Figure 9.2.3) • *CT and MR enterography* demonstrates skip areas of small bowel wall thickening and enhancement, prominent vasa recta in the adjacent mesentery, fibrofatty proliferation, strictures, enteroenteric fistula, abscesses, ileocecal and rectosigmoid area commonly involved (Figure 9.2.3) • Extraintestinal manifestations common in children
Ulcerative colitis	• *Double contrast enema:* Very sensitive to identify subtle lesions • Findings include, continuous involvement of long segment of colon retrogradely starting from rectum, mucosal granularity, ulceration, haustral thickening, underdistensibility, shortened and stiff colon, backwash ileitis • *CT abdomen:* Bowel wall thickening, strictures, lymphadenopathy, fibrofatty proliferation and phlegmon and abscess formation
Trauma	• *Plain X-ray abdomen:* Free air under diaphragm • *Contrast enhanced CT scan:* Solid organ laceration, hematomas and intraperitoneal bleeding.
Acute pancreatitis	• *US abdomen:* Diffusely enlarged hypoechoic pancreas, peripancreatic free fluid and fluid collections in pararenal spaces • *CT abdomen*: Pancreatic necrosis (non-enhancing areas), fluid collections, complications of pancreatitis such as thrombosis of splenoportal axis with cavernoma formation and abscess formation
Acute cholecystitis	• US abdomen is the investigation of choice • Imaging findings include, impacted stone in neck region, grossly distended gallbladder, probe tenderness, wall thickening and pericholecystic fluid collection

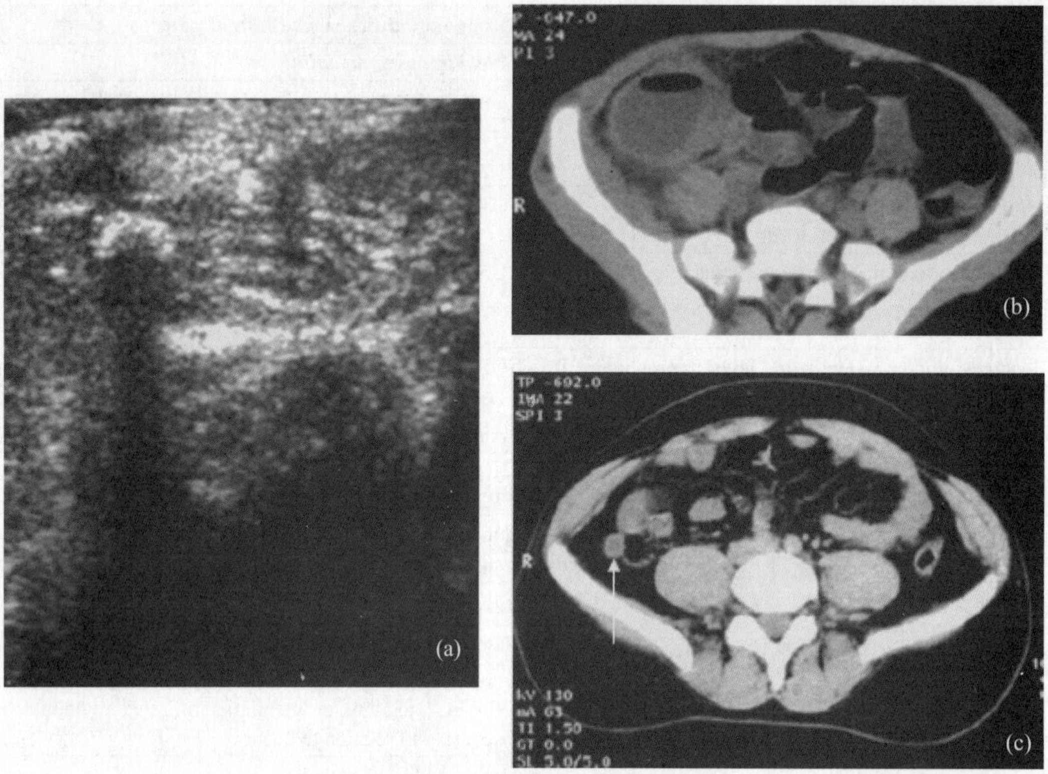

Figure 9.2.1 (a-c): Sonography (a) in acute appendicitis with appendicolith. Appendix is dilated, and thick walled with acoustic shadowing from the calculus. CECT (b and c) shows appendicular abscess with air fluid level (b) and soft tissue ring shadow adjacent to cecum (arrow in c) suggestive of thickened appendix

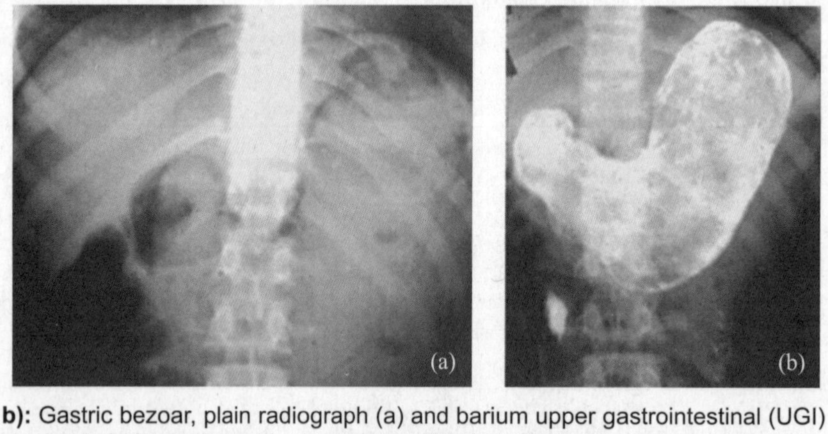

Figure 9.2.2 (a and b): Gastric bezoar, plain radiograph (a) and barium upper gastrointestinal (UGI) study (b) Note typical ill-defined filling defects due to hair masses with air trapped within hair fibers

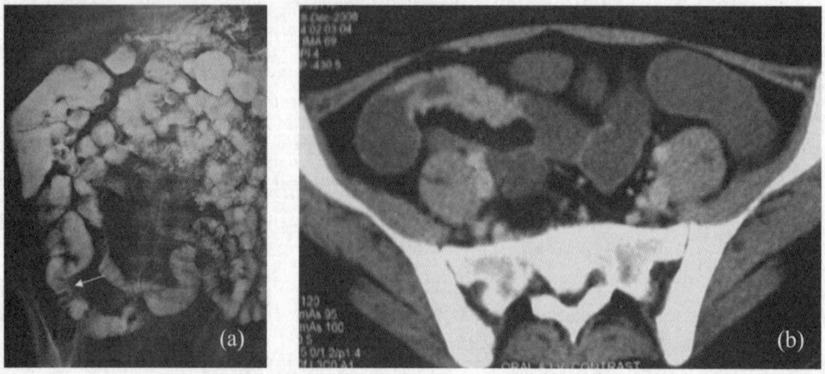

Figure 9.2.3 (a and b): Crohn's disease in an adolescent girl. Barium meal follow through study reveals separation of small bowel loops, mesenteric border shortening and antimesenteric border pseudosacculations (arrow in a). CT enterography study (b) revealed strictures at ileal loops with transverse ulcers and mesenteric fat proliferation

APPROACH TO ADOLESCENT MUSCULOSKELETAL PROBLEMS

1. **Osteochondral Lesions:** MRI allows accurate assessment of the articular cartilage and subchondral surface of bone. On plain radiograph an osteochondral fracture is a crescent-shaped radiolucent defect within which cartilage (radiolucent), degenerative fragmented calcification, or a well-corticated osteochondral body may be evident.
2. **Perthes' Disease:** On plain radiograph imaging findings include collapse of femoral epiphysis with fragmentation and sclerosis. On MRI, features are similar to that of avascular necrosis such as altered signal intensity involving femoral head with double line sign in which an outer band of low signal intensity is associated with an inner border of high signal intensity.
3. **Tumor and Tumor-like Conditions:** Musculoskeletal tumor in adolescent age group can be either benign or malignant. Many other conditions such as bone cyst, fibrous dysplasia, non-ossifying fibroma and fibrous cortical defect can mimic a bone tumor. The choice of ideal investigation is described in Table 9.2.4.
4. **Adolescent Idiopathic Scoliosis:** Imaging evaluation of idiopathic scoliosis involves plain radiographs of the spine. MRI has specific indications (Flowchart 9.2.1).
5. **Arthropathies:** Many arthopathies can present in the adolescent age group and in view of the developmental stages modalities should be chosen with care (Tables 9.2.5 and 9.2.6).

Table 9.2.4: Imaging in bone tumor and tumor-like conditions

Imaging modality	*Utility*
Plain radiograph	Ideal initial investigation modality, characterizes the lesion.
CT	For detecting cortical destruction in bone tumor, chest CT for lung metastases in malignant bone tumor.
MRI	Ideal investigation; detects tumor extent, skip lesions, neurovascular bundle involvement, adjacent muscle group involvement, transphyseal involvement and recurrence. Characterization must be done in conjunction with plain radiograph.

Table 9.2.5: Role of different imaging modalities in arthropathies

Radiography	Ideal initial investigation. In monoarthropathy, it excludes other diseases, such as osteomyelitis or septic arthritis. In polyarticular involvement, affected joint radiography and skeletal survey indicated.
Bone scan	When physical findings do not document definite arthritis, consider bone scanning as a means of identifying a potential focus of osteomyelitis or other abnormalities.
MRI	Inflammatory arthropathy and trauma.
CT	Perform when considering osteoid osteoma in an adolescent with lower extremity pain (often at night) and unremarkable findings on physical examination.

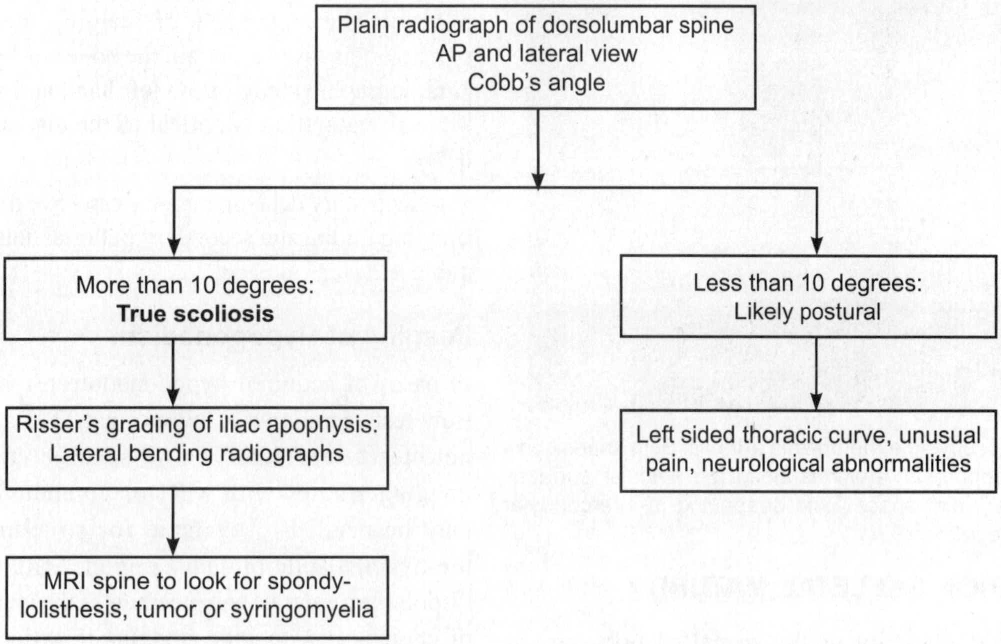

Flowchart 9.2.1: Imaging evaluation in idiopathic adolescent scoliosis

Table 9.2.6: Imaging findings in arthropathies in adolescents	
Juvenile idiopathic arthritis (Figure 9.2.4)	Bilateral symmetrical changes, periarticular osteopenia, ballooning of epiphysis, premature fusion of epiphysis and widening of intercondylar notch in case of knee joint
Juvenile spondyloarthropathies–Ankylosing spondylitis	Bilateral sacroiliac joint widening and irregularity, marginal syndesmophytes, enthesopathy (calcification at tendinous and membranous attachments), facet joint ankylosis, interspinous and supraspinous ligamentous calcification, bony ankylosis
Psoriatic arthropathy	Sacroiliitis, non-marginal syndesmophytes. In psoriatic arthropathy or Reiter's syndrome the erosive changes are asymmetrical and bony ankylosis is less usual. Erosion and periostitis involving interphalangeal joints.
Reactive arthritis	Sacroiliitis, non-marginal syndesmophytes, lower limb commonly involved.
Inflammatory bowel disease (IBD) associated arthritis	Sacroiliitis, non-marginal syndesmophytes.

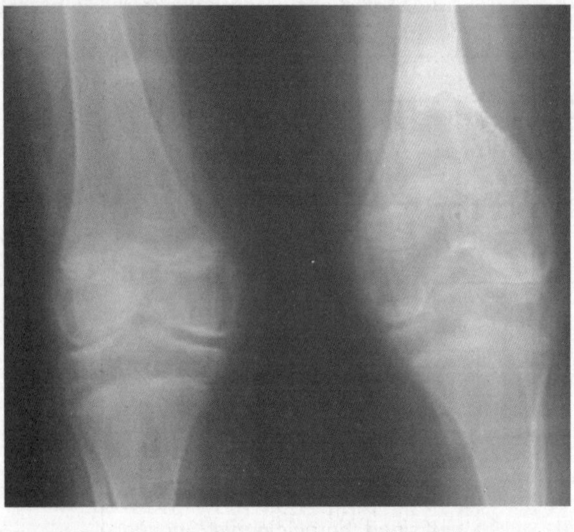

Figure 9.2.4: Juvenile rheumatoid arthritis. Both knees show diffuse osteoporosis, erosions along the articular surfaces with reduced joint spaces and deepening of intercondylar notch on the left side

IMAGING OF SKELETAL MATURITY

The skeletal maturity or the so-called bone age is an important quantitative measure for the clinical diagnosis of endocrinological diseases and growth disorders, particularly in pediatrics. It is also important in medicolegal cases for ascertaining if the person will be put under juvenile category or adult. The methods are discussed in Table 9.2.7.

Table 9.2.7: Imaging methods for skeletal maturity	
Greulich and Pyle's method	Presents a single standardized image for a range of ages of each gender.
Tanner and Whitehouse 2 (TW2) method	More extensive, time consuming; atlas involves the scoring of each carpal bone, the radius and ulna leading to a total score, from which age can be estimated.
Tanner and Whitehouse 3 (TW3) method	Revised version of TW2 method, introduced in 2001, time consuming.
Automated bone age estimation software	Automated analysis of 13 bones: radius, ulna and bones in ray 1, 3 and 5.

IMAGING OF ADOLESCENT UTERUS AND OVARY

Since puberty and related changes are important aspects of adolescence the adolescent girl can present with problems related to the onset of puberty and with menstruation. The primary imaging modality of adolescent uterus and ovary is ultrasonography. The normal physiological appearances of uterus and ovary on US abdomen/pelvis are listed in Table 9.2.8. The common causes of pelvic pain in adolescents and their sonographic features are described in Table 9.2.9.

IMAGING OF DELAYED PUBERTY

Imaging plays a minor role in constitutional delay in puberty. The major role of imaging in constitutional pubertal delay is to ascertain the bone age by radiography. A radiographic study of the left hand and wrist to assess skeletal maturation is critical to the diagnosis of growth delay.

Secondary delay in puberty can have multiple causes. Imaging findings in secondary pubertal delay are listed in Table 9.2.10.

Imaging of Hypogonadism

In cases of acquired hypogonadotropic hypogonadism (low testosterone with low-normal FSH and LH levels) not clearly attributable to a specific cause, pituitary imaging studies with MRI or computed tomography may be needed to evaluate for structural lesions in the hypothalamic-pituitary region. MRI with dynamic Gadolinium contrast enhancement is the imaging modality of choice. The imaging findings in different sellar and pituitary pathologies are listed in Table 9.2.11.

Table 9.2.8: Imaging features of pubertal changes in uterus and ovary		
	Pre-pubertal	***Post-pubertal***
Uterine length	< 4.5 cm	> 4.5 cm
Uterine thickness	<1 cm	> 1 cm
Ovarian volume	< 3 cc	> 3 cc
Uterine body/cervix ratio	< 0.5	About 2
Ovarian appearance	Homogeneous or paucicystic (upto 5 follicles measuring less than 10 mm diameter)	Multicystic (> 6 follicles measuring upto 10 mm) Macrocystic (one or more follicle 10-19 mm diameter) Polycystic (increased stromal echogenicity, more than 10 follicles (3-8 mm) arranged peripherally)

Table 9.2.9: Imaging features of adolescent uterine and ovarian pathologies presenting with pelvic pain	
Hematometra/colpos in cases of cryptomenorrhea (Figure 9.2.5)	*US Pelvis*: Anechoic cystic oblong midline structure posterior to urinary bladder and anterior to rectal gas shadow, with low level internal echoes.
Ectopic pregnancy	*US Pelvis:* Endometrial thickening (owing to decidual reaction), tubal ring sign (cystic structure in the adnexa with echogenic outline, with or without yolk sac and fetal cardiac activity), free fluid in abdomen and pelvis may be seen.
Hemorrhagic ovarian cyst	*US Pelvis:* Cystic lesion with heterogeneous appearance, both hypoechoic and hyperchoic areas, may show fluid-debris levels and posterior enhancement. Hemorrhagic cyst may mimic tubo-ovarian abscess and endometrioma on US pelvis. Clinical features help in differentiating these.
Endometrioma	*US Pelvis:* Cystic lesion in the adnexa with low level internal echoes, may be bilateral. Can mimic hemorrhagic cyst. *MRI Pelvis:* Hypointense signal on T2WI, wall hyperintense on T1W and T1W fat suppressed images.
Ovarian torsion	*US Pelvis:* Ovaries involved in torsion have variable appearance related to hemorrhage, stromal edema and infarction. Ovaries are enlarged, may appear cystic, cystic with septation and cystic with debris. Doppler helps to identify the absence of vascularity.
Ovarian tumors	*US Pelvis*: Solid, solid-cystic areas and cystic lesion with thick septations or solid mural nodule. Common pediatric tumors include teratoma, dysgerminoma, embryonal carcinoma and gonadoblastoma.

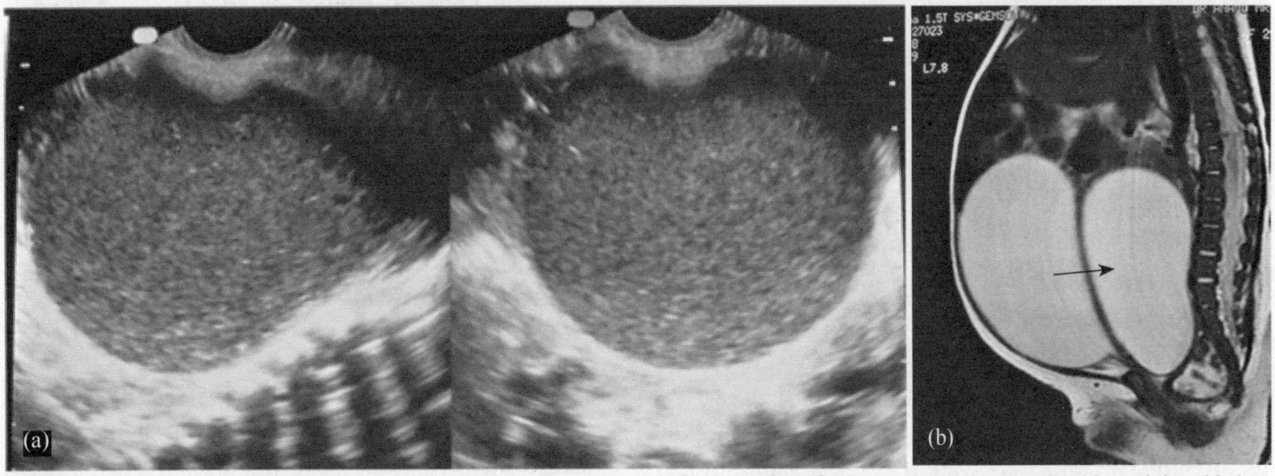

Figure 9.2.5 (a and b): Hematometrocolpos in vaginal atresia. Grey scale US shows a cystic structure in pelvis with low level internal echoes (a). Sagittal T2W MR image shows a bright structure (arrow in b) having a sagittal orientation and lying posterior to the urinary bladder, representing the distended uterus and vagina

Table 9.2.10: Imaging findings in secondary pubertal delay	
Chronic illness	*Pelvic US* in females can monitor pubertal delay
Hypogonadotropic hypogonadism	*Pelvic US*: Uterus, ovaries normal *Testicular US*: Normal *MRI*: Sellar and suprasellar pathologies (vide Table 9.2.11)
Primary gonadal failure	*Gonadal dysgenesis/secondary to trauma or inflammation:* Pelvic and testicular US– streak gonads, ovaries cannot be detected, pre-pubertal appearance of uterus.

Table 9.2.11: Imaging findings in different sellar and pituitary pathologies	
Kallmann syndrome	Absent or hypoplastic olfactory bulbs and tracts
Pituitary hypoplasia/aplasia	Flattened or non-visualized anterior pituitary, empty sella, stretched stalk till sellar floor
Craniopharyngioma (Figure 9.2.6)	Solid or cystic suprasellar mass, hyperintense cyst contents on T1WI, solid components might show enhancement
Hypothalamic glioma	Solid hypothalamic mass, hyperintense on T2WI, shows mild contrast enhancement
Langerhan's cell histiocytosis	Pituitary stalk thickening and enhancement
Septo-optic dysplasia	Absent septum pellucidum, thinning of the optic nerves (may not be apparent on imaging)
Suprasellar germinoma	Solid avidly enhancing mass in the suprasellar location, might show CSF spread

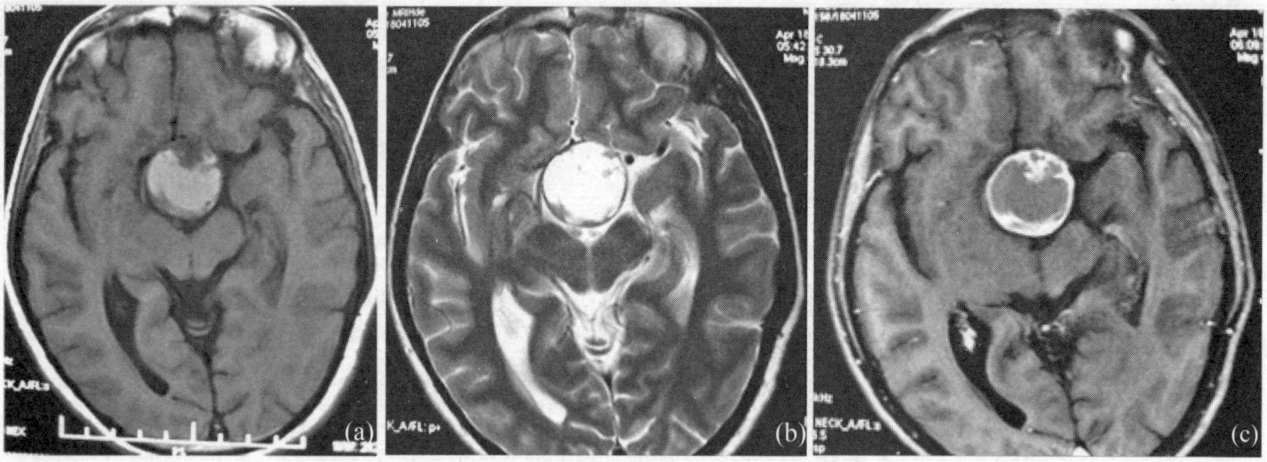

Figure 9.2.6 (a to c): Craniopharyngioma. Axial T1W and T2W MR images (a and b) reveal a hyperintense mass lesion in suprasellar location. Axial contrast enhanced T1W image (c) shows minimal peripheral enhancement

THORACIC IMAGING

Frontal chest radiograph (PA view) is the first and usually the only imaging required in majority patients (most often sufficient for diagnosis, localization of the pathology). However, CT is the preferred next modality for more precise diagnosis. MRI may be useful for mediastinal masses work-up and patients allergic to contrast media. Chest imaging is required for a number of conditions, such as infections, bronchial diseases, interstitial diseases and to identify the cause of hemoptysis. Chest infections are very common in adolescent age group. Chest PA film, one film after completion of the antibiotherapy is sufficient to rule out complications. Radiological resolution is sometimes delayed. Ultrasound is useful for the confirmation of effusion and guided thoracentesis. CT is indicated if parenchymal infiltrates are present, with or without atelectasis not resolving satisfactorily, if there is suspicion of empyema, abscesses, pneumatocele or underlying tumor.

IMAGING OF THYROID NODULE

Ultrasonography

- Sensitive in ascertaining the size and number of thyroid nodules, cannot determine if a nodule is benign or malignant.
- Guide for fine needle aspiration cytology (FNAC) study of nodules if indicated.
- Long-term follow-up of patients with thyroid cancer by detecting small or otherwise inaccessible nodules that could represent recurrence of cancer.

Magnetic Resonance and Computed Tomographic Imaging

These may play adjunctive roles, especially in loco-regional evaluation in thyroid cancer. One should keep in mind that the contrast agent for CT scanning is iodinated and may adversely affect the postoperative ability to treat with 131-I. Non-contrasted CT may be better, if feasible.

IMAGING FOR SINUSITIS

Radiography and non-contrast CT are two most widely used investigational modalities (Table 9.2.12).

SUGGESTED READING

1. ACR American College of Radiology. ACR Appropriateness Criteria. Available at website www.acr.org/Quality-Safety/Appropriateness-Criteria.

Table 9.2.12: Imaging in paranasal sinuses		
Modality	***Techniques***	***Imaging findings***
Paranasal sinus radiography	Open mouth Waters view (occipitofrontal)–Primarily useful for evaluation of maxillary and frontal sinuses, anterior ethmoid and sphenoid sinuses	*Acute sinusitis*: Diffuse opacification, mucosal thickening (> 4 mm), or an air fluid level *Chronic sinusitis*: Osteoblastic response in the affected sinus walls, mucoperiosteal thickening, opacification of sinus cavity, and even reduction of cavity size *Tumor (nasopharyngeal angiofibroma (JNA)*: Opacification of maxillary sinus with bowing of posterior maxillary wall
Non-contrast CT (NCCT)	Multidetector CT with multiplanar reformation in coronal plane	Mucosal thickening, bone sclerosis/erosion, blockage at ostiomeatal unit Can suggest etiology, e.g. bone erosion in fungal sinusitis Can detect extension in tumor (JNA)

2. Birnbaum BA, Jeffrey RB. Jr. CT and sonographic evaluation of acute right lower quadrant abdominal pain. AJR Am J Roentgenol 1998;170(2):361-71.
3. Cohen HL, Haller JO. Abnormalities of puberty and amenorrhoea. Caffey's Paediatric Diagnostic Imaging, 10th edition; Mosby USA 2004; 1939.
4. Herter LD, Golendziner E, Flores JA, Becker E Jr, Spritzer PM. Ovarian and Uterine Sonography in Healthy Girls Between 1 and 13 Years Old: Correlation of Findings with Age and Pubertal Status. AJR Am J Roentgenol 2002;178(6):1531-36.
5. Kim DH, Carucci LR, Baker ME, Cash BD, Dillman JR, Feig BW, *et al.* ACR Appropriateness Criteria Crohn Disease. J Am Coll Radiol 2015;12(10):1048-57.
6. Kuhn JP, Slovis JT, Haller JO. Musculokeletal System in Caffey's Paediatric Diagnostic Imaging, 10th edition; Mosby USA 2004; 1989-2525.
7. Lane MJ, Mindelzun RE. Appendicitis and its mimickers. Semin Ultrasound CT MR 1999;20(2):77-85.
8. Levine MS, Scheiner JD, Rubesin SE, *et al.* Diagnosis of pneumoperitoneum on supine abdominal radiograph. AJR Am J Roentgenol 1991;156:731.
9. Smith MP, Katz DS, Rosen MP, *et al.* For the Expert Panel on Gastrointestinal Imaging. ACR Appropriateness Criteria ® right lower quadrant pain–suspected appendicitis. Am Coll Radiol 2013;10.
10. Yarmish GM, Smith MP, Rosen MP, Baker ME, Blake MA, Cash BD, *et al.* ACR appropriateness criteria right upper quadrant pain. J Am Coll Radiol 2014;11(3):316-22.

10.1 Overview of Drug Administration

Jeeson C Unni, Swati Y Bhave

DRUG ADMINISTRATION IN ADOLESCENTS

There are a variety of routes by which medications can be given to an adolescent. The medications also vary in their form and route of administration (see Table 10.1.1).

EXCIPIENTS

- These are added to liquid medications to provide stability and taste.
- Preparations containing sugar, salt and alcohol need to be identified.
- Permissible alcohol content in medication intended for adolescents > 12 years is 10%, and for 6–12 years is 5%.
- Sugar-free preparations are preferable. The amount of lactose in most medications is too small to produce any symptoms in those with primary or secondary disaccharides deficiency. Nevertheless, they lactose-containing preparations need to be administered cautiously to persons with severe lactose intolerance.
- The adolescents may be occasionally sensitive to oils used as emulsifiers.
- Propylene glycol is generally considered safe but large amounts can cause lactic acidosis, if its elimination is impaired, e.g. in renal failure, in neonates and young children, and in slow metabolizers. It may interact with metronidazole.

PRESCRIBING MEDICATIONS TO ADOLESCENTS

- Adolescents must be involved and made responsible for taking medications.
- Older adolescents should become independent for managing their diseases specially chronic diseases.
- Younger adolescents should be monitored. Younger adolescent who cannot understand, will usually take medicine from someone they trust–a parent or main caretaker.
- If possible, adolescents should know why they need a medicine and should be shown how they can take it.

Table 10.1.1: Different routes and forms of medications

Route	*Liquid*	*Solid*	*Inhaled/sprays*
By mouth	Solutions, suspensions, syrups, elixirs, emulsions, oils	Tablets, capsules, granules, lozenges, chewing tablets, sublingual tablets	Metered dose inhalers, powder devices, compressed air nebulizers
Into the ear	Solutions, suspensions, drops		
Into the eye	Solutions, suspensions, drops, ointments		Sprays
Into the nose	Solutions, suspensions, drops, ointments		
Into the rectum	Enemas–Large and small, water solutions, suspensions, oils, ointments	Suppositories	
On the skin	Solutions, suspensions, drops, ointments, creams, lotions, pastes, shampoos	Powders, soaps	Sprays
Injected–Parenteral, subcutaneous, intramuscular, intravenous, intrathecal or intraosseous	Water solutions, suspensions, oil in water emulsions		

- They must have a proper understanding of what is happening and share in the decision-making as well as the responsibility.
- They must feel in control.
- It is important that those who give medicines know about the medicine and how to give correct dosages.

TIPS TO AVOID ERRORS WHILE GENERATING A PRESCRIPTION

- Take care with calculations–use your head as well as a calculator.
- If possible, always obtain a second independent check of a calculation of dosage.
- Avoid the use of decimal points by prescribing in whole units, i.e. 100 microgram rather than 0.1 mg.
- If a decimal point is required–always use a leading zero, i.e. 0.5 mg.
- Never use a trailing zero, i.e. state 5 mg and not 5.0 mg as the latter can lead to a ten-fold overdose.
- There is no accepted abbreviation for microgram, nanogram or unit. Avoid the use of 'µg' and 'ng' in prescriptions. Replacing unit by 'U' can be misinterpreted as a zero causing a ten-fold overdose.
- Remember to take account of any administration issues such as displacement volume for IV medicines, the correct diluent and administration method.

ORAL MEDICATIONS

- *Liquids:* Some older adolescents prefer liquids.
- Liquids are limited by their short shelf-life. In addition, they are heavy and bulky requiring greater storage space in pharmacy and while transporting.
- Many liquid preparations also require refrigeration.
- Powders for suspension are affected by humidity and need to be mixed with sterile fluids.
- Liquid formulations sometimes have the disadvantage of an unpleasant taste and the accuracy of the dose may be less.
- Taste is a factor that determines compliance with liquid formulations.
- Taste (unpleasant or otherwise) may be masked by adding acceptable flavoring agent or by mixing them in foods or drinks that the adolescent likes.
- Always tell the adolescent if you have put the medicines in food. There is always the possibility that an adolescent could recognize the change in taste of the foodstuff thus served and refuse any further food thinking the medicine would be added again.
- The dosage and absorption of medications may also be affected when it is mixed with food.
- It is important to check literature including drug monographs to ensure that mixing with food does not affect absorption/bioavailability of the drug and advice accordingly.
- Teaspoon size varies and therefore it is not a reliable measure of the desired quantity of liquid medication that an adolescent is prescribed.
- Time spent in explaining (and demonstrating, whenever possible) how a quantity may be measured using a dropper, plastic syringe or medicinal bottle cap with markings for different volumes, is time well spent.

TABLETS

- Tablets are cheaper than most other preparations; one can carry them around easily; and they are stable.
- It is generally felt that adolescents in the school going age can swallow tablets. However, there are exceptions to the rule and many are uncomfortable with swallowing tablets even in late adolescence.
- A liquid 'chaser' could follow immediately after the tablet is swallowed.
- Most tablets can be crushed and most capsules may be emptied to make a suspension in something acceptable.
- But crushing certain tablets to mix them with food or water may change the rate or extent of drug absorption e.g. drugs such as lopinavir/ritonavir used in anti-retroviral therapy (ART).
- Crushing drugs with a narrow therapeutic index, such as levothyroxine could also result in considerable variability between doses.
- It is not advisable to break or crush slow-release or enteric-coated tablets.
- When cutting a tablet, it is necessary to follow specific instructions on the process, including the proper use of a tablet splitter. Splitting tablets is easier when scored tablets are available.
- Whatever method is used to cut or crush a tablet, it is near to impossible to provide an accurate dose where small doses are required.
- Tablets that 'melt' on the tongue in a small amount of saliva or tablets that can be dispersed in a small amount of liquid on a spoon, are easy to administer and ensure accurate dose provided their taste is acceptable.

- It is definitely not advisable to open a capsule and administer the powder, if the reason for having a capsule formulation is to avoid its degradation or neutralization by gastric juices.

Sublingual Administration of Drugs

- This is difficult in young adolescents.
- Advances in pharmaceutical technology have resulted in the development of many different types of tablets, those that melt in the mouth; chewable and oro-dispersible tablets and films.

Administering Through a Nasogastric Tube

- Adolescents with nasogastric (NG) tubes in place should be encouraged to take medicines by mouth.
- This may not be possible if, for example, the tube is in place because of a problem with swallowing.
- Liquid medicines can be given via the tube, provided special precautions are taken to avoid the tube being blocked by the medicine.
- The liquid formulation should flow easily down the tube and the medicine should be 'washed' through with warm water.
- Medicines may be mixed with enteric feeds provided the two are compatible.
- In general, continuous feeding should be discontinued for 15 minutes before giving a medicine down the tube, unless otherwise specified.
- Evening doses of oral medicines are given about half an hour before bedtime.

AEROSOLS

- Giving drugs by inhalation for respiratory conditions delivers the medicine to where it is most needed; uses a lower dose and has fewer side-effects.
- Allowing the adolescent a say in the choice of device to be used improves the chances of success.
- Inhalation therapy is least reliable when the adolescent is not co-operative or is very distressed. The teaching of technique and good care of the devices is essential for success.
- Regular review is necessary to ensure that the devices remain effective and that the adolescents use the system most appropriate to their ability.
- Because products and delivery systems vary, it is important that the manufacturer's directions are followed precisely.
- *Dry powder inhalers:* To use these correctly adolescents need to be able to take a good deep breath in to draw the powder into the airways. They need to be able to hold their breath and not to blow out first.
- *Nebulizers:* The adolescent breathes an aerosol through a facemask or preferably, a mouthpiece. A mouthpiece gives better deposition.
- *Breath-activated inhalers* do not require co-ordination but the adolescent must be able to take a deep breath.
- *Metered dose inhalers* require an adolescent to press and breathe in at the same time. Most school children cannot manage them and their use without spacers is not encouraged. A spacer should always be used if a corticosteroid is being administered via a metered dose inhaler.
- *Spacers with metered dose inhalers (MDI):* The adolescent breathes in and out of a reservoir filled with an aerosol from an MDI. It does not require 'hand-lung' co-ordination. A mouthpiece or facemask may be used. The inspiratory breath must be sufficient to visibly or audibly open the valve. A tidal volume of 10 ml/kg can be used to estimate the number of breaths required to empty the spacer. If necessary the adolescent should be supine and the inhaler and spacer held at 90 (vertical) in order to keep the valve open. Spacers should be cleaned weekly by washing, and standing in air to dry but they should not be wiped. They should be replaced annually.

OPHTHALMIC PREPARATIONS

- Medicines meant for ophthalmic use should be kept sterile.
- An ophthalmic preparation should be discarded 28 days after it is opened as the probability of bacterial contamination is high beyond this period.
- The ideal is to drop the solution or squeeze the ointment into a gully formed by pressure of a finger on the lower lid. Tilt the head back or ask the adolescent to lie down and direct the gaze of the adolescent upwards.
- Avoid touching the eye.
- Massage the ointment into the upper and lower conjunctival sacs with finger massage on the upper and lower lids.
- Eye ointment may be applied either at night (if eye drops used during the day) or 3–4 times daily (if eye ointment used alone).
- One drop is all that is needed; instillation of more than one drop at a time should be discouraged because it

may result in an overflow and wastage of medicine or increase the probability of occurrence of systemic side-effects, and result in an overflow.

- A small amount of eye ointment is applied similarly; the ointment melts rapidly and blinking helps to spread it.
- If multiple drugs are to be instilled, to avoid dilution and overflow it is recommended to maintain an interval of at least 5 minutes between the two; interval may be extended for eye drops with a prolonged contact time, such as gels and suspensions.
- Application of an eye ointment should follow that of eye drops, if both need to be administered at the same time.

Contact Lenses and Ophthalmic Preparations

- Drugs and preservatives in eye preparations can accumulate in hydrogel lenses and can cause adverse reactions.
- Therefore, unless medically indicated, the lenses should be removed before instillation of the eye preparation and not worn during the period of treatment.
- Eye drops may, however, be instilled while patients are wearing rigid corneal contact lenses.
- Ointment preparations should never be used in conjunction with contact lens wear; oily eye drops should also be avoided.

AURAL MEDICATIONS

This is to treat conditions of the external auditory canal, which is not sterile.

Administration of Aural Medications

- Warm the bottle of ear drops if the weather of the room is cold. Rub the bottle back and forth between the palms to let the warmth thus generated heat the bottle. Place the head on one side. Pull the ear backwards and upwards. Place the number of drops prescribed in the ear so that they hit the side of the ear canal and roll into the ear. Wipe any excess drops off the outside of the ear.
- Have the adolescent remain with her/his head tilted or lying on her/his side for a few minutes to allow the drops to flow all the way into the ear.
- Do not put the drops directly into the ear canal without allowing it to hit the side as this could cause pain or dizziness. Gentle massage immediately in front of the ear helps the drops to descend into the ear and relax the adolescent.

DELIVERING INTO THE NOSTRILS

The lining of the nose is very vascular, so the intranasal route offers an alternative to an injection to achieve a systemic effect.

- This is the chosen route for some peptides (e.g. desmopressin).
- Currently however, most nose drops are given for the treatment of local conditions.
- Some adolescents might not like having liquid squirted into the nose.
- Because the nasal passage connects to the throat, there is a tendency for the saline solution to drip down the back of the throat, giving rise to a bad taste.
- When administering nasal drops, the adolescent should lie on his or her back with neck extended and after the drop is instilled the head must be tilted forward.

Instillation of a Nasal Spray

- Make sure to have small towel and tissues on hand!
- In erect position, gently spray one or two nasal drops in one nostril and allow a few seconds for the solution to moisturize the nasal passage and loosen the excess mucus.
- Use a tissue to wipe any drainage from the nose or face.
- Avoid touching the applicator to the nose to prevent the spread of organisms.
- Do the same in the other nostril.
- After spraying both nostrils blow the nose to gently to remove mucus.

TOPICAL MEDICATIONS

Topical application is mainly directed at treating disorders of the skin. However, it can be used as a route for drugs with systemic effect, and it must always be remembered that topical drugs may cause systemic toxicity, particularly if applied to damaged skin.

- Generally the skin is left exposed after topical applications, but a wet dressing may facilitate absorption, and a dry dressing may be used for protection.

- Creams are a semi-solid emulsions with equal amounts of oil and water. They are easy to spread and wash off with water. The active ingredient gets well absorbed and creams promote hydration of the skin.
- Lotions are thinner than creams and feel very light on the skin. The ingredients in lotions are absorbed very quickly. They are preferred for hairy areas.
- Ointments are 80% oil and 20% water. Although the ingredients are not absorbed well quickly, the ointment remains in contact with skin for longer periods due to its occlusive properties. In this manner, ointments promote absorption of the ingredients. This makes them more potent than when packaged as cream or lotion.
- Gels are emulsions that contain oil-in-water. They usually have an alcohol base. They dry into a thin, greaseless, non-staining film. They may be used on hairy areas and when large areas need to be treated. Because they dry the skin they may be used for those with oily skin.
- Pastes are a mixture of powder and ointment (e.g., zinc oxide 20% paste)–powder improves porosity (breathability).
- *Transdermal patch* is a medicated adhesive patch that is placed on skin to deliver a specific dose of medication through the skin and into bloodstream e.g. nicotine, estrogen, testosterone, contraceptives and vaccines.

Tips for Using Topical Medications

- It is important to keep in mind the type of vehicle used for topical medications.
- An occlusive vehicle like an ointment enhances penetration of the active ingredient and improves efficacy.
- The vehicle itself may have a cooling, drying, emollient, or protective action.
- It can also cause side effects by being excessively drying or occlusive.
- The type of preparation used can be determined by the type and site of lesions. For example, greasy ointments should not be preferred for acute weepy dermatitis, and powder in the paste is useful when treating diaper rash.
- Gel or lotion should be preferred for hairy areas.
- The irritation or sensitization potential should also be taken into consideration. Generally, ointments and water-in-oil creams are less irritating, while gels are irritating.
- Ointments do not contain preservatives or emulsifiers, and can be preferred when allergy to preservatives is a concern.

PARENTERAL MEDICATIONS

Drugs may be injected into most of the body spaces. The drugs must be sterile and pyrogen free.

- The skin may be washed and then cleaned with antiseptic (70% isopropyl alcohol) or iodine, an iodophor (e.g. Betadine)–in adolescents not sensitive to the last two mentioned antiseptics.
- If the alcohol is not allowed to evaporate, this may add to the pain of injection. A topical anesthetic cream may also be used. Neither is common practice when insulin is self-administered or when vaccines are given.
- Adolescents, like many adults, may be frightened of needles and their feelings need to be recognized and addressed.
- Adolescents need to be told to lie down for a while after a parenteral drug administration to avoid possible vasovagal syncope (e.g. HPV vaccine).

Subcutaneous (SC) Route

- Small volumes (under 2 ml) of isotonic solutions are usually given into the subcutaneous tissue using short needles with narrow bore and regular bevel.
- The subcutaneous route is used for insulin self-injection and although fat atrophy or hypertrophy can occur, this can be minimized by rotating injection sites, including the outer aspect of the upper arm, and the abdomen. In thinner adolescents it may help to pick up the skin gently between the fingers to create a pocket in which to inject vertically.

Intramuscular (IM) Route

- Most drugs can be injected into muscle but the IM route should be avoided if at all possible.
- In practice the route is used for concentrated and irritating solutions which may cause local pain if injected subcutaneously and which cannot be given other ways.
- In an adolescent who has already received several days of intravenous antibiotics and in whom cannulation has become difficult, two or three days of once a day IM injection to complete the course may be preferable to multiple intravenous cannulation attempts.
- Thin adolescents may be given 1-2 ml and bigger adolescents 1-5 ml using needles of appropriate length for the site chosen.

- The shorter and the narrower the needle, the less pain it will cause.
- Some draw up the fluid with one needle and inject with another, to avoid the solution on the wet needle irritating the needle track.
- Using a single needle saves time and for most drugs leads to no extra reaction.
- Before injecting the solution, the plunger should be slightly withdrawn to check whether the needle has entered a blood vessel. If blood is withdrawn, another site must be chosen.
- However, when IM injections are given at the recommended sites where no large blood vessels exist, pulling back of the syringe to check for blood is not recommended.
- When multi-dose vials are used, the septum must be swabbed with alcohol prior to each withdrawal and the needle should never be left in the stopper in between uses.
- IM injections should not be given to adolescents on anticoagulants or to those with thrombocytopenia.
- As IM injections can damage muscles and leave deep scars, injection sites should be regularly inspected, particularly in the immobile and very sick.
- Auto-disable (AD) syringes are single use, self-locking syringes designed in such a way that these are rendered unusable after single use.

Intravenous (IV) Route

This route is generally chosen when a medicine cannot be given by mouth and one requires faster onset of action.

- Reliable access, often a central vein, should be used for adolescents whose treatment involves irritant or inotropic drugs or who need to receive the medicine over a long period.
- The IV drugs may be given as intermittent bolus, continuous or intermittent infusion. Intravenous administration is used for administering intravenous fluids (maintenance fluids and for correction of fluid, electrolyte and acid-base disturbances), blood and blood products and medications.
- The micro-drip set is useful when drugs and fluids are to be administered at slower rates and in small volumes as the narrow tubing produces smaller drops enabling precise adjustment of slow flow rates.
- Infusion pumps can administer fluids at rates as little as 0.1 ml per hour; administer injections every minute or as repeated boluses; and amounts that vary at different times of the day.
- Fluids can be pumped in at high pressures and hence these pumps may be used for giving accurate amounts of fluids via subcutaneous or epidural routes.

PER-RECTAL ADMINISTRATION

This route is used when drugs cannot be given orally or intravenously or when a local effect is desired.

- Presence of diarrhea, impacted feces and fissure-in-ano are contraindications to the use of this route.
- The adolescent should be lying on his/her side, with legs curled up in a fetal position. The suppository should be gently inserted into the anus, just beyond the anal sphincter. It may be necessary to hold the buttocks together for several minutes to prevent the immediate expulsion of the suppository.

INTRAOSSEOUS (IO) ROUTE

Intraosseous access is resorted to, if vascular access is not rapidly achieved in anyone requiring IV drugs or fluids, especially in a life-threatening emergency. Those trained in the procedure can achieve access successfully in around 80% of attempts, within 1-2 minutes.

- The proximal tibia is the most commonly chosen site for IO catheter insertion.
- The recommended site is the flat area approximately 1 to 2 cm distal to the tibial tuberosity.
- The needle may be angled 10 to 15 degrees caudally to avoid injury to the epiphyseal growth plate.
- Disadvantages of this route include extravasation and rarely osteomyelitis.

ENDOTRACHEAL ROUTE

The endotracheal route may be used for administering drugs when intravenous or intraosseous access is not achieved especially in a life-threatening or serious condition.

- Medications are absorbed through this route but the blood levels attained may not be equivalent to those produced by IV/IO administration.
- Further, for most drugs the optimal doses for endotracheal use are unknown.
- Drugs that can be given by this route include lidocaine, epinephrine, atropine and naloxone.

SUGGESTED READING

1. Buck ML, Wiggins BS, Sesler JM. Intraosseous drug administration in children and adults during cardiopulmonary resuscitation. Ann Pharmacother 2007;41:1679-86.
2. Unni JC, Nair MKC, Menon PSN, Bansal CP, Eds. General information. In: IAP Drug Formulary, 4th Edition. Publication of Indian Academy of Pediatrics 2015;17-25.

Dosages for Medications in Adolescents

10.2

Jeeson C Unni, PSN Menon

ANESTHETICS	
General Anesthetics and Oxygen	
Halothane	*Induction of anesthesia*–Inhaled through calibrated vaporizer–start with 0.5% and increase gradually as required to 2-5% mixed with O_2 or N_2O-O_2. Maintain with 0.5-2% halothane mixed with O_2, O_2-air or N_2O-O_2.
Ketamine	Intermittent 1-4.5 mg/kg as induction followed by maintenance as required–usually ½ induction dose or as IV infusion. IV infusion-induce with 0.5-2 mg/kg followed by maintenance 0.6-2.7 mg/kg/hr. Neuropathic pain for palliative care 0.1-0.3 mg/kg/hr (max 1.5 mg/kg/hr) will suffice. IM 4 mg/kg for diagnostic/pain causing procedures.
Nitrous oxide–N_2O	*Inhalation*–Nitrous oxide is administered with oxygen to avoid the hypoxia which would otherwise occur. Doses may be self-regulated in most cases by the use of a face-mask connected through a demand valve to the cylinder. The valve is operated by the act of inhalation by the patient and closes when the patient ceases to inhale. It should be administered only by personnel trained in its use. Dose adjustments are not necessary in renal or hepatic disease.
Oxygen–O_2	*Hypoxemia and/or respiratory distress, Carbon monoxide poisoning, Shock*–100% by non-rebreather mask initially or endotracheal tube; wean as tolerated. The administration of supplemental oxygen should be considered during **EVERY** pediatric emergency.
Thiopental	IV bolus 4 mg/kg; max 10 mg/kg (facilities for ventilation must) followed in ventilated adolescents only with IV infusion at 2-8 mg/kg/hr. Reduce dose in hepatic disease.
Local Anesthetics	
Bupivacaine	*Caudal block*–15-30 ml of 0.25% or 0.5%. *Epidural block*–10-20 ml of 0.25%-0.5%. *Peripheral nerve block*–5 ml of 0.25% (12.5 mg) or 0.5% (25 mg); max 400 mg/24 hr. *Sympathetic nerve block*–20-50 ml of 0.25% (no epinephrine). The dosage of bupivacaine will depend upon the site of injection and the procedure used. Expert advice should be obtained. Epidural administration should be carried out by, or under the supervision of a consultant anesthetist.
Lidocaine/Lignocaine	*Antiarrhythmic*–Loading dose IV 50-100 mg (50 mg for thin build or those with severely impaired circulation) followed by maintenance dose IV infusion with ECG monitoring. Start with 4 mg/min for 30 min then 2 mg/kg for 2 hours; then 1 mg/min for the rest of the day. Lower conc. further if continued beyond 24 hours. *Ventricular fibrillation or pulseless tachycardia*–IV 50-100 mg. *Local anesthetic*–Local infiltration upto 200 mg–not more frequently than once in 4 hours. *Intraurethral*–3-4 mg/kg prior to catheterization.
Preoperative Medication and Sedation for Short Term Procedures	
Atropine	*Premedication*–SC/IM 300-600 µg as single dose 45 min before procedure for induction in the unpremedicated adolescent. *Sinus bradycardia*–0.5-1 mg every 5 min (maximum 2 mg) *Organophosphorus poisoning*–0.02-0.05 mg/kg every 10-20 min till atropine effect (mydriasis, tachycardia) and then once in 1-4 hours for at least 24 hours.
Diazepam	*Sedation*–IV slowly 10-20 mg. Oral 200-300 µg/kg 45-60 min before procedure. Rectal–10 mg. *Premedication*–Oral–10 mg. *Status epilepticus*–IV bolus 10-20 mg slowly. Repeat after 10 min if required. Start with the smaller dose and increase to higher dose. IV infusion–125 µg/kg/hr. Rectal–10 mg–repeat if required after 5 min. *Anxiolytic (short term)*–Oral–2-10 mg/dose thrice daily. *Suppression of stage IV sleep in parasomnias*–Oral 1.5 mg at bedtime. *Relief of muscle spasm* (post-operative, initial dose for tension and irritability in cerebral spasticity)–10 mg per dose 2 times daily.
Morphine	IV 3-4 mg; may repeat after 5 min if required.

ANALGESICS, ANTI PYRETICS, NON-STEROIDAL ANTI-INFLAMMATORY DRUGS (NSAIDs), DISEASE MODIFYING AGENTS IN RHEUMATOID DISORDERS (DMARDs)	
Non-Opioids and Non-Steroidal Anti-Inflammatory Drugs (NSAIDs)	
Ibuprofen	*Pain/fever*–5-10 mg/kg/dose 3-4 times daily (max 20 mg/kg/day upto 2.4 g/day). *Juvenile idiopathic arthritis and other rheumatic disorders*–30-50 mg/kg/24 hours in 3-4 divided doses –higher doses in systemic JIA.
Paracetamol	325-650 mg every 4-6 hourly.
Acetyl salicylic acid	*Fever*–10-15 mg/kg/dose 4-6 times daily (maximum 4 g/day). *Anti-inflammatory, analgesic dose*– 80-100 mg/kg/day. *Kawasaki disease*–25 mg/kg/dose 4 times daily for 14 days followed by 5 mg/kg once daily for 6-8 weeks. If no evidence of coronary lesions, discontinue. *Anti-platelet dose*–3-5 mg/kg/day, given as a single dose (maximum 75 mg). *Rheumatic fever*–25 mg/kg/dose for 4 doses/day for 2-3 weeks. Then 60 mg/kg/day for total period of 9-12 weeks.
Opioid Analgesics	
Codeine	*Pain*–15-60 mg/dose 4th-6th hourly. Cough–10-20 mg/dose 4th-6th hourly (max 120 mg/24 hours).
Morphine	Given above.
Disease Modifying Agents Used in Rheumatoid Disorders (DMARDs)	
Methotrexate–The most frequently used DMARD	*Juvenile idiopathic arthritis (JIA), juvenile dermatomyositis, vasculitis, uveitis, systemic lupus erythematosus (SLE), localized scleroderma, sarcoidosis*–Oral/SC/IM–10-15 mg/m^2 (increased to max. 25 mg, if needed) once weekly. *Severe acute Crohn's disease*–SC/IM–15 mg/m^2 (max. 25 mg) once weekly followed by maintenance of remission dose oral/SC/IM–15 mg/m^2 (max. 25 mg) once weekly; dose reduced according to response to lowest effective dose. *For all malignant conditions*–Early stage Burkitt's lymphoma, non-Hodgkin's lymphoma, osteogenic sarcoma, some CNS tumors including infant brain tumors, acute lymphoblastic leukemia (IV inj./ infusion); maintenance and remission of acute lymphoblastic leukemia, lymphoblastic lymphoma (oral); and meningeal leukemia, treatment and prevention of CNS involvement of leukemia (intrathecal)–Use doses prescribed in respective protocols. *Severe uncontrolled psoriasis unresponsive to conventional therapy*–Oral–initially 200 µg/kg (max. 10 mg) once weekly increased according to response to 400 µg/kg (max. 25 mg) once weekly.
Sulfasalazine	*JIA*–Oral 10 mg/kg/day 1st week, 20 mg/kg/day 2nd week, 40 mg/kg/day 3rd week, 40-50 mg/kg/day maintenance (max 3 g/day). *Ulcerative colitis/Crohn's disease*–1-2 g/kg/dose 4 times daily and half dose as maintenance. May be used as rectal suppository and enema if these preparations are available.
Hydroxychloroquine	*SLE /JIA*–Oral 5-6.5 mg/kg (max 400 mg) once daily. Adjusted according to plasma levels in severe renal and hepatic impairment.
ANTI-ALLERGICS AND MEDICINES USED IN ANAPHYLAXIS	
Chlorpheniramine	Oral–4 mg 4-6 times daily (max 2 4 mg); IM/IV/SC–10-20 mg once. Repeated upto 4 times daily (max 49 mg in adults).
Dexamethasone	*Croup*–Oral 150 µg/kg/dose twice a day or 600 µg/kg as single daily dose up to max of 12 mg/day. *Anti-emetic with chemotherapy*–IV/oral per dose–4 mg thrice daily until 48 hours after chemotherapy. *Headache of increased intracranial tension (ICT)*–IV/oral 250 µg/kg/dose 2 times daily for 5 days and then reduce the 62.5-125 µg/kg/dose twice daily. *Brain tumor edema*–IV/oral 125-500 µg/kg/dose 2 times daily. *Replacement*–IV/oral 250-500 µg/m^2/dose 2 times daily.
Epinephrine (Adrenaline)	*Cardiac arrest or profound bradycardia, asystole, ventricular fibrillation, or pulseless electrical activity*–Initial dose–IV: 10 µg/kg (0.01 mg/kg); Intraosseous: 10 µg/kg (0.01 mg/kg); Endotracheal: 100 µg/kg (0.10 mg/kg). *Note*: 10 µg/kg=0.1 ml/kg of 1:10000 dilution; 100 µg/kg=0.1ml/kg of 1:1000 dilution. If administered through an endotracheal tube, follow the dose with saline flush or dilute in isotonic saline flush (1 to 5 ml) based on patient size. *Subsequent doses:* Given every 3 to 5 minutes–IV: 100 µg/kg (0.1 mg/kg); Intraosseous: 100 µg/kg (0.1 mg/ kg), Endotracheal: 100 µg/kg (0.1 mg/kg). *Note:* For subsequent doses of epinephrine, a dosage up to 200 µg/kg (0.2 mg/kg) may be given. *Note: Anaphylaxis*–Subcutaneous (SC): 10 µg/kg per dose (maximum 3 doses); IV: 10 µg/kg per dose (10 µg/kg=0.01 ml/kg of 1:1000 dilution or 0.1 ml/kg of a 1:10000 dilution). Repeat the SC dose every 20 minutes while attempting IV access. Some anaphylactic reactions, e.g., latex allergy, require large doses of epinephrine. A continuous infusion of epinephrine may be necessary.

	Continued shock after volume resuscitation–IV infusion: 0.1 to 3.0 µg/kg/min. Start at lowest dose and titrate for desired clinical effect. Preparation of infusion solution: 0.6 mg × body weight (kg) diluted to 100 ml. Infuse at 1 ml/h = 0.1 µg/kg/min using a constant infusion pump. *Note*: Extravasation can result in tissue necrosis injuries. *Status asthmaticus, bronchospasm*–SC: 10 µg/kg per dose (10 µg/kg = 0.01 ml/kg of 1:1000 dilution). Maximum single dose, 300 µg (0.3 ml of 1:1000 dilution). Repeat SC dose every 20 minutes if needed for clinical effect. Total of 3 doses. *Laryngotracheobronchitis:* Racemic epinephrine, 2.25% inhalation solution–20–40 kg: 0.50 ml in 2 ml with normal saline administered by nebulizer; >40 kg: 0.75 ml in 2 ml with normal saline administered by nebulizer. *L-Epinephrine:* An equal volume of 1% L-epinephrine (1:100) is approximately equivalent in biologic activity to 2.25% racemic epinephrine; one can be substituted for the other in equal volumes for inhalation. Alternatively, 5 ml of 1:1,000 L-epinephrine is equivalent to 0.5 ml of 1:100.
Hydrocortisone	See under "Hormones"
Prednisolone	See under "Hormones"
ANTI-DOTES AND OTHER SUBSTANCES USED IN POISONING	
Non-specific	
Activated charcoal	Dose related more to dose of poison (10 times weight of poison is given) than age/weight of child. If amount of toxin unknown, either give as single dose within 1 hour of ingestion of poison or as multiple doses 4th hourly till toxicity abates or side effects of charcoal become evident–by weight 1 g/kg.
Specific	
Atropine sulfate	Given above.
Deferasirox	Start with 20 mg/kg orally once daily calculated to nearest whole tab. Adjust dose in increments of 5-10 mg/kg every 3-6 months based on ferritin levels (max 30 mg/kg/day) since there is limited experience at higher doses.
Deferiprone	25 mg/kg/dose rounded to the nearest 250 mg dose 3 times daily (max 100 mg/kg/day).
Pralidoxime	*Organophosphorus poisoning*–Following resuscitation measures, and 2-4 mg atropine inj., 1-2 g IM or IV as 5% soln. over 5-10 min. or infusion in 100 ml sodium chloride over 15-30 min. Repeat therapy if required.
Calcium gluconate	*Hypocalcemia:* Urgent correction–2 ml/kg of 10% solution IV bolus over 5-10 min (0.3 ml/kg/dose), followed by oral maintenance. If IV maintenance desired for a few days, be careful to avoid extravasation and administer 10% solution at 40 ml/24 hours. *Cardiopulmonary resuscitation*–0.3 ml/kg of 10% solution as single IV bolus. *Parenteral nutrition regimen*–Approximate doses to maintain normal serum calcium–5-10 mmol/24 hours continuous IV over 12-24 hours. *Hyperkalemia*–1-2 ml/kg intravenously.
Naloxone	*Suspected narcotic depression*–IM preferred because it affords more prolonged effect. 0.1 mg/kg may be repeated after 3-4 min (max 2 mg) may be given IV. Repeat doses to maintain opioid reverse. If no response seen after 2 doses, diagnosis of opioid toxicity must be reviewed.
ANTI-CONVULSANTS/ANTI-EPILEPTICS	
Carbamazepine	Initially 200 mg twice daily; increase by 200 mg/day once in a week till effect obtained (usually 1.6-2.4 g/day in 3-4 divided doses).
Sodium valproate	Oral start with 10-15 mg/kg/day in 2 divided doses and maintain at 12.5-15 mg/kg/day.
Phenobarbitone	*Anti-convulsant*–1-3 mg/kg/24 hr oral or IV in 2 divided doses or as single daily dose.
Phenytoin	*Status epilepticus*–Loading dose–15-18 mg/kg IV (not to exceed 1-3 mg/kg/min). *Antiepileptic*–Oral/IV–16 years: 6-7 mg/kg/24 hours once daily or in 2 divided doses, > 16 years 300-600 mg/24 hr once daily or in 2 divided doses. *Arrhythmias*–Loading dose 1.25 mg/kg IV once in 5 min until desired effect or total dose 15 mg/kg. *Maintenance*–250 mg 3-4 times daily.
Clobazam	*Initially orally*–10 mg/dose 2 times daily followed by maintenance of 10-15 (max 30) mg/dose in 2 doses.

ANTI-INFECTIVE MEDICINES	
Anthelminthics–Intestinal Anthelminthics	
Albendazole	*Whipworm, trichuriasis, pinworm, threadworm, hookworm, roundworm, ascariasis*–400 mg. Single dose. May be repeated after 2-3 weeks for pinworm, threadworm. *Ancylostomiasis*–400 mg single dose. *Strongyloidosis (Strongyloides stercoralis)*–400 mg twice daily for 3 days, repeated after 3 weeks. More effective than mebendazole. *Enterobiasis*–100-200 mg single dose, repeated after 4 weeks. *Trichinosis*–2-12 years 400 mg daily once for 5 days. Repeat if necessary. *Tapeworm*– 400 mg daily once for 3 days. *Neurocysticercosis*–In neurocysticercosis, albendazole is used in dose of 15 mg/kg for 3-4 weeks. A short course of 8 days is also found to be effective depending upon location of cyst. 7.5 mg/kg upto maximum of 400 mg twice daily for 14-28 days. Take with food. Repeat if necessary. Under steroid and anticonvulsant cover and in readiness for shunting for raised intracranial pressure. *Hydatid disease, echinococcosis*–15 mg/kg daily for 4 weeks. Repeat the dose after 14 days, if required for next such 3 doses. *Cutaneous larva migrans*–400 mg daily once for 5 days. *Toxocariasis*–400 mg twice daily for 5 days. Steroid cover in symptomatic cases; especially if there is ocular involvement. *Filariasis*–It has adjuvant value to DEC or ivermectin in lymphatic filariasis. A single dose in combination has been used in mass programmes.
Mebendazole	100 mg 2 times daily for 3 consecutive days. Better than albendazole for trichuris infestation. *Hydatid disease*–200-400 mg bid or tid for 3-4 weeks, less effective than albendazole. Reduction in dose for hepatic impairment.
Pyrantel pamoate	11 mg/kg/day as single dose. Repeat after two weeks (max 1 g). In heavy hookworm infestation give for two successive days.
Praziquantel	*Schistosomiasis hematobium (S mansoni)*–Oral 40 mg/kg/day as single dose or in 2 divided doses with food for 1 day. *S japonicum*–60 mg/kg/day in 3 divided doses with food 1 day. *Liver fluke*–60 mg/kg/day in 2 divided doses with food for 3 days. *Lung fluke (Paragonimus westermani)*–75 mg/kg/day 3 divided doses with food for 3 days. *Intestinal fluke (Fasciolopsis buski)*–75 mg/kg/day in 3 divided doses with food for 1 day. *Beef, pork and fish tapeworm*–25 mg/kg/day as single dose with light breakfast for 1 day. *Dwarf tapeworm*–25 mg/kg/day as single dose with light breakfast for 1 day. *Neurocysticercosis*–50 mg/kg/day in 3 divided doses with food for 15-21 days. Give steroids to reduce severity of adverse reactions. *Echinococcosis*–40 mg/kg/day once in a week with food in combination with albendazole as adjunct to surgery and for inoperable cysts. No dosage adjustment for renal failure and hepatic failure.
Anti-Filarials	
Diethylcarbamazine	*Filariasis and loiasis*–Oral 300 µg/kg/dose on day 1 and increased over 3 days to 2 mg/kg/dose daily for 3 weeks. *Tropical pulmonary eosinophilia*–Oral 6 mg/kg/day in 3 divided doses for 21 days. *Toxocariasis (Visceral larva migrans)*–Oral 160 µg/kg/dose on day 1 and 2 and increased over 3 days to 2 mg/kg/dose 3 times and given for further 7-10 days.
Anti-Schistosomals and Anti-Trematode Drugs	
Praziquantel	Given above
Anti-Bacterials	
Beta-Lactam Antibiotics	
Amoxicillin	Oral 20-50 mg/kg/day in 2 or 3 divided doses (maximum of 500 mg 2-3 times daily). *Uncomplicated gonorrhoea*–3 g with 1 g probenecid.
Co-amoxiclav (Amoxicillin + Clavulanic acid)	Dosed on amoxycillin content. 20-45 mg/kg in 2-3 divided doses–give at the start of a meal. IV: Reconstitute a 600 mg vial with 10 ml water for injections (final volume 10.5 ml) and a 1.2 g vial with 20 ml (final volume 20.9 ml). Give by slow IV injection (over 3-4 minutes, within 20 minutes of reconstitution) or infuse over 30-40 minutes and complete infusion within 4 hours of reconstitution. For infusion the reconstituted injection can be diluted to 5 times its volume in NaCl 0.9%. Do not infuse in glucose solutions, as co-amoxiclav is less stable in infusions containing glucose.
Ampicillin	500 mg/dose; IV/IM 25 mg/kg/dose (max1g/dose); IV infusion 100 mg/kg/dose (maximum 3 g/dose)–all given 4 times daily.

Benzyl penicillin	25 mg/kg/dose 4 times daily. In severe infection and meningitis 50 mg/kg/dose 6 times daily to maximum single dose of 2.4 g and daily dose of 14.4 g/day. In moderate renal failure (creatinine cl 10-50 ml/minute/1.73 m^2), dosage interval may be increased to 8-12 hours and in severe renal failure (<10 ml/minute/1.73 m^2) to every 12 hours.
Benzathine penicillin	*Group A streptococcal URI*–12 lakh (L) units as single dose. *Prophylaxis of rheumatic fever*–<27 kg 6 lakh units; >=27 kg–1.2 lakh units every 21 days. *Congenital syphilis*–50,000 units/kg/dose (max 24 L units) once a week for 3 weeks. Early syphilis in adolescents–24 L units as single dose in 2 injection sites. If present for > 1 year–24 L units as single dose in 2 injection sites once weekly for 3 doses.
Phenoxymethyl penicillin	2 g/day (severe infection 3 g/day) in 4 divided doses. *Pneumococcal infection prophylaxis*–Half the above daily dose in 2 divided doses. *Rheumatic fever prophylaxis*–500 mg/day in 2 divided doses.
Cloxacillin	IV/IM 50-100 mg/kg/day in 4 divided doses (max single dose 1 g–may be doubled in severe infection). Oral–1g in 4 divided doses. Doses may be doubled in severe infection. Renal failure–cr cl (<10 ml/minute/1.73 m^2) increase dosage interval to 8th hourly.
Cephalexin	250-500 mg 4 times daily (maximum 4 g/24 hours. Reduce dose in severe renal impairment cr cl (<10 ml/minute/1.73m^2) by reducing dose frequency. Removed by dialysis thus an additional dose may be required after dialysis.
Cefixime	400 mg/24 hr in 1-2 divided doses.
Cefotaxime	1-3 g 2 times daily. Dosage adjustment in renal impairment. Due to extra-renal elimination it is only necessary to reduce dose in severe renal impairment cr cl (<10 ml/minute/1.73 m^2). A normal single dose should be given as a loading dose then the daily dose should be halved without a change in frequency.
Ceftriaxone	50-75 mg/kg once daily IV/IM. *Meningitis*–Loading dose 75 mg/kg followed by 80-100 mg/kg/24 hours once or divided 12 hourly. Maximum 4 g/day. In severe renal failure reduce dose to a maximum of 2 g or 50 mg/kg. No dose adjustment required in hepatic impairment. If both hepatic and severe renal impairment monitor serum concentrations. In patients undergoing dialysis no supplemental dose required but serum concentration monitoring advisable.
Ceftazidime	150 mg/kg/24 hr divided 8th hrly. Maximum 6 g/day. Single dose > 1g to be given IV only. Dose adjustment in renal failure–In mild impairment give a dose every 12 hours, in moderate impairment (cr cl 10-50 ml/minute/1.73 m^2) give a dose once daily and in severe impairment (cr cl <10 ml/minute/1.73 m^2) give 50% of dose once daily. Levels may be monitored if clinically indicated. In hemodialysis: The appropriate maintenance dose should be repeated after dialysis. In peritoneal dialysis: 125-250 mg be added to 21 of dialysis fluid, and given in addition to the IV dose.
Cefpodoxime	9 mg/kg/day in 2 divided doses (maximum single dose–200 mg). The dose frequency should be reduced in renal impairment. Cr cl 10-40 ml and <10 ml/minute/1.73m^2–frequency of dosing once in 24 hours and once in 48 hours respectively
Other Anti-Bacterials	
Azithromycin	400 mg (12-14 years) and 500 mg > 14 years. Alternatively, 10 mg/kg/day once on first day followed by 5 mg/kg/day once daily from day 2–day 5. *Group A beta-hemolytic streptococcal (GAS) pharyngitis and tonsillitis (primary prophylaxis of rheumatic fever)*–12.5 mg/kg/day–Single dose for 5 days (Not recommended for secondary prophylaxis of rheumatic fever). *Chlamydial infection such as non-gonococcal urethritis (NGU) or cervicitis due to susceptible strains of Chlamydia trachomatis*–single dose of 1 g orally. *Bacterial endocarditis prophylaxis*–15 mg/kg (single dose max 500 mg) 30-60 minutes before procedure if allergic to penicillin. *Treatment and postexposure pertussis prophylaxis*–For postexposure prophylaxis, administer to close contacts within 3 weeks of exposure, especially in high-risk patients e.g. women in 3rd trimester, 10 mg/kg/day (maximum 500 mg) on day 1, then 5 mg/kg/day (maximum 250 mg) on days 2-5. *Uncomplicated typhoid fever*–Orally–8-10 mg/kg/day once daily for 7 days–1000 mg on first day, followed by 500 mg once daily for 6 days. Children: 10 mg/kg/day once daily for 7 days or 5-day regimen of 20 mg/kg/day. Continued treatment may be needed to prevent relapse in cryptosporidiosis. *Sexually transmitted diseases (STD) caused by Chlamydia trachomatis*–1 g as single dose.

Erythromycin	*General indications*–250-500 mg 4 times daily. IV 12.5 mg/kg/dose 4 times daily or as a continuous infusion. Maximum dose–4 g/day. Replace by oral dosage as soon as possible. *Topical (acne vulgaris)*–Wash and apply twice daily directly to the affected area. *Secondary prevention of rheumatic fever*–When child is sensitive to penicillin–Oral 20 mg/kg/day max 500 mg twice daily (Contraindicated in liver disorder). *Group A beta-hemolytic streptococcal (GAS) pharyngitis (primary rheumatic fever prophylaxis as an alternative to penicillin in children allergic to penicillin)*–40 mg/kg/day in 4 divided doses for 10 days. Cardiology Sub Chapter of IAP does not recommend using erythromycin for this indication. *Uncomplicated urethral, endocervical, or rectal gonorrhea, penicillinase-producing Neisseria gonorrhoeae, or for gonorrhea during pregnancy*–500 mg PO four times per day for 7 days. *Treatment and post-exposure pertussis prophylaxis*–For post-exposure prophylaxis, administer to close contacts within 3 weeks of exposure, especially in high-risk patients (e.g. women in 3rd trimester). Oral 40-50 mg/kg/day PO (max 2 g/day) in four divided doses for 14 days. *Pneumococcal prophylaxis*–1 g/day in 2 divided doses. *Gastric stasis*–Oral/IV 3 mg/kg 4 times daily.
Chloramphenicol	50 mg/kg/day (maximum 1 g/day) in 4 divided doses–double dose for meningitis, septicemia. Ear drops–2-3 drops 2-3 times daily. Eye ointment may be used in the ear. Eye drops–1 drop 4-6 times daily (1-2 hourly in severe infections). In addition, a small amount of ointment may be applied at bedtime. Eye ointment–Apply 4 times daily (1-2 hourly in severe infections). Continue treatment till 48 hours after the eye is clinically normal.
Netilmicin	IV/IM–6 mg/kg/day in 3 divided doses or 7.5 mg/kg as single dose daily. Intraperitoneal 7.5-10 mg/L in peritoneal dialysis fluid.
Gentamicin	3-6 mg/kg/day in 3 divided doses. Plasma levels done after 3-4 doses to achieve predose level of <2 mg/L and 1 hour post dose peak of 5 mg/L. Alternatively 5-7.5 mg/kg/24 hours IV once daily. Plasma levels done 18-24 hours after 1st dose to achieve predose level of <1 mg/L and 1 hour post dose peak of 16-20 mg/L. Once daily dose regimen (not for endocarditis or meningitis) by intravenous infusion–initially 7 mg/kg, then adjusted according to serum-gentamicin concentration. *Intrathecal/ventricular*–Preservative free preparation–1-2 mg/24 hours. *Pseudomonal lung infection in cystic fibrosis*–By inhalation of nebulized solution–160 mg twice daily. 0.3% eye drops–1 drop upto 6 times/day. In severe infections 1 drop every 15-20 min and gradually decreasing frequency as infection gets controlled till 48 hours after healing. 1.5% eye drops for severe eye infection. Ear drops–2-3 drops 3-4 times daily and at night.
Cotrimoxazole–Trimethoprim (TMP) + Sulphamethoxazole (SMX)	6-20 mg TMP/kg/24 hours divided 12th hourly (maximum 160 mg TMP 12th hourly). *Pneumocystis carinii pneumonia*–Oral/IV 15-20 mg TMP/kg/24 hr divided 12th hourly. *P carinii prophylaxis*–Orally 5 mg TMP/kg/24 hours or 3 times/week.
Nitrofurantoin	*Urinary tract infections (UTI)*–200-400 mg/day in 4 divided doses. *UTI prophylaxis*–1-2.5 mg/kg/day in at bedtime or in 2 divided doses (max 100 mg/24 hr).
Ciprofloxacin	15-30 mg/kg/24 hr in 2 divided doses oral or IV (Maximum single dose IV 400 mg and oral 750 mg). *Dose adjustment in renal or liver failure:* In severe impairment (creatinine clearance <20 ml/min/1.73 m^2). Total daily dosage may be reduced by half, although monitoring serum levels provides the most reliable basis for dose adjustment. No adjustment in impaired hepatic function. *Corneal ulcers*–Apply throughout the day and night. First day–2 drops every 15 min for 6 hours followed by 2 drops every 30 min for the rest of the day, 2nd day–2 drops every hour and from 3rd to 14th day–2 drops 4th hourly. *Superficial infections of eye*–1-2 drops 4 times daily till 48 hours after the eye is clinically normal (use for max. of 21 days).
Metronidazole	See under anti-amebic medicines.
Linezolid	IV infusion over 30-120 min–10 mg/kg 8th hourly for 14-28 days. Those with VP shunts achieve variable CSF therapeutic concentrations–600 mg 12th hourly for 14-28 days. Oral: 600 mg 12th hourly for 10-14 days.
Anti-Leprosy Medicines	
Clofazimine	*Multibacillary leprosy* (in combination with dapsone and rifampicin), by mouth–50 mg once daily and 300 mg once a month; Child 10-14 years, 50 mg on alternate days and 150 mg once a month; continue treatment for 12 months. *Type 2 lepra reaction (erythema nodosum leprosum)*–By mouth–200-300 mg daily in 2 or 3 divided doses for a maximum of 3 months; 4-6 weeks treatment may be required before any effect is seen.
Dapsone	*Leprosy*–Oral 1-2 mg/kg/day as single dose in combination with rifampicin. *Blistering skin conditions*–Start at 500 µg/kg/day and increase or decrease as necessary in 12.5 mg increments.
Rifampicin	Discussed under Anti-tuberculosis Medicines.

Anti-Tuberculosis Medicines	
Isoniazid	*Daily therapy*–10 mg/kg/day–range 10-15 mg/kg/day (max 300 mg); Intermittent therapy–15 mg/day–range 12-17 mg/kg/day.
Rifampicin	*Tuberculosis in combination with other drugs*–Oral 10 mg/kg (max 600 mg/day) as single morning dose. *Meningococcal infection prophylaxis and staphylococcal infections*–Oral 10 mg/kg/dose (max 600 mg/dose) 2 times daily for 2 days for meningococcal infection prophylaxis and for 10-14 days for staphylococcal infections. *H influenzae prophylaxis*–20 mg/kg/dose (max 600 mg/dose) once daily for 4 days. *Cholestasis, pruritus*–5-10 mg/kg (max 600 mg) once daily. *Dose adjustment in liver failure*. Avoid altogether, or reduce doses for tuberculosis and prophylaxis to 8 mg/kg daily.
Ethambutol	Daily therapy–20 mg/kg/day–range 15-20 mg/kg/day (max 1500 mg); Intermittent therapy–30 mg/day–range 25-30 mg/kg/day.
Pyrazinamide	Daily therapy–35 mg/kg/day–range 30-40 mg/kg/day (max 2000 mg); <50 kg 1.5 g/day and > 50 kg 2 g/day as single dose or in 2 divided doses (max 2 g/day) for the first 2 months of the standard 6 months regimen. Intermittent therapy–35 mg/day–range 30-40 mg/kg/day.
Streptomycin	IM–Daily therapy–15 mg/kg/day–range 15-20 mg/kg/day (max 1000 mg); Intermittent therapy–15 mg/day–range 15-20 mg/kg.
Anti-Tuberculosis Medicines–Multi-Drug Resistant Tuberculosis (MDR TB)	
Cycloserine	250-500 mg twice daily for 2 weeks and then increased to 500 mg–1 g in divided doses. *MDR TB–Revised National Tuberculosis Control Program (RNTCP)*–16-25 kg: 250 mg; 26-45 kg: 500 mg; >45 kg: 750 mg; respectively, once daily.
Ethionamide	*MDR TB–RNTCP*–16-25 kg: 375 mg; 26-45 kg: 500 mg; >45 kg: 750 mg; respectively, once daily.
Para-amino-salicylic acid (PAS)	14-16 g/day in 2-3 divided doses–*MDR TB–RNTCP*–PAS with 80% bioavailability–16-25 kg: 5 g; 26-45 kg:–10 g; >45 kg: 12 g; respectively, once daily. In case of PAS with 60% bioavailability the dose will be increased to 7 g (16-25 kg); 14 g (26-45 kg) and 16 g (> 45 kg).
Ofloxacin	*MDR TB–RNTCP*–16-25 kg: 400 mg; 26-45 kg: 600 mg; >45 kg: 800 mg; respectively, once daily. *Eye drops*–1 drop 2-4 hourly for 1st 48 hour s and then 4 times daily till 2 days after healing is achieved (max10 days). *Ear drops–Otitis externa*–10 drops to affected ear(s) 2 times daily for 10 days. *Chronic suppurative otitis media (CSOM)*–10 drops to affected ear(s) 2 times daily for 14 days. *Acute otitis media (AOM) with perforation or with tympanostomy tubes*–5 drops to affected ear(s) 2 times daily for 10 days. IV and oral–10-15 mg/kg/day in a single dose or divided twice daily.
Anti-Fungal Medicines	
Fluconazole	*Mucosal candidiasis*–Oral/IV loading dose 6 mg/kg followed by 3 mg/kg once daily for 7-14 days. *Systemic candidiasis and cryptococcosis*–6-12 mg/kg daily once (max 400 mg)–dose dependent on severity of infection. *Prophylaxis of fungal infection in immunocompromised*–3-12 mg/kg once daily (max 400 mg)–dose dependent on extent and duration of neutropenia.
Griseofulvin	500 mg once daily.
Nystatin	*Intestinal and oral candidiasis*–1 ml 3-4 times daily; *oral candidiasis in immunocompromised*–1 ml 4-6 times, *esophageal/intestinal candidiasis*–5 ml or 1 tab 4-6 times daily.
Potassium iodide	*Sporotrichosis*–Saturated solution (1000 mg/ml); 1 drop 3 times daily, increase as tolerated to max of 1 drop/kg or 40-50 drops 3 times daily, whichever is lower–given till several weeks after all lesions have healed. *Thyrotoxicosis*–50-200 mg 3 times daily (1-10 drops 3 times daily).
Anti-Viral Medicines	
Acyclovir	*Herpes simplex*–200 mg 5 times daily for 5-7 days – start within 72 hours of onset for best results. *Genital herpes*–Treatment of initial infection - reduces severity and duration but no effect on frequency of subsequent recurrent infections. Adolescent–400 mg tid; child–10-20 mg/kg/dose qid for 7-10 days. *Episodic therapy for recurrent genital herpes*–Adolescent 800 mg tid for 2 days. *Herpes simplex prophylaxis in the immunocompromised*–Oral–200-400 mg 4 times daily. *Herpes simplex suppression*–Oral–400 mg twice daily or 200 mg 4 times daily. Increased to 400 mg thrice daily if recurrences occur on standard suppressive therapy or for suppression of genital herpes during late pregnancy (from 36 weeks gestation). Therapy interrupted every 6-12 months to reassess recurrence frequency; consider restarting after two or more recurrences. *Local treatment of herpes simplex infections*–Eye–Apply 1 cm ointment 5 times daily (continue for at least 3 days after complete healing). Skin–Apply to lesions every 4 hours (5 times daily) for 5-10 days, starting at first sign of attack. *Chickenpox and Herpes zoster*–Treat within 24 hours. *Immunocompromised and those at special risk*–(Severe cardiovascular/respiratory disease/chronic skin disorder–10 days with at least 7 days of parenteral treatment–800 mg 5 times daily for 7 days (Herpes zoster in the immunocompromised continue for 2 days after crusting of lesions). IV infusion–5 mg/kg 8th hourly for 5 days. At all ages–double dose in encephalitis or immunocompromised (given for 10-14 days in encephalitis, possibly longer if also immunocompromised). To avoid excessive dose in obese –IV dose calculated on the basis of ideal weight for height. *Attenuation of chickenpox if VZ immunoglobulin not indicated*–Oral–10 mg/kg 4 times daily for 7 days starting 1 week after exposure.

Anti-Retrovirals	
Nucleoside/Nucleotide Reverse Transcriptase Inhibitors	
Didanosine (DDI)	Oral–120 mg/m^2/dose 2 times daily and if given with zidovudine 90 mg/m^2/dose 2 times daily. In renal impairment–creatinine clearance (ml/min/1.73 m^2)/dose/frequency–30-59/60% of normal total dose/2 divided doses, 10-29/40% of normal total dose/once daily, <10/30% of normal total dose/once daily. Total daily dose may be given once daily to improve compliance. Dose reduction better when reintroducing following discontinuation due to pancreatitis/neuropathy/hepatic impairment.
Lamivudine (3TC)	Weight >= 40 kg: 300 mg/day. Safe and effective use has not been established in adolescent <40 kg. Patients with renal impairment: CrCl <= 50 ml/min: Lamivudine requires dose adjustment.
Zidovudine (ZDV or AZT)	180 mg/m^2 2 times daily (max 250 mg/dose). IV 120 mg/m^2 4 times daily.
Non-Nucleoside Reverse Transcriptase Inhibitors	
Efavirenz (EFV or EFZ)	32.5-39.9 kg: 400 mg, 25-32.4 kg: 350 mg, 20-24.9 kg: 300, 15-19.9 kg: 250 mg.
Nevirapine (NVP)	*Treatment of HIV infection in combination with other antiretroviral agents*–200 mg PO once daily for the first 14 days, then 200 mg PO twice daily. If mild to moderate rash with constitutional symptoms is observed during the first 14 days of therapy, do not increase the dose until the rash has resolved; if the rash does not resolve by treatment day 28, discontinue nevirapine and use an alternative treatment regimen. Permanently discontinue treatment if severe hepatotoxicity, severe cutaneous reactions, or hypersensitivity reactions occur. Adolescents in early puberty (Tanner I—II) should be dosed using pediatric schedules i.e., 150 mg/m^2 (not to exceed 400 mg) PO once daily for the first 14 days, then 150 mg/m^2 (not to exceed 400 mg) twice daily. *Pregnant; intrapartum*–The addition of single-dose maternal/infant nevirapine to an ongoing highly active combination antiretroviral therapy regimen does not provide additional efficacy in reducing perinatal transmission and may result in nevirapine resistance in the mother, and is therefore not recommended. In patients who are not receiving any antiretroviral treatment prior to labor, administer 200 mg PO as a single dose at the onset of labor.
Protease Inhibitors	
Ritonavir (RTV)	*Low dose ritonavir to increase effect of atazanavir*–Oral–<20 kg: 80-100 mg OD; > 20 kg: 100 mg OD. *Low dose ritonavir to increase effect of darunavir*–Oral–20-30 kg: 50 mg BD; 30-40 kg: 60 mg BD; >40 kg: 100 mg BD. *Low dose ritonavir to increase effect of fosamprenavir*–Oral–25-33 kg: 3 mg/kg twice daily; >33 kg: 100 mg BD. *Low dose ritonavir to increase effect of saquinavir*–Oral–100 mg BD. *Low dose ritonavir to increase effect of tipranavir*–Oral–200 mg BD.
Anti-Amoebic and Anti-Giardiasis Medicines	
Metronidazole	*Anerobic infections and propionic and methylmalonic acidemia*–Oral/IV 7.5 mg/kg/dose (max 400-500 mg) 3 times daily. *Giardiasis*–Oral 40 mg/kg (max 2 g) once daily for 3 days. *Trichomoniasis*–5 mg/kg/dose (max 300-499 mg/day) 3 times daily for 7 days. *Amebiasis (5-10 days) and balantidiasis (5 days)*–Oral 10 mg/kg (max 400-800 g. *H. pylori*–Oral–400 mg/dose 3 times daily for 14 days with either amoxicillin/omeprazole or clarithromycin/omeprazole. Increase dose interval to 12 hours in renal impairment (Cr Cl <20 ml/min/1.73 m^2). Reduce dose in hepatic impairment and avoid in hepatic encephalopathy.
Diloxanide	1.5 g in 3 divided doses.
Anti-Leishmaniasis Medicines	
Sodium stibogluconate	IV/IM–20 mg/kg (max 850 mg) daily once for 20-30 days. Total daily dose may be given in 2 divided doses 12 hours apart.
Anti-Malarial Medicines	
Curative Treatment of Malaria	
Artesunate + Lumefantrine	*Treatment of uncomplicated P. falciparum and other Plasmodium malaria*–15-24 kg initially 2 tablets followed by 5 further doses of 2 tablets each at 8, 24, 36, 48 and 60 hours (total 12 tablets over 60 hours); 25-34 kg initially 3 tablets followed by 5 further doses of 3 tablets each at 8, 24, 36, 48 and 60 hours (total 18 tablets over 60 hours); over 34 kg initially 4 tablets followed by 5 further doses of 4 tablets each at 8, 24, 36, 48 and 60 hours (total 24 tablets over 60 hours). *Renal impairment:* Severe: caution; monitor ECG and plasma potassium. Hepatic impairment: Severe: caution; monitor ECG and plasma potassium. Non-dispersible tablets may be crushed. If the dose is vomited within 1 hour of taking, the dose should be repeated.

Chloroquine	Doses expressed as chloroquin base–*(P. vivax, P. ovale and sensitive P. falciparum)*–Oral/IV Initially 600 mg followed by 300 mg 6-8 hours later and then daily once for 2 days or 10 mg/kg (max 600 mg) for 1st 2 days followed by 5 mg/kg on 3rd day as single daily dose.
Artesunate	4 mg/kg body weight for 3 days. For severe malaria–2.4 mg/kg IV or IM given on admission (time=0), then at 12 hours and 24 hours, then once a day. (Care should be taken to dilute artesunate powder in 5% sodium bicarbonate provided in the pack).
Sulfadoxine + pyrimethamine	Sulfadoxine (25 mg/kg body weight) and pyrimethamine (1.25 mg/kg body weight) [AS+SP] on day 0 for treatment of P falciparum in all parts of India except in the northeastern states.
Quinine	*Severe malaria*–20 mg quinine salt/kg on admission (IV infusion in 5% dextrose/dextrose saline over a period of 4 hours) followed by maintenance dose of 10 mg/kg 8 hourly; infusion rate should not exceed 5 mg/kg per hour. Loading dose of 20 mg/kg should not be given, if the patient has already received quinine. NEVER GIVE BOLUS INJECTION OF QUININE. If parenteral quinine therapy needs to be continued beyond 48 hours, dose should be reduced to 7 mg/kg 8 hourly.
Primaquine	15 mg once daily for 14 days. *For G6PD deficient patients*–30 mg once in a week for 8 weeks.
Doxycycline	*Multidrug resistant P. falciparum (resistant to both chloroquine and sulfadoxine-pyrimethamine) with quinine* at 3.5 mg/kg once a day for 7 days.
Malaria Prophylaxis	
Chloroquine	Doses expressed as chloroquine base–Malaria prophylaxis–300 mg once weekly. Start 1 week before entering and 4 weeks after leaving endemic area.
Doxycycline	*Short-term chemoprophylaxis (less than 6 weeks)*–100 mg daily in adults and 1.5 mg/kg body weight for children more than 8 years old. The drug should be started 2 days before travel and continued for 4 weeks after leaving the malarious area. Doxycycline is contraindicated in pregnant and lactating women and children less than 8 years.
Mefloquine	*Long-term chemoprophylaxis (more than 6 weeks)*–5 mg/kg body weight (up to 250 mg) weekly and should be administered two weeks before, during and four weeks after leaving the area. Mefloquine is contraindicated in cases with history of convulsions, neuropsychiatric problems and cardiac conditions.
Anti-Pneumocystosis and Anti-Toxoplasmosis Medicines	
Pyrimethamine	*Toxoplasmosis in pregnancy*–If toxoplasma infection is diagnosed in early pregnancy and the fetus is not infected, spiramycin is given. If the fetus is found to be infected then pyrimethamine 50 mg once daily, sulfadiazine 1g 3 times daily and calcium folinate (folinic acid) 15 mg 3 times per week are given until delivery. *Ocular toxoplasmosis, reactivation of toxoplasmosis during HIV infection and toxoplasmosis in immunocompromised child with protracted or incapacitating illness*–2 mg/kg loading dose for 2 days followed by 25-100 mg for 6 weeks to prevent relapse in HIV patients followed by maintenance of a quarter to half of starting dose indefinitely.
Spiramycin	*Pregnant women with suspected or confirmed toxoplasma infection*–1.5 g (4.5 million international units) orally twice daily until term if the fetus is not infected.
Co-trimoxazole	See under anti-bacterials.
ANTI-MIGRAINE MEDICINES	
Treatment of Acute Attack of Migraine (Ibuprofen; Paracetamol–As above)	
Sumatriptan	50-100 mg as single dose. May be repeated if migraine recurs (max 300 mg/day). If there is no response, do not repeat for same attack. SC>10 year. 6 mg single dose. May repeat once not less than 1 hour later for a recurrence (max 12 mg/day). If there is no response, do not repeat for same attack.
Migraine Prophylaxis	
Propranolol	20-40 mg/dose 2-3 times daily.
Flunarizine	10 mg daily once. Dose reduction required in liver impairment.
ANTI-NEOPLASTIC, IMMUNOSUPPRESSIVES AND MEDICINES USED IN PALLIATIVE CARE	
Immunosuppressive Medicines	
Azathioprine	*Organ transplantation; to prevent rejection*–Initially 2-5 mg/kg/24 hr IV or oral; maintenance 1-3 mg/kg/24 hr. *Autoimmune disease like lupus arthritis or nephritic syndrome*–1 mg/kg/24 hr for 6-8 weeks. *ITP*–1 to 4 mg/kg/day. 3 to 6 months therapy is needed for maximal response.

Cyclosporin	*Juvenile idiopathic arthritis, collagen disease, vasculitis, uveitis*–Orally 1-2 mg/kg per dose 2 times daily increased gradually upto 3 mg/kg/dose twice daily. *Organ transplant*–Orally 5-7 mg/kg/dose 2 times daily starting 12 hours before transplant and continued for 1-2 weeks postoperatively gradually reducing to maintenance dose of 1-3 mg/kg/dose 2 times daily or 1.5-4 mg/kg/dose 2 times daily when given with other immunosuppressants as part of triple or quadruple regime. *Bone marrow transplant*–6-7.5 mg/kg/dose 2 times daily starting on day prior to transplant. *Psoriasis/atopic dermatitis*–1.25 mg/kg/dose 2 times daily–increased, if no response, after 2 weeks for dermatitis and 4 weeks for psoriasis till 2.5 mg/kg/dose 2 times daily. *Severe ulcerative colitis*–Orally 3-4 mg/kg 2 times daily. *Crohn's disease*–2.5-4.5 mg/kg 2 times daily. *Steroid resistant nephrotic syndrome*–4-6 mg/kg/day in 2 divided doses. Monitor trough levels of cyclosporine to adjust dose.
Cytotoxic Medicines–Always consult the current treatment protocol for details of dosage and scheduling.	
Asparaginase	*As part of combination therapy*– 6000 units/m^2, 3 times/week for 3 weeks. High-dose IM therapy–25,000 units/m^2/dose weekly once for doses. IV therapy–1000 units/kg/24 hr for 10 days; or 200 units/kg/24 hr for 28 days.
Cyclophosphamide	*Induction*–IV 40-50 mg/kg (1.5-1.8 g/m^2) in divided doses over 2-5 days; Orally 1-5 mg/kg/24 hr followed by maintenance IV 10-15 mg/kg (350-550 mg/m^2) once in 7-10 days or 3-5 mg/kg twice in a week. *SLE*–500-750 mg/m^2/month. *Juvenile rheumatoid arthritis/vasculitis*–IV 10 mg/kg once in 2 weeks. *Bone marrow transplant conditioning*–IV 50 mg/kg/24 hr for 3-4 days. *Nephrotic syndrome*–Orally 2-3 mg/kg/24 hours–upto 12 weeks. In steroid dependent NS, use with alternate day prednisolone. Dose not to exceed a dose of 166 mg/kg. *ITP*–1 to 2 mg/kg/day orally. Response occurs in 2 to 10 weeks. Adjust doses for (1) Renal failure–Cr Cl 25-50 ml/min give half dose and if <25 ml/min avoid; (2) Decreased bone marrow function give 33-50% of dose.
Vincristine	1-2 mg/m^2 once a week. Maximum dose in adults is 2 mg weekly. Dosage reductions may be necessary if toxicity is unacceptable. An increase in the severity of side-effects may be seen in patients with liver disease sufficient to decrease biliary excretion. A 50% dosage reduction is recommended in patients with a serum bilirubin level >50 μmol/L.
Vinblastine	*Hodgkin's in children*–IV 2.5-6 mg/m^2/24 hr 1-2/week for 3-6 weeks (max 12.5 mg/m^2/week). Maximum single dose 10 mg. A 50% dose reduction has been suggested in patients with serum bilirubin >50 μmol/L.
Methotrexate	*Severe acute Crohn's disease*–SC/IM–7-18 years–15 mg/m^2 (max. 25 mg) once weekly followed by maintenance of remission dose–Oral/SC/IM–7-18 years–15 mg/m^2 (max. 25 mg) once weekly; dose reduced according to response to lowest effective dose. *JIA, juvenile dermatomyositis, vasculitis, uveitis, SLE, localized scleroderma, sarcoidosis*–Oral/SC/IM –1-18 years – 10-15 mg/m^2 (increased to max. 25 mg, if needed) once weekly. *For all malignant conditions*–Early stage Burkitt's lymphoma, non-Hodgkin's lymphoma, osteogenic sarcoma, some CNS tumors, acute lymphoblastic leukemia (IV inj./infusion); maintenance and remission of acute lymphoblastic leukemia, lymphoblastic lymphoma (oral); and meningeal leukemia, treatment and prevention of CNS involvement of leukemia (intrathecal)–Use doses prescribed in respective protocols. *Severe uncontrolled psoriasis unresponsive to conventional therapy*–Oral–2-18 years–initially 200 μg/kg (max. 10 mg) once weekly increased according to response to 400 μg/kg (max. 25 mg) once weekly.
Mercaptopurine	*Leukemia/lymphoma/T-NHL*–Oral Induction 2.5-5 mg/kg once daily followed by maintenance of 1.5–2.5 mg/kg/day. *Inflammatory bowel disease*– 2-18 years 1-1.5 mg/kg once daily (max initially 50 mg/day may be increased upto 75 mg/day). Dosage should be carefully adjusted according to blood counts.
Daunorubicin	Remission induction in acute lymphoblastic leukemia (ALL) (combination therapy) 25-45 mg/m^2 on day 1 of every week for 4 cycles (max. total dose 300 mg/m^2).
Hormones and Anti-Hormones–Dexamethasone; Hydrocortisone; Prednisolone are discussed elsewhere.	
MEDICINES AFFECTING THE BLOOD	
Anti-Anemia Medicines	
Ferrous salt	*Iron deficiency anemia*–180 mg of elemental iron in 3 divided doses.
Folic acid	Supplementation in folate deficiency; cofactor in metabolic disorders (e.g. homocystinuria)–5-10 mg, once daily for 6 months if cause correctable and lifelong if uncorrectable. *Megaloblastic anemia due to folate deficiency*–5 mg daily once for 4 months. *Hemolytic anemias*–Oral 10 mg once daily. *To limit methotrexate associated side effects when it is used for JIA*–Oral 1 mg once daily. Dose may be omitted on day methotrexate is given. May be given 5 mg weekly or twice weekly.

Hydroxocobalamin (vitamin B12)	*Vitamin B12 deficiency*–IM 250 µg–1 mg 3 times weekly for 2 weeks followed by 250 µg once weekly till blood counts are normal and then 1 mg once in 2-3 months as maintenance dose. *Hydroxocobalamin responsive inborn errors of metabolism*–IM initially 1 mg daily for 5 days and assess response. If responsive continue maintenance at 1 mg once or twice a week. Oral up to 10 mg once or twice weekly. Oral may be started as soon as response to IM is confirmed but some patients do not respond to oral administration.
Medicines Affecting Coagulation	
Vitamin K	*Bleeding disorders:* 1. Asymptomatic patients with mild abnormal coagulation, where vitamin K deficiency is presumed, vitamin K may be given SC. Dose is 1 to 5 mg. 2. Bleeding in a patient due to Vitamin K deficiency: Should be given 2 to 10 mg of vitamin K SC/IV. IM administration of vitamin K should be avoided as it causes pain, hematoma and swelling. If bleeding is severe then fresh frozen plasma (FFP) may be given in the dose of 10 to 20 ml/kg. 3. Patients with life-threatening hemorrhage or intracranial bleed should be given systemic (intravenous) vitamin K 5 to 20 mg. Along with it prothrombin complex concentrates (not available in India) may be given in a dose of 50 units/kg. Immediate benefit may be derived from administration of FFP.
Heparin sodium	*Thromboembolic disease and ECMO*–50 units/kg IV bolus and 15-35 units/kg/hr continuous IV infusion maintenance dose (adjust to target APTT or heparin level). *Catheter patency*–0.5-1 unit/ml as heparin lock. An IV bolus dose of 75-100 units/kg of heparin results in a therapeutic aPTT in 90% of children. Maintenance dose (as IV infusion) 18 units/kg/hour. *Dosage in catheterization lab*–50-100 units/kg bolus IV or through arterial sheath. *Monitoring*–Heparin dosing monograms have been validated in children. Many physicians use anti Xa levels in critically ill children as aPTT may not be very predictive. In relatively stable infants and in older children, aPTT is used for monitoring as it is more easily performed and is widely available. If aPTT is < 60 seconds, dose of heparin should be increased by 10% every 4-6 hours till aPTT is over 60 seconds. If aPTT exceeds 85 seconds, heparin dose should be decreased and if aPTT is > 95 sec, the heparin infusion should be stopped.
Protamine sulfate	1 mg (0.1 ml) for each 100 units mucous heparin or low molecular weight heparin (LMWH) or 80 units lung heparin given at last dose. Maximum dose 50 mg. Administer within 15 minutes—if the delay is longer less protamine is required, as heparin is rapidly excreted (after 30 minutes give approximately half dose).
Warfarin	*Always seek expert advice before starting anticoagulation.* The dosage schedule is as per INR value. Average dose of is 0.09 mg/kg/day and for adults, 0.04-0.08 mg/kg/day. *Monitoring:* Frequent dose adjustments warrant close supervision of international normalized ratio (INR). Vitamin K antagonists have extensive cross-reactivity with several commonly used drugs and dietary agents. Certain "point-of-care" monitors are commercially available, which are considered reliable and acceptable for checking INR in home setting. They are somewhat similar to "glucometers". INR level is affected by cumulative dose of warfarin taken over the last 5-7 days, so testing INR just after a day of change in dose is not useful. *Dosing of Warfarin* Loading dose (Day 1)–0.2 mg/kg (maximum 10 mg); 0.1 mg/kg in presence of hepatic dysfunction. Days 2-4. INR 1.1-1.3, repeat loading dose. INR 1.4-1.9, give 50% of initial loading dose. INR 2.0-3.0, give 50% of initial loading dose. INR 3.1-3.5, give 25% of initial loading dose. INR > 3.5, hold until < 3.5, restart at 50% of previous dose. Maintenance dose (day 5 and beyond). INR 1.1-1.4, increase dose by 20% of previous dose. INR 1.5-1.9, increase dose by 10% of previous dose. INR 2.0-3.0, no change. INR 3.1-3.5, decrease dose by 10% of previous dose. INR > 3.5, hold until < 3.5, restart at 20% of previous dose.
BLOOD PRODUCTS AND PLASMA SUBSTITUTES	
Plasma Fractions for Specific Use	
Human normal immunoglobulin	Measles and polio–IM 750 mg; Hepatitis A 500 mg; Rubella in pregnancy 750 mg.

Factor VIII concentrate	The dose and dosing schedule for factor VIII must be calculated and adjusted according to the needs of the individual patient, taking into account the patient's body weight, the degree of factor VIII deficiency, the site and extent of the bleeding, the titre of inhibitors, the factor VIII level desired and the clinical condition. The required dosage may be estimated using the following formula as a guide: Number of factor VIII units required = Body weight (kg) × desired increase (International units) in factor VIII × 0.5 (% of normal).
Factor IX complex	Dose should always be tailored to clinical effectiveness in each individual. The number of units needed and the duration of treatment depend on the condition being treated. 20-25 units/kg/dose once daily. In Factor VIII inhibitor patients 75-100 units/kg/dose upto 6th hourly.
CARDIOVASCULAR MEDICINES	
Antiarrhythmic Medicines	
Verapamil	Oral 40-120 mg/dose 3 times daily. Slow IV bolus 100-300 μg/kg (max 5 mg) as single dose with ECG monitoring. May repeat after 30 minutes usually lower doses suffice.
Lidocaine	Loading dose IV bolus 50-100 mg (50 mg for thin build or those with severely impaired circulation) followed by maintenance dose IV infusion with ECG monitoring–start with 4 mg/min for 30 min then 2 mg/kg for 2 hours then 1 mg/min for the rest of the day. Lower conc. further if continued beyond 24 hours. *Ventricular fibrillation or pulseless tachycardia*–IV 50-100 mg.
Phenytoin	Loading dose 1.25 mg/kg IV once in 5 min until desired effect or total dose 15 mg/kg. Maintenance–250 mg 3-4 times daily.
Diltiazem	30-60 mg/dose 2-3 times daily.
Sotalol	40 mg/dose (max 80-160 mg) 2 times daily. According to Shi J *et al.* body surface area is the better predictor for sotalol dosing; the recommended dose is 30-70 mg/m^2/day.
Amiodarone	Amiodarone hydrochloride–Given under the direct supervision of cardiologist. The minimum effective dose used at all times. Oral loading dose of 5 mg/kg (maximum 200 mg) 2-3 times daily for 5 days followed by maintenance dose of 5 mg/kg (maximum 200 mg) once daily. IV loading dose of 5 mg/kg (in rare cases upto max of 15 mg/kg may be given) slowly over 30 min followed by maintenance continuous infusion at 5-15 μg/kg/min (maximum 1.2 g in 24 hours). Central line preferred. In cardiopulmonary resuscitation (CPR) for shock resistant ventricular fibrillation and pulseless tachycardia rapid IV bolus of 5 mg/kg may be given. Amiadarone has a long duration of action and may exert effect for weeks or months after discontinuing. Since it is metabolized in liver, its dose must be adjusted in hepatic dysfunction.
Anti-hypertensive Medicines	
Nifedipine	*Hypertensive crisis/angina*–Sublingual/oral (pierce the capsule and pour contents sublingually or into mouth)–250-500 μg/kg as single dose. *Hypertension/angina*–5-20 mg/kg/dose 3 times daily (max 100 mg/day). *Raynaud's phenomenon*–2.5-10 mg 2-4 times daily. Start with low dose at bedtime and gradually increase to avoid postural hypotension.
Atenolol	0.5-2 mg/kg once daily. Adjust according to pulse and BP. May give 2 times daily upto maximum of 100 mg/24 hours.
Enalapril	Oral 2.5-5 mg/24 hours and titrate to max 40 mg/24 hours in 2 divided doses; IV 0.625-1.25 mg/dose 4 times daily (max 20 mg/24 hours).
Lisinopril	*Hypertension*–Oral; initially, 10 mg PO once daily. The usual dosage range is 20-40 mg PO once daily. Lower dosage may be necessary in patients with renal impairment and in those receiving diuretics. In patients with a creatinine clearance of less than 30 ml/min, initiate therapy with 5 mg PO once daily. Maximum daily dose is 80 mg/day. For patients receiving dialysis, the initial recommended dosage is 2.5 mg PO once daily. Maximum 40 mg/day.
Amlodipine	Oral 100-200 μg/kg daily once (5 mg) increased if required to maximum of 10 mg.
Hydralazine	Oral 50 mg in 2 divided doses. Increase if needed to max dose of 7.5 mg/kg/day or 200 mg/day. IV bolus over 20 min–5-10 mg as single dose. May be repeated upto 4-6 times daily. IV infusion–3-5 mg/hr. In hepatic and renal impairment start with small doses or increase interval between doses.
Medicines Used in Heart Failure	
Digoxin	The doses stated are for patients who have not received cardiac glycosides in the preceding 2 weeks. If cardiac glycosides have been given in the 2 weeks preceding commencement, it should be anticipated that optimum loading doses will be less than those stated (levels should be checked before loading). The dosage schedules are meant as guidelines and careful clinical observation and monitoring of serum digoxin levels should be used as a basic for adjustment of dosage. *In myocarditis,* halve loading and maintenance doses, as the myocardium is more sensitive to cardiac glycosides. Check the doses carefully because an overdose can cause death. Maintenance dose should start 12 hours after loading ends. For those > 10 years, use doses at the lower end of the range in early adolescence and/or in underweight children. 10 μg oral load then 2-5 μg/kg/24 hours maintenance dose orally. Impaired renal function–Cr Cl 10-50 ml/min reduce dose to 25-75%, <10 ml/min reduce dose to 10-25% of normal. Age — Total digitalizing dose — Daily maintenance PO : 0.75-1.5 mg — PO: 0.125-0.5 mg IV : 0.5-1.0 mg — IV: 0.1-0.4 mg

Furosemide	Oral 20-40 mg/dose 2-3 times daily. IV bolus 20-40 mg as single dose (max 4 mg/kg). Dose could be repeated every 8 hours. Continuous infusion may be better and safer in acute heart failure and in postoperative setting. The dose does not need to be adjusted in renal or hepatic impairment.
Captopril	The starting dose is 0.1 mg/kg/dose; it is gradually increased to 0.5-1 mg/kg/dose three times a day (increase after every 4 to 5 doses). Maximum dose is 2 mg/kg/dose. BP and renal parameters should be monitored when up titrating the dose. Captopril is the preferred ACEI in young infants, requires dosing every 6-8 hours.
Enalapril	Oral 2.5-5 mg/24 hr and titrate to max 40 mg/24 hr in 2 divided doses; IV 0.625-1.25 mg/dose 4 times daily (max 20 mg/24 hours).
Antithrombotic Medicines–Unfractionated heparin; Low molecular weight heparin (LMWH); Warfarin discussed elsewhere.	
Acetyl salicylic acid	3-5 mg/kg/day, given as a single dose (maximum 75 mg).
Dipyridamol	100-200 mg/dose 3 times daily before food (avoid antacids).
Clopidogrel	0.2 mg/kg/day is sufficient to achieve platelet inhibition level similar to that in adults taking the standard dose of 75 mg/day. 80% of children would also be taking aspirin. When appropriate, tablets were rounded to the nearest one half, one third, or one fourth tablet.
Lipid-Lowering Agents	
Simvastatin	5 mg at night increased at 4-week intervals to 20 mg per night if required. Reduced dose required with concomitant cyclosporine, danazol, fibrates, amiodarone, diltiazem or verapamil–seek specialized advice.
DERMATOLOGICAL MEDICINES (TOPICAL)	
Antifungal Medicines	
Miconazole	Topical on skin apply on affected area 2 times daily for 10 days after lesions have healed. Oral thrush 5-10 ml 2-4 times daily. Use in the mouth after food and retain as long as possible.
Clotrimazole	Apply 2-3 times daily continuing for 14 days after lesions have healed. *Oral thrush*–10-20 drops gently apply to buccal mucosa (covering all lesions) 4 times daily for 5-7 days. *Vaginal candidiasis*–Apply 2% vaginal gel 5 g deep into vagina at bedtime for 6 consecutive nights (not to be used during menstruation). Or alternatively–100 mg vaginal pessaries for 6 days, 200 mg for 3 days or 500 mg single dose at bedtime. *Scalp seborrhea*–Apply to liquid with selenium to scalp, massage gently, leave for 5 min and then rinse well with water–2-3 times/week. *Otomycosis*–Instill 4-5 drops in ear 3-4 times daily till 2 weeks after infection subsides.
Selenium sulfide	Use as shampoo twice weekly for 2 weeks then once weekly for 2 weeks then as necessary.
Anti-Infective Medicines	
Potassium permanganate	Cleansing and deodorizing suppurating eczematous reactions and wounds for wet dressings or baths, use approx. 0.01% (1 in 10 000) solution or 1 granule dissolved in 300 ml (2 ½ glasses) of water.
Framycetin	Apply 1-3 times daily.
Silver sulfadiazine	*Burns:* After cleaning the wound apply over all affected areas to a depth of 3-5 mm, using a sterile gloved hand or sterile spatula. Where necessary, re-apply to any area from which it has been removed by patient activity. Re-apply at least every 24 hours or more frequently if the volume of exudates is large. *Hand burns*–Apply to the burn and enclose the whole hand in a clear plastic bag or glove which is then closed at the wrist. The patient should be encouraged to move the hand and fingers and the dressing should be changed when an excessive amount of exudates has accumulated in the bag. *Leg ulcers/pressure sores:* The cavity of the ulcer should be filled with cream to a depth of at least 3-5 mm, followed by application of an absorbent pad or dressing, with further application of pressure bandaging as appropriate. Dressings should be changed daily, but if less exudates, every 48 hours may be sufficient. *Finger-tip injuries*–Hemostasis of the injury should be achieved prior to the application of a 3-5 mm layer of cream, and then the finger covered with a finger dressing or the finger of a plastic glove. Dressings should be changed every 2-3 days. In all cases, use the contents of the tube or put on one person only. Discard 50 g tubes 7 days after opening. Discard 250 g and 500 g pots 24 hours after opening.
Mupirocin	*Topical cream*–Apply to affected area 3 times daily for up to 10 days; nasal ointment–Apply to the inner surface of each nostril 2-3 times a day for 5-7 days; ointment–Apply to affected area 2-3 times daily for up to 10 days.
Anti-Inflammatory and Antipruritic Medicines	
Hydrocortisone	1% cream for face and in newborn and ointment for skin of other parts of the body–2-3 times daily.
Calamine lotion	Apply to external area as needed.

Medicines Affecting Skin Differentiation and Proliferation	
Benzoyl peroxide	Topical 2.5% 1-3 times daily sparingly for 15 min. Increase strength and duration of exposure as tolerated. If excessive peeling or redness occurs–decrease to alternate day.
Salicylic acid	Remove dead skin by gentle rubbing with pumice stone or emery board before applying daily.
Urea	Wash affected area, rinse off traces of sap and apply sparingly twice daily.
Dithranol	Apply on a daily basis, leaving on for 20-30 minutes depending on the preparation being used, then remove by washing off. Always commence treatment with 0.1% continuing for at least 1 week increasing if necessary to 0.25%, 0.5%, 1% and 2%. Build up gradually over 4 weeks to the highest tolerated strength that gives the best effect. Apply evenly and sparingly to lesions.
Scabicides and Pediculicides	
Gamma benzene hexachloride	Apply to whole body surface below neck. Scrub baths after 12-24 hours. If required one more application may be repeated after a week. *Pediculosis*–Massage scalp with emulsion at night and cover with a piece of cloth. Following morning, head bath should be taken ensuring that medication does not enter eyes.
Permethrin	Single topical application of up to1 tube. If necessary a second application may be given not less than 7 days after the initial application. Apply to whole body excluding head. Wash off after 8-12 hours. If hands or any part are washed, the treatment must be reapplied. *Pediculosis*–Apply to clean damp hair, leave on for 10 minutes, rinse and dry. Not affected by chlorine in swimming pools.
DIURETICS–(Furosemide discussed elsewhere)	
Hydrochlorothiazide	12.5–100 mg/24 hr. *Nephrogenic diabetes insipidus*–Oral 37.5-75 mg/day in 3 divided doses.
Spironolactone	Oral 1-3 mg/kg/day in 2 divided doses. In resistant ascites, up to 9 mg/kg/day have been given with careful serum potassium monitoring. *Hirsutism*–Start with 50 mg in 2 divided doses, gradually increasing to 100 mg; max up to 200 mg daily can be given.
Mannitol	A test dose may be given to assess renal function–200 mg/kg (max 12.5 g) over 3-5 min to produce urine output of 1 ml/kg/hr for 1-3 hours. *Cerebral and ocular edema*–IV over 30 min 0.5-1 g/kg initially followed by maintenance of 0.25-0.5 g/kg every 4-6 hours as required. *Peripheral edema and ascites*–IV infusion over 2-6 hours 1-2 g/kg.
GASTROINTESTINAL MEDICINES	
Antacids and Other Antiulcer Medicines	
Aluminium hydroxide	*Antacid*–4% w/w–5-10 ml 4 times daily and as required between meals and at bedtime. *Hyperphosphatemia*–Tab containing 840 mg 1-3 tabs 4-5 times daily.
Ranitidine	150 mg/dose 2 times daily. Upto 9 mg/kg may be used. IV bolus 1 mg/kg 2-4 times daily IV infusion 125-250 µg/kg/hr. Reduce dose to 50% in severe renal failure.
Lansoprazol	*Gastroesophageal reflux disease (GERD), acid related dyspepsia, duodenal and benign gastric ulcer including those following NSAID therapy*– Children less than 30 kg–0.5-1 mg/kg (max 15 mg) once daily; Children > 30 kg–15 to 30 mg once daily for 8 to 12 weeks.
Antiemetic Medicines	
Domperidone	*Gastroesophageal reflux and gastric stasis*–Oral 200-400 µg/kg/dose 3-4 times daily before food and at night. *Radiotherapy/chemotherapy induced vomiting*–200-400 µg/kg as single dose. Could give once in 4-8 hours.
Promethazine	*Symptomatic relief of allergy*–10-20 mg 2-3 times daily. *Vomiting and nausea* –Oral 1 mg/kg/24 hours in 4 divided doses. *Sedation*–Oral 1-2mg/kg as single dose. *Sedation in ICU*–Slow IV/Oral/deep IM 100-200 mg in 4 divided doses. Start with lower dose and increase gradually depending on response. May use along with chloral hydrate.
Ondansetron	*Nausea and vomiting; chemotherapy induced*–IV 8 mg as single dose just before chemotherapy and repeated 8-12 hourly during therapy and for 24 hours after. Oral following initial IV dosing to get control–8 mg 2-3 times daily for upto 5 days after a course of chemotherapy. *Post-operative nausea and vomiting* –IV slow infusion–4 mg. *Pruritis*–Oral 4-8 mg/dose 2 times daily. *Palliative for nausea/vomiting and pruritis:* IV/SC 5 mg/m^2 continuous over 24 hours
Laxatives	
Milk of magnesia $Mg(OH)_2$	5-10 ml bedtime daily, reducing dose gradually until constipation is relieved.

Lactulose	*Constipation*–Initial dose 30 ml in 2 divided doses. Then adjust according to response. *Hepatic encephalopathy*–Initially 30-50 ml/dose 3 times daily. Then adjust to produce 2-3 soft stools/day.
Sodium picosulfate	5-15 ml as single dose at bedtime.
HORMONES, OTHER ENDOCRINE MEDICINES	
Adrenal Hormones and Synthetic Substitutes	
Hydrocortisone	*Adrenocortical insufficiency; adrenocortical crisis*–50 mg/m²/day stat followed by 100 mg/m²/day in four divided doses. Reduce to 75 mg/m²/day on day 2 and 50 mg/m²/day on day 3. Maintenance dose 8-15 mg/m²/day.
Prednisolone	*Acute asthma*–Oral 1-2 mg/kg in 2-3 divided doses (max 40 mg/day) for 1-5 days and stop without tapering if the episode is controlled. *Croup requiring intubation*–Oral 2 mg/kg/day in 2 divided doses soon after intubation and continued for 24 hours after extubation. *Nephrotic syndrome*–Oral; initially for 4-6 weeks 60 mg/m² (max 80 mg/day) in 2-3 divided doses as single morning dose and after proteinuriais absent for 3 days; maintenance for 4-8 weeks; followed by 40 mg/m² (max 60 mg) as single morning dose on alternate days for 6 weeks. Then taper and stop. Repeat for relapses. *Autoimmune hepatitis*–2 mg/kg (max 40 mg) once daily. *Inflammatory bowel disease*–1-2 mg/kg (max 60 mg/day)–Taper and stop over a few weeks. *JIA, connective tissue disorder, vasculitis*–Up to 2 mg/kg single morning dose or alternate day at lowest dose that controls disease. Avoid if possible as weaning would be difficult. *Ulcerative colitis, Crohn's disease*–Rectal (enema) at bedtime for 2-4 weeks and continued if response is good. *Intractable seizures*–2 mg/kg/day. *Chemotherapy regimens*–Follow doses recommended for given protocol. *Transplant programs*–Each unit has its own protocol. *Adrenal insufficiency including congenital adrenal hyperplasia*–2.5-5 mg/m² in two divided doses. *Thyroid storm*–1-2 mg/kg/day in two divided doses for 2 weeks. *Hypercalcemia due to vitamin D excess*–2 mg/kg/day in two divided doses for 4-6 weeks. *Immune thrombocytopenic purpura (ITP)*–A course of prednisolone 2 mg/kg is given in divided doses. For patients with mucus membrane hemorrhage or extremely low platelet counts, higher doses–4 to 8 mg/kg/day have also been tried. It is gradually tapered off. If there is no response or if the platelets fall again when steroids are discontinued, a repeat 4 weeks course should be given for 4 weeks. Prolonged corticosteroid therapy is not indicated, even if platelet count remains low as it may depress the bone marrow.
Fludrocortisone	*Adrenal insufficiency*– Oral replacement therapy 50-200 µg once daily according to potassium and/or plasma rennin activity levels. *Sweat test*–3 mg/m² single dose on 2 consecutive days prior to sweat test. *Cerebral salt wasting*–Start with 100 µg daily and increase up to 200-300 µg according to response.
Insulins and Other Anti-Diabetic Agents	
Insulins	Dosage should be adjusted according to response. Dose may need to be increased as patients reach the pubertal growth spurt. Usual dose of insulin is 0.7 unit/kg/day in prepubertal children and 1.0 unit/kg/day in midpuberty and 1.2 unit/kg/day by the end of puberty. At the time of diagnosis, larger doses are required up to 2.0 units/kg/day or higher for a few days to enable restoration of body glycogen, protein and fat stores by increased caloric intake. This period rapidly ends within 7-10 days when the child enters the "honeymoon period" with some residual ß-cell function. Exogenous insulin dose will then reduce up to 0.5 units/kg/day or even lower. The honeymoon period ends in a few months and this will manifest itself by increased insulin requirements triggered by wider fluctuations of blood glucose levels. *Insulin Regimens* Although the new insulin preparations are very effective, in the Indian scenario, these insulins should be recommended with care, depending on the family's financial status. In general, a combination of short (regular) and intermediate acting (NPH or lente) insulins is recommended. In the morning before breakfast approximately one half to two-thirds of the total daily dose of insulin is given with a 2:1 ratio of intermediate to short acting. The remaining one-third of the insulin dose is given before the evening meal again in the same proportion of 2:1 intermediate to short acting insulins. The insulin doses can be refined and adjusted according to the blood sugar profiles obtained subsequently by home blood glucose monitoring using a glucometer. Three or more daily injections of insulin may be required in highly motivated older adolescents based on frequent blood glucose monitoring. Such intensive therapy improves glycemic control toward normal, and diminishes the risk of complications. *IV in diabetic emergencies*–0.025-0.1 units/kg/hr adjusted according to blood glucose concentration. *Hyperkalemia*–5-10 units in 25-50 g dextrose (e.g. 500 ml 5% dextrose with 10 units insulin; 500 ml push then 100-250 ml/hour).

Thyroid Hormones and Anti-Thyroid Medicines	
Levothyroxine	Oral; Initial dose–50-100 µg.
Iodine	*Thyrotoxicosis (preoperative)*–0.1-0.3 ml 3 times daily.
Propylthiouracil	*Oral*–100 mg/dose 3 times daily. Dose gradually tapered after child is euthyroid.
IMMUNOLOGICALS	
Sera and Immunoglobulins	
Anti-tetanus immunoglobulin (human)	*Prevention*–A single dose of 250 international units. If there is a risk of heavy contamination or following burns, or more than 24 hours have elapsed since injury, 500 international units should be given. *Treatment of tetanus*–150 IU/kg IM in multiple sites or by IV infusion.
Diphtheria antitoxin	Differs with site. Nasal–IM 10-20,000 units, Tonsillar IM/IV 15-25,000 units, Pharyngeal or laryngeal IM/IV 20-40,000 units, Combined types or delayed diagnosis IV 40-60,000 units, Severe diphtheria e.g. with extensive membrane and or severe edema (bull neck diphtheria) IV or part IV and IM 40-100,000 units.
Rabies immunoglobulin	20 IU/kg IM and infiltration: Half infiltrated around wound with the rest IM. Give at a different site to the vaccine.
Hepatitis B immunoglobulin	Treatment depends on immunization status and whether exposure is significant e.g. percutaneous needle prick, bite, mucocutaneous exposure to blood, unprotected sexual intercourse, etc–A single dose of HBIG (0.06 ml/kg or 5.0 ml for adults) should be given as soon as possible after exposure and within 24 hours if possible.
Vaccines	
Tetanus, diphtheria and Pertussis vaccines–Tdap/Td	IM at 10-12 years.
Human papilloma virus (HPV) vaccine	Only 2 doses of either of the two HPV vaccines for adolescent/pre-adolescent girls aged 9-14 years. For girls 15 years and older, and immunocompromised individuals 3 doses are recommended. For two-dose schedule, the minimum interval between doses should be 6 months. For 3-dose schedule, the doses can be administered at 0, 1-2 (depending on brands) and 6 months.
Mumps, Measles, and Rubella (MMR) vaccine	Ensure that all adolescents have had 2 doses of MMR vaccine; the minimum interval between the 2 doses is 4 weeks.
Varicella vaccine	Ensure that all adolescents without evidence previous varicella infection, have 2 doses of varicella vaccine. For children aged 7 through 12 years, the recommended minimum interval between doses is 3 months (if the second dose was administered at least 4 weeks after the first dose, it can be accepted as valid); for persons aged 13 years and older, the minimum interval between doses is 4 weeks.
Hepatitis A vaccine	Minimum interval between 2 doses is 6 months. If adolescent has had 1 dose, a 2nd dose may be given. If live attenuated hepatitis A vaccine is used a single dose will suffice.
Rabies vaccine	*Pre-exposure*–1 ml on days 0, 7 and 28. Two doses 4 weeks apart may be adequate in those not expecting to handle animals if post-exposure treatment will be readily available. In this case, if exposure continues, a further dose after 6-12 months will be necessary. Boosters may be given every 2-3 years if there is continuing risk and post-exposure treatment is not readily available. After 2-3 boosters, expert advice should be sought before giving more. *Post-exposure*–When an individual has been exposed via a break in the skin or contamination of a mucosal surface to a potentially rabid animal, consideration should be given to post-exposure treatment. Advice should always be sought before starting treatment. *Unimmunized/incompletely immunized (received < 3 doses or had intradermal)*–Low risk 1 ml on 0, 3, 7, 14 and 30 days and in high risk 1 ml on 0, 3, 7, 14 and 30 days plus rabies immunoglobulin. *Fully immunized individual*–1 ml on 0 and 3 days. As an alternative to this regimen, the patient may be offered a single-visit 4-site intradermal regimen consisting of 4 injections of 0.1 ml equally distributed over left and right deltoids and tights. Rabies immune globulin treatment is not necessary in such cases. The same rules apply to persons vaccinated against rabies who have demonstrated neutralizing antibody titres of at least 0.5 IU/ml.
Typhoid conjugate vaccine	1 dose followed by another after 1 year. Currently, two typhoid conjugate vaccines, Typbar-TCV and PedaTyph are available in Indian market. PedaTyph is not yet approved; the recommendation is applicable to Typbar-TCV only. An interval of at least 4 weeks with the MMR vaccine should be maintained while administering this vaccine.
MUSCLE RELAXANTS (PERIPHERALLY-ACTING) AND CHOLINESTERASE INHIBITORS	
Neostigmine	Oral 1 month–15-30 mg/dose repeated at suitable intervals according to response. IM 1-2.5 mg repeated at suitable intervals. Reversal of non-depolarising neuromuscular blockade–IV bolus over 1 min–80 µg/kg with 20 µg/kg of atropine (for drugs other than atracurium) and 50 µg/kg with 20 µg/kg of atropine (for atracurium).

Suxamethonium	IV 1 mg/kg; IM 4 mg.
Vecuronium	IV bolus–80-100 µg/kg as single dose and adjust dose and interval as required. IV infusion 50-80 µg/kg/hr.
Pyridostigmine	Oral initially 30-120 mg. The dose is increased in increments of 25-50% daily till maximum improvement is obtained and given in divided doses at suitable intervals. Usual total daily dose 300 mg-1.2 g.
PSYCHOTHERAPEUTIC MEDICINES	
Medicines Used in Disorders of Attention and Activity	
Methylphenidate	5 mg/dose 1-2 times daily. Increase at weekly increments of 5-10 mg daily. Max 60 mg/day given in 2-4 divided doses. Avoid dosing in the evenings.
Atomoxetine	Start at 0.5 mg/kg/day and dose may be increased after a minimum of 3 days to a target dose of 1.2 mg/kg/day, given once daily or in 2 divided doses in the morning and late afternoon. No additional benefit is seen in doses more than 1.2 mg/kg/day. Do not exceed 1.4 mg/kg/day or 100 mg/day.
Medicines Used in Sleep Disorders (Insomnia, Bedtime Refusal, Sleep Talking, Sleep Walking, Restless Leg Syndrome)	
Melatonin	Oral 2-3 mg 20-30 min before bedtime. May be increased to 4-6 mg if benefit not achieved in 1-2 weeks. Maximum of 10 mg tried. If still no response in 2 weeks, drug is stopped.
Clonazepam	Start with 1 mg bedtime to maintenance of 1-2.5 mg/dose 3 times daily.
Clomipramine	Start with 25 mg/day and gradually increase upto 250 mg/day according to response usually as single dose at bedtime (may give in divided doses).
Medicines Used in Substance Dependence Programmes (Tobacco, Alcohol, Illicit Drugs)	
Topiramate	Oral initially 25 mg followed by maintenance of 100-200 mg. Doses upto 6 mg/kg twice daily have been used. Use starting dose for 2 weeks then increase dose every 2 weeks taking at least 6 weeks to reach maintenance dose. Use with caution in renal failure, titrating dose and intervals between dose adjustments to efficacy and side-effects. Supplemental doses required after dialysis. *Migraine prophylaxis*–Initially 25 mg bedtime for 1 week, increase weekly by 25 mg/day; a dose of 50-100 mg daily in 2 divided doses would suffice (max 200 mg/day).
Bupropion	Orally 150-300 mg (usually 150 mg) once in the morning.
Medicines Used in Depressive Disorders	
Fluvoxamine	25-50 mg after food twice daily or 12-18 years 100 mg once daily–Increasing to max doses of 300 mg/day needs to be under expert supervision.
Fluoxetine	*Depression*–Oral 10 mg once daily, gradually increase over 3 weeks to 20 mg once daily. *Bulimia*–Oral 60 mg once daily. *Obsessive compulsive disorder (OCD) and Anxiety*–Oral 20 mg once daily. Gradually increase by 10-20 mg increments once in 2 weeks if required (max 60 mg/day). *Idiopathic musculoskeletal pain*–20 mg once daily.
Medicines Used in Bipolar Mood Disorders (Mania/Depression)	
Resperidone	*Aggressive behavior, Tourette syndrome*–Oral 0.5-2 mg once daily or in 2 divided doses. *Schizophrenia*–Oral 0.5-2 mg once daily or in 2 divided doses.
Medicines Used in Anxiety Disorders, Panic Disorder–Fluvoxmine, Clonazepam detailed earlier	
Sertraline	50 mg once daily.
Propranolol	*Situational anxiety*–10-20 mg prior to the event.
Medicines Used in Obsessive Compulsive Disorders– Fluvoxamine; Fluoxetine and Clomipramine already detailed above.	
Medicines Used in Psychotic Disorders, Schizophrenia–Resperidone already detailed.	
Olanzapine	5-20 mg once daily. Usual dose is 10 mg daily.
Chlorpromazine	*Schizophrenia, violent behavior, agitation*–25 mg/dose 4 times daily (max 300 mg/day). *Intractable hiccup*–25-50 mg/dose 3-4 times daily. *Nausea and vomiting of terminal illness*–10-25 mg/dose (max 75 mg/ day)–4 times daily.
Haloperidol	*Schizophrenia, mania and tic disorders including tourette syndrome*–0.5-30 mg/day (max 60 mg/day) in 2 divided doses. *Intractable hiccup*–1.5 mg 3 times daily. Adjust according to response.
MEDICINES ACTING ON THE RESPIRATORY TRACT–Prednisolone already detailed	
Budesonide	*Asthma prophylaxis*–Aerosol 200-400 µg and Turbohaler 100-400 µg twice daily to be used regularly. Can use upto 800 µg/day in severe asthmatics. *Nebulizer*–500 µg-1mg 2 times daily–Higher doses may be used. *Croup*–2 mg with nebulizer when required.

Fluticasone	*Inhaled*–50-200 μg, > 16 years 100 μg–1 mg 2 times daily. Starting dose appropriate for severity of disease, adjusted to attain control and then reduced to minimal effective dose according to individual response. *Nebulized*–1 mg 2 times daily for acute exacerbation of asthma. *Intranasal*–100 μg (2 sprays) in each nostril twice daily for allergic rhinitis.
Salbutamol	Oral: 1 month–0.3-0.7 mg/kg/day. Aerosol inhaler upto 100-200 μg single dose on demand. Nebulizer solution, 1.25-2.5 mg 1-2 hourly initially and then 4-6 hourly.
Formoterol fumarate	*Aerosol inhaler/turbohaler in combination with budesonide*–6-12 μg 1-2 times daily; dry powder inhaler–12 μg 1-2 times daily. For regular prophylactic use. Increase upto 24 μg twice in a day in severe obstruction.
Salmeterol	*Along with Fluticasone*–50-100 μg 2 times daily as preventor.
VITAMINS AND MINERALS	
Ascorbic acid	*Scurvy*–Oral initially 500 mg then 100 mg/day for 1 week then 50 mg/day for prophylaxis. *Metabolic indications*–200-400 mg/day. *Transient tyrosinemia*–50-200 mg/day for 1-2 weeks.
Thiamine (Vitamin B1)	*Congenital lactic acidosis*–Oral 100-300 mg once daily.
Vitamin A (retinol)	Oral :10,000 IU daily. Prophylaxis of vitamin A deficiency 100,000 IU once in 6 months as a national program.
Vitamin E (alpha tocopheryl acetate)	200 mg once daily.
Vitamin K	See under drugs affectng coagulation.
Vitamins A and D	5 ml of emulsion of 1 capsule daily orally.
Vitamin D	*Treatment of nutritional rickets*–2000 (for infants) to 5000 (for older children) units cholecalciferol PO daily for 3 months. Single large dose therapy, with 60,000 (in older infants) to 120,000 (in older children) IU orally may also be given initially and followed by an additional dose after 2-3 months if necessary. *Prophylaxis*–400 units daily or 60,000 units once every 2 months for 3-6 months.
Folic acid	Discussed in detail earlier.

Growth Charts 1: Boys 0-18 Years IAP and WHO Combined Growth Charts for Height and Weight

11.1

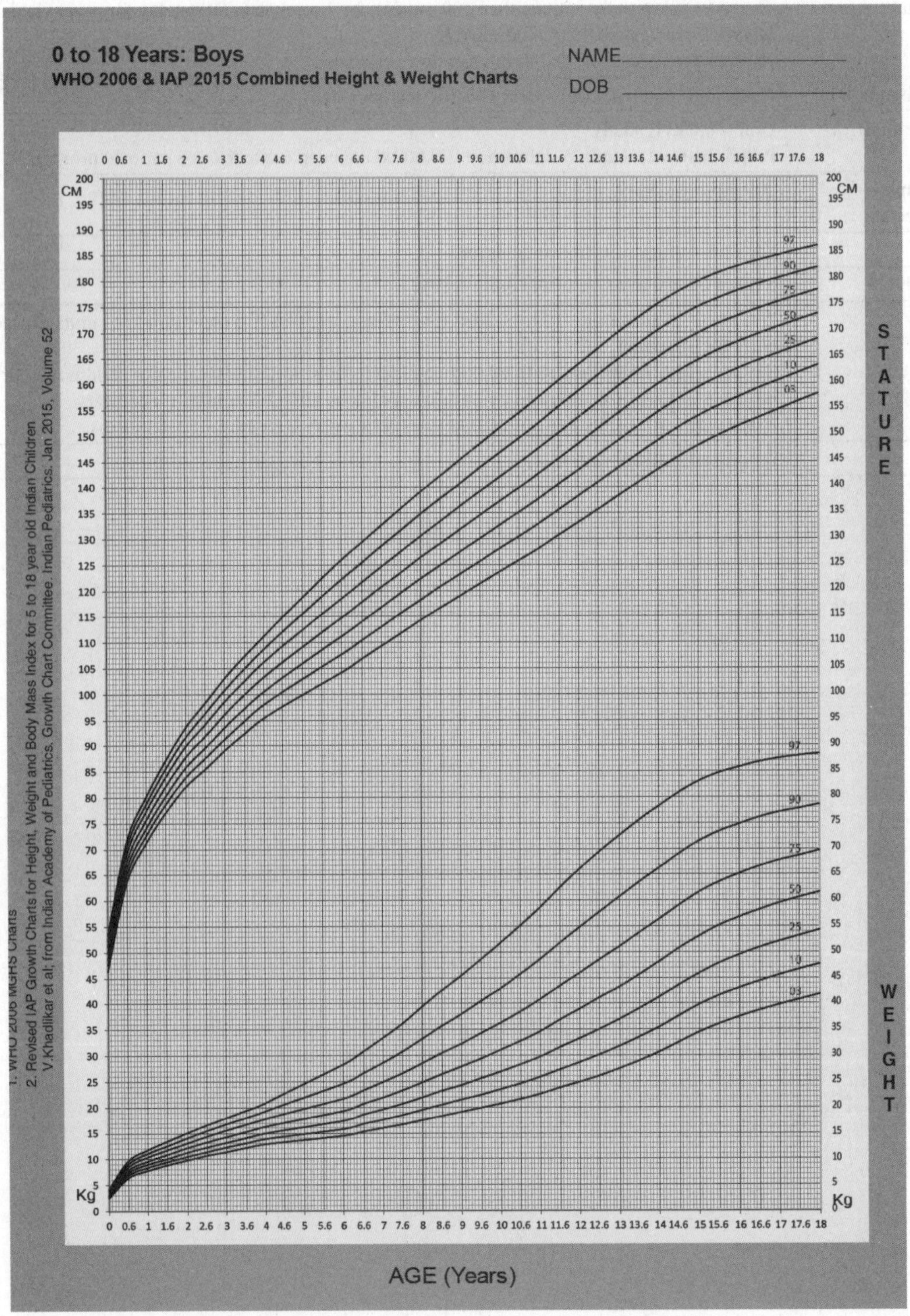

Reproduced with permission from Indian Academy of Pediatrics, Mumbai.

Growth Charts 2: Girls 0-18 Years IAP and WHO Combined Growth Charts for Height and Weight

11.2

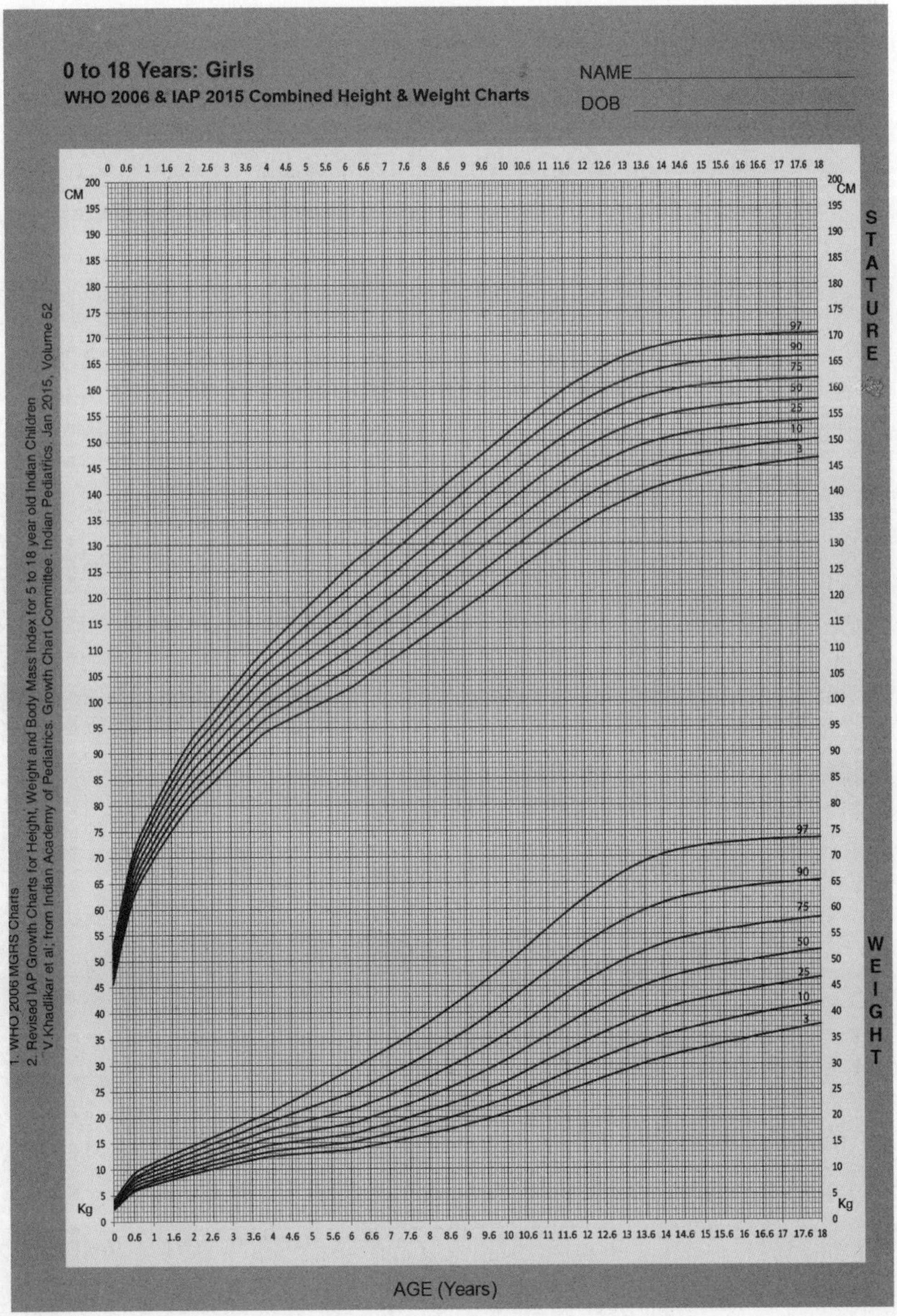

Reproduced with permission from Indian Academy of Pediatrics, Mumbai.

Growth Charts 3: Boys 5-18 Years IAP Growth Charts for Body Mass Index (BMI)

11.3

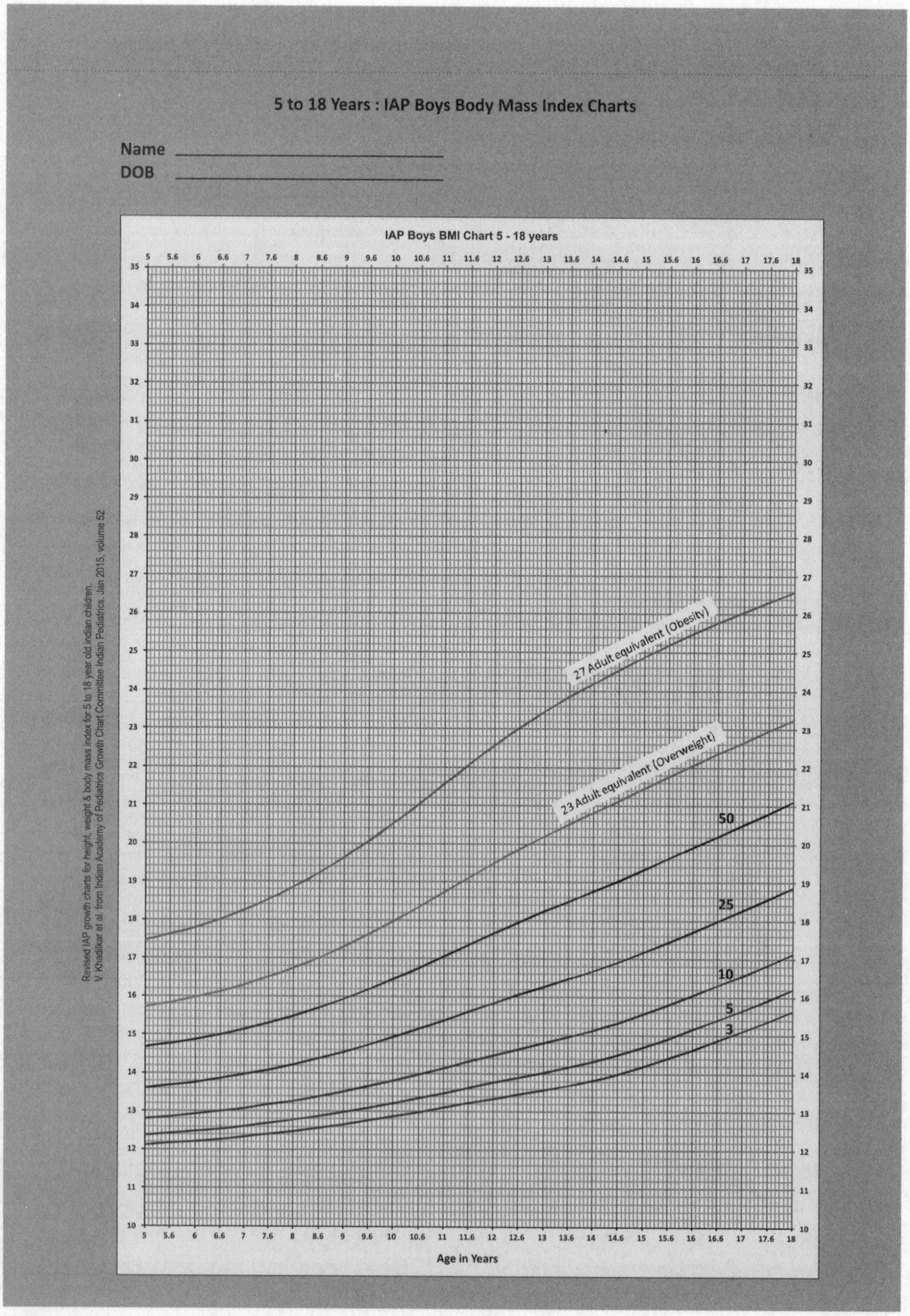

Reproduced with permission from Indian Academy of Pediatrics, Mumbai.

Growth Charts 4: Girls 5-18 Years IAP Growth Charts for Body Mass Index (BMI)

11.4

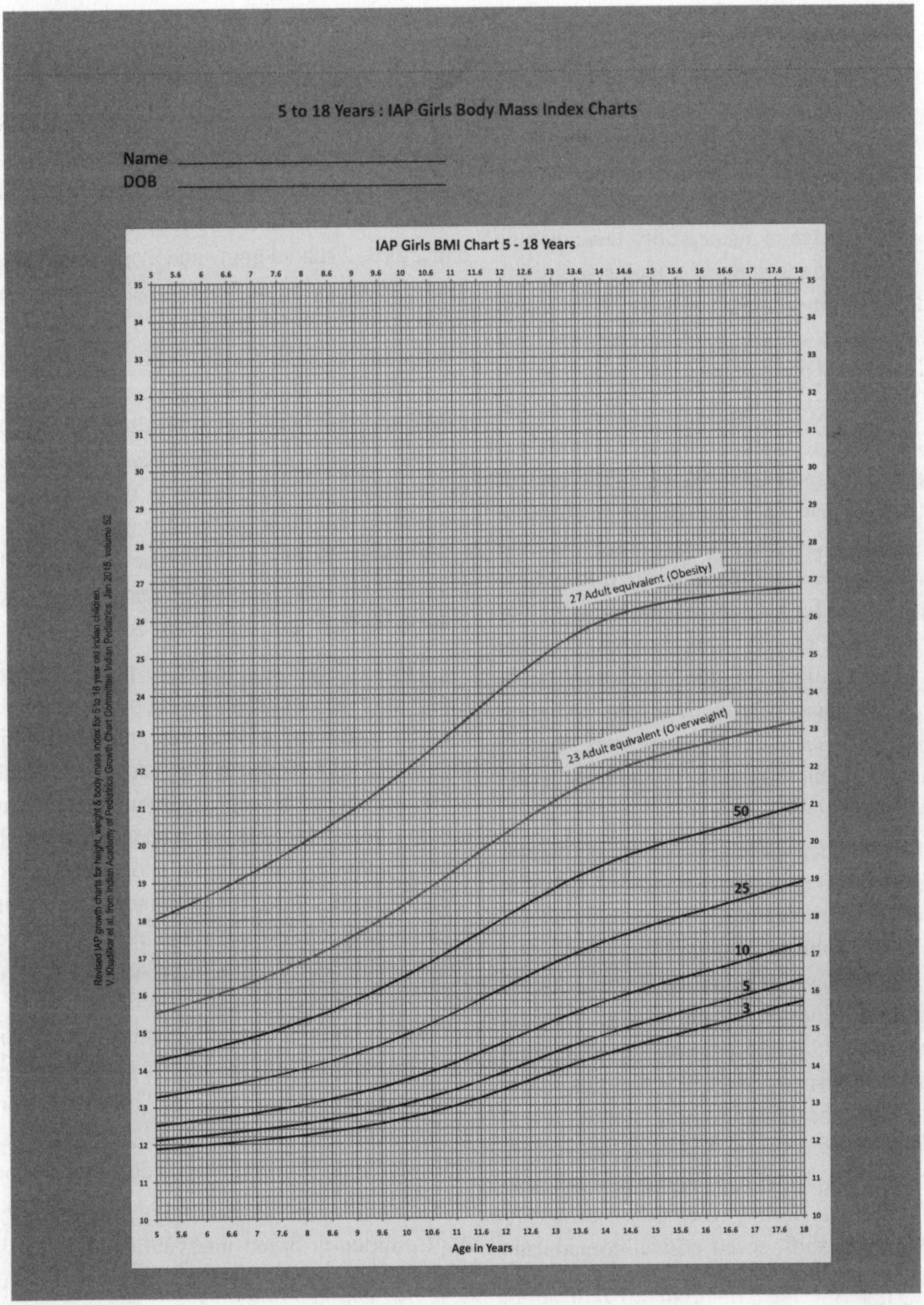

Reproduced with permission from Indian Academy of Pediatrics, Mumbai.

Rashtriya Kishor Swasthya Karyakram

11.5

Harish K Pemde, Kamlesh Harish

Adolescence is fascinating period of life not only for adolescents but also for policy makers and planners. About 22% of India's population is adolescents (10-19 years) and if they are coupled with young adults, then together they (10-24 years) constitute about one-third of our population. India has the largest population of adolescents i.e. 253 million in world. We have to successfully leverage this demographic dividend for sustainable, inclusive growth and all round development of the nation. We need to underline the fact that investments in adolescents will have an immediate, direct and positive impact on India's health goals and on the newly planned *sustainable development goals*.

Ministry of Health and Family Welfare, Government of India has come forward to fulfill the health and development needs of adolescents and framed a new adolescent health strategy culminating into a new national health program for adolescents–Rashtriya Kishor Swasthya Karyakram (RKSK). This program presents holistic management of health needs of adolescents and looks for convergence of various sectors including education, women and child development, and labor as well as the other important stakeholders including parents and civil society organizations.

The vision and objectives of new Adolescent Health Strategy (Table 11.5.1) indicate a paradigm shift in health care policy of Government of India. This program focuses on community based health promotion and preventive care along with strengthening health care facility based care during both health and illness. It also moves from one-size-fits-all approach to customized programing addressing specific needs of adolescents. RKSK is the first major health program where healthy individuals (adolescents) are being approached directly by field level health care providers for not only promoting their health but also ensuring that they remain healthy when they grow up. To achieve this paradigm shift, seven critical components (Table 11.5.2) have been identified. To achieve the aims of new adolescent health strategy six strategic priorities have also been identified (Table 11.5.3).

The new adolescent health program (RKSK) has dual focus i.e. on strengthening clinic-based care and on developing community-based interventions. The latter includes the provision of 4 peer educators (PE) (2 boys and 2 girls; 2 school going and 2 out-of-school) for every 1000-2000 population. The PEs will be trained in common adolescent health related issues. They will work in close association to ASHAs and ANMs. The latters will act as their mentors and as links between PEs/adolescents and health services. Adolescent Health Day (AHD) will be organized every quarter. PEs, health workers, and other stakeholders will participate in these AHDs. Relevant adolescent health topics and common issues will be taken up as themes during these days. Specific media interventions will target adolescents, parents, school and college teachers, and other stakeholders.

These efforts are likely to produce demands for health care services that are supposed to be adolescent friendly. Informed adolescents and PEs will need that their health related concerns are addressed adequately, and whenever needed appropriate promotive, preventive, and curative health services are available to them. Provision of counselors exclusively for adolescents in adolescent friendly health clinics is perhaps the most important step in promoting adolescent health care in facilities. These counselors will be trained to manage routine psychosocial and adolescence related concerns, and to provide counseling services to adolescents. These counselors can also support physicians in providing therapeutic counseling to adolescent clients. These counselors will act as first-point-of-contact in health care facilities and they will coordinate between various departments and experts for providing needed health care to adolescents.

Community based interventions will serve all the targeted adolescents for information and commodities

Table 11.5.1: Vision and objectives of new adolescent health strategy

Vision

All adolescents in India are able to realize their full potential by making informed and responsible decisions related to their health and well-being.

Objectives

The adolescent health strategy aims at achieving the following:

1. Increase the availability and access to information about adolescent health.
2. Increase accessibility and utilization of quality adolescents counseling and health services.
3. Forge multi-sectoral partnerships to create safe and supportive environments for adolescents.

Table 11.5.2: Critical components (7Cs) of new adolescent health strategy

1. **Coverage:** Dedicated programing for 10 to 19 years with universal coverage i.e. urban and rural; in school and out of school; married and un-married including the vulnerable and underserved subgroups.
2. **Content:** Six strategic priorities–Nutrition, Reproductive and Sexual Health, Mental Health, Preventing Injuries and Violence (including Gender Based Violence), Substance Misuse and Non-Communicable Diseases. Life-skills education is identified as a key intervention.
3. **Communities:** Peer educators/mentors (both girls and boys)–selected, trained and mentored by the teachers in an institutional setting and jointly by ASHAs and AWWs in community based settings. Creating an enabling environment at Aanganwadi Centers (AWCs), SABLA-Kishori Samooh, Teen Clubs and VHNSC and creating new spaces like organizing the quarterly Adolescent Health Day.
4. **Clinics (Health Facilities):** Strengthening Adolescent Friendly Health Clinics–walk in services at Sub-Center level and a dedicated weekly Adolescent Clinic at the Primary Health Center. Dedicated adolescent health counselors will be available from block/CHC onwards. Specialty clinics are planned at District and Medical Colleges. Relevant capacity building of service providers across levels and departments. The strategy also proposes to include Adolescent Health specific additions/modifications in curriculum of undergraduate and postgraduate medical and nursing courses.
5. **Counseling:** Channels of information provision at every level of adolescent universe, for instance: peers, nodal/school teachers, ground level health service providers. This service is also aimed at influencers, care givers and families who act as gatekeepers and stakeholders.
6. **Communication:** Communication intervention at every level. Health professionals to act as advocates on behalf of young people and as providers to young people and their caregivers/parents using methods and language deemed appropriate by the adolescents themselves.
7. **Convergence:** Intra-ministerial (with existing programmes of the Ministry of Health and Family Welfare) and relevant inter-ministerial convergence.

Table 11.5.3: Six strategic priorities of new adolescent health strategy

1. **Improve nutrition**
   - Reduce the prevalence of malnutrition among adolescent girls and boys.
   - Reduce the prevalence of iron-deficiency anemia (IDA) among adolescent girls and boys.
2. **Improve sexual and reproductive health (SRH)**
   - Improve knowledge, attitudes and behavior, in relation to SRH.
   - Reduce teenage pregnancies.
   - Improve birth preparedness, complication readiness and provide early parenting support for adolescent parents.
3. **Enhance mental health**
   - Address mental health concerns of adolescents.
4. **Prevent injuries and violence**
   - Promote favorable attitudes for preventing injuries and violence (including GBV) among adolescents.
5. **Prevent substance misuse**
   - Increase adolescents' awareness of the adverse effects and consequences of substance misuse.
6. **Address NCDs**
   - Promote behavior change in adolescents to prevent NCDs such as hypertension, stroke, cardiovascular diseases and diabetes.

Abbreviations: GBV–Gender based violence; NCDs–Non-communicable diseases.

such as sanitary napkins, iron and folic acid (IFA) tablets and non-clinical contraception, and addressing common issues through periodic Adolescent Health Days.

An important component of the strategy is provision for capacity building through (i) inclusion of adolescent health in pre-service curriculum of medical and nursing courses, and (ii) in-service training of various health care workers through training programs and through e-learning and distance learning courses.

IMPLICATIONS FOR PRACTICING PHYSICIANS

To begin with, RKSK is being launched in some districts of every state. This program will also be promoted in lay media and by using IEC activities. These efforts will create or enhance the awareness about adolescent health among adolescents and parents both. Availability of services in public sector will certainly be a boon for adolescents and their parents. However, a large proportion of our population depends on private providers for health care needs. Adolescents and their parents are no exceptions and some of them will look for a competent provider in private sector too.

When adolescents become aware of their specific developmental needs, they would certainly look for a provider who is friendly to him/her, is competent enough to look after him/her, and at the same time can fulfill the needs of privacy and confidentiality. Thus, every physician needs to learn the nuances of adolescent health and medicine. This is a historic opportunity and physicians cannot afford to lose the momentum.

WHO List of Technical Resources on Adolescent Health

11.6

Rajesh Mehta

2015

- Building an adolescent-competent workforce–Policy brief
- Core competencies in adolescent health and development for primary care providers including a tool to assess the adolescent health and development component in pre-service education of health care providers
- Global standards for quality health care services for adolescents

2014

- Adolescent HIV testing, counseling and care–Implementation guidance for health providers and planners
- Health for the world's adolescents: A second chance in the second decade
- MCA highlights 2012-13: Progress report–WHO's Department of Maternal, Newborn, Child and Adolescent Health
- Options for linking health interventions for adolescents with HPV vaccination

2013

- Compilation of WHO recommendations on maternal, newborn, child and adolescent health
- Comprehensive cervical cancer prevention and control–A healthier future for girls and women
- Preconception care to reduce maternal and childhood mortality and morbidity–Meeting report and packages of interventions: WHO HQ, February 2012

2012

- Making health services adolescent friendly–Developing national quality standards for adolescent friendly health services
- MCA highlights 2010-11: Progress report–WHO's Department of Maternal, Newborn, Child and Adolescent Health

2011

- Preventing early pregnancy and poor reproductive outcomes among adolescents in developing countries–WHO guidelines
- Strengthening the adolescent component of HIV/AIDS and reproductive health programmes–A training course for public health managers

2010

- Adolescent Job Aid–A handy desk reference tool for primary level health workers
- Second global consultation on service provision for adolescents living with HIV–Consensus statement
- Strengthening the health sector response to adolescent health and development–Flyer

2009

- A qualitative review of psychosocial support interventions for young people living with HIV
- Analytic case studies: Initiatives to increase the use of health services by adolescents
- Generating demand and community support for sexual and reproductive health services for young people–A review of the literature and programmes
- IMAI one-day orientation on adolescents living with HIV–Participants manual, Facilitator guide
- Promoting adolescent sexual and reproductive health through schools in low income countries–An information brief
- Quality assessment guidebook–A guide to assessing health services for adolescent clients

2008

- Global Guidance Briefs on HIV interventions for young people
- More Positive Living–Strengthening the health sector response to young people living with HIV
- Strengthening the health sector response to care, support, treatment and prevention for young people living with HIV 13-17 November 2006 Blantyre, Malawi

2007

- Adolescent pregnancy: unmet needs and undone deeds–A review of the literature and programmes
- Adolescents, social support and help-seeking behavior–An international literature review and programme consultation with recommendations for action
- CAH progress report 2006
- Concerted WHO efforts to address adolescent health and development–Leaflet
- Helping parents in developing countries improve adolescents' health
- Married adolescents: No place of safety
- Summaries of projects in developing countries assisting the parents of adolescents
- The adolescent with a chronic condition

2006

- Guidelines for adaptation of the WHO orientation programme on adolescent health for health care providers in Europe and Central Asia
- Orientation programme on adolescent health for health–care providers
- Pregnant adolescents–Delivering on global promises of hope
- Preventing HIV/AIDS in young people–A systematic review of the evidence from developing countries

2005

- Psychosocial support for children and adolescents
- Sexually transmitted infections among adolescents–The need for adequate health services

INDEX

Q

R